MW00846700

Designing Clinical Research

FIFTH EDITION

Designing Clinical Research

FIFTH EDITION

Warren S. Browner, MD, MPH

Chief Executive Officer, Sutter Health California Pacific Medical Center
Clinical Professor of Epidemiology & Biostatistics
University of California, San Francisco

Thomas B. Newman, MD, MPH

Professor Emeritus of Epidemiology & Biostatistics, and Pediatrics
University of California, San Francisco

Steven R. Cummings, MD

Executive Director, San Francisco Coordinating Center
California Pacific Medical Center Research Institute
Professor Emeritus of Medicine, and Epidemiology & Biostatistics
University of California, San Francisco

Deborah G. Grady, MD, MPH

Deputy Editor, JAMA Internal Medicine
Professor Emeritus of Medicine, and Epidemiology & Biostatistics
University of California, San Francisco

Alison J. Huang, MD, MAS

Professor of Medicine, Urology, and Epidemiology & Biostatistics
University of California, San Francisco

Alka M. Kanaya, MD

Professor of Medicine, and Epidemiology & Biostatistics
University of California, San Francisco

Mark J. Pletcher, MD, MPH

Professor of Epidemiology & Biostatistics, and Medicine
University of California, San Francisco

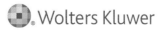

Philadelphia • Baltimore • New York • London
Buenos Aires • Hong Kong • Sydney • Tokyo

Acquisitions Editor: Joe Cho
Development Editor: Ariel S. Winter
Editorial Coordinator: Sean Hanrahan
Editorial Assistant: Maribeth Wood
Marketing Manager: Kristen Watrud
Production Project Manager: David Saltzberg
Design Coordinator: Steve Druding
Manufacturing Coordinator: Beth Welsh
Prepress Vendor: S4Carlisle Publishing Services

Fifth edition

Copyright © 2023 Wolters Kluwer.

Copyright © 2013 by LIPPINCOTT WILLIAMS & WILKINS, a WOLTERS KLUWER business. © 2007 by Lippincott Williams & Wilkins, a Wolters Kluwer business. 2001 Lippincott Williams & Wilkins. 1998 Williams & Wilkins. All rights reserved. This book is protected by copyright. No part of this book may be reproduced or transmitted in any form or by any means, including as photocopies or scanned-in or other electronic copies, or utilized by any information storage and retrieval system without written permission from the copyright owner, except for brief quotations embodied in critical articles and reviews. Materials appearing in this book prepared by individuals as part of their official duties as U.S. government employees are not covered by the above-mentioned copyright. To request permission, please contact Wolters Kluwer at Two Commerce Square, 2001 Market Street, Philadelphia, PA 19103, via email at permissions@lww.com, or via our website at shop.lww.com (products and services).

9 8 7 6 5 4 3 2 1

Printed in Singapore

Library of Congress Cataloging-in-Publication Data

Names: Browner, Warren S. author.
Title: Designing clinical research / Warren S. Browner, Thomas B. Newman,
    Steven R. Cummings, Deborah G. Grady, Alison J. Huang, Alka M. Kanaya,
    Mark J. Pletcher.
Description: 5th edition. | Philadelphia: Wolters Kluwer Health, [2023] |
    Preceded by Designing clinical research / Stephen B. Hulley ... [et al.].
    4th ed. 2013. | Includes bibliographical references and index.
Identifiers: LCCN 2021043257 (print) | LCCN 2021043258 (ebook) | ISBN
    9781975174408 (paperback) | ISBN 9781975174422 (ebook)
Subjects: MESH: Epidemiologic Methods | Research Design
Classification: LCC RA651 (print) | LCC RA651 (ebook) | NLM WA 950 | DDC
    614.4072—dc23
LC record available at https://lccn.loc.gov/2021043257
LC ebook record available at https://lccn.loc.gov/2021043258

This work is provided "as is," and the publisher disclaims any and all warranties, express or implied, including any warranties as to accuracy, comprehensiveness, or currency of the content of this work.

This work is no substitute for individual patient assessment based upon healthcare professionals' examination of each patient and consideration of, among other things, age, weight, gender, current or prior medical conditions, medication history, laboratory data and other factors unique to the patient. The publisher does not provide medical advice or guidance and this work is merely a reference tool. Healthcare professionals, and not the publisher, are solely responsible for the use of this work including all medical judgments and for any resulting diagnosis and treatments.

Given continuous, rapid advances in medical science and health information, independent professional verification of medical diagnoses, indications, appropriate pharmaceutical selections and dosages, and treatment options should be made and healthcare professionals should consult a variety of sources. When prescribing medication, healthcare professionals are advised to consult the product information sheet (the manufacturer's package insert) accompanying each drug to verify, among other things, conditions of use, warnings and side effects and identify any changes in dosage schedule or contraindications, particularly if the medication to be administered is new, infrequently used or has a narrow therapeutic range. To the maximum extent permitted under applicable law, no responsibility is assumed by the publisher for any injury and/or damage to persons or property, as a matter of products liability, negligence law or otherwise, or from any reference to or use by any person of this work.

shop.lww.com

MKO122

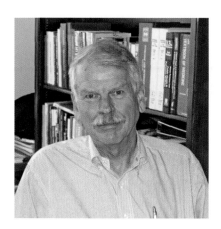

To Stephen Hulley, MD, MPH, who conceived, delivered, and parented the four previous editions of this book, creating a palimpsest that still shines through.

To our families, for tolerating our obsessions with arcane concepts and pressing deadlines.

And to our teachers, colleagues, and students, for inspiring us to dig deeper and explain things better.

Contents

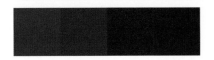

Contributing Authors

Daniel Dohan, PhD
Professor, Philip R. Lee Institute for Health Policy Studies
University of California, San Francisco

Michael A. Kohn, MD, MPP
Professor Emeritus of Epidemiology & Biostatistics
University of California, San Francisco

Bernard Lo, MD
Professor Emeritus of Medicine
Director Emeritus, Program in Medical Ethics
University of California, San Francisco

Introduction

This fifth edition of *Designing Clinical Research* (DCR) marks the 35th anniversary of the book's publication—and the first edition whose preparation has not been led by our fearless mentor, Steve Hulley, about whom more later. What started as a collection of handouts for a small seminar has become the most widely used textbook in its field, having sold over 150,000 copies.

From its inception, DCR has been aimed at clinical investigators at the outset of their careers, who may have taken a class in epidemiology at some point in their education and remember some of the concepts, but more likely do not. Indeed, many of us (SRC, WSB, TBN, and DGG) started our own academic careers four decades ago in a similar position: We were interested in clinical research, had attended journal clubs that discussed (and criticized) published articles during our training, but were clueless about how to go about designing a study. At the time, most academic health centers had little to offer.

Fortunately, Steve Hulley recognized that although epidemiology was the basic science for clinical research, many studies were designed and led by investigators whose epidemiologic training and understanding were slim-to-none. At the time, subspecialty fellows interested in basic research were trained in laboratory techniques before they began a project at a lab bench, while those interested in clinical research were left mostly on their own or even advised to choose a more traditional career path. Steve filled that gap by developing and teaching a course on how to design clinical research studies, then by leading a fellowship program sponsored by the Andrew W. Mellon Foundation to train a cohort of "clinical epidemiologists" (complete with brass name tags for our newly minted specialty), and finally by mentoring his freshly trained protégés as we fledged. All of this took place at the University of California, San Francisco (UCSF), a health sciences campus then and still best-known for its deep commitment to—and success in—basic research.

From the beginning, DCR has represented the next phase of Steve's vision, namely, to spread the word beyond the Bay Area. Many readers are now health sciences students and practitioners around the world (DCR has been translated into Arabic, Chinese, Japanese, Korean, Spanish, and Portuguese) starting their careers in clinical research (or at least considering it). They have come to appreciate how epidemiologic principles can guide the many judgments involved in designing studies that inform evidence-based clinical practice.

While staying true to its original mission to be a primer, not an encyclopedia, the fifth edition of DCR has modernized (some might say "Finally!") our approach to understanding causal effects. To reflect advances in how epidemiologists think, we now include an introduction to counterfactual models and directed acyclic graphs. We resisted making this change for many years: The material, located at the core of the book, is challenging intellectually. We hope readers will find that the swim—a deeper understanding of how epidemiologists estimate causal effects—was worth the walk down a long pier.

We've added new chapters on community-engaged research and on qualitative studies to reflect the growing importance of these approaches to clinical research. We moved the exercises to the ends of the chapters, in the hope that they will be more noticeable there, while leaving the answers at the end of the book. We've used **red font** to highlight concepts defined in the glossary, which has been expanded. Almost all of the figures have been redesigned, using consistent colors to represent various aspects of study design (eg, indigo for interventions, purple for predictors, and ocher for outcomes). More important, we enlisted three "junior" authors—all of whom are more senior than the rest of us were when we started working on the book's first edition. In part, that reflects the tremendous growth of clinical research since 1988: There are many more well-trained clinical investigators and they have risen through the ranks of academia. Our hope is that subsequent editions will get a similar refresh.

The fifth edition is accompanied by the DCR website at https://dcr-5.net, which contains materials for teaching DCR, including links to a detailed syllabus for the 4- and 7-week DCR workshops that we present to trainees each year at UCSF. In addition, there are useful tools for investigators, including an excellent interactive sample size calculator at www.sample-size.net.

Many things about the book have *not* changed. Just as Steve Hulley intended, the fifth edition of DCR is still aimed squarely at clinical researchers at the beginning of their careers. We avoid jargon and technical terms as much as possible. We focus on the important stuff, like how to find a good research question and how to develop an efficient, effective, and ethical study design. For example, the chapters on estimating sample size enable readers with no training in statistics to make these calculations on their own, without needing to wrestle with formulas. The material on causal reasoning uses simple examples and graphics to explain a complex topic. We still use feminine pronouns in the first part of the book and masculine in the second, and now use plural pronouns in the last, to empower all clinical investigators. However, DCR still does not address the important areas of how to analyze, present, and publish the findings of clinical research—topics that our readers can pursue with other books (1-4).

Finally, a few words of advice. A career as an independent clinical researcher requires surmounting the twin hurdles of becoming the first author of an important paper and the principal investigator on a peer-reviewed grant. DCR can help you achieve those goals, especially when combined with another essential ingredient—a research mentor who cares about you and your career. We strongly suggest that, after purchasing (or borrowing) this book, you find a more senior colleague who can support you through the intricacies of designing and executing a clinical research project.

As access to training has improved, the competition has gotten stiffer and the "time to independence" longer. Perseverance is as important as creativity. All of us have received countless rejection letters from journals and funding agencies. It can be discouraging reading that your work and ideas have merit—just not enough or not soon enough. While it may sometimes seem as if many of the most interesting questions have been answered, that is an illusion. Preventable diseases still occur frequently, while how to prevent others remains unknown. Potential treatments and innovative diagnostic tests are being developed daily. Large proportions of people—and their health-related concerns—have been underrepresented systematically in research. With so much opportunity, the pursuits of truth and justice can be a lifelong calling.

REFERENCES

1. Vittinghoff E, Glidden DV, Shiboski SC, et al. *Regression Methods in Biostatistics: Linear, Logistic, Survival, and Repeated Measures Models.* 2nd ed. Springer-Verlag; 2012.
2. Katz MH. *Multivariable Analysis: A Practical Guide for Clinicians and Public Health Researchers.* 3rd ed. Cambridge University Press; 2011.
3. Newman TB, Kohn MA. *Evidence-Based Diagnosis: An Introduction to Clinical Epidemiology.* 2nd ed. Cambridge University Press; 2020.
4. Browner WS. *Publishing and Presenting Clinical Research.* 3rd ed. Lippincott Williams & Wilkins; 2012.

Acknowledgments

We are grateful to the University of California, San Francisco, especially the Department of Epidemiology & Biostatistics, for providing us with a nurturing home during the past 40 years; to our colleagues in clinical research at UCSF, the California Pacific Medical Center Research Institute, and throughout the world; and to the team at Wolters Kluwer for helping us assemble this new edition. Special thanks to Anita Stewart for her help with self-reported measurements, to Frank Harrell for inspiring us to include Bayesian approaches, and to John Boscardin and Martina Steurer for their assistance with some of the figures.

We are also grateful to our colleagues who are working to improve the world; in appreciation, part of the royalties from this book will be donated to organizations that work to promote health regionally or globally, including Physicians for Social Responsibility (www.psr.org), Americares (www.americares.org), and the Institute on Aging (ioaging.org).

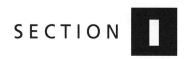

Basic Ingredients

CHAPTER 1

Getting Started: The Anatomy and Physiology of Clinical Research

Warren S. Browner, Thomas B. Newman, and Mark J. Pletcher

This chapter introduces clinical research from two viewpoints, developing themes that run throughout the book. One is the anatomy of research—the tangible elements of a study plan, such as the research question, design, participants, measurements, sample size calculation, and so forth. An investigator's goal is to design these components in a fashion that will make the project feasible and efficient and that will enhance the validity of the study's findings.

The other theme is the physiology of research—how it works. Studies are useful to the extent that they yield valid conclusions about what happened in the study and then about how those conclusions generalize to the larger world. The goal is to minimize any errors that might threaten those processes.

Separating the two themes is artificial in the same way that the anatomy of the human body doesn't make much sense without some understanding of its physiology. But the separation has the advantage of simplifying our thinking about a complex topic.

■ ANATOMY OF RESEARCH: WHAT IT'S MADE OF

The structure of a research project is set out in its protocol, the written plan of the study. Protocols are well known as devices for seeking grant funds and Institutional Review Board (IRB) approval, but they also have a vital scientific function: helping the investigator organize her research in a logical, focused, and efficient way. Table 1.1 outlines the components of a protocol. We introduce the whole set here, expand on each component in the ensuing chapters of the book, and return to put the completed pieces together in Chapter 20.

Research Question

The research question[1] is the objective of the study, the uncertainty the investigator wants to resolve. Research questions often begin with a general concern that must be narrowed down to a concrete, researchable issue. Consider, for example, the general question of whether caffeine affects cognitive function. Although a good place to start, this question must be focused further before planning efforts can begin. Often, this involves breaking the question into more specific components and singling out one or two of these to build the protocol around. Here are a few examples of possible research questions:

- Are the effects of caffeine on cognitive function short-term, long-term, or both?
- Does chronic caffeine use reduce the risk of developing dementia?
- How is caffeine consumption best measured?
- Are there harmful effects from consuming caffeine?
- Does it matter whether caffeine is consumed in coffee? Tea? Caffeinated soft drinks?

---

[1]Terms in red are defined in the Glossary.

TABLE 1.1 ANATOMY OF RESEARCH: THE STUDY PLAN

DESIGN COMPONENTS	PURPOSE
Research question(s)	What question(s) will the study address?
Background and significance	Why are these questions important?
Design	How is the study structured?
Type of study	
Participants	Who are they, and how will they be selected?
Selection criteria	
Sampling design	
Variables	What measurements will be made?
Predictor variables	
Confounding variables	
Outcome variables	
Statistical issues	How large is the study, and how will it be analyzed?
Hypotheses	
Sample size	
Analytic approach	

There are, of course, many more potential research questions about this topic; the investigator's task is to choose one that is **feasible, important, novel,** and **ethical** to study. These attributes have an easy-to-remember acronym—FINE—as discussed in Chapter 2.

Background and Significance

Developing a meaningful research question requires becoming knowledgeable about the areas to be studied. Often, talking with experts and doing a thorough literature review will lead the investigator to modify the research question. So the first step in designing a clinical research project is determining what is—or is not—already known about the topic at hand. That's followed by pondering how to add to that current knowledge. This step involves thinking long and hard, and talking with colleagues and mentors, about the important but as-yet unanswered questions.

These thoughts will eventually be synthesized and summarized in a brief background and significance section that provides the rationale for the study. In this section, the investigator cites relevant previous research (especially her own and that of her colleagues), emphasizing the problems with that research and the uncertainties that remain. She also specifies how the findings of her proposed study will help resolve these uncertainties, by leading to new scientific knowledge, changing clinical practice, or influencing practice guidelines or health policy.

Design

There is no best design for all research questions. Rather, the investigator must determine the type of design that will work best for the chosen research question and her available resources. A fundamental decision is whether to apply an **intervention** and examine its effects in a **clinical trial** or simply to make measurements on the study **participants** in an **observational study** (Table 1.2). Among clinical trial options, the **randomized blinded trial** is usually the most desirable design, but nonrandomized or unblinded designs may occasionally be all that are feasible for some interventions.

TABLE 1.2 EXAMPLES OF CLINICAL RESEARCH DESIGNS TO FIND OUT WHETHER CAFFEINE CONSUMPTION REDUCES THE RISK OF DEMENTIA

EPIDEMIOLOGIC DESIGN	KEY FEATURE	EXAMPLE
Observational Designs		
Cross-sectional study	A group examined at one point in time	The investigator interviews a group of participants about current and past caffeine intake and correlates results with scores on a test of cognitive function.
Cohort study	A group (usually without the outcome) identified at the beginning of the study and followed over time	She measures caffeine consumption in a group of participants with normal cognitive function and examines them at follow-up visits to see if those who consume caffeine are less likely to develop dementia.
Case-control study	Two groups selected based on the presence or absence of an outcome	She compares past caffeine intake in a group of people with dementia (the "cases") with that in a group with normal cognitive function (the "controls").
Clinical Trial Design		
Randomized blinded trial	Two groups created by a random process and a blinded intervention	She randomly assigns participants with normal cognitive function to receive caffeine supplements or a placebo that is identical in appearance and then follows both treatment groups for several years to observe the incidence of dementia.

Among observational studies, two common designs are **cross-sectional studies**, in which observations are made on a single occasion, and **cohort studies**, in which observations are made in a group of participants who are followed over time. This latter group of studies can be further divided into **prospective cohort** studies—which begin in the present and follow participants into the future—and **retrospective cohort** studies—which examine information collected in the past—although these distinctions are not always hard and fast. A third common observational design is the **case-control study**, in which the investigator compares a group of people who have developed the **outcome** of interest (the **cases**) with another group that has not (the **controls**).

Each research question requires a judgment about which design is the most efficient way to get a reliable answer. The randomized blinded trial is often held up as the best design for establishing causality and determining the efficacy of an intervention, but there are many situations for which an observational study is a better choice or the only feasible option: It would not be easy to randomly assign people to stop or start drinking coffee, for example. The relatively low cost of case-control studies and their suitability for rare outcomes make them attractive for some questions. These issues are discussed in Chapters 8 through 14, each dealing with a particular set of designs.

A typical sequence for studying a topic begins with observational studies of a type often called **descriptive**. These studies explore the lay of the land—for example, describing distributions of health-related characteristics and diseases in the **population**:

- What is the frequency of caffeine consumption among adults 70 years of age and older?
- What proportion of older adults have abnormal cognitive function?

Studies of medical tests, such as whether serum levels of a new **biomarker** correlate with cognitive dysfunction, are a special form of descriptive studies (see Chapter 13).

Descriptive studies are usually followed or accompanied by **analytic studies** that evaluate **associations**, usually to permit **inferences** about **cause-effect** relationships:

- Is the average amount of caffeine consumed per day associated with performance on tests of cognitive function?
- Are people with dementia less likely to have a history of regular caffeine consumption than are controls with normal cognitive function?

The final step is often a clinical trial to establish the effects of an intervention:

- Do older adult volunteers who are randomly assigned to take caffeine supplements have a lower risk of developing dementia than those who are assigned to take a placebo?

Clinical trials usually occur relatively late in a series of research studies about a given question, because they tend to be more difficult and expensive, may be more likely to expose participants to harm, and usually address a narrowly focused question that arose from the findings of observational studies.

It is useful to characterize a study in a single sentence that summarizes the design and research question. If the study has two major phases, the design for each should be mentioned.

- This is a **cross-sectional study** of the association between caffeine consumption and cognitive function in 60- to 74-year-old people, followed by a **prospective cohort study** of whether caffeine use is associated with a lower rate of subsequent cognitive decline.

Some designs do not easily fit into the categories listed previously, and describing them with the right level of detail in a single sentence can be challenging. It is worth the effort, however: A concise description of the research question and design clarifies the investigator's thoughts and is useful for orienting colleagues and consultants.

Study Participants

Two major decisions must be made in choosing the **sample** of study participants (Chapter 3). The first is to describe the **kinds of people you wish to study**, specifying the **inclusion** and **exclusion criteria** that will define your study participants. The second decision concerns how you will recruit an appropriate number of people from an accessible subset of this population to participate in the study. For example, a case-control study of caffeine use and dementia might begin (after securing IRB approval) by reviewing electronic health records at your institution to identify patients with a diagnosis of dementia or cognitive dysfunction and then contacting them and appropriate controls to see if they are interested in participating.

Variables

Another major set of decisions in designing any study concerns the choice of which **variables** to measure (Chapter 4). A study of caffeine consumption, for example, might ask about different types of beverages and "stay alert" pills that contain varying levels of caffeine and include questions about portion size, frequency, and timing of intake.

In an analytic study, the investigator studies the associations among variables to predict outcomes and to draw inferences about cause and effect. When considering the association between two variables, the one that occurs first—or is more likely on biologic grounds to be causal—is called the **predictor variable**; the other is called the **outcome variable**.[2] Most observational studies have many predictor variables (eg, age, sex, race/ethnicity, smoking history, caffeine intake) and several outcome variables (eg, cognitive function, quality of life).

---

[2]Predictors are sometimes termed **independent** variables and outcomes **dependent** variables, but the meaning of these terms is less self-evident. Predictor variables can be **exposures**, **risk factors** or **protective factors**, **treatments** or **interventions**, or **test results**, terms that we use throughout the book when appropriate.

Clinical trials examine the effects of an intervention, which is a special kind of predictor variable that the investigator manipulates, such as treatment with caffeine capsules (or matching placebos). This design allows her to use **randomization** to minimize the influence of **confounding** variables—other predictors of the outcome, such as smoking or educational level, that also influence caffeine intake and may confuse the interpretation of the findings. Confounding, a particularly thorny topic, is discussed in detail in Chapter 10.

Statistical Issues

The investigator must develop plans for estimating the **sample size** as well as for managing and analyzing the study data. This generally involves specifying a **research hypothesis** (Chapter 5), a version of the research question that provides the basis for testing the **statistical significance** of the findings:

- **Hypothesis:** Adults 60 to 74 years of age who consume an average of at least two cups of coffee per day (or an equivalent amount of caffeine) have better cognitive function than those with lower levels of consumption.

The research hypothesis also allows the investigator to calculate the sample size—the number of participants needed to find a statistically significant difference in outcomes between the study groups with reasonable probability, given that one exists, an attribute known as **power** (Chapter 5). Purely descriptive studies (eg, "What proportion of people with normal cognitive function drink coffee daily?") do not involve tests of statistical significance and thus do not require a hypothesis; instead, the number of participants needed to produce acceptably narrow **confidence intervals** for means, proportions, or other descriptive statistics can be calculated.

■ PHYSIOLOGY OF RESEARCH: HOW IT WORKS

The goal of clinical research is to improve our understanding of the real world from the findings of the study (see the lower half of Figure 1.1). First, the findings of the study must be interpreted, a process that depends on **internal validity**, the degree to which the study's results reflect what happened in the study. Next, the investigator makes inferences from the study conclusions to enhance our understanding of the real world. This process depends on **external validity** (or **generalizability**), the fidelity with which those conclusions apply to people and events outside the study.

When an investigator plans a study, she reverses the process, working from left to right in the upper half of Figure 1.1 with the goal of maximizing the validity of these inferences at the end of the study. She designs a study plan in which the choice of research question, participants, and measurements enhances the external validity of the study and facilitates its implementation to maximize internal validity. In the following sections, we address design and then implementation before turning to the errors that threaten the validity of these inferences.

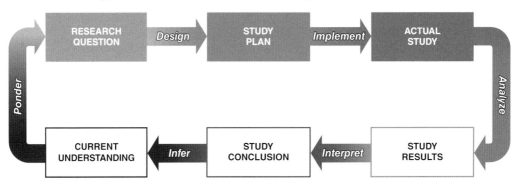

■ **FIGURE 1.1 The basic structure of clinical research.** At each step, choices and errors affect the inferences that can be made from the completed study.

Designing the Study

Consider this simple descriptive research question about caffeine and cognitive function:

- What is the average daily caffeine consumption among adults 70 years of age or older with normal cognitive function?

This question cannot be answered with perfect accuracy because it would be impossible to study the entire **target population** of all older adults, never mind that methods of measuring caffeine consumption and cognitive function are imperfect. Rather, the investigator must settle for a related question that *can* be answered:

- What is the self-reported average daily caffeine consumption ascertained from a mailed questionnaire sent to patients cared for at the investigator's institution who are at least 70 years of age and who do not have a diagnosis of dementia or cognitive dysfunction recorded in their electronic medical records?

The transformation from research question to study plan is illustrated in Figure 1.2. One major component of this transformation is the choice of a **sample** of participants to represent the population. Because there are almost always practical barriers to studying the target population as a whole, the group specified in the protocol must usually be a sample of that population. Using the investigator's institution to identify potential participants is a compromise that makes the study feasible, but it has the disadvantage that it may produce a different pattern of caffeine use than in the general population, even if everyone returns the **questionnaire**. More important, the absence of a recorded diagnosis of dementia or cognitive dysfunction certainly does not ensure that someone has normal cognitive function.

The other major component of the transformation is the choice of variables to represent the phenomena of interest. The variables specified in the study plan are usually proxies for these phenomena. For example, the decision to use a self-report questionnaire to assess caffeine consumption in the prior month is a fast and inexpensive way to collect information. However, it is unlikely to be perfectly accurate because people usually cannot remember exactly how much caffeine they drank the previous month and because that month may not reflect their usual pattern of caffeine consumption.

In short, each of the differences in Figure 1.2 between the research question and the study plan represents a choice to make the study more feasible and efficient. This increase in practicality, however, comes with a cost: the risk that those choices may produce a less relevant conclusion because the study answered a question that differed somewhat from the research question.

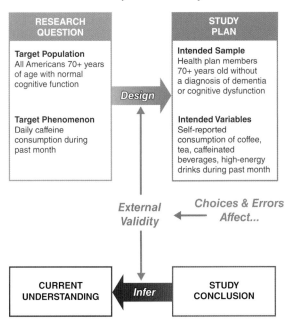

■ **FIGURE 1.2 Choices and errors made in the design of the study affect its external validity.** If the intended sample and variables do not sufficiently represent the target population and the phenomena of interest, the ability to draw inferences to improve our understanding of the problem is reduced.

Implementing the Study

The implementation of the study plan affects the fidelity with which the actual study follows that plan. At issue here is the problem of a wrong answer to the research question because the way the sample was drawn—or the measurements were made—differed substantially from how they were designed (Figure 1.3).

The actual sample of study participants is almost always different from the intended sample. Plans to study all eligible clinic patients without dementia or cognitive dysfunction, for example, could be disrupted by incomplete diagnoses in the electronic medical record, wrong addresses for the mailed questionnaires, and refusals to participate. Those who are reached and agree to participate may have a different pattern of caffeine consumption than those not reached or not interested. In addition to these problems, the actual measurements can differ from the intended measurements. If the format of the questionnaire is unclear, participants may get confused and check the wrong box, or they may simply omit a question by mistake.

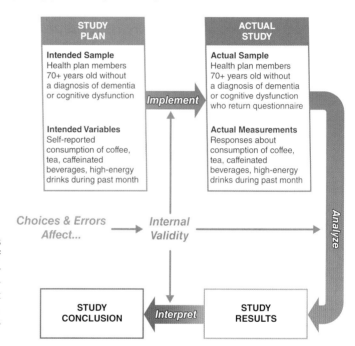

■ **FIGURE 1.3 Choices and errors made in the implementation of the study affect its internal validity.** If the actual sample and measurements do not sufficiently represent the intended sample and variables, the ability to draw valid conclusions from the study's findings is reduced.

Causal Inference

Many studies aim to establish a cause-effect association—that is, a predictor *causes* an outcome—in order to identify clinical or public health interventions that may improve health. For example, if caffeine use causes a decrease in the risk of developing dementia, then perhaps we should recommend it widely. A special kind of validity problem arises in studies that attempt to establish causal inference. If a cohort study finds an association between caffeine intake and dementia, does this represent cause and effect, or is caffeine intake only related to a confounding exposure (say, reading the morning newspaper) that protects against dementia? Reducing the likelihood of confounding and other rival explanations is one of the major challenges in designing an observational study (Chapter 10).

The Errors of Research

Recognizing that no study is entirely free of errors, the goal is to maximize the validity of any inferences made from what was observed in the study. Some erroneous inferences can be addressed in the analysis phase of research, but a better strategy is to focus on design and implementation (Figure 1.4), preventing errors from occurring in the first place.

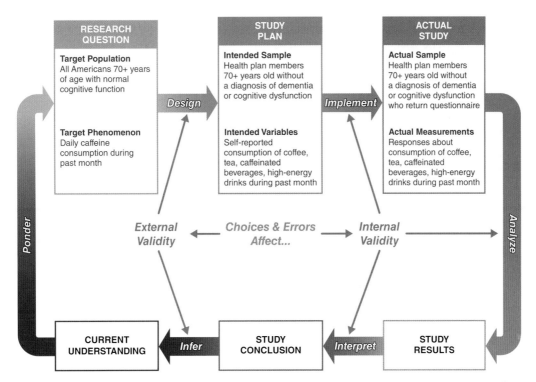

■ FIGURE 1.4 The physiology of research. Choices and errors made in the design and implementation of the study affect its internal and external validity.

The two main kinds of mistakes that interfere with research inferences are called **random error** and **systematic error**. The distinction is important because the strategies for minimizing them are quite different.

Random error is a mistake due to *chance*—meaning that there is no known cause or predictable pattern to the error. Random error can distort a measurement in either direction. For example, if the true prevalence of daily caffeine consumption is exactly 40% among the several thousand members of the health plan 70 years of age and older, a well-designed sample of 100 patients from that accessible population might contain exactly 40 patients who consume caffeine each day. It's quite likely, however, that the sample would contain a slightly different number, such as 38, 39, 41, or 42. Occasionally, chance would produce a substantially different number, such as 32 or 49. Among the many techniques for reducing the influence of random error, the simplest is to increase the sample size. The use of a larger sample diminishes the likelihood of a substantially wrong result by increasing the **precision** of the estimate—the degree to which the observed prevalence approximates 40% each time a sample is drawn. But increasing the sample size also increases the cost of a study; fortunately, there are other ways to reduce random error, including using better instruments to make measurements (Chapter 4).

Systematic error is a wrong result due to bias—sources of variation that distort the study findings in one direction. An illustration is the decision (Figure 1.2) to study patients in a local health plan, where the recording of the diagnoses of dementia and cognitive dysfunction may have been influenced by the plan's efforts to avoid (or encourage!) overcoding. Increasing the sample size has no effect on systematic error. The best way to improve an estimate's **accuracy** (the degree to which it approximates the true value) is to reduce the size of potential biases—a topic to which much of this book is devoted. In addition, the investigator can seek additional information to assess the importance of possible biases, such as using a second sample drawn from another setting.

The examples of random and systematic error in the preceding two paragraphs are components of **selection bias**, which threatens inferences from the study participants to the population. Both random and systematic errors can also contribute to **measurement error**, threatening the

TABLE 1.3 APPROACHES TO CONTROLLING RANDOM AND SYSTEMATIC ERRORS IN THE DESIGN AND IMPLEMENTATION PHASES OF A STUDY

TYPE OF ERROR	SOLUTION
Random	Improve precision of measurements (Chapter 4)
	Increase sample size (Chapters 5 and 6)
Systematic	Improve accuracy and validity of measurements (Chapter 4)
	Choose a better design (Chapters 8-14)
Random and systematic	Quality control (Chapter 18)

inferences from the study measurements to the phenomena of interest. An illustration of *random* measurement error is the variation in responses that occurs when a questionnaire is administered on several occasions. An example of *systematic* measurement error is misestimation of the amount of caffeine consumption due to problems in the questionnaire (eg, failing to ask about energy drinks). Strategies for controlling these errors are presented in Chapters 3 and 4.

As summarized in Table 1.3, getting the best possible answer to the research question is a matter of designing, implementing, and interpreting the study to minimize the magnitude of potential errors.

■ TRANSLATIONAL RESEARCH

Translational research refers to studies that translate basic science discoveries into clinical practice or that expand clinical research findings into broad-scale public health or community-based programs. These studies should be designed in the same way as other clinical research studies, although the number of investigators is often larger and the process itself more complex and iterative. Successful translational research requires collaborations among investigators along the spectrum of research, all of whom should be prepared to revise their plans: It's not unusual for a treatment that looks promising in laboratory animals to cause adverse effects when tested in people, or for a screening test that works in an academic clinic to be cumbersome to apply or less accurate in a community setting. The earlier those collaborations begin, the more likely that the investigators will be able to pose an important research question, develop a worthwhile study plan, and avoid setbacks that could have been anticipated.

Translating from Laboratory to Clinical Research

A host of tools—including DNA sequencing, gene expression arrays, molecular imaging, proteomics, and metabolomics—have moved from basic science laboratories into clinical investigation. Compared with ordinary clinical research, successful translation of tests and treatments discovered in bench research usually requires personal laboratory experience or a collaborator with those skills. Bench-to-bedside research necessitates a thorough understanding of the underlying basic science. Many clinical researchers believe that they can master this knowledge easily—just as many laboratory-based scientists believe clinical research does not require special training and expertise. But the skill sets for basic and clinical research barely overlap, and conceiving good translational research questions requires expertise and close collaboration in more than one area.

For example, suppose a gene that regulates circadian rhythm in mice has been identified and a clinical investigator with expertise in sleep disturbances wants to study whether variants in the human homolog of that gene affect sleep patterns in people. To develop a meaningful research question about the potential effects of that gene, she will need collaborators who are familiar with the biology of the gene and its protein product(s), as well as the advantages and limitations of the various methods of genotyping. Similarly, suppose a laboratory-based investigator has found a unique pattern of gene expression in lymph nodes obtained from women with breast cancer. To study whether that pattern is useful prognostically, she should collaborate with investigators who understand the importance of test-retest reliability, sampling and blinding, and the effects of prior probability of disease on the applicability and clinical utility of her discovery. Finally, a research team interested in testing a new medication may need scientists familiar with molecular biology, pharmacokinetics and pharmacodynamics, phase I and II clinical trials, and practice patterns in the relevant field of medicine.

Translating from Clinical to Population Research

Designing studies to apply findings from clinical research to larger and more diverse populations may also require additional expertise, such as in identifying high-risk or underserved groups, understanding the difference between screening and diagnosis, and knowing how to implement changes in health care delivery systems. On a practical level, this kind of research usually needs access to large groups of participants, such as those enrolled in health plans or the residents of an entire county. Support and advice from a department chair, the chief of the medical staff at an affiliated hospital, the leader of a managed care organization, or the director of the local health department may be helpful when planning these studies.

Some investigators take a shortcut when designing this type of translational research, for example, planning to expand on results seen in their own specialty clinic by enrolling participants from similar practices at other university medical centers, rather than involving practitioners in the community. This is a bit like translating Aristophanes into modern Greek—it will still not be very useful for English-speaking readers. Testing research findings in larger and more diverse populations often requires partnerships with community members and adapting methods to fit nonacademic organizations, as discussed in Chapter 15.

■ DESIGNING THE STUDY

Study Plan

The process of developing the study plan begins with a one-sentence research question that specifies the main predictor and outcome variables and the target population. Three versions of the study plan are then produced in sequence, each larger and more detailed than the preceding one.

- Study outline (Table 1.1 and Appendix 1A). This one-page summary of the design serves as a standardized checklist to remind the investigator to address all the components. The sequence has an orderly logic that helps clarify the investigator's thinking on the topic.
- Study protocol. This expansion on the study outline usually ranges from 5 to 15 pages. It is used to plan the study and to apply for IRB approval and grant support. The protocol parts are discussed throughout this book and summarized in Chapter 20.
- Operations manual. Studies that enroll participants and collect data also develop a comprehensive manual that includes specific procedural instructions, questionnaires, data collection forms, and other materials. Even studies that use precollected data, such as from an electronic health record, must specify exactly how those data will be used. The manual ensures a uniform and standardized approach to carrying out the study with good quality control (Chapter 18).

The research question and study outline should be written out at an early stage. Putting thoughts in writing leads the way from vague ideas to specific plans and provides a concrete basis for getting advice from colleagues and consultants. It is a challenge to do it—ideas are easier to talk about than to write down—but the rewards are a faster start and a better project. Although some early-stage investigators are understandably impatient to begin their study without taking the time to spell out detailed plans, this often leads to a poorly conceived project and subsequent delays.

Appendix 1A is an example of a study outline. This kind of outline deals more with the anatomy of research (Table 1.1) than with its physiology (Figure 1.4), so the investigator must remind herself to think carefully about minimizing the errors that may result when it is time to draw inferences from the study findings. A study's virtues and problems can be revealed by explicitly considering how the question the study is likely to answer differs from the research question, given the plans for acquiring participants and making measurements, and the likely problems of implementation.

With the study outline in hand and the intended inferences in mind, the investigator can proceed with the details of her protocol. This iterative process includes getting advice from colleagues, drafting specific recruitment and measurement methods, considering scientific and ethical appropriateness, modifying the study question and outline as needed, pretesting specific recruitment and measurement methods, making more changes, getting more advice, and so forth.

Trade-offs

Regrettably, errors are an inherent part of all studies. The main issue is whether the errors will be large enough to make the conclusions of the study unreliable. When designing a study, the investigator is in much the same position as a labor union official bargaining for a new contract. The union official begins with a wish list—shorter hours, higher wages, better benefits, and so forth. She must then make concessions, holding on to the things that are most important and relinquishing those that are not essential or realistic. At the end of the negotiations comes a final, but vital, step: She looks at the best contract she could negotiate and decides if it is worth signing.

The same sort of concessions must be made by an investigator when she transforms the research question to the study plan and considers potential problems in implementation. On one side are the issues of internal and external validity; on the other, feasibility. Compromises are always necessary. But once a study plan has been formulated, the investigator should examine it afresh to decide whether it adequately addresses the research question and whether it can be implemented with acceptable levels of error. This last step of deciding whether the study as designed is worth pursuing—the equivalent of the union negotiator determining whether to agree to the proposed contract—is, unfortunately, sometimes omitted. Or its answer is no, and there is a need to begin the process anew. But take heart! Good scientists distinguish themselves not so much by their uniformly good research ideas as by their alacrity in turning over those that won't work and moving on to better ones.

■ SUMMARY

1. The **anatomy** of research is the set of tangible elements that make up the study plan: the **research question** and its significance, and the **design, study participants**, and **measurement approaches**. The challenge is to design elements that balance feasibility with the need to produce valid study conclusions.

2. The **physiology** of research is how the study works. The study findings are used to draw conclusions about measurable phenomena in an accessible population (**internal validity**) in order to apply those conclusions to other situations, people, and events (**external validity** or generalizability). The challenge here is to design and implement a study plan with adequate control over two major threats to validity—**random error** (chance) and **systematic error** (bias)—and that adds to our current knowledge about the research question.

3. In designing a study, the investigator may find it helpful to consider Figure 1.4, the relationships between the **research question** (what she wants to answer), the **study plan** (what the study is designed to answer), and the **actual study** (what the study will actually answer, given the errors of implementation that can be anticipated).

4. A good way to develop the study plan is to begin with a one-sentence version of the research question that specifies the main variables and target population and expand this into a one-page outline that sets out the study elements in a standardized sequence. Later, the **study plan** will be expanded into the **protocol** and the **operations manual**.

5. Good judgment by the investigator and advice from colleagues are needed for the many trade-offs involved and for determining the overall viability of the project.

APPENDIX 1A
Outline of a Study

This is the brief study plan for a project carried out by Michael Jung, MD, MBA, which began while he was an anesthesia resident at UCSF, mentored by Jina Sinskey, MD. Most beginning investigators find observational studies easier to do, but in this situation a randomized clinical trial of modest size and scope was feasible. The study results were published in a high-impact journal (1).

■ PERIOPERATIVE VIRTUAL REALITY FOR PEDIATRIC ANESTHESIA

Background and Significance

Perioperative pediatric anxiety is a common and important aspect of the psychological impact of anesthesia and surgery on children. Prior research has shown that the incidence of high anxiety at induction can be as high as 50% in children who present for surgery and general anesthesia (2). Audiovisual distraction, including virtual reality (VR), has the potential to be a safe, noninvasive, nonpharmacologic modality to reduce anxiety.

Specific Aim

To conduct a randomized controlled trial to examine the effect of immersive audiovisual distraction with a VR headset on perioperative anxiety in pediatric patients presenting for elective surgery and general anesthesia.

Methods

Overview of Design

In this prospective, randomized, controlled, parallel group study, children scheduled for elective surgery and general anesthesia will be randomly allocated to either a VR group or a control (no VR) group. Group VR patients will undergo audiovisual distraction with VR during induction of general anesthesia in the operating room. A validated instrument, the Modified Yale Preoperative Anxiety Scale (mYPAS), will be used to assess anxiety.

Study Participants

The target population for this research project is children ages 5 to 12 years old presenting for elective surgery and general anesthesia; the accessible population consists of similar children seen at the UCSF Benioff Children's Hospital.

Measurements

The predictor variable is the intervention (ie, VR headset or no headset). The primary outcome is perioperative pediatric anxiety (measured as mYPAS score), which will be ascertained three times: in the preoperative holding area, on entering the operating room, and during induction of general anesthesia.

Randomization and Blinding

Randomization will use a computer-generated random assignment table, incorporated into a programmed study application (Redcap) and concealed from the study recruitment personnel. A time-stamped entry including medical record number and consent completion are entered for randomization. Given the nature of the VR headset (a patient is either wearing it or not), blinding will not be used.

Data Analysis

The predictor variable is dichotomous: VR headset or no VR headset. The outcome variable (mYPAS score at induction) is a continuous variable ranging from 0 to 100, which will be compared between groups using a t test. Categorical outcomes will be analyzed with chi-squared analysis. A significance level of 0.05 will be used.

Sample Size Estimates

Based on a prior investigation of preoperative anxiety in children ages 5 to 12 years old (3), mean $\pm$ SD mYPAS scores in the control group will be 30.1 $\pm$ 8.4. Recruiting 31 participants per group would yield a power of 80% ($\beta = 0.20$) to detect a 20% difference in mYPAS scores at induction between the two groups.

REFERENCES FOR APPENDIX 1A

1. Jung MJ, Libaw JS, Ma K, Whitlock EL, Feiner JR, Sinskey JL. Pediatric distraction on induction of anesthesia with virtual reality and perioperative anxiolysis: a randomized controlled trial. *Anesth Analg.* 2021;132(3):798-806.
2. Kain ZN, Mayes LC, Caldwell-Andrews AA, Karas DE, Mcclain BC. Preoperative anxiety, postoperative pain, and behavioral recovery in young children undergoing surgery. *Pediatrics.* 2006;118(2):651-658.
3. Moura LA, Dias IM, Pereira LV. Prevalence and factors associated with preoperative anxiety in children aged 5-12 years. *Rev Lat Am Enfermagem.* 2016;24:e2708.

APPENDIX 1B
Exercises for Chapter 1. Getting Started: The Anatomy and Physiology of Clinical Research

1. The Early Limited Formula (ELF) study was carried out in two academic medical centers in California with the goal of encouraging breastfeeding by newborn babies who had lost ≥5% of their body weight in the first 36 hours after birth. In this randomized clinical trial, the ELF intervention consisted of teaching parents to syringe-feed 10 mL of formula after each breastfeeding until the onset of mature milk production; control parents were taught infant soothing techniques. The proportion of mothers who reported exclusive breastfeeding at 3 months to a blinded interviewer was 79% in the ELF group, compared with 42% in the control group ($P = 0.02$) (1).
   For each of the following statements, indicate (a) whether it is an internal validity or external validity inference; (b) whether you think it is a valid inference; and (c) any reasons why it might *not* be valid.
   a. For the women in this study, provision of ELF increased breastfeeding rates at 3 months.
   b. Provision of ELF to infants born in a Boston community hospital who have ≥5% weight loss in the first 36 hours will likely lead to higher breastfeeding rates at age 6 months.
   c. Based on the results of this study, an international effort to provide formula to most newborns is likely to enhance successful breastfeeding and improve the health of the newborns and their mothers.
2. For each of the following summaries drawn from published studies, write a single sentence that specifies the design and the research question, including the main predictor and outcome variables, and the intended sample.
   a. Investigators in Winston-Salem, North Carolina, surveyed a random sample of 2228 local high school students about their frequency of watching wrestling on television in the previous 2 weeks, and 6 months later asked the same students about fighting at school and on dates. The adjusted odds of reporting fighting with a date increased by 14% for each episode of wrestling the students reported having watched 6 months before (2).
   b. To assess whether the amount of breastfeeding protects women against ovarian cancer, investigators surveyed 493 Chinese women with newly diagnosed ovarian cancer and 472 other hospitalized women, all of whom had breastfed at least one child. They found a dose-response relationship between total months of breastfeeding and reduced risk of ovarian cancer. For example, women who had breastfed for at least 31 months had an odds ratio of 0.09 (95% CI: 0.04 to 0.19), compared with women who had breastfed less than 10 months (3).
   c. To see whether an association between dietary saturated fat intake and reduced sperm concentration in infertile men extended to the general population, Danish investigators collected semen samples and food frequency questionnaires from consenting young men at the time of their examination for military service. They found a significant dose-response relation between self-reported dietary saturated fat intake and reduced sperm concentrations (eg, 41% [95% CI 4%, 64%] lower sperm concentration in the highest quartile of saturated fat intake compared with the lowest) (4).

d. Embolic stroke in atrial fibrillation may be preventable by occluding the left atrial appendage. Investigators studied patients with atrial fibrillation undergoing cardiac surgery for another indication (5). They occluded the left atrial appendage during surgery for half of the patients (randomly selected) and did not for the other half. In the 2379 patients in the occlusion group, 114 (4.8%) had a stroke or systemic embolism, compared with 168 (7.0%) of 2391 without occlusion ($P < 0.001$).

REFERENCES

1. Flaherman VJ, Aby J, Burgos AE, Lee KA, Cabana MD, Newman TB. Effect of early limited formula on duration and exclusivity of breastfeeding in at-risk infants: an RCT. *Pediatrics.* 2013;131(6):1059-1065.
2. DuRant RH, Champion H, Wolfson M. The relationship between watching professional wrestling on television and engaging in date fighting among high school students. *Pediatrics.* 2006;118:e265-e272.
3. Su D, Pasalich M, Lee AH, Binns CW. Ovarian cancer risk is reduced by prolonged lactation: a case-control study in southern China. *Am J Clin Nutr.* 2013;97:354-359.
4. Jensen TK, Heitmann BL, Jensen MB, et al. High dietary intake of saturated fat is associated with reduced semen quality among 701 young Danish men from the general population. *Am J Clin Nutr.* 2013;97:411-418.
5. Whitlock RP, Belley-Cote EP, Paparella D, et al. Left atrial appendage occlusion during cardiac surgery to prevent stroke. *New Engl J Med.* 2021;384:2081-2091.

Conceiving the Research Question and Developing the Study Plan

Steven R. Cummings and Alka M. Kanaya

The research question is the uncertainty that the investigator wants her study to resolve. There are many good research questions, and even as we succeed in answering some, we remain surrounded by others. For example, among older adults, loneliness is strongly associated with a decline in functional status and an increase in mortality (1). But this finding leads to new questions: Can we diminish loneliness among the elderly by providing a structured in-home support program? Would this type of program prevent functional decline? What types of interventions work best: peer, family, or group support? Can a program be effective if conducted remotely by phone or video? Is loneliness also associated with declines in cognitive function?

The challenge in finding a research question is defining an important one that has not been answered and that can be transformed into a feasible, ethical, and valid study plan. This chapter presents strategies for accomplishing this.

■ ORIGINS OF A RESEARCH QUESTION

For an established investigator, the best research questions usually emerge from the findings and problems she has observed in her own prior studies and in those of other scientists in the field. A new investigator has not yet developed this base of experience. Although a fresh perspective sometimes allows a creative person to conceive new approaches to old problems, lack of experience is largely an impediment.

A good way to begin is to clarify the difference between a research question and a *research interest*. Consider this research question:

- **Does providing a regular basic income reduce depression among middle-aged adults?**

This might be asked by someone whose research interest involves social determinants of health, depression prevention or management, or health policy interventions. The distinction between research questions and research interests matters because it may turn out that although a specific question cannot be transformed into a viable study plan, the investigator can still address her research interest by asking a different question.

Of course, it's impossible to formulate a research question if you are not even sure about your research interest. If you find yourself in this boat, you're not alone: Many new investigators have not yet discovered a topic that excites them and that is amenable to a feasible study plan. You can begin by considering what sorts of research studies have piqued your interest when you read them. Or perhaps you recall a patient whose treatment seemed inadequate or inappropriate: What could have been done differently that might have improved her outcome? Or you question current practices, for example, whether physical exams for all new patients, as required by many payers, will reduce the risk of diseases or the cost of care during the next few years.

Investigators often have several potential research questions. Being involved in more than one project at a time is helpful: When one is stalled (eg, while waiting to hear back from the Institutional Review Board (IRB) or a collaborator), you can be working on another. But having too many projects spreads limited time and resources, so a wise approach is to prioritize the top few on the basis of how well they meet the characteristics of a good question, reviewed further on. Your attention may necessarily focus on a research question that has a time-sensitive opportunity, such as a funding deadline. Keep a list of ideas to return to as your bandwidth allows. Sharing your questions with other investigators, fellows, or students may allow you to participate in a study as a coinvestigator or mentor.

Expertise

It is important to become an expert in the area of study. Scholarship is foundational to successful research. A new investigator should conduct a thorough search of published literature in the areas pertinent to the research question and read important papers critically. Carrying out a systematic review may be a good next step for developing and establishing expertise in a research area, and the underlying literature review can serve as background for grant proposals and research reports.

Recent advances may be known to active investigators in a field long before they are published. Mastery of a subject entails staying abreast of multiple sources of information, including getting alerts about relevant literature through PubMed and journals, participating in scientific meetings, building relationships with experts in the field, and even following thought leaders on social media platforms (eg, Twitter). It is helpful to consult the website ClinicalTrials.gov to see if protocols like the one you are envisioning have already been registered. Although the website is concerned primarily with clinical trials, observational studies are sometimes included. Similarly, if you are planning a systematic review, many of these are registered on the *Prospero* website (https://www.crd.york.ac.uk/prospero/#aboutpage).

Addressing a Medical or Public Health Need

Impactful research results may arise from a need for better treatments, tests, or health services. Recognizing opportunities for feasible solutions is most likely to grow out of personal experience with the relevant conditions, populations, and programs. This is often an opportunity to generate novel and impactful research.

Being Alert to New Ideas and Techniques

It is helpful to attend conferences at which new work is presented. At least as important as the formal presentations are the opportunities for informal conversations with other scientists during poster sessions and breaks. An investigator who overcomes any reticence to engage a speaker at a coffee break may find the experience richly rewarding—and, occasionally, she will acquire a new senior colleague. For a speaker whose work seems especially relevant, it may be worthwhile to review her recent publications and then contact her to arrange a meeting during the conference.

A skeptical attitude toward prevailing beliefs can stimulate good research questions. For example, it was widely believed that lacerations that extend through the dermis required sutures to assure rapid healing and a satisfactory cosmetic outcome. However, Quinn et al. noted personal experience and evidence from case series that wounds of moderate size repair themselves regardless of whether wound edges are approximated (2). They carried out a randomized trial in which patients with uncomplicated hand lacerations less than 2 cm in length received tap water irrigation and a 48-hour antibiotic dressing. One group was randomly assigned to have their wounds sutured; the other group did not receive sutures. Participants in the suture group reported more painful and time-consuming treatments in the emergency room, but blinded assessment revealed similar time-to-healing and cosmetic results.

The application of new technologies often generates insights into, and questions about, familiar clinical problems, which in turn can generate new paradigms (3). Advances in genetic, molecular, imaging, and digital health technologies, for example, have spawned translational research studies that have led to treatments and tests that have changed clinical medicine. An example is the use of deuterated creatine (D_3Cr), a biomarker for muscle mass measurement that is more accurate and less expensive than dual energy x-ray absorptiometry scans (4). D_3Cr measurements can be applied to study whether muscle mass predicts outcomes after elective surgery and as a more accurate way to study whether exercise improves skeletal muscle mass. Taking a new concept, technology, or finding from one field and applying it to a problem in another can lead to innovative research questions.

Clinical experience is a rich source of questions about potential causes of, and ways to treat, a disease. Careful observations of patients may lead to recognition of new risk factors for conditions, rare genetic syndromes, or complications of treatment. Detailed descriptions of the discovery might be published as a case report or case series, alerting others to recognize additional cases. For example, clinicians observed unusual femoral fractures in nine patients who had been treated for many years with alendronate, a treatment for osteoporosis (5). This eventually led to large epidemiologic studies confirming that longer use of alendronate leads to an increased risk of these atypical fractures (6).

Collaborations with other investigators commonly generate new ideas and questions to pursue. This is particularly true when the scientist brings expertise or methods from a different field. Such collaborators can be an ongoing source of innovations and ideas as a member of a research team.

Teaching is also an excellent source of inspiration. Ideas for studies often occur while preparing presentations or during discussions with inquisitive students, who often ask for explanations about standard practices or beliefs that reveal uncertainty or lack of evidence that points to the need for research.

There is a major role for creativity in the process of conceiving research questions, imagining new methods to address old questions, and playing with ideas. Some creative ideas come to mind during informal conversations with colleagues over lunch; others arise from discussing recent research or your own ideas in small groups. Many inspirations are solo affairs that strike while preparing a lecture, showering, perusing social media, or just sitting and thinking. The trick is to put an unresolved problem clearly in view and allow the mind to run freely around it. Deliberate exposure to diverse scientific disciplines—journal articles, presentations at meetings outside your special interests—sometimes leads to new ideas that can cross-fertilize your research area with new measurements or concepts.

Fear of criticism or of having unusual ideas can inhibit creativity and quash the pursuit of novel questions that challenge current paradigms. Seek the support of colleagues who enjoy imagining new ideas. There is also a need for tenacity, returning to a troublesome problem repeatedly until a resolution is reached.

■ CHARACTERISTICS OF A GOOD RESEARCH QUESTION

The characteristics of a research question that lead to a good study plan are that it be Feasible, Important, Novel, and Ethical (which form the mnemonic *FINE*; Table 2.1).

Feasible

It is best to know the practical limits and problems of studying a question early on, before wasting much time and effort along unworkable lines.

- Number of participants. Many studies do not achieve their intended purposes because they cannot enroll enough participants. Estimate the sample size requirements for a study early on (Chapters 5 and 6). Consider how many participants are likely to be available for the study, the number who would be excluded or refuse to enroll, and the number who would be lost to follow-up. Even careful planning often produces estimates that are overly optimistic.

TABLE 2.1 "FINE" CRITERIA FOR A GOOD RESEARCH QUESTION AND STUDY PLAN

Feasible

> Adequate number of participants
> Adequate technical expertise
> Affordable in time and money
> Fundable

Important

> May lead to improvements in clinical care or public health
> Contributes to an investigator's reputation for rigorous and valuable research

Novel

> New findings
> Confirms, refutes, or extends previous findings
> May lead to innovations in concepts of health and disease, medical practice, or methodologies for research

Ethical

> Meets the criteria set by the Institutional Review Board
> Addresses health equity

Before devoting effort to developing other details, the investigator should ensure that there are enough eligible and willing participants. It is sometimes necessary to carry out a pilot **survey** or a review of stored electronic data to be sure. If the number of participants appears insufficient, the investigator can consider several strategies: expanding the inclusion criteria, eliminating unnecessary exclusion criteria, lengthening the time frame for enrolling participants, acquiring additional sources of participants, developing more precise measurement approaches, inviting colleagues to join in a multicenter study, and using a different study design.

- **Essential expertise.** The investigators must have the skills, equipment, and experience needed to design the study, recruit the participants, measure the variables, and manage and analyze the data. It may be valuable to collaborate with an expert or assemble a team with the skills and experience to shore up technical expertise that is unfamiliar to the investigator. For example, it is often wise to include a statistician as a member of the research team from the beginning of the planning process to provide advice about sample size and analytic methods. When a new measurement method is needed, such as an assay of a new biomarker, expertise in the best methods should be sought.

- **Availability of appropriate data.** If addressing your question would rely on secondary data sets (Chapter 16), it is important to know the availability and limitations of information in potentially relevant data sets.

- **Cost in time and money.** Estimate the costs of each component of a project, bearing in mind that the time and money needed will generally exceed the amounts projected at the outset. If the projected costs exceed the available funds, the only options are to consider a less expensive design or to develop additional sources of funding. Early recognition of a study that is too expensive or time-consuming can lead to modification or abandonment of the plan before a great deal of effort is expended.

- **Scope.** Problems often arise when an investigator attempts to accomplish too much, making many measurements at repeated contacts with a large group of participants in an effort to answer too many research questions. The solution is to narrow the scope of the study and focus only on the most important goals. Many scientists find it difficult to give up the opportunity to answer interesting side questions, but the reward may be a better answer to the main question at hand.

- **Fundability.** Few investigators have the personal or institutional resources to fund their own research projects, particularly if participants need to be enrolled and followed or expensive measurements must be made. The most elegantly designed research proposal will not be feasible if no one will pay for the study to be carried out. Identifying potential sources of funding is discussed in Chapter 20.

Important

There are many motivations for pursuing a particular research question: the exhilaration of getting at the truth of a matter, because it is a logical next step in building a career, or because it will provide support to sustain your line of research.

- **Significance.** The best motivation for pursuing a research question is to improve health and well-being. So, imagine the possible results of the study and consider how each one might advance scientific knowledge, influence clinical practice or public health policy, or guide further research. Then confirm that you are not the only one who believes that the question is important. Speak with mentors, outside experts, and representatives of potential funders such as National Institutes of Health (NIH) program officers before devoting substantial energy to developing a research plan or grant proposal that peers and funding agencies believe will not change practice. Significance—a criterion that is scored separately on grant proposals—often drives the overall impact score for a project.
- **Furthers your career.** Another important consideration is whether pursuit of a particular research question will contribute to your career. Will the study build new skills, develop collaborations, or provide funding to expand your team? Will the results generate respect for the value or rigor of your research? In contrast, spending time on a question that will take years to produce a result that is likely to have little impact or visibility will slow the development of your career. Although tempting in some respects, pursuing studies to add papers to a CV or promotion packet may result in a body of work that has little impact on science or health.

Novel

A study that merely reiterates what is already established is not worth the effort and cost and is unlikely to receive funding. The novelty of a proposed study can be determined by reviewing the literature, consulting with experts who are familiar with as-yet unpublished research, and looking for abstracts of funded projects in your area of interest on the NIH Research Portfolio Online Reporting Tools (RePORT) website (http://report.nih.gov/categorical_spending.aspx) and the ClinicalTrials.gov website. Reviews of studies submitted to the NIH give weight to whether a proposed study is innovative such that a successful result could shift paradigms of research or clinical practice through the use of new concepts, methods, or interventions (Chapter 20). Although novelty is an important criterion, a research question need not be totally original—it can be worthwhile to ask whether a previous observation can be replicated, whether the findings in one population also apply to others, or whether a new measurement method can clarify the relationship between known risk factors and a disease. A confirmatory study is particularly useful if it avoids the weaknesses of previous studies or if the prior result was unexpected.

Ethical

Ethical research involves more than just avoiding unethical behavior or causing harm. It also includes promoting equity and the well-being of participants and the public.

- **Human subjects research.** A good research question must be answerable by an ethical study. If the study poses unacceptable risks, especially for vulnerable groups, or invades privacy (Chapter 7), the investigator must seek other ways to answer the question. If there is uncertainty about whether the study (or an aspect of it) is ethical, discuss the concern at an early stage with a representative of the IRB.

- **Health equity.** Institutional and other structural barriers are a major driver of health disparities. Research should not contribute to greater inequities but rather address and lessen these disparities. One step toward improving health equity is to make an extra effort to include participants of diverse backgrounds and experiences (eg, by gender, race/ethnicity, socioeconomic status, or English language proficiency). Another is to involve traditionally understudied participants in designing and disseminating the research. Research frameworks that build on a partnership with community members to dismantle systemic inequities are discussed in Chapter 15.

■ DEVELOPING THE STUDY PLAN

It helps to summarize the research question and study design in a single sentence at an early stage. Some studies are descriptive (eg, "A cross-sectional study of the prevalence of peanut allergy among Texas kindergarteners"), but most aim to determine whether a predictor is associated with or causes an outcome (eg, "A cohort study to estimate the effect of phototherapy on breastfeeding at 2 months among term newborns in Northern California").

The next step is to create a brief (one-page) outline of the **study plan**, which should describe the importance of the study, the design, the study participants and how they will be selected, how many participants will be needed, and what measurements will be made (see Appendix 1A in Chapter 1). This requires some self-discipline, but it forces the investigator to clarify her ideas and identify specific problems that need attention. The outline also provides a basis for obtaining specific suggestions from mentors and colleagues.

The development of a study plan is an *iterative process* of making incremental improvements in the study's design, such as revising the selection criteria or reestimating the sample size, reviewing modifications with colleagues, and pretesting key features, if appropriate. As the protocol takes shape, pilot studies to ensure the availability and willingness of enough participants may lead to changes in the recruitment plan. Concurrently, the investigator may also be building a team to help with the measurements, statistical plan, proposal for funding (Chapter 20), and, if all goes well, conducting the study.

Primary and Secondary Questions

Many studies have more than one research question. Clinical trials often address the effect of the intervention on more than one outcome. For example, the Women's Health Initiative was designed to determine whether reducing dietary fat intake would reduce the risk of breast cancer, but an important secondary hypothesis was to examine its effect on coronary events (7). Almost all cohort and case-control studies look at several risk factors for each outcome. The advantage of designing a study with several research questions is the efficiency that can result, with several answers emerging from a single study. The disadvantages are the increased complexity of the study's design and implementation and of drawing statistical inferences when there are multiple hypotheses (Chapter 5). A sensible strategy is to establish a **primary research question** around which to focus the study plan and sample size estimate. Adding **secondary research questions**, measurements, or biologic samples enables a study to address more than one question and to create a database and bank of specimens for analyses, articles, and preliminary work to support proposals to answer the next questions.

■ CHOOSING AND WORKING WITH A MENTOR

Nothing substitutes for experience in guiding the many judgments involved in conceiving a research question and fleshing out a study plan. Therefore, an essential strategy for a new investigator is to apprentice herself to an **experienced primary mentor** who has the time and interest to work with her regularly. A team, with co-mentors from different disciplines, is often necessary to help a new investigator develop expertise in both the content and the research approach, acquire the skills to carry out a project, and develop into an independent investigator.

Choose a mentor carefully. Talk with others who have served as mentees, review a potential mentor's CV to see if she has published or obtained grants with previous mentees, and meet potential mentors to understand how they like to work and what they expect from mentees.

A good mentor will be available for regular meetings and informal discussions about your ideas. A mentor may open doors to networking and funding opportunities, encourage the development of independent work, and include a new investigator on grant proposals and manuscript projects whenever appropriate. Good relationships of this sort can also lead to tangible resources, such as help from research or administrative assistants; access to clinical populations, data sets, and specimen banks; specialized laboratories and office space; statistical support; and financial resources and a research team—not to mention lifelong friendships.

On the other hand, a bad mentor can be a barrier to success by reacting critically to new ideas in a way that inhibits creativity. A bad mentor takes credit for findings that arise from a new investigator's work or assumes the lead role on publishing or presenting her findings. Mentoring relationships are also subject to social and interpersonal dynamics of gender, race/ethnicity, and power. If the junior investigator feels that the mentoring relationship is abusive, then she should seek help from other senior colleagues or, if there is concern for harassment, discrimination, or retaliation, from the Title IX officer at her institution. More commonly, many mentors are simply too busy or distracted to pay attention to a new investigator's needs. In either case, once discussions with the mentor have proved fruitless, we recommend finding a way to move on to a more appropriate advisor, perhaps by involving a neutral senior colleague or other members of the mentoring team.

Sometimes, a mentor may give you a project or manuscript to finish (often from a previous mentee) because the mentor lacks the time or interest. This might be an excellent opportunity to publish as a lead author, but it can also be an exercise in frustration that does not further your career or expertise. (There may be a good reason why a previous mentee abandoned the project.) Although it may be uncomfortable, a new investigator should discuss the potential value to her training and career and decline the opportunity if there would be little benefit. This may be a scenario where a mentoring team can serve as a check on any dubious tasks or projects.

■ SUMMARY

All studies should start with a research question that addresses what the investigator would like to know. The goal is to find one that can be developed into a good study plan.

1. Expertise is essential to developing research questions that are worth pursuing. A **systematic review** of research pertinent to an area of research interest is a good place to start. Attending conferences, meeting other scientists, and following areas of interest on social media extend the investigator's expertise beyond what is already published.
2. Good research questions arise from **speaking with colleagues**, **critical thinking** about clinical practices and problems, **applying new methods** to old issues, and **considering ideas** that emerge from teaching, daydreaming, and the tenacious pursuit of solutions to vexing problems.
3. Before committing much time and effort to writing a proposal or carrying out a study, the investigator should consider whether the research question and study plan are "FINE": **feasible**, **important**, **novel**, and **ethical**. Those who fund research give priority to proposals that may have innovative and significant impacts on science and health.
4. Early on, the research question should be developed into a one-page written **study outline** that specifically describes the importance of the study, the design, the study participants, the number that will be needed, and the measurements that will be made.

5. Developing the research question and study plan is an iterative process that includes consultations with advisors and colleagues and building a team that can assist with measurements, statistical aspects of the study, and writing proposals for funding.

6. Most studies have more than one question, and it is useful to focus on a single primary question in designing and implementing the study. Adding secondary questions and measurements, and storing biologic specimens, can build a resource for additional articles and preliminary studies for the next research questions.

7. A new investigator must choose one or two senior scientists to serve as her mentor(s): experienced investigators who will take time to meet, provide resources and connections, encourage creativity, and promote the independence and visibility of their junior scientists.

REFERENCES

1. Perissinotto CM, Cenzer IS, Covinsky K. Loneliness in older persons: a predictor of functional decline and death. *Arch Intern Med*. 2012;172(14):1078-1083.

2. Quinn J, Cummings S, Callaham M, et al. Suturing versus conservative management of lacerations of the hand: randomized controlled trial. *BMJ*. 2002;325:299-301.

3. Kuhn TS. *The Structure of Scientific Revolutions*. University of Chicago Press; 1962.

4. Cawthon P, Orwoll ES, Peters KE, et al. Strong relation between muscle mass determined by D3-creatine dilution, physical performance, and incidence of falls and mobility limitations in a prospective cohort of older men. *J Gerontol A Biol Sci Med Sci*. 2019;74(6):844-852.

5. Goh SK, Yang KY, Koh JS, et al. Subtrochanteric insufficiency fractures in patients on alendronate therapy: a caution. *J Bone Joint Surg Br*. 2007;89(3):349-353.

6. Black DM, Geiger EJ, Eastell R, et al. Atypical femur fracture risk versus fragility fracture prevention with bisphosphonates. *N Engl J Med*. 2020;383(8):743-753.

7. Howard BV, Van Horn L, Hsia J, et al. Low-fat dietary pattern and risk of cardiovascular disease: the Women's Health Initiative Randomized Controlled Dietary Modification Trial. *JAMA*. 2006;295(6):655–666.

APPENDIX 2A
Exercises for Chapter 2. Conceiving the Research Question and Developing the Study Plan

1. Consider the research question: "What is the relationship between marijuana use and health?" First, convert this into a more specific version that includes study design, predictor and outcome variables, and target population. Then discuss whether the research question and design you have chosen meet the FINE criteria (Feasible, Important, Novel, Ethical). Rewrite the question and design to resolve any problems in meeting these criteria.

2. Consider the research question: "Does acetaminophen (paracetamol) cause asthma?" Put yourself back in the year 2000, when this question was starting to be asked, and provide one-sentence descriptions of two observational studies and one clinical trial to address this research question. Make sure each description specifies the study design, predictor and outcome variables, and target population. Then, for each, consider whether the research question and design you have chosen meet the FINE criteria.

3. Use the ideas in this chapter and your own interests to conceive a research question and devise a one-page outline of a study you might carry out. Does it meet the FINE criteria? Discuss different designs, target populations and samples, and variables to optimize your study.

CHAPTER 3

Choosing the Study Participants: Specification, Sampling, and Recruitment

Warren S. Browner, Thomas B. Newman, and Mark J. Pletcher

T he study plan must specify a **sample** that can be studied at an acceptable cost in time and money yet is both large enough to control random error and representative enough to allow valid interpretations and inferences about how well the study results generalize to the **target population**. That said, generalizability is rarely a simple yes-or-no matter. Rather, it is a complex qualitative judgment that depends on the investigator's choice of whom to study and how to sample them.

We will come to the issue of choosing the appropriate *number* of study **participants** in Chapters 5 and 6. In this chapter, we address the process of specifying and **sampling** the *kinds* of participants who will be both representative and feasible to enroll (Figure 3.1). We also discuss strategies for recruiting these people into the study.

Not all clinical research focuses on individuals; some studies involve families, work groups, hospital units, towns, or other units of observation. However, this chapter primarily draws upon examples in which the participants are people.

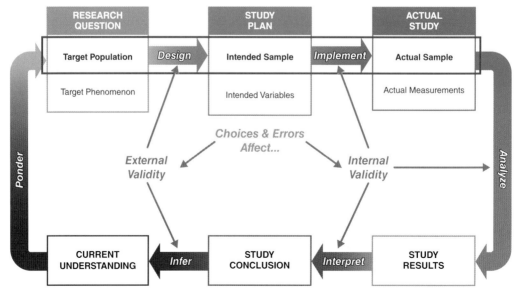

■ **FIGURE 3.1** This chapter focuses on the items within the red box: choosing a sample of study participants that represents the target population for the research question.

■ BASIC TERMS AND CONCEPTS

Populations and Samples

A population is a complete set of people with a set of specified characteristics. In lay usage, geographic characteristics are commonly used to define a population—for example, the population of Clark County, Nevada. In research, clinical and demographic characteristics are used to define a **target population**, the large set of people beyond the study to which the results will be generalized, such as teenagers with asthma. The **accessible population** is a geographically and temporally defined subset of the target population that is available for study—say, teenagers with asthma cared for in the investigator's community in a given year. (The term "patient population" is sometimes used in clinical parlance as a rough synonym for the accessible population.)

A **sample** is a defined subset of the accessible population. The **intended sample** is the subset of the accessible population that the investigator seeks to include in the study (such as teenagers with asthma cared for at the three medical centers that agree to provide access to their electronic medical records), whereas the *actual* sample consists of the participants who join the study (such as those who agree to enroll).

Generalizing the Study Findings

The classic Framingham Study (1) was an early approach to designing a study to allow inferences from findings observed in a sample to be applied to a target population (Figure 3.2).

The sampling design called for identifying all the families in Framingham, Massachusetts, with at least one person aged 30 to 59 years, listing the families by address, and then asking age-eligible persons in the first two of every group of three families to participate. (This design is not as tamperproof as choosing each participant by a random process, as

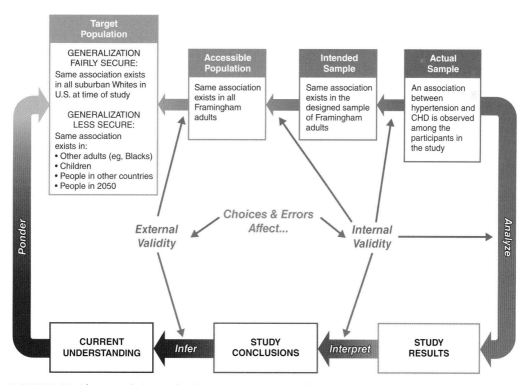

■ **FIGURE 3.2** After a study is completed, interpretations and inferences are made when generalizing from the results in the study participants to the target population(s). This process moves from right to left.

discussed later in this chapter.) The sampling scheme raises a few concerns. One-third of the Framingham residents selected for the study refused to participate; instead, the investigators accepted other age-eligible residents who volunteered (1). Because volunteers are often healthier than those who decline participation, the characteristics of the actual sample undoubtedly differed from those of the intended sample. More important, Framingham's population was not representative of the United States, or even Massachusetts, as it comprised mainly middle-class Whites.

Every sample, however, has some errors; the issue is how those errors affect the interpretations and inferences that can be made from the study results. The sampling errors in the Framingham Study do not seem large enough to invalidate the conclusion that risk relationships observed in the study—for example, that hypertension is a risk factor for coronary heart disease (CHD)—can be generalized to all the residents of Framingham. The next concern is the validity of generalizing the finding that hypertension is a risk factor for CHD from the accessible population of Framingham to target populations elsewhere. This inference is more subjective. The town of Framingham was selected in part because it seemed typical of similar communities elsewhere and was convenient to the investigators, whose university home was 25 miles away in Boston. The validity of generalizing the risk relationships observed in the Framingham Study to other populations relies on a set of assumptions, many of which cannot be verified. As it has turned out, subsequent studies have found that the association between hypertension and CHD is similar in Framingham residents and many other populations, including inner city Blacks. However, hypertension is much more common in the latter group, illustrating that descriptive studies of the *distributions* of many characteristics often do not generalize to other populations as well as studies of *associations* do.

Steps in Designing the Protocol for Acquiring Study Participants

The inferences in Figure 3.2 are presented from right to left, the sequence used for interpreting the findings of a completed study. An investigator who is planning a study reverses this sequence, beginning on the left (Figure 3.3). She begins by specifying the clinical and demographic characteristics of the target population that will serve the research question well. She then uses *geographic* and *temporal criteria* to specify a study sample that is representative and practical.

■ SELECTION CRITERIA

Suppose an investigator wants to study the efficacy of low-dose testosterone supplements (as compared with placebo) for enhancing libido in postmenopausal women. She should begin by identifying the characteristics of the target population to whom the results would be applied—and then design her sample to include participants who are as similar as possible to that ideal (Table 3.1). Collectively, these attributes are known as the **selection** (or **entry**) **criteria.**

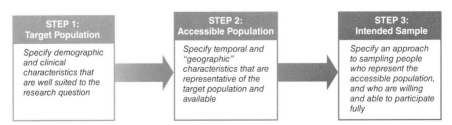

■ **FIGURE 3.3** As a study is designed, the investigator proceeds from left to right as she develops the protocol for choosing the study participants. The word "geographic" is used somewhat loosely; for example, it may refer to members of a health plan or even users of a social media platform.

TABLE 3.1 DESIGNING SELECTION CRITERIA FOR A CLINICAL TRIAL OF LOW-DOSE TESTOSTERONE VERSUS PLACEBO TO ENHANCE LIBIDO IN MENOPAUSE

DESIGN FEATURE	EXAMPLE
Inclusion criteria (be specific) describing who will be studied:	
Clinical characteristics of primary relevance to the research question	Women concerned about decreased libido Have a sexual partner
Demographic focus	Age 50-59 years
Geographic (administrative) focus Temporal focus	Patients attending clinic at the investigator's hospital between January 1 and December 31 of specified year
Exclusion criteria (be parsimonious) describing subsets of the population that will not be studied because of:	
A high likelihood of being lost to follow-up	Substance abuse Plans to move out of state
An inability to provide good data	Disoriented or cognitively impaired Has a language barrier[a]
Being at high risk of possible adverse effects	History of myocardial infarction or stroke

[a]Alternatives to excluding those with a language barrier (when these subgroups are sizeable and important to the research question) would be collecting nonverbal data or using bilingual staff and questionnaires.

Establishing Selection Criteria

Inclusion criteria define the main characteristics of the target population that pertain to the research question and study design. In our example, the research question is most relevant for women who have concerns about decreased libido. In addition, having a sexual partner is likely critical for measuring the effects of testosterone supplementation. Age is often a crucial factor; in this example, one investigator might decide to focus on women in their fifties, speculating that in this group the benefit-to-harm ratio of the drug might be optimal, whereas another might make a different decision and focus on older women.

Many cohort studies recruit participants who are at higher-than-average risk of developing the study outcome because it reduces the necessary size of the sample (see Chapter 5). For example, a study to determine the risk factors for osteoporotic fractures might enroll women 65 years of age and older, because their fracture risk is greater than those in younger women or men; this was exactly the strategy used in the Study of Osteoporotic Fractures! (2). Similarly, a clinical trial of a new treatment to reduce the risk of colon cancer might enroll participants with a history of colonic polyps.

A study's inclusion criteria often involve trade-offs between scientific and practical goals. For example, although patients at the investigator's own hospital are often a ready source of participants, peculiarities of local referral patterns might interfere with the ability to generalize the results to other populations. When deciding about inclusion criteria, the important goals are to make decisions that are sensible, that can be used consistently throughout the study, and that can be described clearly to others who must decide to whom the published conclusions apply. In some circumstances, it's also important to consider how the inclusion criteria can redress previous biases or decisions that led to underrepresentation of certain groups. For example, while the Study of Osteoporotic Fractures originally included only the highest risk group (namely, White women), subsequent cohorts enrolled Black women as well as men (3, 4).

Exclusion criteria define limited exceptions to the broad brushstrokes of the inclusion criteria and should be used parsimoniously. They should generally be limited to characteristics that might interfere with the ability to provide **informed consent**, the quality of the data, the acceptability of a randomized treatment, or the success of follow-up efforts (Table 3.1). Difficulty with English, major psychological problems such as substance abuse, and serious illness may be such examples. Clinical trials differ from observational studies in being more likely to have exclusions mandated by concern for the safety of an intervention in certain participants, such as women who are or might become pregnant.

Of course, it's easy to convert some inclusion criteria (say, being older than age 70 years and a nonsmoker) to exclusion criteria (say, not enrolling anyone 69 years of age or younger, or who smokes), and vice versa. When there is a choice, we prefer inclusion criteria—they describe the characteristics of those in the study. Indeed, a good general rule is to have as *few* exclusion criteria as possible.

Many clinical trials develop inclusion and exclusion criteria to identify those most likely to benefit from the study treatment—and least likely to have adverse effects. This may involve excluding participants for whom prior therapies have made their disease more difficult to treat. Sometimes, clinical trials enroll only participants who have already responded well to other medications and thus appear likely to benefit from the new treatment. In both these situations, a better choice would be to include participants who most need a new therapy because they have previously failed others: they represent a likely target population for that treatment.

Some studies are designed primarily to learn something about the biology of a disease (such as its characteristics and causes), whereas others are designed primarily to guide pragmatic treatment decisions (such as whether to use a medical or surgical approach) (5). These different purposes can affect decisions about selection criteria. For example, an investigator interested primarily in measuring the precise physiologic effects of testosterone supplementation might define a narrow sample by excluding women who take any other medications. In contrast, another investigator might enroll a sample with few exclusions so that study results would apply more generally.

Specifying the clinical characteristics for selecting participants often involves difficult judgments about how to define those criteria. How, for example, would an investigator put into practice the criterion that the participants be in "good health"? She might, for example, decide not to include those with any self-reported illnesses, but this would likely exclude large numbers of potential participants, such as those with osteoarthritis, who may be perfectly suitable for the research question at hand. That's why an investigator should specify the justification for each of the study's inclusion and exclusion criteria to ensure they are all necessary and appropriate.

Finally, an investigator should avoid having selection criteria that might be caused by one of the outcomes being studied (eg, a study of the risk factors for lung cancer should not have recent weight loss as an inclusion or exclusion criterion). This concern is covered in greater detail in the discussion about "conditioning on shared effects" in Chapter 10.

Clinical Versus Representative Populations

When recruiting participants with a specific disease, hospitalized or clinic patients may be easy to find, but selection factors that determine who comes to the hospital or clinic may have an important effect. For example, a specialty clinic at an academic medical center attracts patients with serious forms of the disease, giving a distorted impression of the disease's features and prognosis. Sampling from community-based practices may be a better choice.

Samples often include participants who have been recruited by mail or e-mail, or by advertising on the internet or mass media. They are not fully representative of the general population, however, because some kinds of people are more likely than others to be contacted or to participate (as the preelection polls in the United States in 2016 and 2020 made clear). True **population-based samples**—such as National Health and Nutrition Examination Survey (NHANES), a representative sample of US residents—are difficult and expensive to recruit, but useful for guiding public health and clinical practice (6).

The size and diversity of a sample can be increased by collaborating with colleagues in other locations; by using preexisting data sets such as NHANES and Medicare records; or by obtaining access to data from public health agencies, health care organizations, and medical insurance companies. These data sets have come into widespread use in clinical research and are often more representative of national populations and less time-consuming to "enroll" (see Chapter 16).

For a variety of reasons, ranging from inconvenience to lack of community involvement to systemic racism, some segments of the population, such as members of ethnic minorities or those who are poor, have been underrepresented in research, making it difficult to estimate the effects of a treatment or exposure in these groups with adequate precision. These deficits can lead—and have led—to health disparities; responsible investigators should plan to devote extra resources to recruiting participants from these groups.

Having a sample that represents a diverse population enables the investigator to look at whether the results of the study differ among various groups, such as men and women or by race/ethnicity. Unless it's a specific aim of the study, however, any single study may not have enough participants in those groups to detect such differences unless they are large. But reporting the results in key subgroups—when combined with other studies that also report their results in that fashion—may make it possible to identify such differences in a **systematic review** or **meta-analysis**.

■ SAMPLING

Often, the potential number of people who meet the selection criteria is too large to study, and a sample (subset) of the accessible population must be chosen. This is not true, of course, for a study that uses existing data that are available in an electronic format; in this situation, the investigator may be able to study the entire accessible population after getting the necessary approvals.

There are two major categories of sampling approaches, one that involves having a defined probability for choosing each participant from the population and one that does not. Not surprisingly, these are called **probability** and **nonprobability samples**. Because the validity of drawing inferences from any sample depends on how well it represents the accessible population, this requires a subjective judgment with nonprobability samples.

Probability Samples

Probability sampling, the gold standard for statistical inferences, uses a random process to give each member of the accessible population a specified chance of being included in the sample (Figure 3.4). This provides a rigorous basis for estimating the fidelity with which phenomena observed in the sample represent those in the accessible population and for computing statistical significance and confidence intervals. The approach usually requires a **sampling frame**—a listing of all people (or clusters; see later) in the accessible population who might be included in the study. It has several versions.

- A **simple random sample** is selected from the sampling frame using a random process in which every participant has the same probability of being selected. For example, an investigator studying the outcomes of cataract surgery might identify all patients who underwent the procedure in her health system during the period of study. Suppose there were 2500 such patients, of whom the investigator has the resources to interview only 100. After

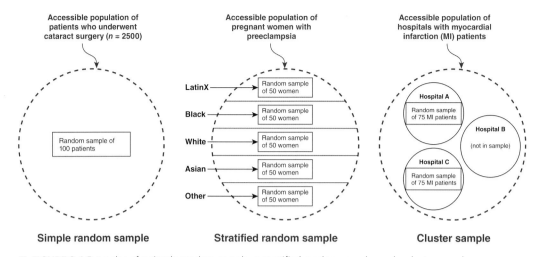

■ **FIGURE 3.4** Examples of a simple random sample, a stratified random sample, and a cluster sample.

enumerating the patients from 1 to 2500, a random number from 0 to 1 would be assigned to each of them; this can be done easily using the spreadsheet function RAND(). The sample is then sorted from the lowest random number to the highest, and the investigator selects the first 100 patients in the sorted list. If some of those who are selected do not participate, they would be replaced by those with the next lowest random numbers.

- A **systematic sample** differs from a simple random sample in that the sample is selected by a periodic process (eg, the Framingham approach of taking the first two out of every three families from a list of town families ordered by address). Systematic sampling is susceptible to errors caused by natural periodicities in the population, and it allows the investigator to predict and perhaps manipulate those who will be in the sample. It offers no logistic advantages over simple random sampling, and in clinical research it is rarely a better choice.

- A **stratified random sample** begins by dividing the population into subgroups according to characteristics such as sex or age and then taking a random sample from each of these "strata." The stratified subsamples can be weighted to draw disproportionately from subgroups that are less common in the population but of special interest to the investigator. In studying the incidence of preeclampsia in pregnancy, for example, the investigator could stratify the population by self-identified race/ethnicity and then sample equal numbers from each stratum. Less common races would then be relatively overrepresented, yielding incidence estimates of comparable precision for each one.

- A **cluster sample** is a random sample of natural groupings (clusters) of individuals in the population. Cluster sampling is useful when the population is widely dispersed or when it is impractical to list and sample from all its elements. Consider, for example, trying to interview patients with lung cancer selected randomly from a statewide registry. Patients could be studied at lower cost by choosing a random sample of the hospitals at which the patients were diagnosed and interviewing the cases from those facilities.

Community surveys often use a two-stage cluster sample: A random sample is drawn from city blocks *enumerated* on a map, and a subsample of the addresses in those blocks is selected for study by a second random process. Cluster sampling has the disadvantage that naturally occurring groups are often more homogeneous than the population; a city block, for example, tends to have people of similar socioeconomic status. This means that the effective sample size (after adjusting for within-cluster similarities) will be somewhat smaller than the number of participants, and the statistical methods used to analyze the data—and to estimate the sample size (Chapter 6)—must take the clustering into account.

Nonprobability Samples

Probability samples are ideal, but they can be inconvenient or costly, or even impossible if a sampling frame cannot be constructed. By contrast, nonprobability samples—which do not involve a random selection process—are typically easier to identify.

- A **consecutive sample** enrolls potential participants who meet the entry criteria in some sort of order, such as the first 50 who are identified. The advantage of this approach is that it does not require prior enumeration of the accessible population, but it has potential drawbacks in terms of generalizability. This approach works best when **recruitment** extends over a period long enough to include seasonal variations or other temporal changes that are important to the research question.
- A **convenience sample** consists of participants who were selected because they were easy for the investigator to identify and enroll. Although access and feasibility are inevitable considerations for any study involving engagement with human beings, investigators should be aware that favoring convenience over rigor will diminish the scientific value of their study; indeed, the term "convenience sample" is sometimes used pejoratively. Probability sampling is preferable whenever feasible.

Comments on Sampling

The use of descriptive statistics and tests of statistical significance to draw inferences about the accessible population from observations in the study assumes that probability sampling has been used. In clinical research, however, enrolling a probability sample of the accessible population may not be possible. Thus, the decision about whether the proposed sampling design is satisfactory usually requires that the investigator make a judgment: for the research question at hand, will the conclusions drawn from observations in the study sample be similar to the conclusions that would result from studying a true probability sample of the accessible population? And beyond that, will the conclusions apply to the target population?

It's important not to confuse **random sampling**, used to determine which members of an accessible population are selected for a study, with **randomization** (or random assignment), which is used, for instance, to determine whether a participant in a clinical trial receives the active treatment or placebo (see Chapter 11). They both share the benefits of using random numbers when making inferences, but few studies employ both techniques. (A notable exception—albeit one that does not involve clinical research—involves social media companies that assess how well various "enticements" work by selecting random users to see randomly assigned versions of advertisements.) (7)

Many journals require that the sampling scheme for a study—including the number of potential participants lost at each stage of recruitment and follow-up—be included in a diagram. It's worth preparing the study plan with that requirement in mind.

■ RECRUITMENT

The *feasibility* of recruiting study participants helps to determine the sampling approach. Recruitment has two main goals: One is to enroll a sample that adequately represents the accessible population to minimize the prospect of getting the wrong answer to the research question due to systematic error (bias). The other is to obtain a sufficient sample size to minimize the prospect of getting the wrong answer due to random error (chance).

Achieving a Representative Sample

The approach to recruiting a **representative sample** begins in the design phase with wise decisions about choosing the target and accessible populations, as well as the type of sampling. It ends with implementation, guarding against errors in applying the entry criteria to prospective study participants, and enhancing successful retention strategies as the study progresses.

A common error occurs when the actual sample of recruited participants does not reflect the accessible population due to differential rates of enrollment. People who volunteer for research studies are usually healthier, more educated, and less likely to smoke, for example, than those who decline. Blacks tend to enroll at lower rates than others, perhaps in part to previous studies that were overtly racist (see Chapter 7). Volunteer bias may be even more extreme when researchers use digital methods of engaging participants (8). Higher-touch recruitment strategies that emphasize relationship-building between research staff and potential participants are typically required to enroll a diverse sample. Comprehensive approaches to enrolling a diverse and representative sample are discussed further in the chapter on community-engaged research (Chapter 15).

Especially for descriptive studies (like election polls), *nonresponse*[1] is another major concern. The proportion of participants selected for the study who agree to be enrolled (the **response rate**) influences the validity of inferring that the enrolled sample represents the accessible population. People who are difficult to reach and those who refuse to participate once they are contacted tend to be different from those who enroll. The level of nonresponse that will compromise the generalizability of the study depends on the nature of the research question and on the reasons for not responding. However, a nonresponse rate of only 25%, a good achievement in many settings, can seriously distort the estimate of the prevalence of a disease when the disease itself affects the likelihood that someone will respond.

The degree to which **nonresponse bias** may influence the conclusions of a study can sometimes be estimated by acquiring additional information on a sample of nonrespondents, which requires more resources and specific approval from the Institutional Review Board (IRB). For example, a study that recruits participants via social media might obtain publicly available information on nonrespondents. Or a study that recruits participants by mail from a list of clinic patients might offer a random sample of nonrespondents a financial incentive to answer a few additional questions over the phone.

The best way to deal with nonresponse bias, however, is to minimize the number of nonrespondents by using repeated contact attempts and a variety of methods (mail, e-mail, telephone). Among those contacted successfully, refusal to participate can be minimized by improving the efficiency and attractiveness of the study, by choosing a design that avoids invasive and uncomfortable tests, by using brochures and individual discussion to allay anxiety and discomfort, by providing incentives such as reimbursing the costs of transportation and providing the results of tests, and by circumventing language barriers with bilingual staff and translated questionnaires. Another option is to include an incentive for completing the study.

Recruiting Sufficient Numbers of Participants

Falling short in recruitment is one of the most common problems in clinical research. Indeed, as some colleagues wrote:

> However, as time progresses, the initial enthusiasm for recruitment gradually fades. In the face of the harsh realities of research, such as slow recruitment, negative emotions often become dominant. Researchers may experience feelings of despair, self-blame, guilt, a sense of failure, worthlessness, loneliness, frustration and subclinical depression; sometimes even paranoia sets in (9).

---

[1]Concern with nonresponse in the process of *recruiting* participants for a study (the topic of this chapter) is chiefly a concern in descriptive studies that have a primary goal of estimating distributions of variables. Nonresponse during *follow-up* is a major issue in prospective studies that follow participants over time, particularly in a clinical trial of an intervention that may alter the response rate (Chapter 11).

These are strong words, but they reflect an underlying truth: In planning a study, it is best to assume that the number of participants who meet the entry criteria and agree to enter the study will be fewer, sometimes by several fold, than the number projected at the outset. There are several approaches to this problem: Estimate the magnitude of the recruitment problem empirically with a pretest; plan the study with a sample size that is larger than believed necessary; and make contingency plans should the need arise for additional participants. While recruitment is ongoing it is important to monitor progress in meeting the recruitment goals and tabulate reasons for falling short. Understanding why potential participants are lost to the study at various stages can lead to strategies for reducing these losses.

Sometimes, recruitment involves selecting participants who are already known to the members of the research team (eg, in a study of a new treatment in patients attending the investigator's clinic). Here, the chief concern is to present the opportunity for participation in the study fairly, making clear the advantages and disadvantages. In discussing participation, the investigator must recognize the ethical dilemmas that arise when her role as the patient's physician might conflict with her interests as an investigator (Chapter 7). Indeed, an investigator should almost always ask a disinterested colleague to obtain informed consent when considering the enrollment of one of her own patients in a study that presents any potential risk or inconvenience.

More often, recruitment involves enrolling potential participants who are not known to the research team. It is helpful if at least one member of the team has previous experience with the various ways to contact prospective participants. These include screening in work settings or public places such as shopping malls; sending out large numbers of solicitations (via e-mail or snail mail) using listings such as driver's license holders; advertising on the internet or social media; inviting referrals from clinicians; carrying out retrospective record reviews; and examining lists of patients seen in clinic and hospital settings. Some of these approaches involve concerns with privacy invasion that must be considered by an IRB.

Special populations, such as frail or disabled persons, may require additional recruitment techniques, such as home visits or free transportation. This kind of outreach is particularly important when the inability to come to a clinic appointment for an examination may influence the generalizability of the study.

It may also be helpful to prepare for recruitment by getting the support of relevant organizations. For example, the investigator can meet with hospital administrators to discuss a clinic-based sample; the local medical society to enlist support for a mailing to physicians; and community leaders and the county health department to plan a community screening operation. Written endorsements can be included as an appendix to applications for funding. It may also be useful to create a favorable climate in the community by giving public lectures or participating in community advocacy events and by advertising through social and mass media, fliers, websites, and mailings.

But our best advice to new investigators concerning recruitment is simple: **avoid it when possible**. Once you have clarified your research question and plan, first determine whether another research team has already enrolled a sample and made measurements that might suffice to answer your question—and then contact them to see if you can access and analyze their data (see Chapter 16) or even add a new measurement at a subsequent study visit. This step, which requires becoming an expert in the literature and then having the courage to reach out to investigators you may not know, can save years of effort.

■ SUMMARY

1. Most clinical research is based, philosophically and practically, on the use of a **sample to represent a population**.
2. The advantage of sampling is efficiency: It allows the investigator to **draw inferences** about a large population by examining a subset at relatively low cost in time and effort. The disadvantages are the errors it introduces: if the sample is not sufficiently representative for the

research question, the findings may not generalize well to the target population, and if it is not large enough, the findings may not sufficiently minimize the role of chance.

3. In designing a sample, the investigator begins by conceptualizing the target population with a specific set of **inclusion criteria** that establish the clinical and demographic characteristics of participants who are well suited to the research question, with a parsimonious set of **exclusion criteria** that eliminate participants who are unethical or inappropriate to study.

4. She then selects an **accessible population** that is geographically and temporally convenient.

5. The next step is to design an **approach to sampling** from that accessible population. Probability sampling strategies are optimal when a listing of the accessible population is available. Selecting participants purely on the basis of convenience may yield a biased sample.

6. Finally, the investigator must design and implement strategies for **recruiting** and **retaining** participants who are sufficiently representative of the target population.

REFERENCES

1. Framingham Heart Study. *Epidemiological background and design: The Framingham Heart Study*. https://framingham heartstudy.org/fhs-about/history/epidemiological-background

2. Cummings SR, Nevitt MC, Browner WS, et al. Risk factors for hip fracture in white women. Study of Osteoporotic Fractures Research Group. *N Engl J Med*. 1995;332(12):767-773.

3. Cauley JA, Lui LY, Ensrud KE, et al. Bone mineral density and the risk of incident nonspinal fractures in black and white women. *JAMA*. 2005;293(17):2102-2108.

4. Orwoll E, Blank JB, Barrett-Connor E, et al. Design and baseline characteristics of the osteoporotic fractures in men (MrOS) study—a large observational study of the determinants of fracture in older men. *Contemp Clin Trials*. 2005;26(5):569-585.

5. Thorpe KE, Zwarenstein M, Oxman AD, et al. A pragmatic-explanatory continuum indicator summary (PRECIS): a tool to help trial designers. *J Clin Epidemiol*. 2009;62(5):464-475.

6. Centers for Disease Control and Prevention, NCHS. *National Health and Nutrition Examination Survey*. https://www.cdc.gov/nchs/nhanes/index.htm

7. Bakshy E., Eckles D, Yan E, et al. Social influence in social advertising: evidence from field experiments. In: *Proceedings of the 13th ACM Conference on Electronic Commerce (EC '12)*. ACM; 2012: 146-161. https://research.fb.com/wp-content/uploads/2016/11/social-influence-in-social-advertising-evidence-from-fieldexperiments.pdf

8. Guo X, Vittinghoff E, Olgin JE, Marcus GM, Pletcher MJ. Volunteer participation in the Health eHeart Study: a comparison with the US population. *Sci Rep*. 2017;7(1):1956.

9. Patel M, Doku V, Tennakoon L. Challenges in recruitment of research participants. *Adv Psych Treatment*. 2003;9:229-238.

APPENDIX 3A
Exercises for Chapter 3. Choosing the Study Participants: Specification, Sampling, and Recruitment

1. An investigator is interested in the following research question: "What are the factors that cause people to start smoking?" She decides on a cross-sectional sample of high school students, invites eleventh graders in her suburban high school to participate, and studies those who volunteer.
   a. Discuss the suitability of this sample for the target population of interest.
   b. Suppose that the investigator decides to avoid volunteer bias by designing a 25% random sample of the entire eleventh grade, but that the actual sample turns out to be 70% female. If it is known that equal numbers of boys and girls are enrolled in the eleventh grade, then the disproportion in the sex distribution represents an error in drawing the sample. Could this have occurred through random error, systematic error, or both? Explain your answer.

2. An investigator is considering designs for surveying rock concert patrons to determine their attitudes toward wearing earplugs during concerts to protect their hearing. Name the following sampling schemes for selecting individuals to fill out a brief questionnaire, commenting on feasibility and whether the results will be generalizable to all people who attend rock concerts.
   a. As each patron enters the theater, she is asked to throw a virtual die (on the investigator's cell phone). All patrons who throw a 6 are invited to fill out the questionnaire.
   b. As each patron enters the theater, she is asked to throw a virtual die. Men who throw a 1 and women who throw an even number are invited.
   c. Tickets to the concert are numbered and sold at the box office in serial order, and each patron whose ticket number ends in 1 is invited.
   d. After all the patrons are seated, five rows are chosen at random by drawing from a shuffled set of cards that has one card for each theater row. All patrons in those five rows are invited.
   e. The first 100 patrons who enter the theater are invited.
   f. Some tickets were sold by mail and some at the box office just before the performance. Whenever there were five or more people waiting in line to buy tickets at the box office, the last person in line (who had the most time available) was invited.
   g. When patrons began to leave after the performance, those who seemed willing and able to fill out the questionnaire were invited.

3. Edwards et al. (1) reported on the burden of infection caused by human metapneumovirus (HMPV) among children <5 years old. The participants were children in counties surrounding Cincinnati, Nashville, and Rochester, NY, during the months of November to May from 2003 to 2009, who sought medical attention for acute respiratory illness or fever. Consenting inpatients were enrolled Sunday through Thursday, outpatients 1 or 2 days per week, and emergency department patients 1 to 4 days per week. The authors combined the proportion of children testing positive at each site with nationwide data (from the National Ambulatory Medical Care Survey and the National Hospital Ambulatory Care Survey) on the population frequency of visits for acute respiratory illness or fever to estimate the overall burden of

HMPV in the United States. They estimated HMPV was responsible for 55 clinic visits and 13 emergency department visits per 1000 children annually.

a. What was the target population for this study?

b. What was the accessible population, and how suitable was it for generalizing to the target population?

c. What was the sampling scheme, and how suitable was it for generalizing to the accessible population?

d. Describe in general terms how the sampling scheme would need to be taken into account when calculating confidence intervals for the HMPV rates they calculate.

REFERENCE

1. Edwards KM, Zhu Y, Griffin MR, et al. Burden of human metapneumovirus infection in young children. *N Engl J Med.* 2013;368:633-643.

Planning the Measurements: Precision, Accuracy, and Validity

Steven R. Cummings, Thomas B. Newman, and Alison J. Huang

Measurements describe phenomena in terms that can be analyzed statistically, and the validity of a study depends on how well the variables designed for—and measured in—the study represent the phenomena of interest (Figure 4.1), for example, how well does parental recall of birth weight measure actual birth weight? (1) These concepts are important for all types of measurements, including physical examinations, laboratory tests, and scores from questionnaires.

This chapter begins by considering how the choice of measurement **scale** influences the information content of the measurement. We then turn to the central goal of maximizing test **accuracy** by designing measurements that are relatively **precise** (free of random error) and **unbiased** (free of systematic error), thereby enhancing the appropriateness of drawing inferences from these measurements to the phenomena of interest. We address the concept of **validity**, a qualitative relative of accuracy, before concluding with some considerations for clinical and translational research, noting especially the advantages of storing specimens for later measurements.

The topics discussed in this chapter apply to the study's predictor and outcome variables, as well as to the study's **covariates**, the remaining set of measured variables. The measurement methods for some covariates will not require detailed planning, because many can be borrowed from previous research. But the investigator will almost always need to give special attention to the study's main predictor(s) and outcome(s)—and possibly a few others—tailoring their measurements to the specific needs of the study.

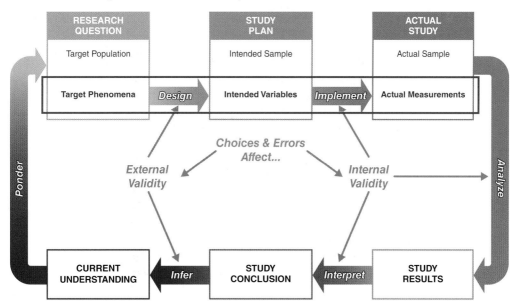

■ **FIGURE 4.1** This chapter focuses on the items within the red box: designing measurements that represent the phenomena of interest for the research question.

■ MEASUREMENT SCALES

Table 4.1 presents a simplified classification of measurement scales and the information they contain. The classification is important because some types of variables are more informative than others, adding power or reducing sample size requirements, and revealing more detailed distribution patterns.

Categorical Variables: Dichotomous, Nominal, and Ordinal

Phenomena that are not suitable for quantification are measured by classifying them in categories. **Categorical variables** with two possible values (eg, dead or alive) are termed **dichotomous**. Categorical variables with more than two categories (**polychotomous**) can be further characterized according to the type of information they contain. Among these, **nominal variables** have categories that are not ordered; type A blood, for example, is neither more nor less than type B blood. Nominal variables tend to have an absolute qualitative character that makes them straightforward to measure. In contrast, **ordinal variables** do have an order, such as severe, moderate, and mild pain. The additional information is an advantage over nominal variables, but because ordinal variables do not specify a numerical or uniform difference or ratio of one category to the next, the information content is less than that of numerical variables.

Numerical Variables: Continuous and Discrete

Numerical variables can be quantified with a number that expresses how much or how many. A **continuous variable**, such as the blood hemoglobin level, quantifies how much on a scale that has a theoretically infinite number of values, although the method used to measure it will likely generate only some of those values. In contrast, a **discrete variable** has a countable number of

TABLE 4.1 MEASUREMENT SCALES

TYPE OF MEASUREMENT	CHARACTERISTICS OF VARIABLE	EXAMPLE	DESCRIPTIVE STATISTICS	STATISTICAL POWER
Categorical				
Dichotomous	Two categories	Vital status (alive or dead)	Counts, proportions	Low
Nominal	Unordered categories	Gender identity; blood type	Same as above	Low
Ordinal	Ordered categories with intervals that are not quantifiable	Degree of pain (none, mild, moderate, severe); social class	In addition to the above: medians	Intermediate
Numeric				
Continuous	Infinite number of values	Weight; hemoglobin level	In addition to the above: means, standard deviations	High
Discrete or count[a]	Limited number of values (typically integers)	Number of pregnancies; number of sexual partners	Same as ordinal when there are few possible values; same as continuous when there are many	High if the variable takes on many possible values, especially if the average is near the middle

[a]Count variables are discrete variables that can only be whole numbers (0, 1, 2, 3, …).

values usually expressed as a positive or negative integer, such as the change in the number of people living in a household during a pandemic. Discrete variables that are well distributed over many possible values, say, six or more, can resemble continuous variables in statistical analyses and be equivalent for the purpose of designing measurements.

Choosing a Measurement Scale

A good general rule is to prefer continuous over categorical variables when there is a choice, because the additional information they contain improves statistical efficiency. In a study comparing the antihypertensive effects of several treatments, for example, measuring blood pressure in millimeters of mercury allows the investigator to observe the magnitude of the change in every participant, whereas measuring it as hypertensive versus normotensive limits the assessment. The continuous variable contains more information, and the result is a study with more power and/or a smaller sample size (Chapters 5 and 6).

Continuous variables also allow for more flexibility than categorical variables in fitting the data to the nature of the variable or the shape of the association, especially when the relationship might have a complex pattern. For example, a study of the association of body mass index (BMI) with mortality may be able to detect a U-shaped pattern, with higher mortality in those with low and high levels of BMI compared with intermediate levels (2) and may be able to describe threshold values where mortality begins to change. And a study of predictors of low-birth-weight babies should record actual birth weight rather than above or below the conventional 2500 g threshold for low birth weight; this leaves analytic options open, such as to change the cutoff that defines low birth weight, to develop an ordinal scale with several categories of birth weight (eg, <1500, 1500 to 1999, 2000 to 2499, and ≥2500 g), or to use the continuous measurement.

Similarly, when there is the option of designing the number of response categories in an ordinal scale, as in a question about satisfaction with care, it is often useful to provide a half-dozen categories that range from "strongly agree" to "strongly disagree." These results can later be collapsed into a dichotomy (agree and disagree), but the reverse would not be possible.

Many characteristics, such as pain or quality of life, are difficult to describe with categories or numbers, but quantifying them is essential to answering important research questions. This is illustrated by the Short Form (SF)-36, a standardized questionnaire for assessing quality of life that produces discrete numerical ratings of eight dimensions, including physical, social, and emotional function and general well-being (3). The process of classification and measurement, if done well, can increase the objectivity of our knowledge, reduce bias, and provide more detailed communication.

■ PRECISION

The precision of a variable is the degree to which it is reproducible, with nearly the same value each time it is measured. A beam scale can measure body weight with great precision, whereas measuring balance by timing how long a participant keeps her feet together with eyes closed may produce values that vary from one observer or one occasion to another. Precision has a very important influence on the power of a study. The more precise a measurement, the greater the statistical power at a given sample size to test hypotheses about that measurement (Chapter 5).

Precision (also called **reproducibility**, **reliability**, and **consistency**) is a function of random error (chance variability); the greater the error, the less precise the measurement. There are three main sources of random error in making measurements.

- **Observer variability** is due to the observer and includes such things as choice of words in an interview and skill in using a mechanical instrument.

- **Instrument variability** is due to the instrument and includes changing environmental factors (eg, temperature), differences between batches of reagents, and so on.
- **Participant variability** is due to intrinsic variability in characteristics of study participants unrelated to variables under study that may influence the measurement, such as variability in measurements of strength, due to time of day, time since last food intake, or effort.

Assessing Precision

Precision is assessed as the reproducibility of repeated measurements, comparing measurements made either by the same person (within-observer reproducibility) or different people (between-observer reproducibility). It can also be assessed within or between instruments. The reproducibility of continuous variables is often expressed as either the within-participant **standard deviation** or the coefficient of variation (within-participant standard deviation divided by the mean).[1] For categorical variables, percent agreement, the interclass correlation coefficient, and the **kappa** statistic are often used (4-6).

Strategies for Enhancing Precision

There are five approaches to minimizing random error and increasing the precision of measurements (Table 4.2):

1. **Standardizing the measurement methods.** All study protocols should include detailed instructions for making the measurements. These may include written directions with pictures or a short video on how to prepare the environment and the participant, how to carry out and record the measurement, how to **calibrate** the instrument, and so forth (Appendix 4A). This set of materials, part of the **operations manual**, is essential for most studies. Even when there is only a single observer, specific written guidelines for making each measurement will help ensure that her performance is uniform over the duration of the study and serve as the basis for describing the methods when the results are published.

2. **Training and certifying the observers.** Training will improve the consistency of measurement techniques, especially when several observers are involved. It is often desirable to test mastery of the techniques specified in the operations manual and to certify that observers have achieved the prescribed level of performance (Chapter 18). When multiple observers make measurements for a study (eg, determining whether a physical finding is present or whether a death was caused by breast cancer), it is helpful to measure and take steps to optimize their interrater reliability (eg, using Kappa; see Chapter 13).

3. **Refining the instruments.** Mechanical and electronic instruments can be engineered to reduce variability. Similarly, questionnaires and interviews should go through multiple iterations to increase clarity and avoid potential ambiguities (Chapter 17).

4. **Automating the instruments.** Variations in the way human observers make measurements can be eliminated with automatic devices and self-response questionnaires.

5. **Repetition.** The influence of random error from any source is reduced by repeating the measurement and using the mean of two or more readings. For example, taking the average of two measurements of leg strength will improve the precision of a measurement that is prone to variability in effort from test to test. Precision will be substantially increased by this strategy, the primary limitations being the added cost and practical difficulties of repeating the measurements as well as the possibility of systematic changes in the measurement with

---

[1]When there are two measurements of a continuous variable per participant, it may be tempting to express their agreement using a correlation coefficient. However, because the correlation coefficient is extremely sensitive to outliers, a better approach is a "Bland-Altman" plot (4), in which the difference between the two measurements is plotted as a function of their mean. If the absolute value of the difference between the measurements tends to increase linearly with the mean, the coefficient of variation is a better way to summarize variability than the within-participant standard deviation.

TABLE 4.2 STRATEGIES FOR REDUCING RANDOM ERROR, WITH ILLUSTRATIONS FROM A STUDY OF ANTIHYPERTENSIVE TREATMENT

STRATEGY TO REDUCE RANDOM ERROR	SOURCE OF RANDOM ERROR	EXAMPLE OF RANDOM ERROR	EXAMPLE OF STRATEGY TO PREVENT THE ERROR
1. Standardizing the measurement methods in an operations manual	Observer	Variation in blood pressure (BP) measurement due to variable rate of cuff deflation (often too fast)	Specify that the cuff be deflated at 2 mm Hg/s
	Participant	Variation in BP due to variable length of quiet sitting before measurement	Specify that participant sit in a quiet room for 5 minutes before BP measurement
2. Training and certifying the observer	Observer	Variation in BP due to variable observer technique	Train observer in standard techniques
3. Refining the instrument	Instrument and observer	Variation in BP due to noisy manometer	Purchase new high-quality manometer and periodically test accuracy
4. Automating the instrument	Observer	Variation in BP due to variable observer technique	Use automatic BP measuring device
	Participant	Variation in BP due to participant's emotional reaction to observer	Use automatic BP measuring device
5. Repeating the measurement	Observer, participant, and instrument	All measurements and all sources of variation	Use mean of two or more BP measurements

repetition, for example, due to tiring on strength tests or improved test-taking for tests of cognitive ability.

For each measurement in the study, the investigator must decide how vigorously to pursue each of these strategies. This decision can be based on the importance of the variable, the magnitude of the potential problem with precision, and the feasibility and cost of the strategy. In general, standardizing and training should always be used, and repetition is guaranteed to improve precision when it is feasible and affordable.

■ ACCURACY

The accuracy of a variable is the degree to which it represents the true value. Accuracy depends on both maximizing precision and minimizing bias (Table 4.3). When serum bilirubin was measured using instruments that had been miscalibrated, for example, the results were precise but biased (7). This concept is further illustrated in Figure 4.2. Accuracy and precision do often go hand in hand and many of the strategies for increasing precision also improve accuracy.

TABLE 4.3 THE PRECISION AND ACCURACY OF MEASUREMENTS

	PRECISION	ACCURACY
Definition	The degree to which a variable has nearly the same value when measured several times	The degree to which a variable approximates the true value
Best way to assess	Comparison among repeated measures	Comparison with a "gold standard"
Value to study	Increase power to detect effects	Increase validity of conclusions
Threatened by	Random error (chance) contributed by	Random and systematic error (bias) contributed by
	The observer	The observer
	The participant	The participant
	The instrument	The instrument

Unlike precision, accuracy is affected by **bias** (systematic error); the greater the error, the less accurate the variable. The three main classes of random error noted in the earlier section on precision each have corresponding biases here.

- **Observer bias** is a distortion, conscious or unconscious, in the perception or reporting of the measurement by the observer. It may represent systematic errors in the way an instrument is operated, such as a tendency to round blood pressure measurements down to a nearest zero mm Hg or to use leading questions when interviewing a participant.
- **Instrument bias** can result from faulty function of a mechanical instrument. A scale that has not been calibrated recently may have drifted downward, producing consistently low body weights.
- **Participant bias** is a distortion of the measurement by the study participant, for example, in reporting an event; it is also called "respondent or recall bias." Patients with breast cancer who believe that alcohol is a cause of their cancer, for example, may exaggerate the alcohol intake they report.

The accuracy of a measurement is best assessed by comparing it, when possible, to a "**gold standard**"—a reference measurement carried out by a technique that is believed to best represent the true value of the characteristic. What measurement to designate as the gold standard can be a difficult judgment, drawing on previous work in the field and a consensus of experts.

For measurements on a continuous scale, the degree of accuracy can be expressed as the mean difference between the measurement under investigation and the gold standard across study participants. For measurements on a dichotomous scale, accuracy in comparison with a gold standard can be described in terms of sensitivity and specificity (Chapter 13). For

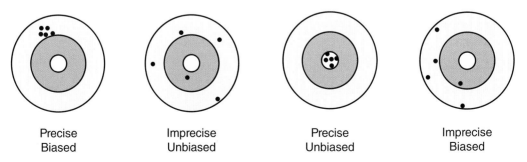

| Precise | Imprecise | Precise | Imprecise |
| Biased | Unbiased | Unbiased | Biased |

■ **FIGURE 4.2** The difference between imprecision and bias.

measurements on categorical scales with more than two response options, the percent correct on each can be calculated.

Strategies for Enhancing Accuracy

The major approaches to increasing accuracy include the first four strategies listed earlier for precision, and three additional ones (Table 4.4):

1. Standardizing the measurement methods.
2. Training and certifying the observers.

TABLE 4.4 STRATEGIES FOR REDUCING SYSTEMATIC ERROR, WITH ILLUSTRATIONS FROM A STUDY OF ANTIHYPERTENSIVE TREATMENT

STRATEGY TO REDUCE SYSTEMATIC ERROR	SOURCE OF SYSTEMATIC ERROR	EXAMPLE OF SYSTEMATIC ERROR	EXAMPLE OF STRATEGY TO PREVENT THE ERROR
1. Standardizing the measurement methods in an operations manual	Observer	Consistently high diastolic blood pressure (BP) readings due to using the point at which sounds become muffled	Specify the operational definition of diastolic BP as the point at which sounds cease to be heard
	Participant	Consistently high readings due to measuring BP right after walking upstairs to clinic	Specify that participant sit in quiet room for 5 min before measurement
2. Training and certifying the observer	Observer	Consistently high BP readings due to failure to follow procedures specified in operations manual	Trainer checks accuracy of observer's reading by repeating the measurement
3. Refining the instrument	Instrument	Consistently high BP readings with standard cuff in participants with very large arms	Use extra-wide BP cuff in obese or very muscular patients
4. Automating the instrument	Observer	Conscious or unconscious tendency for observer to read BP lower in group randomized to active drug	Use automatic BP measuring device
	Participant	BP increase due to proximity of attractive technician	Use automatic BP measuring device
5. Making unobtrusive measurements	Participant	Tendency of participant to overestimate compliance with study drug	Measure study drug level in urine
6. Calibrating the instrument	Instrument	Consistently high BP readings due to manometer being out of adjustment	Calibrate every month
7. Blinding	Observer	Conscious or unconscious tendency for observer to read BP lower in active treatment group	Use double-blind placebo to conceal study group assignment
	Participant	Tendency of participant who knew she was on active drug to overreport side effects	Use double-blind placebo to conceal study group assignment

3. Refining the instruments.
4. Automating the instruments.
5. **Making unobtrusive measurements.** It is sometimes possible to design measurements that the participants are not aware of, thereby eliminating the possibility that they will consciously bias the variable. For example, an evaluation of the effect of placing a hand sanitizer and a hand hygiene poster in a hospital cafeteria utilized observers who blended in with cafeteria customers (8).
6. **Calibrating the instrument.** The accuracy of many instruments, especially those that are mechanical or electrical, can be increased by periodic **calibration** with a gold standard.
7. **Blinding.** This classic strategy does not improve the overall accuracy of the measurements, but it can eliminate differential bias that affects one study group more than another. In a double-blind clinical trial, if blinding is successful the participants and observers do not know whether active medicine or placebo has been assigned, and any inaccuracy in measuring the outcome will be the same in the two groups.

The decision on how vigorously to pursue each of these seven strategies for each measurement rests, as noted earlier for precision, on the judgment of the investigator. The considerations are the potential impact that the anticipated degree of inaccuracy will have on the conclusions of the study, and the feasibility and cost of the strategy. The first two strategies (standardizing and training) should always be used, calibration is needed for any instrument that has the potential to change over time, and blinding is essential whenever feasible.

■ VALIDITY

Validity resembles accuracy, but we think of it as adding a qualitative dimension to considering how well a measurement represents the phenomena of interest. For example, blood levels of creatinine and cystatin C, two chemicals excreted by the kidneys, might be equally *accurate* (eg, within 1% of the true level), but cystatin C may be more *valid* as a measure of kidney function because creatinine levels are also influenced by the amount of muscle (9).

Validity is often not amenable to assessment with a gold standard, particularly for measurements aimed at subjective and abstract phenomena such as pain or quality of life. Several constructs are used to address the validity of these measurement approaches.

- **Content validity** examines how well the measurement represents all aspects of the phenomena under study. For example, the SF-36 questionnaire includes questions on social, physical, and emotional functioning, general health, mental health, and bodily pain to assess quality of life (3).
- **Face validity** describes whether the measurement seems inherently reasonable, such as assessing frailty by muscle weakness, feeling exhausted, weight loss, and slow usual walking speed (10).
- **Construct validity** is the degree to which a certain measurement matches what one would expect from theory; for example, a measurement of social isolation should be able to separate individuals who have few or no friendships and who do not participate in social activities from those who have many friends and participate in several social activities.
- **Predictive validity** is the ability of the measurement to predict an outcome; for example, how well the measurement of frailty predicts admission to long-term care.
- **Criterion-related validity** is the degree to which a new measurement, such as a new biochemical test of muscle mass, correlates with measurements of muscle strength.

The general approach to measuring subjective and abstract phenomena is to begin by searching the literature and consulting with experts in an effort to find a suitable instrument (typically a questionnaire) that has already been validated. Using such an instrument has the advantage of making the results of the new study comparable to earlier work in the area and may simplify and strengthen the process of applying for grants and publishing the results. Its disadvantages, however, are that the validation process may have been suboptimal and that an instrument taken off the shelf may be outmoded or not optimal for the research question.

If existing instruments are not suitable for the needs of the study, then the investigator may decide to develop a new measurement approach and validate it herself. This can be an interesting challenge and even lead to a worthwhile contribution to the literature, but it generally requires a lot of time and effort. It is fair to say that the process is often less conclusive than the word "validation" connotes.

■ OTHER FEATURES OF MEASUREMENT APPROACHES

Measurements should be sensitive[2] enough to detect differences in a characteristic that are important to the investigator. Just how much sensitivity is needed depends on the research question. For example, for a trial of whether a treatment improves heart function, measuring the distance that a participant is able to walk in 6 minutes is likely to be more sensitive to change in cardiac performance than a self-reported rating of shortness of breath after walking one block.

An ideal measurement is specific, representing only the characteristic of interest. For example, an echocardiographic measurement of the contractile function of the heart would be more specific to the effect of a treatment on heart failure than the 6-minute walking distance, which is also influenced by lung function and the fatigability of leg muscles.

Measurements should be appropriate to the objectives of the study. A study of stress as an antecedent to myocardial infarction, for example, would need to consider what kind of stress (psychological or physical, acute or chronic) was of interest before setting out the operational definitions for measuring it.

Measurements should provide an adequate distribution of responses in the study sample. A measure of functional status is most useful if it produces values that range from high in some participants to low in others. A major reason for pretesting is to ensure that the actual responses do not all cluster around one end of the possible range of responses, also described as "floor and ceiling effects."

Whenever possible, measurements should be designed in a way that minimizes subjective judgments. Objectivity is achieved by reducing the involvement of the observer and the participant and by using automated instruments. One danger in these strategies, however, is the consequent tunnel vision that limits the scope of the observations and the ability to discover unanticipated phenomena. This can be addressed by including some open-ended questions, and an opportunity for acquiring subjective and qualitative data, in addition to the quantitative measurements.

In designing a study, there is a tendency to keep adding items that are not central to the research question but that could be of interest. It is true that additional measurements enable investigators to use the data to answer additional questions. However, it is important to keep in mind the value of efficiency and parsimony. The full set of measurements should be designed to collect useful data at an affordable cost in time and money with acceptable burden on participants. Collecting too much information is a common error that can tire participants, overwhelm the team making the measurements, and clutter data management and analysis. The result may be a more expensive study that is paradoxically less successful in answering the main research questions.

■ MEASUREMENTS ON STORED MATERIALS

Some measurements can be made only during contact with the study participants, but many can be carried out later on biologic specimens banked for chemical, genetic, or other analyses or on images from radiographic and other procedures filed electronically (Table 4.5).

---

[2]We'll define sensitivity and specificity more formally as characteristics of diagnostic tests in Chapter 13. Here, they have the same general meaning: sensitivity relates to how good the measurement is at finding what you want to find, whereas specificity is about how good it is at avoiding finding what you don't want to find.

TABLE 4.5 EXAMPLES OF MEASUREMENTS THAT CAN BE MADE ON STORED MATERIALS

TYPE OF MEASUREMENT	EXAMPLES	BANK FOR LATER MEASUREMENT
Medical history	Diagnoses, laboratory test results, medications, operations, symptoms, physical findings; application of natural language processing	Electronic medical records
Biochemical measures	Markers of inflammation, levels of cell-free DNA, microbiome profile	Serum, plasma, urine, stool
Genetic/molecular tests	Whole genome sequencing, DNA methylation	Whole blood or tissue specimens
Imaging	Body composition, bone structure, artificial intelligence analyses to predict disease or outcomes	X-rays, computerized tomography, and other methods

One advantage of such storage is the opportunity to reduce the cost of the study by making measurements only on individuals who turn out during follow-up to have an outcome of interest and a sample of others, such as by doing a **nested case-control study** (Chapter 9). Archiving biologic specimens and images also has the advantage that scientific advances after the study has begun may lead to new ideas and measurement techniques that can then be employed, funded by new grants. Specimens should be collected carefully, frozen quickly, and archived in a way—at very low temperatures (–70 °C or even –190 °C) that preserves them for future assays. This approach allows for the application of increasingly sophisticated types of measurements, such as proteomics or expression of genes in individual cells. Investigators should consider archiving several types of specimens such as plasma, urine, white blood cells, or stool samples for quantifying species of bacteria, to anticipate development of a wide array of future assays. It is also important to obtain informed consent from participants that covers a wide scope of future potential uses of the specimens.

■ SUMMARY

1. Variables are either **numerical** or **categorical**. Numerical variables are **continuous** (quantified on an infinite scale) or **discrete** (quantified on a finite scale such as integers); categorical variables are **nominal** (unordered) or **ordinal** (ordered). Those that have only two categories are termed **dichotomous**.
2. Variables that contain more information provide greater power and/or allow smaller sample sizes, according to the following hierarchy: **continuous variables > discrete numerical variables > ordinal variables > nominal** and **dichotomous variables**.
3. The **precision** of a measurement (ie, the reproducibility of replicate measures) is another major determinant of power and sample size. Precision is reduced by **random error** (chance) from three sources of variability: the observer, the participant, and the instrument.
4. Strategies for **increasing precision** that should be part of every study are to **define** and **standardize methods** in an **operations manual** and to train and certify observers. Other strategies that are often useful are **refining** and **automating** the instruments and **repetition**—using the mean of repeated measurements.
5. The accuracy of a measurement is the degree to which it approximates a gold standard. Accuracy is reduced both by **imprecision** (random error) and **bias** (systematic error) from the same three sources: the observer, participant, and instrument.

6. The strategies for minimizing bias include all those listed for precision (except repetition). In addition, bias can be reduced by making **unobtrusive measures** and by **calibrating instruments**. In comparisons between groups, blinding reduces differential bias.

7. **Validity** is the degree to which a measurement represents the phenomena it is intended to measure. It can sometimes be assessed by comparison to a **gold standard**. For abstract and subjective variables where there is no gold standard, it is assessed by **content validity**, **face validity**, **construct validity**, **predictive validity**, and **criterion-related validity**.

8. Individual measurements should be **sensitive, specific, appropriate**, and **objective**, and they should produce a **range of values**. In the aggregate, they should be broad but parsimonious, serving the research question at moderate cost in time and money and not placing undue burden on participants.

9. Investigators should consider **storing biologic samples, images, and other materials** for later measurements that can take advantage of new technologies as they are developed and the efficiency of nested case-control designs.

REFERENCES

1. Kassem Z, Burmeister C, Johnson DA, et al. Reliability of birth weight recall by parent or guardian respondents in a study of healthy adolescents. *BMC Res Notes*. 2018;11:878.
2. Jiang M, Zou Y, Xin Q, et al. Dose-response relationship between body mass index and risks of all-cause mortality and disability among the elderly: a systematic review and meta-analysis. *Clin Nutr*. 2019;38(4):1511-1523.
3. Ware JE, Gandek B Jr. Overview of the SF-36 health survey and the international quality of life assessment project. *J Clin Epidemiol*. 1998;51:903-912. A description of the SF-36 is available at https://www.rand.org/health-care/surveys_tools/mos/36-item-short-form.html
4. Bland JM, Altman DG. Measurement error and correlation coefficients. *BMJ*. 1996;313:41-42; also, Measurement error proportional to the mean. *BMJ*. 1996;313:106.
5. Newman TB, Kohn M. *Evidence-Based Diagnosis: An Introduction to Clinical Epidemiology*. 2nd ed. Cambridge University Press; 2020: Chapter 5, 110-143.
6. Cohen J. A coefficient of agreement for nominal scales. *Educ Psychol Meas*. 1960;20:37-46.
7. Kuzniewicz MW, Greene DN, Walsh EM, McCulloch CE, Newman TB. Association between laboratory calibration of a serum bilirubin assay, neonatal bilirubin levels, and phototherapy use. *JAMA Pediatr*. 2016;170(6):557-561.
8. Filion K, Kukanich KS, Chapman B, et al. Observation-based evaluation of hand hygiene practices and the effects of an intervention at a public hospital cafeteria. *Am J Infect Control*. 2011;39:464-470.
9. Peralta CA, Shlipak MG, Judd S, et al. Detection of chronic kidney disease with creatinine, cystatin C, and urine albumin-to-creatinine ratio and association with progression to end-stage renal disease and mortality. *JAMA*. 2011;305:1545-1552.
10. Xue QL, Tian J, Fried LP, et al. Physical frailty assessment in older women: can simplification be achieved without loss of syndrome measurement validity? *Am J Epidemiol*. 2016;183(11):1037-1044.

APPENDIX 4A
Operational Definition of a Measurement of Grip Strength

The **operations manual** describes the method for conducting and recording the results of all the measurements made in the study. This example describes the use of a dynamometer to measure grip strength. To standardize instructions from examiner to examiner and from participant to participant, the protocol includes a script of instructions to be read to the participant verbatim.

■ PROTOCOL FOR MEASURING GRIP STRENGTH WITH THE DYNAMOMETER

Grip strength will be measured in both hands. The handle should be adjusted so that the participant holds the dynamometer comfortably. Place the dynamometer in the right hand with the dial facing the palm. The participant's arm should be flexed 90° at the elbow with the forearm parallel to the floor.

1. Demonstrate the test to the participant. While demonstrating, use the following description: "This device measures your arm and upper body strength. We will measure your grip strength in both arms. I will demonstrate how it is done. Bend your elbow at a 90° angle, with your forearm parallel to the floor. Don't let your arm touch the side of your body. Lower the device and squeeze as hard as you can while I count to three. Once your arm is fully extended, you can loosen your grip."
2. Allow one practice trial for each arm, starting with the right if she is right-handed. On the second trial, record the kilograms of force from the dial to the nearest 0.5 kg.
3. Reset the dial. Repeat the procedure for the other arm.

The arm should not contact the body. The gripping action should be a slow, sustained squeeze rather than an explosive jerk.

APPENDIX 4B
Exercises for Chapter 4. Planning the Measurements: Precision, Accuracy, and Validity

1. Classify the following variables as dichotomous, nominal, ordinal, continuous, or discrete numerical. Could any of them be modified to increase power, and, if so, how?
   a. History of heart attack (present/absent)
   b. Age
   c. Education (college degree or more/less than college degree)
   d. Race
   e. Number of alcohol drinks per day
   f. Depression (none, mild, moderate, severe)
   g. Percent occlusion of coronary arteries
   h. Hair color
   i. Obese (body mass index $\geq$ 30 kg/m^2)/nonobese (body mass index $<$ 30 kg/m^2)

2. An investigator is interested in the research question: "Does intake of fruit juice at age 6 months predict body weight at age 1 year?" She plans a prospective cohort study, measuring body weight using an infant scale. Several problems (listed further on) are noted during pretesting. Are these problems due to imprecision (random error), bias (systematic error), or both? Is the problem mainly due to observer, participant, or instrument variability, and what can be done about it?
   a. The 10-kg reference weight used to calibrate the scale has a true weight of 10.2 kg.
   b. Weighing the 10-kg reference on the scale repeatedly gives a mean $\pm$ standard deviation of 10.01 $\pm$ 0.2 kg.
   c. Some babies are frightened, and when they try to squirm off the scale, the observer must hold them on to complete the measurement.
   d. The pointer on the scale swings up and down wildly for babies who don't lie still.
   e. Some of the babies arrive for the examination immediately after being fed, whereas others are hungry; some of the babies are weighed with wet diapers.

3. The investigator is interested in studying the effect of resident work-hour limitations on surgical residents. One area she wishes to address is burnout, and she plans to assess it with two questions (answered on a 7-point scale) from a more extensive questionnaire: (a) "How often do you feel burned out from your work?" and (b) "How often do you feel you've become more callous toward people since you started your residency?"
   The investigator sets out to assess the validity of these questions for measuring burnout. For each of the following descriptions, name the type of validity being assessed:
   a. Residents with higher burnout scores were more likely to drop out of the program in the following year.
   b. A small group of residents are asked to review the items and report that these seem like reasonable questions to ask to address burnout.
   c. Burnout scores increase during the most arduous rotations and decrease during vacations.
   d. A previous study of more than 10,000 medical students, residents, and practicing physicians showed that these two items almost completely captured the emotional exhaustion and depersonalization domains of burnout as measured by the widely accepted (but much longer) Maslach Burnout Inventory (1).

REFERENCE

1. West CP, Dyrbye LN, Sloan JA, Shanafelt TD. Single item measures of emotional exhaustion and depersonalization are useful for assessing burnout in medical professionals. *J Gen Intern Med.* 2009;24(12):1318-1321.

Getting Ready to Estimate Sample Size: Hypotheses and Underlying Principles

Warren S. Browner, Thomas B. Newman, and Mark J. Pletcher

After an investigator has decided whom and what she is going to study and the design to be used, she must decide how many participants to sample. Or perhaps she already knows the number of potential participants and wants to determine whether there are enough to make the study worthwhile. Even the most rigorously executed study may fail to contribute meaningfully to answering the research question if the **sample size** is too small. On the other hand, a study with too large a sample will be more difficult and costly than necessary and may even find differences that are too small to be meaningful clinically. The goal of sample size planning is to estimate an *appropriate number* of participants for a given study design.

It's worth understanding how to do sample size estimates even if a study's sample size is *fixed* or *preset*, for instance, because the participants have already been enrolled or the data collected. As you will see shortly, in those situations what will matter will be how well that sample size can answer the research question.

This material appears early in the book for a very important reason. Our experience has shown that many new investigators put a lot of effort into designing studies that turn out to be impractical for a simple reason: They require sample sizes that exceed the investigator's capacity. It's much better to recognize that problem early in the design process, when there is still time to revise or even reconsider the research question and plan. Fortunately, even a simple one-page research plan—if it includes a clear **research hypothesis**, as discussed further on—usually provides enough information to make an initial sample size estimate.

Although a useful guide, sample size calculations give a deceptive impression of statistical objectivity. They are only as accurate as the data and estimates on which they are based, which are often just informed guesses. *Sample size planning* is best thought of as a mathematical way of making a ballpark estimate. It often reveals that the research design is not feasible or that different **predictor** or **outcome variables** are needed. Therefore, sample size should be estimated early in the design phase of a study, when major changes are still possible.

Before setting out the specific approaches to calculating sample size for several common research designs in Chapter 6, we will spend some time considering the *underlying principles*. Readers who find some of these principles confusing will enjoy discovering that sample size planning does not require their total mastery. However, just as a recipe makes more sense if the cook is somewhat familiar with the ingredients, sample size calculations are easier if the investigator is acquainted with the basic concepts. Even if you plan to ask a friendly biostatistician for help calculating your study's sample size, understanding how the process works will allow you to participate in considering the assumptions and estimates involved in the calculations.

■ HYPOTHESES

The process begins by restating your research question as a research hypothesis that summarizes the main elements of the study—the sample and the predictor and outcome variables. For example, suppose your research question is whether people who do crossword puzzles are less likely to develop dementia. Your research hypothesis would need to specify the sample (eg, people living in a retirement community who have normal cognitive function), the predictor variable (doing crossword puzzles at least once a week on average), and the outcome variable (an abnormal score on a standard test of cognitive function after 2 years of follow-up).

Hypotheses per se are not needed in **descriptive studies** that describe how characteristics are distributed in a population, such as the prevalence of abnormal cognitive function in the retirement community. (This does not mean, however, that you won't need to do a sample size estimate for a descriptive study, but that the methods for doing so, described in Chapter 6, are different.) Hypotheses are needed for **analytic studies**, which will use tests of statistical significance to compare findings among groups, such as the research question we posed about crossword puzzles and dementia. Because most **observational studies** and all **experiments** address research questions that involve making comparisons, most studies need to specify at least one hypothesis. If any of the following terms appear in the research question, then the study is not simply descriptive, and a research hypothesis should be formulated: greater than, less than, more likely than, associated with, compared with, related to, similar to, correlated with, predicts, causes, and leads to.

Characteristics of a Good Research Hypothesis

A good hypothesis must be based on a good research question. It should also be simple, specific, and stated in advance.

Simple Versus Complex

A **simple hypothesis** contains one predictor variable and one outcome variable:

> Among patients with Type II diabetes, a sedentary lifestyle is associated with an increased risk of developing proteinuria.

> (In this example, "sedentary lifestyle" is the predictor variable, and the development of proteinuria is the outcome variable; both are dichotomous.)

A **complex hypothesis** contains more than one predictor variable:

> Among patients with Type II diabetes, a sedentary lifestyle and alcohol consumption are associated with an increased risk of developing proteinuria.

Or it contains more than one outcome variable:

> Among patients with Type II diabetes, alcohol consumption is associated with increased risks of developing proteinuria and neuropathy.

Complex hypotheses like these are not readily tested with a single statistical test and are more easily approached as two or more simple hypotheses. Sometimes, however, a combined predictor or outcome variable can be used:

> Among patients with Type II diabetes, alcohol consumption is associated with an increased risk of developing a microvascular complication (ie, proteinuria, neuropathy, or retinopathy).

In this last example, the investigator has decided that what matters is whether a participant develops a complication, not what type of complication occurs.

Specific Versus Vague

A *specific* hypothesis leaves no ambiguity about the participants and variables or about how the test of statistical significance will be applied. It uses concise operational definitions that summarize the nature and source of the participants and how variables will be measured:

> Prior use of tricyclic antidepressant medications for at least 6 weeks is more common in patients hospitalized for myocardial infarction at Longview Hospital than in controls hospitalized for pneumonia.

This is a long sentence, but it communicates the nature of the study in a clear way that minimizes any opportunity for testing something a little different once the study findings have been examined. It would be incorrect to substitute, during the analysis phase of the study, a different measurement of the predictor, such as self-reported depression, without considering the issues of **multiple hypothesis testing** and data manipulation (topics we discuss at the end of the chapter). Usually, to keep the research hypothesis concise, some details are made explicit in the study plan rather than being stated in the research hypothesis.

It is often obvious from the research hypothesis whether the predictor variable and the outcome variable are dichotomous, continuous, or categorical. If it is not clear, then the type of variables can be specified:

> Among nonobese men 35 to 59 years of age, at least weekly participation in a bowling league is associated with an increased risk of developing obesity (body mass index > 30 kg/m^2) during 10 years of follow-up.

Again, if the research hypothesis gets too cumbersome, the definitions can be left out, if they are clarified in the study plan.

In Advance Versus After-the-Fact Hypotheses

The research hypothesis should be stated explicitly in writing **a priori**, in advance of the study. This will keep the research effort focused on the primary objective, create a stronger basis for interpreting the study, and prevent searching through the data to find a "positive" result. Hypotheses formulated after examination of the data—so-called **post hoc hypotheses**—are a form of multiple hypothesis testing that can lead to overinterpreting the importance of the findings. Misrepresenting a hypothesis as having been made in advance, rather than after-the-fact, is a form of **scientific misconduct**.

The Null and Alternative Hypotheses

Warning: If you have never had any formal training in statistics, or have forgotten what you did learn, the next few paragraphs may not make sense the first time(s) you read them. Try to work through the terminology even if it seems cumbersome or confusing.

The process begins by restating the research hypothesis to one that proposes that there is no difference between the groups being compared. This restatement, called the **null hypothesis**, will become the formal basis for testing statistical significance when you analyze your data at the end of the study. By assuming that the null hypothesis is true—that there really is no association in the population—the statistical tests you use will help to estimate the probability that the association observed in your study may be due to chance alone.

For example, suppose your research question is whether drinking nonpurified water from wells is associated with an increased risk of developing peptic ulcer disease (perhaps because of a greater likelihood of *Helicobacter pylori* contamination). You are doing a case-control study that will compare cases of peptic ulcer disease with controls selected from the same clinic who have lower gastrointestinal ailments. Your null hypothesis—that there is no association between the predictor and outcome variables in the population—would be:

> Cases of peptic ulcer disease have the same likelihood of drinking nonpurified well water as do controls.

The proposition that there *is* an association ("Cases of peptic ulcer disease have a greater likelihood of drinking nonpurified well water than do controls.") is called the **alternative hypothesis**. The alternative hypothesis cannot be tested directly; it is accepted by default if the test of statistical significance rejects the null hypothesis (see later).

■ UNDERLYING STATISTICAL PRINCIPLES

A research hypothesis, such as that 15 minutes or more of exercise per day is associated with a lower mean fasting blood glucose level in middle-aged women with diabetes, is either true or false in the real world. Because an investigator cannot study all middle-aged women with diabetes, she must test the hypothesis in a sample of that target population. As noted in Figure 1.5, there will always be a need to draw inferences about phenomena in the population from events observed in the sample. Unfortunately, by chance alone, sometimes what happens in a sample does not reflect what would have happened if the entire population had been studied.

In some ways, the investigator's problem resembles that faced by a jury judging a defendant (Table 5.1). The absolute truth about whether the defendant committed the crime cannot usually be determined. Instead, the jury begins by presuming innocence: The defendant did not commit the crime. The jury must then decide whether there is enough evidence to **reject the presumed innocence** of the defendant; the standard is known as **beyond a reasonable doubt**. A jury can err, however, by convicting an innocent defendant or failing to convict a guilty one.

In similar fashion, the investigator starts by presuming the null hypothesis of no association between the predictor and outcome variables in the population. On the basis of the data collected in her sample, she uses statistical tests to determine whether there is enough evidence to **reject the null hypothesis** in favor of the alternative hypothesis that there is an association in the population.

TABLE 5.1 THE ANALOGY BETWEEN JURY DECISIONS AND STATISTICAL TESTS

JURY DECISION	STATISTICAL TEST
Innocence: The defendant did not counterfeit money.	**Null hypothesis:** There is no association between regular exercise and mean fasting blood glucose levels in middle-aged women with diabetes.
Guilt: The defendant did counterfeit money.	**Alternative hypothesis:** There is an association between regular exercise and mean fasting blood glucose levels in middle-aged women with diabetes.
Standard for rejecting innocence: Beyond a reasonable doubt.	**Standard for rejecting null hypothesis:** Level of statistical significance (alpha, α).
Correct judgment: Convict a counterfeiter.	**Correct inference:** Conclude that there is an association between exercise and mean fasting glucose levels when one does exist in the population.
Correct judgment: Acquit an innocent person.	**Correct inference:** Conclude that there is no association between exercise and mean fasting glucose levels when one does not exist.
Incorrect judgment: Convict an innocent person.	**Incorrect inference (type I error):** Conclude that there is an association between exercise and mean fasting glucose levels when there is actually none.
Incorrect judgment: Acquit a counterfeiter.	**Incorrect inference (type II error):** Conclude that there is no association between exercise and mean fasting glucose levels when there is actually one.

Type I and Type II Errors

Like a jury, an investigator may reach a wrong conclusion. Sometimes, by chance alone, a sample is not representative of the population, and the results in the sample do not reflect reality in the population, leading to an erroneous inference. A **type I error (false-positive)** occurs if an investigator rejects a null hypothesis that is actually true in the population; a **type II error (false-negative)** occurs if the investigator fails to reject a null hypothesis that is actually false in the population. Although type I and type II errors can never be avoided entirely, the investigator can reduce their likelihood by increasing the sample size (the larger the sample, the less likely that it will differ substantially from the population) or by adjusting the design or the measurements in other ways that we will discuss.

In this chapter and the next, we deal only with ways to reduce type I and type II errors due to *chance* variation, also known as random error. False-positive and false-negative results can also occur because of **bias**, but errors due to bias are not usually referred to as type I and type II errors. Such errors are troublesome, because they may be difficult to detect and cannot usually be quantified using statistical methods or avoided by increasing the sample size. (See Chapters 3, 4, and 8 to 13 for ways to reduce errors due to bias.)

Effect Size

The likelihood that a study will be able to detect an association between a predictor and an outcome variable in a sample depends on the actual magnitude of that association in the population. If it is large (eg, a 20 mg/dL difference in fasting glucose), it will be easy to detect in the sample. Conversely, if the size of the association is small (a difference of 2 mg/dL), it will be hard to detect in the sample.

Unfortunately, the investigator almost never knows the exact size of the association; one of the purposes of the study is to estimate it! Instead, the investigator must choose the size of the association in the population that she wishes to detect in the sample. That quantity is known as the **effect size**. Selecting an appropriate effect size is perhaps the most difficult aspect of sample size planning (1). The investigator should try to find data from prior studies in related areas to make an informed guess about a reasonable effect size. Alternatively, she can choose the smallest effect size that in her opinion would be clinically meaningful (say, a 10 mg/dL reduction in the fasting glucose level).

Of course, from the public health point of view, even a reduction of 2 or 3 mg/dL in fasting glucose levels might be important, especially if it were easy to achieve. The choice of the effect size is always arbitrary, and considerations of feasibility are often paramount. Indeed, when the number of available or affordable participants is limited, the investigator may have to work backward (Chapter 6) to determine the effect size she will be able to detect given the number of participants she is able to study and then ask whether that effect size is reasonable.

Many studies have several effect sizes, because they measure several different predictor and outcome variables. When designing a study, the sample size should be determined using the desired effect size for the most important hypothesis; the detectable effect sizes for the other hypotheses can then be estimated. If there are several hypotheses of similar importance, then the sample size for the study should be based on whichever hypothesis needs the largest sample.

Alpha (α), Beta (β), and Power

After a study is completed, the investigator uses statistical tests to try to reject the null hypothesis in favor of its alternative, in much the same way that a prosecuting attorney tries to convince a jury to reject innocence in favor of guilt. Depending on whether the null hypothesis is true or false in the target population, and assuming that the study is free of bias, four situations are possible (Table 5.2). In two of these, the findings in the sample and reality in the population are concordant, and the investigator's inference will be correct. In the other two situations, either a type I or a type II error has been made, and the inference will be incorrect.

TABLE 5.2 TRUTH IN THE POPULATION VERSUS THE RESULTS IN THE STUDY SAMPLE: THE FOUR POSSIBILITIES

| | TRUTH IN THE POPULATION | |
RESULTS IN THE STUDY SAMPLE	ASSOCIATION BETWEEN PREDICTOR AND OUTCOME	NO ASSOCIATION BETWEEN PREDICTOR AND OUTCOME
Reject null hypothesis	Correct	Type I error
Fail to reject null hypothesis	Type II error	Correct

The investigator establishes the tolerability of making type I and type II errors by chance alone in advance of the study. The maximum probability of committing a type I error (rejecting the null hypothesis when it is actually true) by chance is called **alpha**, also known as the **level of statistical significance**.

If, for example, a study of the effects of regular exercise on fasting blood glucose levels is designed with an alpha of 0.05, then the investigator has set 5% as the maximum chance of incorrectly rejecting the null hypothesis if it is true (and inferring that regular exercise and fasting blood glucose levels are associated in the population when, in fact, they are not). This is the level of reasonable doubt that the investigator will be willing to accept when she uses statistical tests to analyze the data after the study is completed.

The probability of making a type II error (failing to reject the null hypothesis when it is actually false) is called **beta**. The quantity [1 – beta] is called **power**, the probability of correctly rejecting the null hypothesis in the sample if the actual effect in the population equals the specified effect size.

If beta is set at 0.10, then the investigator has decided that she is willing to accept a 10% chance of missing an association of the specified effect size if it exists. This is equivalent to a power of 0.90, that is, a 90% chance of correctly rejecting the null hypothesis. For example, suppose that regular exercise really does lead to an average reduction of 20 mg/dL in fasting glucose levels among diabetic women in the population. If the investigator replicated the study with the same 90% power on numerous occasions, we would expect that in 90% of those studies she would correctly reject the null hypothesis (at the specified level of alpha) and conclude that exercise is associated with fasting glucose levels. This does not mean that the investigator would be unable to detect a smaller effect in the population, say, a 15 mg/dL reduction; it means simply that she will have less than a 90% likelihood of doing so.

Ideally, alpha and beta would be set close to zero, minimizing the possibility of false-positive and false-negative results. Reducing them, however, requires increasing the sample size or one of the other strategies discussed in Chapter 6. **Sample size planning aims at choosing a sufficient number of participants to keep alpha and beta at an acceptably low level without making the study unnecessarily expensive or difficult.**

Many studies set alpha at 0.05 and beta at 0.20 (a power of 0.80). These are arbitrary values, and others are sometimes used: The conventional range for alpha is between 0.01 and 0.10, and that for beta is between 0.05 and 0.20. In general, the investigator should use a low alpha when the research question makes it particularly important to avoid a type I (false-positive) error—for example, in testing the efficacy of a potentially dangerous medication. She should use a low beta (and a small effect size) when it is especially important to avoid a type II (false-negative) error—for example, in reassuring the public that living near a toxic waste dump is safe. Finally, a study that is relatively easy to do—and without any risk or inconvenience to participants (say, because the data have already been collected)—may be reasonable to pursue even if its power is substantially less than 0.80.

Sides of the Alternative Hypothesis

An alternative hypothesis can be either one-sided or two-sided. A **one-sided alternative hypothesis** specifies the direction of the association between the predictor and outcome variables. For example, the hypothesis that drinking well water *increases* the risk of peptic ulcer disease is a one-sided hypothesis. A **two-sided alternative hypothesis** states only that there is an association; it does not specify the direction, such as "Drinking well water is associated with a different risk of peptic ulcer disease—either increased or decreased—than drinking other types of water."

One-sided alternative hypotheses may be appropriate in unusual circumstances when only one direction of an association would be clinically important or biologically meaningful. An example is the one-sided hypothesis that a new drug for hypertension is more likely to cause rashes than a placebo; the possibility that the drug causes fewer rashes than the placebo is not usually worth testing (however, it might be if the drug had anti-inflammatory properties!). In those rare situations in which an investigator is interested only in one of the sides of the alternative hypothesis (eg, a noninferiority trial designed to determine whether a new antibiotic is no less effective than one in current use; see Chapter 12), sample size can be calculated accordingly. A one-sided hypothesis, however, should never be used just to reduce the sample size.

It is important to keep in mind the difference between the research hypothesis, which is usually one-sided, and the alternative hypothesis that is used when planning sample size, which is almost always two-sided. For example, suppose the research hypothesis is that recurrent use of antibiotics during childhood is associated with an increased risk of inflammatory bowel disease. That hypothesis specifies the direction of the anticipated effect, so it is one-sided. Why use a two-sided alternative hypothesis when planning the sample size? The answer is that most of the time, both sides of the alternative hypothesis (ie, greater risk or lesser risk) are interesting, and the investigators would want to publish the results no matter which direction was observed in the study. Statistical rigor requires the investigator to choose between one- and two-sided hypotheses before analyzing the data; switching from a two-sided to a one-sided alternative hypothesis to reduce the *P* value (see further on) is not correct. In addition—and this is probably the real reason that two-sided alternative hypotheses are much more common—most grant and manuscript reviewers expect two-sided hypotheses and are extremely critical of a one-sided approach in the absence of very strong justification.

P Values—and Their Limitations

Now it's time to return to the *null hypothesis,* whose purpose will finally become clear. The null hypothesis has only one function: to act like a straw man. It is assumed to be true so that it can be rejected as false with a statistical test. When the data are analyzed, a statistical test is used to determine the **P value**, which is the probability of seeing—by chance alone—an effect[1] as big as or bigger than that seen in the study if the null hypothesis actually were true.

The key insight is to recognize that if the null hypothesis is true, and there really is no difference between the groups being compared in the population, then *chance* is the only way that an unbiased study could have found a difference in the sample. (Ways to address bias are discussed in Chapter 10.)

If the *P* value is small, then the null hypothesis of no difference can be rejected in favor of its alternative, namely, that there is a difference. By "small" we mean a *P* value that is less than alpha, the predetermined level of statistical significance. However, a *nonsignificant result* (ie, one with a

---

[1]We have sacrificed a bit of statistical purity in the interest of readability. *P* values are computed by calculating the value of a *test statistic* (such as the *t* test) that has a known distribution under the null hypothesis. The *P* value is the probability of obtaining a value of this test statistic at least as extreme as was obtained in the study, assuming the null hypothesis is true. Because more than one test statistic can sometimes be computed for a study, there may be more than one possible *P* value for the observed effect size. Thus, it is important to specify in advance the statistical test that will be used to avoid the appearance of "P-hacking": trying several statistical approaches to the data to find one that yields the desired result.

P value greater than alpha) does not mean that there is no association in the population. Rather, it indicates that the association observed in the sample could have occurred *by chance alone.* For example, a P value of 0.56 indicates that an association similar in size to that seen in the study would occur more than half the time by chance alone if there were no association in the population.

When a two-sided statistical test is used, the P value includes the probabilities of committing a type I error in each of the directions (eg, erroneously concluding that there is a greater risk or a lesser risk), which is about twice as great as the probability in either direction alone. So a one-sided P value of 0.05, for example, is usually the same as a two-sided P value of 0.10. (Some statistical tests are asymmetric, which is why we said "usually.")

To illustrate, suppose an investigator finds that women who played intercollegiate sports were twice as likely to undergo total hip replacements later in life as those who did not play sports, but—perhaps because the number of participants in the study was modest—this apparent effect had a P value of "only" 0.08. This means that even if athletic activity and hip replacement were not associated in the population, there would be an 8% probability of finding an association at least as large as the one observed by the investigator by chance alone. If the investigator had used a two-sided alternative hypothesis and set the significance level at a two-sided alpha of 0.05, she would have to conclude that the association in the sample was "not statistically significant." It might be tempting to switch to a *one*-sided P value and report it as "P = 0.04." A much better choice, however, would be to report her results with the 95% confidence interval and comment that "these results, although suggestive of an association, did not achieve statistical significance (P = 0.08)." This solution preserves the integrity of the original two-sided hypothesis design, while acknowledging that statistical significance is not an all-or-none situation.

To be sure, some epidemiologists and statisticians argue against setting an arbitrary criterion when designing a study for deciding whether a P value will be statistically significant (2, 3). However, proposed alternatives (4)—such as estimating the cost and value of the information that a study will provide—rely on their own assumptions and are not yet very useful when designing a study, especially one that must undergo peer review before being funded. At least for now, the methods we outline in this chapter and the next remain the standards in clinical research and provide a good foundation for more advanced approaches.

That said, investigators should *never* just report that a result is "statistically significant at P < 0.05." **What matters much more is the magnitude of the association between the predictor and outcome variables and how precisely that association can be estimated, usually expressed as a confidence interval (5).**

Type of Statistical Test

The formulas used to calculate sample size are based on mathematical assumptions, which differ for each statistical test. Before the sample size can be calculated, the investigator must decide on the statistical approach to analyzing the data. That choice depends mainly on the type of predictor and outcome variables in the study. Table 6.1 lists some common statistics used in data analysis, and Chapter 6 provides simplified approaches to estimating sample size for studies that use these statistics.

■ ADDITIONAL POINTS

Variability

It is not simply the size of an effect that is important; its **variability** also matters. Statistical tests depend on being able to show a difference between the groups being compared. The greater the variability (or spread) in the outcome variable among the participants, the more likely it is that the values in the groups will overlap and the more difficult it will be to demonstrate an overall difference between them. Because measurement error contributes to the overall variability, less precise measurements require larger sample sizes (6).

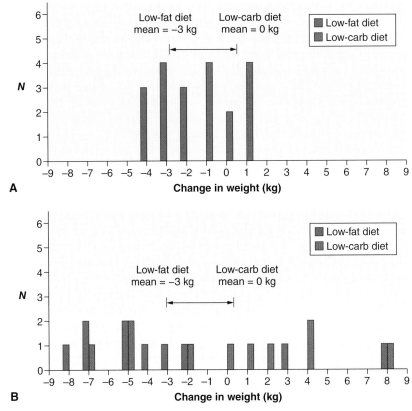

■ **FIGURE 5.1 A:** *Weight loss achieved by two diets.* All participants on the low-fat diet lost from 2 to 4 kg, whereas weight change in those on the low-carbohydrate (carb) diet varied from −1 to +1 kg. There is no overlap between the groups, and it is therefore reasonable to conclude that the low-fat diet is better at achieving weight loss (as would be confirmed with a two-sample paired *t* test, which has a *P* value < 0.001). **B:** *Weight loss achieved by two diets.* There is substantial overlap in weight change in the two groups. Although the effect size is the same (3 kg) as in **A**, there is little evidence that one diet is better than the other (as would be confirmed with a two-sample paired *t* test, which has a *P* value of 0.19).

Consider a study of the effects of two diets (low fat and low carbohydrate) in achieving weight loss in a trial of 40 participants. If all those on the low-fat diet lost about 3 kg and all those on the low-carbohydrate diet lost little, if any, weight (an effect size of 3 kg), it is likely that the low-fat diet is really better (Figure 5.1A). On the other hand, if the average weight loss were still 3 kg in the low-fat group and 0 kg in the low-carbohydrate group but there was a great deal of overlap between the two groups (the situation in Figure 5.1B), the greater variability would make it more difficult to detect a difference between the diets, and a larger sample size would be needed.

When one of the variables used in the sample size estimate is continuous (eg, change in body weight in Figure 5.1), the investigator will need to estimate its variability to estimate the sample size. (See the section on the *t* test in Chapter 6 for details.) Often, variability is accounted for by the other parameters used in the sample size estimates, so it need not be specified.

Multiple and Post Hoc Hypotheses

When more than one hypothesis is tested in a study, the likelihood that at least one will achieve statistical significance by chance alone increases. For example, if 20 independent hypotheses are tested at an alpha of 0.05, the likelihood is substantial (64%; $[1 − 0.95^{20}]$) that at least one hypothesis will be statistically significant by chance alone. Some statisticians advocate adjusting the level of statistical significance when more than one hypothesis is tested in a study. This keeps the overall probability of accepting any one of the alternative hypotheses, when all the findings are due to chance, at the specified level. For example, genomic studies that look for an association between thousands of genotypes and a disease need to use a much smaller alpha than 0.05, or they risk identifying many false-positive associations.

One approach, called the **Bonferroni correction**, after the Italian mathematician Carlo Emilio Bonferroni, is to divide the significance level (say, 0.05) by the number of hypotheses tested. If there were four hypotheses, for example, each would be tested at an alpha of 0.0125 (ie, 0.05 ÷ 4). This requires substantially increasing the sample size over that needed for testing each hypothesis at an alpha of 0.05. Thus, for any particular hypothesis, the Bonferroni approach reduces the chance of a type I error at the cost of either increasing the chance of a type II error or requiring a greater sample size. If the results of a study are still statistically significant after the Bonferroni adjustment, that loss of power is not a problem. However, a result that loses statistical significance after Bonferroni adjustment, thus failing to support an association that was actually present in the population (a type II error), is more problematic.

Especially in these cases, the issue of what significance level to use depends more on the **prior probability** of each hypothesis than on the number of hypotheses tested. For this reason, our view is that the Bonferroni approach to multiple hypothesis testing is generally too stringent. There is an analogy with the use of diagnostic tests that may be helpful (7, 8). When interpreting the results of a diagnostic test, a clinician considers the likelihood that the patient being tested has the disease in question. For example, a modestly abnormal test result in a healthy person (a serum alkaline phosphatase level that is 15% greater than the upper limit of normal) is probably a false-positive test that is unlikely to have much clinical importance. Similarly, a *P* value of 0.05 for an unlikely hypothesis is probably also a false-positive result.

However, an alkaline phosphatase level that is 10 or 20 times greater than the upper limit of normal is unlikely to have occurred by chance (although it might be a laboratory error). So too a very small *P* value (say, <0.001) is unlikely to have occurred by chance (although it could be due to bias). It is hard to dismiss very abnormal test results as being false-positives or to dismiss very low *P* values as being due to chance, even if the prior probability of the disease or the hypothesis was low.[2] However, bias can explain even very small *P* values, a topic we return to in Chapter 9.

Moreover, the number of tests that were ordered, or hypotheses that were tested, is not always relevant. The interpretation of an elevated serum uric acid level in a patient with a painful and swollen joint should not depend on whether the physician ordered just a single test (the uric acid level) or obtained the result as part of a panel of 20 tests. Similarly, when interpreting the *P* value for testing a research hypothesis that makes good sense, it should not matter that the investigator also tested several unlikely hypotheses. What matters most is the reasonableness of the research hypothesis being tested: that it has a substantial prior probability of being correct. (Prior probability, in this "**Bayesian**" approach, is often a subjective judgment based on evidence from other sources.) Hypotheses that are formulated during the design of a study usually meet this requirement; after all, why else would the investigator put the time and effort into planning and doing the study?

What about *unanticipated* associations that appear during the collection and analysis of a study's results? This process is sometimes called **hypothesis generation** or, less favorably, "data-mining" or going on a "fishing expedition." The many informal comparisons that are made during data analysis are a form of multiple hypothesis testing. A similar problem arises when variables are redefined during data analysis or when results are presented for subgroups of the sample. Significant *P* values for post hoc hypotheses—those that were not considered during the design of the study—are all too often due to chance. They should be viewed with great skepticism and labeled clearly as data generated and are best considered as a source of potential

---

[2]The exception is some genetic studies, in which millions or even billions of associations may be examined.

research questions for future studies. Under no circumstances should an investigator claim or imply that a post hoc hypothesis was conceived at the time the study was designed.

There are times when an investigator fails to specify a particular hypothesis in advance, although that hypothesis seems reasonable when it is time for the data to be analyzed. This might happen, for example, if a new risk factor is identified while the study is going on. In that sort of situation, the important issue is whether there is a reasonable prior probability—based on evidence from other sources—that the hypothesis is true (7, 8). Still, such a hypothesis should be labeled as being post hoc.

It's often tempting to concoct a hypothesis to fit an unlikely result that emerges during data analysis, but there is little to no statistical rigor attached to doing so. Indeed, as the physicist Richard Feynman pointed out, almost any observation may seem remarkable in hindsight: "You know, the most amazing thing happened to me tonight…I saw a car with the license plate ARW 357. Can you imagine? Of all the millions of license plates in the state, what was the chance that I would see that particular one tonight?" (9).

There are, however, some advantages to formulating more than one hypothesis when planning a study. The use of *multiple unrelated hypotheses* increases the efficiency of the study, making it possible to answer more questions with a single research effort and to discover more of the true associations that exist in the population. For example, a cohort study of the effect of dietary predictors, such as red meat intake, on the risk of colorectal cancer might also look at cardiovascular outcomes, assuming it is easy to gather the additional data.

It may also be a good idea to formulate several *related* hypotheses; if the findings are consistent, the study conclusions are made stronger. Studies in patients with heart failure, for example, have found that the use of angiotensin-converting enzyme inhibitors is beneficial in reducing cardiac admissions, cardiovascular mortality, and total mortality. Had only one of these hypotheses been tested, the inferences from these studies would have been less definitive. Even so, testing several related and restated hypotheses introduces another problem. Suppose that when those hypotheses are tested at the end of the study only one turns out to be statistically significant, whereas tests of the other hypotheses are not even close to being significant. Then the investigator must decide (and try to convince editors and readers) whether the significant result, the nonsignificant results, or both sets of results are correct.

Primary and Secondary Hypotheses

Some studies, especially large, randomized trials, specify some hypotheses as *secondary*. This usually happens when there is one **primary hypothesis** around which the study has been designed but the investigators are also interested in other research questions that are of lesser importance. For example, the primary outcome of a trial of zinc supplementation might be seeing a practitioner for an upper respiratory tract infection; a secondary outcome might be self-reported days missed from work or school. If the study is being done to obtain approval for a pharmaceutical agent, the primary outcome is what will matter most to the regulatory body. Stating a few **secondary hypotheses** in advance increases the credibility of the results when those hypotheses are tested, but the more secondary hypotheses there are, the less credible each one becomes.

A good rule, particularly for clinical trials, is to establish in advance as many hypotheses as make sense but specify just one as the primary hypothesis, which can be tested statistically without argument about whether to adjust for multiple hypothesis testing. More important, having a primary hypothesis helps to focus the study on its main objective and provides a clear basis for the main sample size calculation.

■ SUMMARY

1. Sample size planning is an important part of the design of both analytic and descriptive studies. The **sample size** should be estimated early in the process of developing the study plan so that appropriate modifications can be made.

2. Analytic studies and experiments need a **hypothesis** that specifies, for the purpose of subsequent statistical tests, the anticipated association between the main predictor and outcome variables. Purely descriptive studies, lacking comparison, do not require a hypothesis.

3. Good hypotheses are **specific** about the population that will be sampled and the variables that will be measured, **simple** (there is only one predictor and one outcome variable), and **formulated in advance**.

4. The **null hypothesis**, which proposes that the predictor variable is not associated with the outcome, is the basis for tests of statistical significance. The **alternative hypothesis** proposes that they are associated. Statistical tests attempt to reject the null hypothesis of no association in favor of the alternative hypothesis, namely, that there is an association.

5. An alternative hypothesis is either **one-sided** (only one direction of association will be tested) or **two-sided** (both directions will be tested). One-sided hypotheses should be used only in unusual circumstances, when only one direction of the association is clinically or biologically meaningful.

6. For analytic studies and experiments, the sample size is an estimate of the number of participants required to detect an association of a **given effect size** and **variability** at a specified likelihood of making **type I** (false-positive) and **type II** (false-negative) **errors**. The maximum likelihood of making a type I error is called **alpha**; that of making a type II error, **beta**. The quantity (1 – beta) is **power**, the chance of observing an association of a given effect size in a sample if one is actually present in the population.

7. It is often desirable to establish more than one hypothesis in advance, but the investigator should specify a **single primary hypothesis** as a focus and for sample size estimation. Interpretation of findings from **testing multiple hypotheses** in the sample, including unanticipated findings that emerge from the data, is based on a judgment about the **prior probability** that they represent real phenomena in the population.

REFERENCES

1. Van Walraven C, Mahon JL, Moher D, et al. Surveying physicians to determine the minimal important difference: implications for sample-size calculation. *J Clin Epidemiol*. 1999;52:717-723.
2. Goodman SN. Toward evidence-based medical statistics. 1: the P value fallacy. *Ann Intern Med*. 1999;130:995-1004.
3. Goodman SN. Toward evidence-based medical statistics. 2: the Bayes factor. *Ann Intern Med*. 1999;130:1005-1013.
4. Bacchetti P. Current sample size conventions: flaws, harms, and alternatives. *BMC Med*. 2010;8:17.
5. Daly LE. Confidence limits made easy: interval estimation using a substitution method. *Am J Epidemiol*. 1998;147:783-790.
6. McKeown-Eyssen GE, Tibshirani R. Implications of measurement error in exposure for the sample sizes of case-control studies. *Am J Epidemiol*. 1994;139:415-421.
7. Browner WS, Newman TB. Are all significant P values created equal? The analogy between diagnostic tests and clinical research. *JAMA*. 1987;257:2459-2463.
8. Newman TB, Kohn, MA. *Evidence-Based Diagnosis: an Introduction to Clinical Epidemiology*. 2nd ed. Cambridge University Press; 2020: 285-289.
9. Feynman R, Leighton R, Sands M. *Six Easy Pieces: Essentials of Physics Explained by Its Most Brilliant Teacher*. Basic Books; 2011.

APPENDIX 5A
Exercises for Chapter 5. Getting Ready to Estimate Sample Size: Hypotheses and Underlying Principles

1. Define the concepts in **red font**.

   An investigator is interested in designing a study with sufficient **sample size** to determine whether body mass index is associated with stomach cancer in women between 50 and 75 years of age. She is planning a case-control study with equal numbers of cases and controls. The **null hypothesis** is that there is no difference in mean body mass index between cases of stomach cancer and controls; she has chosen an **alternative hypothesis** with two sides. She would like to have a **power** of 0.80, at a **level of statistical significance** (alpha) of 0.05, to be able to detect an **effect size** of a difference in body mass index of 1 kg/m^2 between cases and controls. Review of the literature indicates that the **variability** of body mass index among women is a standard deviation of 2.5 kg/m^2.

2. Which of the following is likely to be an example of a type I error? A type II error? Neither?

   a. A randomized trial finds that participants treated with a new analgesic medication had greater mean declines in their pain scores during a study than did those treated with placebo ($P = 0.03$).

   b. A 10-year study reports that 110 participants who smoke do not have a greater incidence of lung cancer than 294 nonsmokers ($P = 0.31$).

   c. An investigator concludes that "our study is the first to find that use of alcohol reduces the risk of diabetes in men less than 50 years of age ($P < 0.05$)."

CHAPTER 6

Estimating Sample Size: Applications and Examples

Warren S. Browner, Thomas B. Newman, and Mark J. Pletcher

Chapter 5 introduced the basic principles that underlie estimating sample sizes. This chapter presents several cookbook techniques for using those principles. The first section deals with sample size estimates for an **analytic study or experiment**, including some special issues that apply to these studies, such as multivariable analysis. The second section considers studies that are primarily **descriptive**. Subsequent sections deal with studies that have a **fixed or preset sample size**, strategies for **maximizing power**, and the approach to estimating a sample size when there appears to be **insufficient information** from which to work. The chapter concludes with **common errors to avoid**. Chapter appendices include lookup tables for several basic methods of estimating sample size.

We always teach new investigators to make their own sample size estimates. You can do this using the tables in this chapter, statistical software, or a dedicated tool like www.sample-size.net (developed for the University of California San Francisco [UCSF] Training in Clinical Research Program). Even if your study design requires a more complicated statistical approach than those covered in this chapter or you plan to submit a research proposal to an agency that requires you to have biostatistical support, it's worthwhile estimating a "back of the envelope" sample size before you consult with a biostatistician. Most of the time, you will be pleasantly surprised how close your estimate comes!

■ SAMPLE SIZE TECHNIQUES FOR ANALYTIC STUDIES AND EXPERIMENTS

There are several variations on the recipe for estimating sample size in an analytic study or experiment, but they all have certain steps in common:

1. State the **null hypothesis** and either a one- or two-sided **alternative hypothesis**.
2. Select the appropriate **statistical test** from Table 6.1 based on the type of predictor variable and outcome variable in those hypotheses.
3. Choose a reasonable **effect size** (and estimate the **variability** of the measurement, if necessary).
4. Set **alpha** and **beta**. Specify a two-sided alpha unless the alternative hypothesis is clearly one-sided.
5. Use the appropriate table in the appendix, an online calculator, or a statistical package to estimate the sample size.

Even if the exact value of one or more of the ingredients is uncertain, it is important to estimate the sample size early in the design phase. Waiting too long to estimate the sample size can lead to a rude awakening: It may be necessary to start over with new ingredients, which may require redesigning the entire study. That is why this topic is covered early in this book.

Not all analytic studies will fit neatly into one of the three main categories of sample size estimation that follow. A few of the more common exceptions are discussed in the section called "Other Considerations and Special Issues."

TABLE 6.1 SIMPLE STATISTICAL TESTS FOR USE IN ESTIMATING SAMPLE SIZE[a]

PREDICTOR VARIABLE	OUTCOME VARIABLE	
	Dichotomous	Continuous
Dichotomous	Chi-squared test[b]	t test
Continuous	t test	Correlation coefficient

[a]See section on "Other Considerations and Special Issues" for what to do about categorical (nominal and ordinal) variables, or if planning to analyze the data with another type of statistical test.

[b]The chi-squared test is always two-sided; a one-sided equivalent is the Z statistic.

The *t* Test

The **t test** (sometimes called "Student's t test," after the pseudonym of its developer) is commonly used to determine whether the mean value of a continuous variable in one group differs significantly from that in another group. Although the t test assumes that the distribution (spread) of the variable in each of the two groups approximates a normal (bell-shaped) curve, it can be used to estimate sample sizes for most continuous variables unless the number of participants is small (fewer than 30 to 40) or there are extreme outliers.

The t test is usually used to compare continuous *outcome* variables in a cohort study or experiment. For example, it can be used to compare birth weights of babies born to mother treated with two different antidepressants. However, it can also be used when you have a continuous *predictor* variable in a case-control study; in this situation, it compares the mean value of the predictor variable in cases with that in controls.

To estimate the sample size for a study in which the mean values of a continuous variable will be compared using a t test (see Examples 6.1a and 6.1b), the investigator must

1. State the null hypothesis and specify whether the alternative hypothesis is one- or two-sided.
2. Choose the effect size (E), expressed as the difference in the mean values of the continuous variable between the study groups.
3. Estimate variability in the continuous variable, expressed as its anticipated standard deviation (S).
4. Calculate the standardized effect size (E/S), defined as the effect size divided by the standard deviation.
5. Set alpha and beta.

Example 6.1a Estimating Sample Size When Using the *t* Test in a Cohort Study

Problem: The research question is whether adding ipratropium bromide to albuterol alone improves asthma control. The investigator plans a randomized trial of the effect of these drugs on FEV_1 (forced expiratory volume in 1 second) after 2 weeks of treatment. A previous study has reported that the mean FEV_1 in persons with asthma treated with albuterol was 2.0 L, with a standard deviation of 0.5 L. The investigator would like to be able to detect a difference of 10% or more in mean FEV_1 between the two treatment groups. How many patients are required in each group (albuterol plus ipratropium and albuterol alone) at alpha (two-sided) = 0.05 and power = 0.80?

Solution: The ingredients for the sample size calculation are as follows:

Null hypothesis: Mean FEV_1 after 2 weeks of treatment is the same in asthmatic patients treated with albuterol alone as in those treated with albuterol plus ipratropium.

Alternative hypothesis (two-sided): Mean FEV_1 after 2 weeks of treatment is different in asthmatic patients treated with albuterol alone from what it is in those treated with albuterol plus ipratropium.

Mean FEV1 with albuterol alone: 2.0 L; mean FEV1 with albuterol plus ipratropium: 2.2 L; effect size = 0.2 L (= 2.2 – 2.0 = 10% of 2.0).

Standard deviation of FEV1 = 0.5 L.

Standardized effect size = effect size ÷ standard deviation = 0.2 L ÷ 0.5 L = 0.40.

Alpha (two-sided) = 0.05; beta = 1 – 0.80 = 0.20. (Recall that beta = 1 – power.)

Looking across from a standardized effect size of 0.40 in the leftmost column of Table 6A and down from alpha (two-sided) = 0.05 and beta = 0.20, **100 patients are required per group.** This is the number of patients in each group who need to complete the study; even more will need to be enrolled to account for dropouts. If this sample size is not feasible, the investigator might reconsider the study design or perhaps settle for only being able to detect a larger effect size. See the section on the *t* test for paired samples (Example 6.8) for a potential solution.

Example 6.1b Estimating Sample Size When Using the *t* Test in a Case-Control Study

Problem: The research question is whether plasma dihydrotestosterone levels are associated with the risk of developing seminoma (a type of testicular cancer). The investigator plans a case-control study comparing dihydrotestosterone levels in new cases of seminoma with controls selected from the same community. The mean dihydrotestosterone level in men is about 1.5 nmol/L, with a standard deviation of 0.5 nmol/L. (Because seminomas are rare, we can assume these same values apply to controls.) The investigator would like to be able to detect a difference of 20% or more in mean levels between the cases and controls. How many participants are required in each group at alpha (two-sided) = 0.05 and power = 0.80?

Solution: The ingredients for the sample size calculation are as follows:

Null hypothesis: Mean serum dihydrotestosterone level is the same in cases of seminoma as it is in controls.

Alternative hypothesis (two-sided): Mean serum dihydrotestosterone level differs in men with seminoma compared with controls.

Mean serum dihydrotestosterone level in controls = 1.5 nmol/L; mean serum dihydrotestosterone level in cases = 1.8 nmol/L; effect size = 0.3 nmol/L (= 1.8 – 1.5 = 20% of 1.5).

Standard deviation of dihydrotestosterone level = 0.5 nmol/L.

Standardized effect size = effect size ÷ standard deviation = 0.3 ÷ 0.5 = 0.6.

Alpha (two-sided) = 0.05; beta = 1 – 0.80 = 0.20. (Recall that beta = 1 – power.)

Looking across from a standardized effect size of 0.60 in the leftmost column of Table 6A and down from alpha (two-sided) = 0.05 and beta = 0.20, **45 cases and 45 controls are required.**

As discussed in Chapter 5, choosing the effect size can be difficult. When using the *t* test, all that is needed for sample size estimation (along with alpha and beta) is a single value: the standardized effect size. This unitless number, however, is somewhat divorced from clinical reality. To choose a standardized effect size with clinical meaning, it's often advisable to begin by specifying the anticipated mean values of the variable in the two groups that will be compared, then determine the difference between those means (the effect size), and finally divide that difference by the variable's standard deviation. Although specifying the group means themselves is not required—only the difference between them—doing so helps to ground the process.

The standard deviation of a variable, which reflects a combination of true population variation and measurement error, is critical: The greater it is, the larger the sample size must be for a given effect size. Most often, the standard deviation can be estimated from previous studies in the literature or consultation with experts, but there are times when an investigator cannot obtain any meaningful information about a variable's standard deviation, for instance, because she is using a new questionnaire or instrument (see "How to Estimate Sample Size When There Is Insufficient Information").

It is often useful to use the *change* in a continuous measurement (eg, change in bodyweight during a study) as an outcome variable. That's because the standard deviation of the change in a variable is usually smaller than the standard deviation of the variable itself; therefore, the sample size will also be smaller, as discussed in the section "Use Paired Measurements" (p. 79) and Example 6.8 later in this chapter.

Once the investigator has chosen alpha, beta, and a standardized effect size, the sample size can be estimated. We recommend using www.sample-size.net or another web-based tool or statistical package for this purpose, but you can also use a lookup table like Table 6A if you have equal-sized groups. To use Table 6A, look down its leftmost column for the standardized effect size. Next, read across the table to the chosen values for alpha and beta to determine the sample size required *per group*. Scanning Table 6A and the other lookup tables in the appendix will give you a sense of how your choices influence the sample size.

There is a convenient shortcut (1) for estimating the sample size using the *t* test when more than about 30 participants will be studied and power is set at 0.80 (beta = 0.20) and alpha (two-sided) at 0.05:

$$\text{Sample size (per equal-sized group)} = 16 \div (\text{standardized effect size})^2$$

In Example 6.1a, the shortcut estimate of the sample size would be $16 \div (0.4)^2 = 100$ per group, the same as that obtained from the lookup table or by using an online calculator.

The Chi-Squared Test

The **chi-squared** (χ^2) **test** can be used to compare the proportions of participants who have a dichotomous outcome (or predictor) in each of two groups. The chi-squared test is always two-sided; an equivalent test for one-sided hypotheses is the one-sided **Z test**.

In a cohort study, cross-sectional study, or experiment, the effect size is specified by the difference between P_0, the proportion of participants expected to have the outcome in one group (ie, the risk of the outcome), and P_1, the proportion expected in the other group. For example, in a cohort study comparing the effects of exposure to herbicides on the risk of developing non-Hodgkin lymphoma, P_0 would be the proportion of those unexposed to herbicides who develop non-Hodgkin lymphoma, and P_1 would be the proportion of those exposed to herbicides who do so. Variability is a function of P_0 and P_1, so it need not be specified separately.

Case-control studies differ slightly: the effect size is specified by the difference between P_1, the proportion of cases expected to have the exposure, and P_0, the proportion of controls expected to have the exposure. For example, in a case-control study of whether being a vegan is protective against colon cancer, P_1 would be the proportion of cases of colon cancer who are vegan, and P_0 would be the proportion of controls who are vegan. Again, variability is a function of P_0 and P_1, so it need not be specified.

To estimate the sample size for a study that will be analyzed with the chi-squared test or Z test to compare two proportions (Examples 6.2a and 6.2b), the investigator must

1. State the null hypothesis and decide whether the alternative hypothesis should be one- or two-sided.
2. Estimate the effect size (and its variability) in terms of P0 and P1, the proportions being compared in the two groups.
3. Set alpha and beta.

Example 6.2a Estimating Sample Size When Using the Chi-Squared Test in a Cohort Study

Problem: The research question is whether people who practice Tai Chi have a lower risk of developing back pain than those who jog for exercise. A review of the literature suggests that the 2-year risk of back pain is about 30% in joggers. The investigator hopes to be able to show that those who practice Tai Chi have at least a 10% absolute reduction in that risk. At alpha (two-sided) = 0.05 and power = 0.80, how many participants will need to be studied to determine whether the 2-year incidence of developing back pain is 20% (or less) in those who do Tai Chi?

Solution: The ingredients for the sample size calculation are as follows:

Null hypothesis: The incidence of back pain is the same in those who jog and those who practice Tai Chi.

Alternative hypothesis (two-sided): The incidence of back pain differs in those who jog and those who practice Tai Chi.

P_1 (incidence in those who jog) = 0.30; P_0 (incidence in those who practice Tai Chi) = 0.20; effect size = 0.10 (= |0.30 − 0.20|).

Alpha (two-sided) = 0.05; beta = 1 − 0.80 = 0.20.

Looking across from 0.20 (the *smaller* of P_0 and P_1) in the leftmost column in Table 6B.1 and down from 0.10 (the effect size), the middle number for alpha (two-sided) = 0.05 and beta = 0.20, the **required sample size is 313 in each group** who complete the study.

Example 6.2b Estimating Sample Size When Using the Chi-Squared Test in a Case-Control Study

Problem: The research question is whether eating sushi during the third trimester of pregnancy is associated with the risk of placenta previa (a rare outcome). The investigator wants to be able to detect an odds ratio of 2.5 or greater at alpha (two-sided) = 0.05 and power = 0.80, with an equal number of cases and controls. She estimates, on the basis of an online survey, that about 25% of pregnant women eat sushi during the third trimester of pregnancy. How many cases of placenta previa (and an equal number of pregnant women with uncomplicated pregnancies as controls) will she need to study?

Solution: The ingredients for the sample size calculation are as follows:

Null hypothesis: The proportion of women with placenta previa who ate sushi during the third trimester of pregnancy is the same as the proportion of control women who did so.

Alternative hypothesis (two-sided): The proportion of women with placenta previa who ate sushi during the third trimester of pregnancy differs from the proportion of control women who did so.

Because the outcome is rare, P_0, **the prevalence of eating sushi in controls,** will be almost the same as the prevalence of eating sushi among all pregnant women. Thus, P_0 = 0.25. P_1, **the prevalence of eating sushi in women with placenta previa,** is calculated from P_0 and the odds ratio using the equation on p. 70. Thus, P_1 = (2.5 × 0.25) ÷ [(1 − 0.75) + (2.5 × 0.25)] = 0.45 (approximately). The **effect size = 0.20** (= |0.45 − 0.25|).

Alpha (two-sided) = 0.05; beta = 1 − 0.80 = 0.20.

Looking across from 0.25 in the leftmost column in Table 6B.1 and down from 0.20, the middle number for alpha (two-sided) = 0.05 and beta = 0.20 is the **required sample size of 98 cases and 98 controls.**

Appendix 6B gives the sample size requirements for several combinations of alpha and beta and a range of values of P_0 and P_1 when the groups being compared are the same size. To estimate the sample size, look down the leftmost column of Tables 6B.1 or 6B.2 for the smaller of P_0 and P_1 (if necessary, rounded to the nearest 0.05 in Table 6B.1, or 0.01 in Table 6B.2). Next, read across for the difference between P_0 and P_1. Based on the chosen values for alpha and beta, the table gives the sample size required per *equal-sized* group.

When the group sizes are not equal, the lookup table in Appendix 6B will not suffice, and a calculation will be required. For example, in Example 6.2b, it will likely be much easier to find controls (women without placenta previa) than cases (women with placenta previa). Choosing multiple controls for each case will reduce the number of cases needed. In this situation, the sample size can be estimated at www.sample-size.net, using the "Proportions-Sample size" calculator, entering alpha (0.05) and beta (0.20), and then specifying the proportion of participants (q_1) in Group 1 (the cases) as, say, 0.25 (which would result in a 1:3 ratio of cases to controls). At $P_1 = 0.45$ and $P_0 = 0.25$, only 63 cases and 190 controls are needed. Although the total sample size is bigger $[(63 + 190) > (98 + 98)]$, the recruitment is likely more feasible.

Using the Risk Ratio or Odds Ratio to Estimate P_0 and P_1

Often, it is useful to think about the effect size in terms of the **risk ratio** (or **relative risk**) of the outcome. In a cohort study, cross-sectional study, or experiment, it is straightforward to convert between the risk ratio and the two proportions (P_0 and P_1), because the relative risk is just P_1 divided by P_0. For example, suppose an investigator is studying whether adolescents who use social media excessively (say, more than 5 hours a day) are twice as likely as less frequent users to develop depression. If she believes that 6% of less frequent users of social media become depressed ($P_0 = 0.06$), she would specify that 12% of excessive users would become depressed ($P_1 = 0.12$).

For a case-control study, the situation is more complex. Rather than using the risk ratio—which cannot be calculated directly in a case-control study (see Appendix 9B)—it is necessary to use the **odds ratio (OR)**, which is defined in terms of P_0 (the proportion of controls with the exposure) and P_1 (the proportion of cases with the exposure):

$$OR = \frac{P_1 \times (1 - P_0)}{P_0 \times (1 - P_1)}$$

To estimate the sample size, the investigator would specify the odds ratio (OR) and P_0; then P_1 is

$$P_1 = \frac{OR \times P_0}{(1 - P_0) + (OR \times P_0)}$$

For example, in the case-control study of social media use and depression, if the investigator expects that 15% of controls (those who are not depressed) will use social media excessively ($P_0 = 0.15$) and wishes to detect an odds ratio (OR) of 2 associated with excessive use, then

$$P_1 = \frac{2 \times 0.15}{(1 - 0.15) + (2 \times 0.15)} = \frac{0.3}{1.15} = 0.26$$

Estimating P_0 and P_1 from the Overall Risk

Although most investigators can specify the risk ratio that they want to detect in a cross-sectional or cohort study, the risks of the outcome in those with the predictor (P_1) and those without the predictor (P_0) may not be clear. However, when an investigator can determine the overall risk of an outcome in the intended sample (P), it's straightforward to estimate P_1 and P_0 for a given risk ratio (RR).

If the two groups that will be compared (ie, those with and those without the predictor) are of equal size, the formulas for determining P_0 and P_1 are simple:

$$P_0 = \frac{2 \times P}{RR + 1} \text{ and } P_1 = RR \times P_0$$

For example, suppose you are doing a prospective cohort study to determine whether a predictor (say, levels of sun exposure at or below the median) leads to a 1.5-fold increase in the risk of hip fracture among older women (thus RR = 1.5). You anticipate that about 1% of the women in your study will have a hip fracture during follow-up; thus $P = 0.01$. Then $P_0 = (2 \times 0.01) \div (1.5 + 1) = 0.008$, and $P_1 = 1.5 \times 0.008 = 0.012$. As a quick check, P should equal the average of P_0 and P_1 when the groups sizes are equal.

More commonly, the groups being compared will be unequal in size, so the formulas must include the proportion of the sample in the unexposed group, called q_0:

$$P_0 = \frac{P}{(RR + q_0 \times (1 - RR))} \text{ and } P_1 = RR \times P_0$$

For example, suppose the predictor (eg, having the lowest decile of sun exposure) occurs in 10% of the sample; thus, the proportion in the unexposed group, q_0, is 0.90. Then $P_0 = 0.01 \div [1.5 + (0.90 \times -0.5)] = 0.00952$ and $P_1 = 1.5 \times 0.00952 = 0.0143$. In this situation, P should equal the *weighted* average of P_0 and P_1.

The Correlation Coefficient

Although the **correlation coefficient** (r) is not used frequently in sample size calculations for clinical research, it can be used when the predictor and outcome variables are both continuous. The correlation coefficient, which measures the strength of the linear association between the two variables, varies between -1 and $+1$. The closer the absolute value of r is to 1, the stronger the association; the closer to 0, the weaker the association. Height and weight in adults, for example, are highly correlated in some populations, with $r \approx 0.9$. Such high values, however, are uncommon; many biologic associations have much smaller correlation coefficients. (Negative values of r indicate that as one variable increases, the other decreases, as, for example, blood lead level and IQ in children.)

Correlation coefficients are common in some fields of clinical research, such as behavioral medicine, but using them to estimate the sample size has a disadvantage: Correlation coefficients have little intuitive meaning. When squared (r^2), a correlation coefficient represents the proportion of the spread (**variance**) in an outcome variable that results from its linear association with a predictor variable, and vice versa. Although small values of r, such as those ≤ 0.3, may be statistically significant if a sample is large enough, they may not be very meaningful clinically or scientifically, since they "explain" at most 9% (0.3^2) of the variance.

An alternative—and often preferred—way to estimate the sample size for a study in which the predictor and outcome variables are both continuous is to dichotomize one of the two variables (say, at its median) and use the t test calculations instead. This has the advantage of expressing the effect size as a difference between two groups.

If you do choose to estimate sample size for a study using a correlation coefficient (Example 6.3), you must

1. State the null hypothesis, and decide whether the alternative hypothesis is one- or two-sided.
2. Estimate the effect size as the absolute value of the correlation coefficient (r) that the investigator would like to be able to detect. (Variability is a function of r and is already included in the table.)
3. Set alpha and beta.

In Appendix 6C, look down the leftmost column of Table 6C for the effect size (r). Next, read across the table to the chosen values for alpha and beta, yielding the *total* sample size required. Table 6C yields the appropriate sample size when the investigator wishes to reject the null hypothesis that there is no association between the predictor and the outcome variables (eg, $r = 0$). If the investigator wishes to determine whether the correlation coefficient in the study differs from a value other than zero (eg, $r = 0.4$), she should use the calculator at www.sample-size.net.

Example 6.3 Estimating Sample Size When Using the Correlation Coefficient in a Cross-Sectional Study

Problem: The research question is whether urinary cotinine levels (a measure of the intensity of current cigarette smoking) are correlated with bone density in smokers. A previous study found a modest correlation ($r = -0.3$) between reported smoking (in cigarettes per day) and bone density (in g/cm^3); the investigator anticipates that urinary cotinine levels will be at least as well correlated. How many smokers will need to be enrolled, at alpha (two-sided) = 0.05 and beta = 0.10?

Solution: The ingredients for the sample size calculation are as follows:

Null hypothesis: There is no correlation between urinary cotinine level and bone density in smokers.

Alternative hypothesis: There is a correlation between urinary cotinine level and bone density in smokers.

Effect size (r) = absolute value of $r = |-0.3| = 0.3$.

Alpha (two-sided) = 0.05; beta = 0.1.

Using Table 6C, reading across from $r = 0.30$ in the leftmost column and down from alpha (two-sided) = 0.05 and beta = 0.10, **113 smokers will be required.**

■ OTHER CONSIDERATIONS AND SPECIAL ISSUES

Dropouts

Each sampling unit must be available for analysis; participants who are enrolled in a study but in whom outcome status cannot be ascertained (such as **dropouts**) do not count in the sample size. If the investigator anticipates that any of her participants will not be available for follow-up (as often happens), she should estimate the proportion that will be lost and increase the size of the *enrolled* sample accordingly. If, for example, the investigator estimates that 20% of her sample will be lost to follow-up, then the sample size should be increased by a factor of $(1 \div [1 - 0.20])$ or 1.25.

Categorical and Count Variables

Recall that categorical variables can be either ordinal (in which the different categories have a logical order, such as no, mild, moderate, or severe pain) or nominal (in which there is no order, like blood type). Although there are mathematical reasons why estimating a sample size for an ordinal variable using a t test may not be appropriate, in practice an ordinal variable can be treated as a continuous variable if the number of categories is relatively large (six or more), the observations are well spread across the categories, and averaging the values of the variable makes sense.

In other situations, the best strategy is to change the research hypothesis slightly by dichotomizing the categorical variable. As an example, suppose a researcher is studying whether proficiency in speaking English (assessed as little-to-none, some, capable, fluent, and native) is associated with wait time in an emergency department. In this situation, the investigator could estimate the sample size as if the predictor were dichotomous (eg, some proficiency or less versus capable or more).

Similar considerations apply for **count variables**. Although there are formal techniques for estimating sample size (2), if a count variable is well distributed over six or more values, then the t test can be used to approximate the sample size; if not, the values can be dichotomized at or near the median, and the sample size can be estimated with a chi-squared test.

Survival Analysis

When an investigator wishes to compare two groups in terms of how long they live or stay free of an adverse event (such as cancer recurrence), **survival analysis** is an appropriate technique for analyzing the data (3, 4). Although the outcome variable, say months until recurrence in women with advanced breast cancer, *appears* to be continuous, the t test is not appropriate (because the outcome will be missing in those who are alive at the end of the study without a recurrence). Similarly, an investigator might want to compare the *rate* of developing an outcome (say, per 100 person-years of follow-up) in two groups. In both situations, a reasonable approximation of the required sample size can be made by estimating the proportions of participants expected to have the outcome in the two groups within a certain time period and using the chi-squared test to estimate the sample size.

However, if the outcome—say, mortality in a study of advanced pancreas cancer—is expected to occur in most of the participants, a better strategy (because it minimizes the total sample size) is to estimate the sample size on the basis of the proportions of those in each group who are expected to have the outcome when about *half* of the total outcomes have occurred. For example, in a study comparing disease-free survival in patients with advanced pancreas cancer treated with standard versus experimental treatment, in which about 60% of the participants in the standard treatment group are expected to have died by 2 years, compared with 40% of those who received an experimental treatment, the sample size can be estimated using survival at two years as the dichotomous outcome.

A tool like www.sample-size.net can be used to obtain a more refined estimate of the sample size when survival analysis is planned.

Clustered Samples

Some research designs involve the use of **clustered samples**, in which participants are sampled in groups (Chapter 12). Consider, for example, a study of whether a continuing medical education intervention for clinicians improves the rate of smoking cessation among their patients. Suppose that 20 physician practices are randomly assigned to the group that receives the intervention and 20 practices are assigned to a control group. One year later, the investigators plan to review the charts of a random sample of 50 patients who had been smokers at baseline in each practice to determine how many have quit smoking. Does the sample size equal 40 (the number of practices) or 2000 (the number of patients)? The answer, which lies somewhere in between those two extremes, depends on how similar the patients within each practice are (in terms of their likelihood of smoking cessation) compared with the similarity among all the patients. Estimating this quantity often requires doing a small study, unless another investigator has previously done so. There are several techniques for estimating the required sample size for a study using clustered samples (5-7), but they are challenging and usually require the assistance of a statistician.

Matching

For a variety of reasons, an investigator may choose to use a matched design (Chapter 10). The techniques in this chapter, which ignore any matching, nevertheless provide reasonable estimates of the required sample size unless the exposure (in a matched case-control study) or outcome (in a matched cohort study) is strongly correlated with the matching variable. More precise estimates, which require the investigator to specify the correlation between exposures or outcomes in matched pairs, can be made using standard approaches (8) or statistical software.

Multivariable Adjustment and Other Special Statistical Analyses

When designing an observational study, an investigator may decide that one or more variables will confound the association between the predictor and the outcome (Chapter 10) and plan to use statistical techniques to adjust for these **confounders** when she analyzes her results. When this **adjustment** is included in testing the primary hypothesis, the estimated sample size needs to take this into account.

Analytic approaches that adjust for confounding variables often increase the required sample size (9, 10). The magnitude of this increase depends on several factors, including the prevalence of the confounder, the strength of the association between the predictor and the confounder, and the strength of the association between the confounder and the outcome. These effects are complex, and no general rule covers all situations.

Statisticians have developed **multivariable adjustment** methods, such as linear and **logistic regression**, that allow the investigator to adjust for confounding variables. One widely used statistical technique, **Cox proportional hazards** analysis, can also adjust for differences in length of follow-up to estimate a **hazard ratio** as the measure of association. If one of these techniques is going to be used to analyze the data, there are corresponding approaches for estimating the required sample size (3, 11-14). Sample size techniques are also available for other designs, such as studies of potential genetic risk factors or candidate genes (15-17), economic studies (18-20), dose-response studies (21), or studies that involve more than two groups (22). Again, the Internet is a useful resource for these more sophisticated approaches.

It is usually easier, at least for novice investigators, to begin by estimating the sample size assuming a simpler method of analysis, such as the chi-squared test or the *t* test. It's also a good way to check the results obtained when using more sophisticated methods. Suppose, for example, an investigator is planning a case-control study of whether birth weight (a continuous variable) is associated with the occurrence of pediatric brain tumors (a time-to-event variable). Even if the eventual plan is to analyze the data with Cox proportional hazards analysis, a ball-park sample size can be estimated with the *t* test. It turns out that the simplified approaches usually produce sample size estimates that are similar to those generated by more sophisticated techniques. An experienced biostatistician should be consulted, however, if a grant proposal that involves substantial costs is being submitted for funding: Reviewers will expect you to use a sophisticated approach even if they realize that the sample size estimates are based on guesses about the risk of the outcome, the effect size, and so on. Having your sample size estimated by a statistician also conveys the message that you have access to the collaborators who will be needed to manage and analyze the study's data. Indeed, a biostatistician will contribute in many other ways to the design and execution of the study. But she will surely appreciate working with a clinical investigator who has thought about the issues, gathered information on the necessary parameters, and has made an initial attempt to estimate the sample size.

Equivalence and Noninferiority Trials

Sometimes, the goal of a study is to *rule out* a substantial association between the predictor and the outcome variables. An **equivalence trial** tests whether a new drug has pretty much the same efficacy as an established drug. This situation poses a challenge when planning sample size, because the desired effect size is zero or very small. A **noninferiority trial** is a one-sided version of this design that examines whether the new drug is at least not substantially worse than the established drug (Chapter 12).

Sample size calculations for these designs are complex (23-26), and the advice of an experienced statistician will be helpful. A *rough estimate* of the sample size can be made by specifying substantial power (say, 0.90 or 0.95) to reject the null hypothesis when the effect size is small enough that it would not be clinically important (eg, a difference of 5 mg/dL in mean fasting glucose levels). One problem with equivalence and noninferiority trials, however, is that the additional power and the small effect size often require a very large sample size; of the two designs, noninferiority trials have the advantage of being one-sided, permitting either a smaller sample size or a smaller alpha.

Another problem with these designs involves the loss of the usual safeguards that are inherent in the paradigm of the null hypothesis, which protects a conventional study that compares an active drug with a placebo against type I errors (falsely rejecting the null hypothesis). The paradigm ensures that many problems in the design or execution of a study, such as imprecise measurements or excessive loss to follow-up, make it *harder* to reject the null hypothesis. Investigators in a conventional study, who are trying to reject a null hypothesis, have a strong incentive to do the best possible study. For a noninferiority study, however, in which the goal is to find no difference, those safeguards do not apply: Studies that are poorly designed and executed tend to blur any distinctions between the groups being compared, making it easier to miss a difference that might exist.

■ SAMPLE SIZE TECHNIQUES FOR DESCRIPTIVE STUDIES

Estimating the sample size for descriptive studies, including studies of diagnostic tests, is also based on somewhat different principles. Such studies do not rely on tests of statistical significance. Therefore, the concepts of power and the null and alternative hypotheses do not apply. Instead, the investigator estimates descriptive statistics, such as means and proportions; the size of the study then determines the precision of these estimates. Often, however, descriptive studies (What is the prevalence of depression among elderly patients in a medical clinic?) are also used to ask analytic questions (What are the predictors of depression among these patients?). In this situation, sample size should be estimated for the analytic study as well to avoid the common problem of having inadequate power for what turns out to be the research question of greater interest.

Estimates from descriptive studies are commonly reported with their **confidence intervals**, a range of values about the sample mean or proportion. A confidence interval is a measure of the precision of a sample estimate. The investigator sets the confidence level, such as 95% or 99%. An interval with a greater confidence level (say, 99%) is wider, and therefore more likely to include the true population value, than an interval with a lower confidence level (say, 90%).

The width of a confidence interval depends on the sample size. For example, an investigator might wish to estimate the mean score on the U.S. Medical Licensing Examination in a group of medical students who were taught using an alternative web-based curriculum. From a sample of 50 students, she might estimate that the mean score in the population of all students is 215, with a 95% confidence interval from 205 to 225. A smaller study, say with 20 students, might estimate a similar mean score, but its estimate would almost certainly be less precise and thus have a wider 95% confidence interval.

When estimating sample size for descriptive studies, the investigator specifies the desired level and width of the confidence interval. The sample size can then be determined from Appendix 6D or 6E, or with an online calculator.

Continuous Variables

When the variable of interest is continuous, a confidence interval around the mean value of that variable is often reported. To estimate the sample size for that confidence interval (Example 6.4), the investigator must

1. Estimate the standard deviation of the variable of interest.
2. Specify the desired precision (total width) of the confidence interval.
3. Select the confidence level for the interval (eg, 95%, 99%).

To use Appendix 6D, standardize the total width of the interval (divide it by the standard deviation of the variable), then look down the leftmost column of Table 6D for the expected standardized width. Next, read across the table to the chosen confidence level for the required sample size.

Example 6.4 Estimating Sample Size for a Descriptive Study of a Continuous Variable

Problem: The investigator seeks to determine the mean reading grade level among third graders in an urban area, with a 95% confidence interval of ±0.25 grades. A previous study found that the standard deviation of reading grades in a similar city was 1.4 grades.
    Solution: The ingredients for the sample size calculation are as follows:
    Standard deviation of variable (SD) = 1.4 grades.
    Total width of interval = 0.5 grades (0.25 grades above and 0.25 grades below the mean). The standardized width of interval = total width ÷ SD = 0.5 ÷ 1.4 = 0.35.
    Confidence level = 95%.
    Reading across from a standardized width of 0.35 in the leftmost column of Table 6D and down from the 95% confidence level, **the required sample size is 126 third graders.**

Dichotomous Variables

In a descriptive study of a dichotomous variable, results can be expressed as a confidence interval around the estimated proportion of participants with one of the values. This includes studies of the **sensitivity** or **specificity** of a diagnostic test, which may appear at first glance to be continuous variables but are actually proportions (Chapter 13). To estimate the sample size for that confidence interval, the investigator must

1. Estimate the expected proportion with the variable of interest in the population. (If more than half of the population is expected to have the characteristic, then plan the sample size on the basis of the proportion expected *not* to have the characteristic.)
2. Specify the desired precision (total width) of the confidence interval.
3. Select the confidence level for the interval (eg, 95%).

In Appendix 6E, look down the leftmost column of Table 6E for the expected proportion with the variable of interest. Next, read across the table to the chosen width and confidence level, yielding the required sample size.
    Example 6.5 provides a sample size calculation for studying the sensitivity of a diagnostic test, which yields the required number of participants with the disease. (When studying the specificity of the test, the investigator must estimate the required number of participants who do *not* have the disease.) Several of the other parameters—such as **receiver operating characteristic (ROC) curves**, **likelihood ratios**, and reliability—that are discussed in Chapter 13 have specific techniques for estimating sample size (27-29).

Example 6.5 Estimating Sample Size for a Descriptive Study of a Dichotomous Variable

Problem: The investigator wishes to determine the sensitivity of a new diagnostic test for thyroid cancer. Based on a pilot study, she expects that 80% of patients with thyroid cancer will have positive tests. How many such patients will be required to estimate a 95% confidence interval for the test's sensitivity of 0.80 ± 0.05?

Solution: The ingredients for the sample size calculation are as follows:

Expected proportion = 0.20. (Because 0.80 is more than 0.5, sample size is estimated from the proportion expected to have a falsely negative result, ie, 0.20.)

Total width = 0.10 (0.05 below and 0.05 above the expected proportion).

Confidence level = 95%.

Reading across from 0.20 in the leftmost column of Table 6E and down from a total width of 0.10, the middle number (representing a 95% confidence level) yields **the required sample size of 246 patients with thyroid cancer.**

■ WHAT TO DO WHEN SAMPLE SIZE IS FIXED

Study planning involves making difficult choices, often provoked by the realization that an initial sample size estimate is unattainable, unaffordable, or both. For many investigators, the next step is to estimate the effect size that corresponds to a realistic sample size and decide whether it's worth pursuing the study. **Experienced investigators often start at this step.**

In other situations, such as when doing a secondary data analysis, the sample size may have been determined before you design your study. Even when you are designing a study from scratch, it's common to find that the number of participants who are available or affordable for study is limited. Indeed, **investigators often "work backward" from a fixed or realistic sample size** to determine the effect size that they will have a reasonable power to detect. That's part of the reason why it's silly to treat a sample size estimate as if it were carved into stone.

When an investigator must work backward from a preset (or maximum affordable) sample size (Example 6.6), she estimates the effect size that can be detected at a given power (usually 80%). Less commonly, she estimates the power to detect a given effect. The investigator can use the sample size tables in the chapter appendices, interpolating when necessary, or use statistical software and sample size calculators such as www.sample-size.net that can estimate the detectable effect size from a fixed sample size.

Example 6.6 Estimating the Detectable Effect Size When Sample Size Is Fixed

Problem: An investigator is studying whether a 6-week meditation program for new mothers of twins reduces stress (on a 0 to 30 scale), as compared with a control group that receives a pamphlet describing relaxation. She estimates that she will have access to 200 new mothers of twins during her fellowship; based on a small pilot study, she estimates that about half of those mothers (ie, 100) might be willing to participate in and complete the study. If the **standard deviation of the stress score** is expected to be 5 points in both the control and the treatment groups, what size difference will the investigator be able to detect between the two groups, at **alpha (two-sided)** = 0.05 and **beta** = 0.20?

Solution: In Table 6A, reading down from alpha (two-sided) = 0.05 and beta = 0.20 (the rightmost column in the middle triad of numbers), 45 participants per group are required to detect a **standardized effect size** of 0.6, which is equal to 3 points (0.6 × 5 points). The investigator (who will have about 50 participants per group) will be able to **detect a difference slightly smaller than 3 points between the two groups.**

A general rule is that a study should have a power of 80% or greater to detect a reasonable effect size. There is nothing magical about 80%: Sometimes, an investigator gets lucky and finds a statistically significant result even when she had limited power to do so. After all, even a power of 50% provides a 50-50 chance of observing a statistically significant effect in the sample when one is actually present in the population. Thus, it may be worthwhile to pursue studies that have less than 80% power if the cost of doing so is small, such as when analyzing data that have already been collected. And there are some studies—for example, one showing that a novel treatment for long-standing refractory pulmonary hypertension reduces pulmonary arterial pressures by more than 50%—in which a sample size of two or three participants would suffice to indicate that further study (on safety and effects on clinical outcomes) is warranted.

The investigator should keep in mind, however, that she might face the difficulty of interpreting (and publishing) a study that *fails* to find an association because of insufficient power: The wide confidence intervals will reveal the possibility of a substantial effect size. It's also important to recognize that an underpowered study that had a statistically significant result may be criticized because reviewers and editors are skeptical as to whether the investigator really intended to look for that particular association or whether she tested scores of hypotheses and cherry-picked the one result that had a significant *P* value.

■ STRATEGIES FOR MINIMIZING SAMPLE SIZE AND MAXIMIZING POWER

When the estimated sample size is greater than the number of participants that can be studied realistically, the investigator should proceed through several steps. First, the calculations should be checked, because it is easy to make mistakes. Next, the ingredients should be reviewed. Is the effect size unreasonably small or the variability unreasonably large? Is alpha or beta too small? Is the confidence level too high or the desired width of the interval too narrow?

These technical adjustments can be useful, but it is important to realize that statistical tests ultimately depend on the information contained in the data. Many changes in the ingredients, such as reducing power from 90% to 80%, do not improve the quantity or quality of the data that will be collected. There are, however, several strategies for reducing the required sample size—or for increasing power for a given sample size—that increase the information content of the collected data. Many of these strategies involve modifications of the research hypothesis, so the investigator should consider whether the new hypothesis still answers the research question that she wishes to study.

Use Continuous Variables

When continuous variables are an option, they usually permit smaller sample sizes than dichotomous variables. Blood pressure, for example, can be expressed either as millimeters of mercury (continuous) or as the presence or absence of hypertension (dichotomous). The former permits a smaller sample size for a given power or a greater power for a given sample size.

Example 6.7 Use of Continuous Versus Dichotomous Variables

Problem: Consider a controlled trial to determine the effect of a new activity program (versus usual care) on patient satisfaction among elderly nursing home residents. Previous studies found that patient satisfaction (on a 0 to 100 scale) is approximately normally distributed, with a mean of 65 and a standard deviation of 10, and that about 10% of residents have poor or very poor satisfaction (defined as a score of 49 or less). The new activity program is thought to be worthwhile if it can increase mean satisfaction by 5 points after 3 months. This change in the mean value corresponds to a reduction in the proportion whose satisfaction is poor or very poor to about 5%.

One design might treat satisfaction as a dichotomous variable (poor or very poor versus fair or better). Another might use all the information contained in the measurement and treat satisfaction as a continuous variable. How many participants would each design require at alpha (two-sided) = 0.05 and beta = 0.20?

Solution: The ingredients for the sample size calculation using a *dichotomous outcome variable* (poor or very poor versus fair or better) are as follows:

Null hypothesis: The proportion of elderly nursing home residents whose satisfaction is poor or very poor after 3 months of an activity program is the same as the proportion whose satisfaction is poor or very poor after 3 months of usual care.

Alternative hypothesis: The proportion of elderly nursing home residents whose satisfaction is poor or very poor after 3 months of an activity program differs from the proportion whose satisfaction is poor or very poor at the same time among those receiving usual care.

P_0 (proportion poor or very poor in usual care) = 0.10; P_1 (in activity group) = 0.05. Effect size = 0.05 (= 0.10 − 0.05).

Alpha (two-sided) = 0.05; beta = 0.20.

Using Table 6B.1, reading across from 0.05 in the leftmost column and down from an expected difference of 0.05, the middle number (for alpha [two-sided] = 0.05 and beta = 0.20), this design would require 473 participants per group.

The ingredients for the sample size calculation using a *continuous outcome variable* (satisfaction on a 0 to 100 scale) are as follows:

Null hypothesis: Mean satisfaction in elderly nursing home residents after 3 months of an activity program is the same as mean satisfaction after 3 months of usual care.

Alternative hypothesis: Mean satisfaction in elderly nursing home residents after 3 months of an activity program differs from the mean satisfaction after 3 months of usual care.

Mean satisfaction after 3 months of usual care = 65; mean satisfaction after 3 months of an activity program = 70; effect size = 5 (= 70 − 65).

Standard deviation of satisfaction score = 10

Standardized effect size = effect size ÷ standard deviation = 5 ÷ 10 = 0.5.

Alpha (two-sided) 0.05; beta = 0.20.

Using Table 6A, reading across from a standardized effect size of 0.50, with alpha (two-sided) = 0.05 and beta = 0.20, this design would require about 64 participants in each group. (In this example, the shortcut sample size estimate from p. 68 of 16 ÷ (standardized effect size)^2, or 16 ÷ $(0.5)^2$, gives the same estimate of 64 participants per group.) The bottom line is that the use of a continuous outcome variable will require a substantially smaller sample size, albeit one that answers a different research question.

Use Paired Measurements

In some experiments or cohort studies with a continuous outcome variable, **paired measurements** can be made in each participant—one at baseline, the other at the conclusion of the study. The outcome variable is then the *change* between this pair of measurements. In this situation, a *t* test on the paired measurements can be used to compare the mean value of this change in the two groups. This technique often permits a smaller sample size, because comparing each participant with herself removes the baseline between-participant part of the variability of the outcome variable. However, when the pair of measurements are not at least moderately correlated, those benefits are outweighed by the added variability from using two measurements instead of one. The breakeven point is a correlation of 0.5, as can be seen from the following mathematical formula:

$$SD_{paired} = SD_{single} \sqrt{2 \times (1 - correlation_{baseline, follow-up})}$$

For example, if the standard deviation of a single weight measurement (SD_{single}) is 13 kg and the correlation between the measurements made at baseline and follow-up is 0.8, then the standard deviation of the paired measurement (SD_{paired}) is 8.2 kg.

$$8.2 = 13\sqrt{2 \times (1 - 0.8)}$$

Sample size for this type of t test is estimated in the usual way (Example 6.8), except that the standardized effect size (E/S in Table 6A) is the anticipated mean difference in the *change* in the variable divided by the standard deviation *of those changes*.

Although using paired measurements makes sense in terms of sample size and efficiency, it can be hard to find information about the standard deviation of the change score (or the correlation between baseline and follow-up measurements, so that the standard deviation can be calculated). See the section on "How to Estimate Sample Size When There is Insufficient Information" (p. 82) for some suggestions.

Example 6.8 Use of the *t* Test with Paired Measurements

Problem: Recall Example 6.1, in which the investigator studying the treatment of asthma was interested in determining whether FEV_1 will be 200 mL higher after adding ipratropium bromide compared with albuterol alone. Sample size calculations indicated that 100 participants per group were needed, more than are likely to be available. Fortunately, a colleague points out that asthmatic patients have great differences in their FEV_1 values even *before* treatment. These between-patient differences account for much of the variability in FEV_1 after treatment, therefore obscuring the effect of treatment. She suggests using a (two-sample) paired t test to compare the *changes* in FEV_1 in the two groups. Data available from electronic health records finds that the standard deviation of the change in FEV_1 after starting a new bronchodilator therapy is about 250 mL. How many participants would be required per group, at alpha (two-sided) = 0.05 and beta = 0.20, if we use the same effect size (0.2 L = 200 mL) as in Example 6.1?

Solution: The ingredients for the sample size calculation are as follows:

Null hypothesis: The change in mean FEV_1 after 2 weeks of treatment is the same in asthmatic patients treated with albuterol alone as in those treated with albuterol plus ipratropium.

Alternative hypothesis: The change in mean FEV_1 after 2 weeks of treatment differs in asthmatic patients treated with albuterol alone from that in those treated with albuterol plus ipratropium.

Effect size = 200 mL.
Standard deviation of the outcome variable = 250 mL.
Standardized effect size = effect size ÷ standard deviation = 200 mL ÷ 250 mL = 0.8.
Alpha (two-sided) = 0.05; beta = 1 − 0.80 = 0.20.

Using Table 6A, this design would require only about 26 participants per group, a much smaller sample size than the 100 per group in Example 6.1.

A Brief Technical Note

This chapter always refers to two-sample t tests, which are used when comparing the mean values of continuous variables in two groups of participants. A two-sample t test can be unpaired if the variable itself is being compared between two groups (Example 6.1) or paired if the variable is the change in a pair of measurements (Example 6.8).

A third type of t test, the one-sample paired t test, compares whether the mean change in a pair of measurements within a single group differs from zero change. This type of analysis is common in time-series designs (Chapter 12), a before-after approach to examining treatments that are difficult to randomize, such as studying the effect of elective hysterectomy—a decision few women are willing to leave to a coin toss—on quality of life measured on a 0 to 10 scale. (That said, the absence of a comparison group makes it difficult to know what would have happened had the participants been left untreated.) When planning a study that will be analyzed with a one-sample paired t test, the total sample size is half of the sample size *per group* listed in Appendix 6A. For example, at alpha = 0.05 (two-sided) and beta = 0.2, detecting a 0.5 standard deviation difference ($E/S = 0.5$) would require 64/2 = 32 participants. Appendix 6F presents additional information on the use and misuse of one- and two-sample t tests.

Use More Precise Variables

Because they reduce variability, more precise variables permit smaller sample sizes. Even a modest change in precision can have a substantial effect on sample size. For example, when using the t test to estimate sample size, a 20% decrease in the standard deviation of the outcome variable results in a 36% decrease in the sample size. Techniques for increasing the precision of a variable, such as making measurements in duplicate, are presented in Chapter 4.

Use Unequal Group Sizes

Because an equal number of participants in each of two groups usually gives the greatest power for a given total number of participants, Tables 6A, 6B.1, and 6B.2 in the appendices assume equal sample sizes in the two groups. Often, however, the distribution of participants is not equal in the two groups, or it is easier or less expensive to recruit participants for one group than the other. It may also turn out, for example, that an investigator wants to estimate sample size for a cohort study comparing the 20% who smoke cigarettes with the 80% who do not. Or, in a case-control study, the number of persons with the disease may be small, but it may be possible to sample a much larger number of controls. In general, the gain in power when the size of one group is increased to twice the size of the other is considerable; tripling and quadrupling one of the groups provide progressively smaller gains. Sample sizes for unequal groups can be computed using sample size calculators in statistical software or on the web.

There is a useful approximation (30) for estimating sample size for case-control studies of dichotomous risk factors and outcomes that use c controls per case (Example 6.9). If n represents the number of cases that would have been required for one control per case (at a given alpha, beta, and effect size), then the approximate number of cases (n') that will be required with cn' controls is

$$n' = \frac{c+1}{2c} \times n$$

For example, if $c = 2$ controls per case, then $[(2 + 1) \div (2 \times 2)] \times n = 3/4 \times n$, and only 75% as many cases are needed. As c gets larger, n' approaches 50% of n (when $c = 10$, for example, $n' = 11/20 \times n$).

Example 6.9 Use of Multiple Controls Per Case in a Case-Control Study

Problem: An investigator is studying whether exposure to household insecticide is a risk factor for aplastic anemia. The original sample size calculation indicated that 25 cases would be required, using one control per case. Suppose that the investigator has access to only 18 cases. How should the investigator proceed?

Solution: The investigator should consider using multiple controls per case (after all, she can find many patients who do not have aplastic anemia). **By using three controls per case,** for example, the *approximate* number of cases that will be required is $[(3 + 1) \div (2 \times 3)] \times 25 = 17$.

Use a More Common Outcome

When planning a study of a dichotomous outcome, the more frequently that outcome occurs (up to when about 50% of people have the outcome), the greater the power. So changing the definition of an outcome is one of the best ways to increase power: If an outcome occurs more often, there is more of a chance to detect its predictors. Indeed, **power depends more on the number of those who have the outcome than on the total number in the study.** Studies with rare outcomes, like breast cancer in healthy women, require very large sample sizes to have adequate power.

One of the best ways to have an outcome occur more frequently is to enroll participants at greater risk for developing that outcome (such as women with a family history of breast cancer). Others are to extend the follow-up period, so that there is more time to accumulate outcomes, or to loosen the definition of what constitutes an outcome (eg, by including ductal carcinoma in situ). All these techniques (Example 6.10), however, may change the research question, so they should be used with caution.

Example 6.10 Use of a More Common Outcome

Problem: Suppose an investigator is comparing the efficacy of an antiseptic gargle versus a placebo gargle in preventing upper respiratory infections. Her initial calculations indicated that her anticipated sample of 200 volunteer college students was inadequate, in part because she expected that only about 20% of her participants would have an upper respiratory infection during the 3-month follow-up period. Suggest a few changes in the study plan.

Solution: Here are a few possible solutions: (a) **study a sample of pediatric interns and residents,** who are likely to experience a greater incidence of upper respiratory infections than college students; or (b) **do the study in the winter,** when these infections are more common; or (c) **follow the sample for a longer period,** say 6 or 12 months; or (d) intentionally expose the participants to rhinovirus (with their knowledge and agreement, of course!). All of these solutions involve modification of the research hypothesis, but they seem to reasonably maintain relevance to the overall research question about the efficacy of antiseptic gargle.

■ HOW TO ESTIMATE SAMPLE SIZE WHEN THERE IS INSUFFICIENT INFORMATION

Often, the investigator finds that she is missing one or more of the ingredients for the sample size calculation and becomes frustrated in her attempts to plan the study. This is an especially frequent problem when the investigator is using an instrument of her own design (such as a new questionnaire comparing quality of life in women with stress versus urge incontinence). How should she go about deciding what fraction of a standard deviation of the scores on her instrument would be clinically significant?

The first strategy is an extensive search for previous and related findings on the topic and on similar research questions. Roughly comparable situations and mediocre or dated findings may be good enough. For example, are there data on quality of life among patients with other urologic problems or even with a somewhat related condition, like having a colostomy? If the literature review is unproductive, she should contact other investigators about their judgment on what to expect and whether they are aware of any unpublished results that may be relevant.

Another alternative is to recognize that for continuous variables that have a roughly bell-shaped distribution, the standard deviation can be estimated as one-quarter of the difference between the high and low ends of the range of values that occur commonly, ignoring extreme values. For example, if most people have a serum sodium level between 135 and 143 mEq/L (an 8 mEq/L range), the standard deviation of serum sodium would be about 2 mEq/L ($1/4 \times 8$ mEq/L).

If there is still no information available, she may consider doing a **pilot study** or obtaining a data set for a secondary analysis to obtain the missing ingredient(s) before embarking on the main study. Indeed, a pilot study is recommended for almost all studies that involve new instruments, measurement methods, or recruitment strategies. It saves time in the long run by enabling an investigator to do a better job planning and implementing the main study: being familiar with a key measurement is always a good thing.

When a variable is categorical, or the mean and standard deviation of a continuous variable remain in doubt, it's always possible to dichotomize that variable. Categories can be lumped into two groups, and continuous variables can be split at their mean, median, or a clinically mean-ingful cutoff point. For example, dividing quality of life into "better than the median" or "the median or less" avoids having to estimate its standard deviation in the sample—although one still has to estimate what proportions of participants would be above the overall median in each of the two groups being studied. The chi-squared test can then be used to make a reasonable, albeit somewhat high, estimate of the sample size.

Sometimes, however, the investigator must choose the detectable effect size based on a value that she considers to be *clinically meaningful.* In that situation, the investigator should vet her choice with colleagues in the field. For example, suppose that an investigator is studying a new invasive treatment for severe refractory gastroparesis, a condition in which at most 5% of patients improve spontaneously. If the treatment is shown to be effective, her gastroenterologist colleagues indicate that they would be willing to treat up to five patients to produce a sustained benefit in just one of them. (Because the treatment is expensive and has substantial side effects, they don't think that number would be more than five.) A **number needed to treat** (NNT) of 5 corresponds to an absolute **risk difference** of 20% (NNT = 1/risk difference), so the investigator should estimate the sample size on the basis of a comparison of $P_0 = 5\%$ versus $P_1 = 25\%$ (ie, 59 participants per group at a power of 0.80 and a two-sided alpha of 0.05).

If all this fails, the investigator should just make an *educated guess* about the likely values of the missing ingredients, estimating the required sample (or effect) size under several different assumptions. The process of thinking through the problem and imagining the findings will often result in a reasonable estimate, and that is what sample size planning is about. This is a better option than just deciding, in the absence of any rationale, to design a study to have 80% power at a two-sided alpha of 0.05 to detect a standardized effect size of, say, 0.5 between the two groups (n = 64, per group, by the way). Very few grant reviewers will accept that sort of arbitrary decision.

■ COMMON ERRORS TO AVOID

Many inexperienced investigators (and some experienced ones!) make mistakes when planning sample size. A few of the more common ones follow:

1. A frequent error is estimating the sample size late during the design of the study. Do it early in the process, when fundamental changes can still be made.
2. When planning a clinical trial or cohort study, don't assume that the outcome will occur as frequently in the study as it does in the target population: participants in studies tend to be healthier than average. For example, in the Study of Osteoporotic Fractures, we estimated that the risk of hip fracture among participants would be only two-thirds of that seen in the population—a prediction that turned out to be close to true.
3. Dichotomous variables can appear to be continuous when they are expressed as a percentage or rate. For example, vital status (alive or dead) might be misinterpreted as a continuous variable when expressed as percent alive. Similarly, in a cohort study, a dichotomous outcome can appear to be continuous (eg, stroke rate per 100 person-years). For all of these, the outcome itself is

actually dichotomous (yes/no, true/false, etc.) and an appropriate simple approach in planning sample size would be the chi-squared test.

4. The sample size estimates the number of participants with outcome data, not the number who need to be enrolled. The investigator should always plan for dropouts and participants with missing data.

5. The tables at the end of the chapter assume that the two groups being studied have equal sample sizes. If the group sizes are not equal, as is often true, then the calculators on the web (eg, www.sample-size.net) or in statistical software packages should be used.

6. When using the t test to estimate the sample size, the standard deviation of the outcome variable is a key factor. Therefore, if the outcome is the change in a continuous variable, the investigator should use the standard deviation of that change rather than the standard deviation of a one-time measurement.

7. Be aware of clustered data. If there appear to be two "levels" of sample size (eg, one for physicians and another for patients), clustering is a likely problem, and the tables in the appendices do not apply.

8. If you find yourself having difficulty estimating a sample size for your study, be sure that your research hypothesis meets the criteria discussed in Chapter 5 (simple, specific, and stated in advance).

9. Remember that there is nothing magical (never mind biblical) about using an alpha of 0.05—it's just a widely accepted convention.

■ SUMMARY

1. When estimating **sample size for an analytic study**, the following steps need to be taken:
   a. **state the null and alternative hypotheses**, specifying the number of sides;
   b. select a **statistical test** that could be used to analyze the data, based on the types of predictor and outcome variables (the chi-squared test if both are dichotomous, the t test if one is dichotomous and one continuous, and the correlation coefficient if both are continuous);
   c. estimate the **effect size** (and the **variability** of the measurements, if necessary); and
   d. specify appropriate values for **alpha** and **beta**, based on the importance of avoiding type I and type II errors.

2. Other considerations in calculating sample size for analytic studies include adjusting for **potential dropouts**; strategies for dealing with **categorical variables**, **survival analysis**, **clustered samples**, **multivariate adjustment**; and special statistical approaches to **equivalence** and **noninferiority trials**.

3. The steps for estimating sample size for descriptive studies, which do not have hypotheses, are to (a) **estimate the proportion** of participants with a dichotomous outcome **or the standard deviation** of a continuous outcome; (b) specify the **desired precision** (width of the confidence interval); and (c) specify the **confidence level** (eg, 95%).

4. When sample size is predetermined, the investigator can **work backward** to estimate the detectable effect size or, less commonly, the study's power.

5. **Strategies to minimize sample size** include using continuous variables, more precise measurements, paired measurements, and more common outcomes, as well as increasing the number of controls per case in case-control studies.

6. When there seems to be not enough information to estimate the sample size, the investigator should **review the literature** in related areas and **consult with colleagues** to help choose an effect size that is clinically meaningful.

7. **Errors** to avoid include **estimating sample size too late**, **misinterpreting proportions** expressed as percentages, not taking **missing participants and data** into account, and not addressing **clustered or paired data** appropriately.

REFERENCES

1. Lehr R. Sixteen S-squared over D-squared: a relation for crude sample size estimates. *Stat Med*. 1992;11:1099-1102.
2. Li H, Wang L, Wei L, Quan H. Sample size calculation for count data in comparative clinical trials with nonuniform patient accrual and early dropout. *J Biopharm Stat*. 2015;25(1):1-15.
3. Barthel FM, Babiker A, Royston P, Parmar MK. Evaluation of sample size and power for multi-arm survival trials allowing for non-uniform accrual, non-proportional hazards, loss to follow-up and cross-over. *Stat Med*. 2006;25(15):2521-2542.
4. Ahnn S, Anderson SJ. Sample size determination in complex clinical trials comparing more than two groups for survival endpoints. *Stat Med*. 1998;17(21):2525-2534.
5. Kerry SM, Bland JM. Trials which randomize practices II: sample size. *Fam Pract*. 1998;15:84-87.
6. Hemming K, Girling AJ, Sitch AJ, et al. Sample size calculations for cluster randomised controlled trials with a fixed number of clusters. *BMC Med Res Methodol*. 2011;11:102.
7. Jahn-Eimermacher A, Ingel K, Schneider A. Sample size in cluster-randomized trials with time to event as the primary endpoint. *Stat Med*. 2013;32(5):739-751.
8. Edwardes MD. Sample size requirements for case–control study designs. *BMC Med Res Methodol*. 2001;1:11.
9. Drescher K, Timm J, Jöckel KH. The design of case–control studies: the effect of confounding on sample size requirements. *Stat Med*. 1990;9:765-776.
10. Lui KJ. Sample size determination for case–control studies: the influence of the joint distribution of exposure and confounder. *Stat Med*. 1990;9:1485-1493.
11. Latouche A, Porcher R, Chevret S. Sample size formula for proportional hazards modelling of competing risks. *Stat Med*. 2004;23(21):3263-3274.
12. Novikov I, Fund N, Freedman LS. A modified approach to estimating sample size for simple logistic regression with one continuous covariate. *Stat Med*. 2010;29(1):97-107.
13. Vaeth M, Skovlund E. A simple approach to power and sample size calculations in logistic regression and Cox regression models. *Stat Med*. 2004;23(11):1781-1792.
14. Dupont WD, Plummer WD Jr. Power and sample size calculations for studies involving linear regression. *Control Clin Trials*. 1998;19:589-601.
15. Murcray CE, Lewinger JP, Conti DV, et al. Sample size requirements to detect gene-environment interactions in genome-wide association studies. *Genet Epidemiol*. 2011;35(3):201-210.
16. Wang S, Zhao H. Sample size needed to detect gene-gene interactions using linkage analysis. *Ann Hum Genet*. 2007;71(Pt 6):828-842.
17. Witte JS. Rare genetic variants and treatment response: sample size and analysis issues. *Stat Med*. 2012;31(25):3041-3050.
18. Willan AR. Sample size determination for cost-effectiveness trials. *Pharmacoeconomics*. 2011;29(11):933-949.
19. Glick HA. Sample size and power for cost-effectiveness analysis (Part 2): the effect of maximum willingness to pay. *Pharmacoeconomics*. 2011;29(4):287-296.
20. Glick HA. Sample size and power for cost-effectiveness analysis (Part 1). *Pharmacoeconomics*. 2011;29(3):189-198.
21. Patel HI. Sample size for a dose-response study. *J Biopharm Stat*. 1992;2:l-8.
22. Day SJ, Graham DF. Sample size estimation for comparing two or more treatment groups in clinical trials. *Stat Med*. 1991;10:33-43.
23. Guo JH, Chen HJ, Luh WM. Sample size planning with the cost constraint for testing superiority and equivalence of two independent groups. *Br J Math Stat Psychol*. 2011;64(3):439-461.
24. Zhang P. A simple formula for sample size calculation in equivalence studies. *J Biopharm Stat*. 2003;13(3):529-538.
25. Stucke K, Kieser M. A general approach for sample size calculation for the three-arm 'gold standard' non-inferiority design. *Stat Med*. 2012;31(28):3579-3596.
26. Julious SA, Owen RJ. A comparison of methods for sample size estimation for non-inferiority studies with binary outcomes. *Stat Methods Med Res*. 2011;20(6):595-612.
27. Obuchowski NA. Sample size tables for receiver operating characteristic studies. *AJR Am J Roentgenol*. 2000;175(3):603-608.
28. Simel DL, Samsa GP, Matchar DB. Likelihood ratios with confidence: sample size estimation for diagnostic test studies. *J Clin Epidemiol*. 1991;44:763-770.
29. Sim J, Wright CC. The kappa statistic in reliability studies: use, interpretation, and sample size requirements. *Phys Ther*. 2005;85(3):257-268.
30. Jewell NP. *Statistics for Epidemiology*. Chapman and Hall; 2004:68.

APPENDIX 6A
Sample Size Required per Equal-Sized Group When Using the *t* Test to Compare Means of Continuous Variables

TABLE 6A SAMPLE SIZE *PER GROUP* FOR COMPARING TWO MEANS

ONE-SIDED $\alpha =$		0.005			0.025			0.05		
TWO-SIDED $\alpha =$		0.01			0.05			0.10		
E/S^a $\beta =$	0.05	0.10	0.20	0.05	0.10	0.20	0.05	0.10	0.20
0.10	3565	2978	2338	2600	2103	1571	2166	1714	1238
0.15	1586	1325	1040	1157	935	699	963	762	551
0.20	893	746	586	651	527	394	542	429	310
0.25	572	478	376	417	338	253	347	275	199
0.30	398	333	262	290	235	176	242	191	139
0.40	225	188	148	164	133	100	136	108	78
0.50	145	121	96	105	86	64	88	70	51
0.60	101	85	67	74	60	45	61	49	36
0.70	75	63	50	55	44	34	45	36	26
0.80	58	49	39	42	34	26	35	28	21
0.90	46	39	32	34	27	21	28	22	16
1.00	38	32	26	27	23	17	23	18	14

[a]E/S is the standardized effect size, computed as E (expected effect size, i.e., the difference between the group means) divided by S (SD of the outcome variable). To estimate the sample size, read across from the *standardized effect size* and down from the specified values of alpha (α) and beta (β) for the required sample size in each group. For a one-sample *t* test, the *total* sample size is one-half of the number listed.

■ CALCULATING VARIABILITY

Variability is usually reported as either the standard deviation or the **standard error of the mean** (SEM). For the purposes of sample size calculation, the standard deviation of the variable is most useful. Fortunately, it is easy to convert from one measure to another: The standard deviation is simply the standard error times the square root of N, where N is the number of participants whose values were averaged. Suppose a study reported that the weight loss in 25 persons on a low-fiber diet was 10 ± 2 kg (mean ± SEM). The standard deviation would be $2 \text{ kg} \times \sqrt{25} = 10$ kg.

■ APPROACH FOR OTHER VALUES

For values of E/S that do not appear in this table, or when the groups being compared are not of equal size, please use the calculator at www.sample-size.net.

APPENDIX 6B
Sample Size Required per Equal-Sized Group When Using the Chi-Squared Statistic or Z Test to Compare Proportions of Dichotomous Variables

TABLE 6B.1 SAMPLE SIZE *PER GROUP* FOR COMPARING TWO PROPORTIONS

UPPER NUMBER: $\alpha = 0.05$ (ONE-SIDED) OR $\alpha = 0.10$ (TWO-SIDED); $\beta = 0.20$

MIDDLE NUMBER: $\alpha = 0.025$ (ONE-SIDED) OR $\alpha = 0.05$ (TWO-SIDED); $\beta = 0.20$

LOWER NUMBER: $\alpha = 0.025$ (ONE-SIDED) OR $\alpha = 0.05$ (TWO-SIDED); $\beta = 0.10$

SMALLER OF P_0 AND P_1[a]	ABSOLUTE DIFFERENCE BETWEEN P_1 and P_0									
	0.05	0.10	0.15	0.20	0.25	0.30	0.35	0.40	0.45	0.50
0.05	381	129	72	47	35	27	22	18	15	13
	473	159	88	59	43	33	26	22	18	16
	620	207	113	75	54	41	33	27	23	19
0.10	578	175	91	58	41	31	24	20	16	14
	724	219	112	72	51	37	29	24	20	17
	958	286	146	92	65	48	37	30	25	21
0.15	751	217	108	67	46	34	26	21	17	15
	944	270	133	82	57	41	32	26	21	18
	1252	354	174	106	73	53	42	33	26	22
0.20	900	251	121	74	50	36	28	22	18	15
	1133	313	151	91	62	44	34	27	22	18
	1504	412	197	118	80	57	44	34	27	23
0.25	1024	278	132	79	53	38	29	23	18	15
	1289	348	165	98	66	47	35	28	22	18
	1714	459	216	127	85	60	46	35	28	23
0.30	1123	300	141	83	55	39	29	23	18	15
	1415	376	175	103	68	48	36	28	22	18
	1883	496	230	134	88	62	47	36	28	23
0.35	1197	315	146	85	56	39	29	23	18	15
	1509	395	182	106	69	48	36	28	22	18
	2009	522	239	138	90	62	47	35	27	22
0.40	1246	325	149	86	56	39	29	22	17	14
	1572	407	186	107	69	48	35	27	21	17
	2093	538	244	139	90	62	46	34	26	21

(continued)

TABLE 6B.1 SAMPLE SIZE *PER GROUP* FOR COMPARING TWO PROPORTIONS (*continued*)

0.45	1271	328	149	85	55	38	28	21	16	13
	1603	411	186	106	68	47	34	26	20	16
	2135	543	244	138	88	60	44	33	25	19
0.50	1271	325	146	83	53	36	26	20	15	—
	1603	407	182	103	66	44	32	24	18	—
	2135	538	239	134	85	57	42	30	23	—
0.55	1246	315	141	79	50	34	24	18	—	—
	1572	395	175	98	62	41	29	22	—	—
	2093	522	230	127	80	53	37	27	—	—
0.60	1197	300	132	74	46	31	22	—	—	—
	1509	376	165	91	57	37	26	—	—	—
	2009	496	216	118	73	48	33	—	—	—
0.65	1123	278	121	67	41	27	—	—	—	—
	1415	348	151	82	51	33	—	—	—	—
	1883	459	197	106	65	41	—	—	—	—
0.70	1024	251	108	58	35	—	—	—	—	—
	1289	313	133	72	43	—	—	—	—	—
	1714	412	174	92	54	—	—	—	—	—
0.75	900	217	91	47	—	—	—	—	—	—
	1133	270	112	59	—	—	—	—	—	—
	1504	354	146	75	—	—	—	—	—	—
0.80	751	175	72	—	—	—	—	—	—	—
	944	219	88	—	—	—	—	—	—	—
	1252	286	113	—	—	—	—	—	—	—
0.85	578	129	—	—	—	—	—	—	—	—
	724	159	—	—	—	—	—	—	—	—
	958	207	—	—	—	—	—	—	—	—
0.90	381	—	—	—	—	—	—	—	—	—
	473	—	—	—	—	—	—	—	—	—
	620	—	—	—	—	—	—	—	—	—

The one-sided estimates use the Z statistic.

[a]P_0 represents the proportion of participants expected to have the outcome in one group, P_1 in the other group. (In a case-control study, P_1 represents the proportion of cases with the predictor variable, P_0 the proportion of controls with the predictor variable.) To estimate the sample size, read across from the smaller of P_0 and P_1 and down from the absolute value of the expected difference between P_1 and P_0. The three numbers represent the sample size required in each group for the specified values of alpha (α) and beta (β).

Additional detail for P_0 and P_1 between 0.01 and 0.10 is provided in Table 6B.2.

■ APPROACH FOR OTHER VALUES

For values of P_0 and P_1 that do not appear in this table or in Table 6B.2, or when the groups being compared are not of equal size, please use the calculator at www.sample-size.net.

TABLE 6B.2 SAMPLE SIZE *PER GROUP* FOR COMPARING TWO PROPORTIONS, THE SMALLER OF WHICH IS BETWEEN 0.01 AND 0.10

UPPER NUMBER: $\alpha = 0.05$ (ONE-SIDED) OR $\alpha = 0.10$ (TWO-SIDED); $\beta = 0.20$

MIDDLE NUMBER: $\alpha = 0.025$ (ONE-SIDED) OR $\alpha = 0.05$ (TWO-SIDED); $\beta = 0.20$

LOWER NUMBER: $\alpha = 0.025$ (ONE-SIDED) OR $\alpha = 0.05$ (TWO-SIDED); $\beta = 0.10$

SMALLER OF P_0 AND P_1	ABSOLUTE DIFFERENCE BETWEEN P_1 and P_0									
	0.01	0.02	0.03	0.04	0.05	0.06	0.07	0.08	0.09	0.10
0.01	2019	700	396	271	204	162	134	114	98	87
	2512	864	487	332	249	197	163	138	120	106
	3300	1125	631	428	320	254	209	178	154	135
0.02	3205	994	526	343	249	193	157	131	113	97
	4018	1237	651	423	306	238	192	161	137	120
	5320	1625	852	550	397	307	248	207	177	154
0.03	4367	1283	653	414	294	224	179	148	126	109
	5493	1602	813	512	363	276	220	182	154	133
	7296	2114	1067	671	474	359	286	236	199	172
0.04	5505	1564	777	482	337	254	201	165	139	119
	6935	1959	969	600	419	314	248	203	170	146
	9230	2593	1277	788	548	410	323	264	221	189
0.05	6616	1838	898	549	380	283	222	181	151	129
	8347	2308	1123	686	473	351	275	223	186	159
	11,123	3061	1482	902	620	460	360	291	242	206
0.06	7703	2107	1016	615	422	312	243	197	163	139
	9726	2650	1272	769	526	388	301	243	202	171
	12,973	3518	1684	1014	691	508	395	318	263	223
0.07	8765	2369	1131	680	463	340	263	212	175	148
	11,076	2983	1419	850	577	423	327	263	217	183
	14,780	3965	1880	1123	760	555	429	343	283	239
0.08	9803	2627	1244	743	502	367	282	227	187	158
	12,393	3308	1562	930	627	457	352	282	232	195
	16,546	4401	2072	1229	827	602	463	369	303	255
0.09	10,816	2877	1354	804	541	393	302	241	198	167
	13,679	3626	1702	1007	676	491	377	300	246	207
	18,270	4827	2259	1333	893	647	495	393	322	270
0.10	11,804	3121	1461	863	578	419	320	255	209	175
	14,933	3936	1838	1083	724	523	401	318	260	218
	19,952	5242	2441	1434	957	690	527	417	341	285

The one-sided estimates use the Z statistic.

■ APPROACH FOR OTHER VALUES

For values of P_0 and P_1 that do not appear in this table or in Table 6B.1, or when the groups being compared are not of equal size, please use the calculator at www.sample-size.net.

APPENDIX 6C
Total Sample Size Required When Using the Correlation Coefficient (*r*)

TABLE 6C SAMPLE SIZE FOR DETERMINING WHETHER A CORRELATION COEFFICIENT DIFFERS FROM ZERO

ONE-SIDED $\alpha =$	0.005			0.025			0.05		
TWO-SIDED $\alpha =$	0.01			0.05			0.1		
$\beta =$	0.05	0.10	0.20	0.05	0.10	0.20	0.05	0.10	0.20
r^{a}									
0.05	7118	5947	4663	5193	4200	3134	4325	3424	2469
0.10	1773	1481	1162	1294	1047	782	1078	854	616
0.15	783	655	514	572	463	346	477	378	273
0.20	436	365	287	319	259	194	266	211	153
0.25	276	231	182	202	164	123	169	134	98
0.30	189	158	125	139	113	85	116	92	67
0.35	136	114	90	100	82	62	84	67	49
0.40	102	86	68	75	62	47	63	51	37
0.45	79	66	53	58	48	36	49	39	29
0.50	62	52	42	46	38	29	39	31	23
0.60	40	34	27	30	25	19	26	21	16
0.70	27	23	19	20	17	13	17	14	11
0.80	18	15	13	14	12	9	12	10	8

[a]To estimate the total sample size, read across from *r* (the expected correlation coefficient) and down from the specified values of alpha (α) and beta (β).

■ APPROACH FOR OTHER VALUES

For values of *r* that do not appear in this table, please use the calculator at www.sample-size.net.

APPENDIX 6D
Sample Size for a Descriptive Study of a Continuous Variable

TABLE 6D SAMPLE SIZE FOR COMMON VALUES OF *W/S*[a]

W/S	CONFIDENCE LEVEL		
	90%	95%	99%
0.10	1083	1537	2665
0.15	482	683	1180
0.20	271	385	664
0.25	174	246	425
0.30	121	171	295
0.35	89	126	217
0.40	68	97	166
0.50	44	62	107
0.60	31	43	74
0.70	23	32	55
0.80	17	25	42
0.90	14	19	33
1.00	11	16	27

[a]*W/S* is the standardized width of the confidence interval, computed as *W* (desired total width) divided by *S* (standard deviation of the variable). To estimate the total sample size, read across from the *standardized width* and down from the specified confidence level.

■ APPROACH FOR OTHER VALUES

For values of *W/S* that do not appear in this table, please use the calculator at www.sample-size.net.

APPENDIX 6E
Sample Size for a Descriptive Study of a Dichotomous Variable

TABLE 6E SAMPLE SIZE FOR PROPORTIONS

UPPER NUMBER: 90% CONFIDENCE LEVEL

MIDDLE NUMBER: 95% CONFIDENCE LEVEL

LOWER NUMBER: 99% CONFIDENCE LEVEL

EXPECTED PROPORTION (P)[a]	TOTAL WIDTH OF CONFIDENCE INTERVAL (W)						
	0.10	0.15	0.20	0.25	0.30	0.35	0.40
0.10	98	44	—	—	—	—	—
	138	61	—	—	—	—	—
	239	106	—	—	—	—	—
0.15	139	62	35	22	—	—	—
	196	87	49	31	—	—	—
	339	151	85	54	—	—	—
0.20	174	77	44	28	19	14	—
	246	109	61	39	27	20	—
	426	189	107	68	47	35	—
0.25	204	91	51	33	23	17	13
	288	128	72	46	32	24	18
	499	222	125	80	55	41	31
0.30	229	102	57	37	25	19	14
	323	143	81	52	36	26	20
	559	249	140	89	62	46	35
0.40	261	116	65	42	29	21	16
	369	164	92	59	41	30	23
	639	284	160	102	71	52	40
0.50	272	121	68	44	30	22	17
	384	171	96	61	43	31	24
	666	296	166	107	74	54	42

[a]To estimate the sample size, read across the *expected proportion* (P) who have the variable of interest and down from the desired *total width* (W) of the confidence interval. The three numbers represent the sample size required for 90%, 95%, and 99% confidence levels.

■ APPROACH FOR OTHER VALUES

For values of P that do not appear in this table, please use the calculator at www.sample-size.net.

APPENDIX 6F
Use and Misuse of *t* Tests

Two-sample *t* tests, a primary focus of this chapter, are used when comparing the mean values of a variable in two groups. The two groups can be defined by a dichotomous predictor variable—say, active drug versus placebo in a randomized trial, or presence versus absence of a risk factor in a cohort study—or they can be defined by a dichotomous outcome variable, as in a case-control study. A two-sample *t* test can be *unpaired*, if measurements obtained on a single occasion are being compared between two groups, or *paired*, if the change in measurements made at two points in time in each participant (say, before and after an intervention) are being compared between the groups. A third type of *t* test, the one-sample paired *t* test, compares the mean change in measurements made at two points in time within participants in a single group to zero (or some other specified change).

Table 6F illustrates the misuse of one-sample paired *t* tests in a study designed for a **between-group** comparison—a randomized blinded trial of the effect of a new sleeping pill on quality of life (measured on a 0 to 10 scale). In situations like this, some investigators have performed (and published!) findings with two separate one-sample *t* tests—one each in the treatment and placebo groups—which is inappropriate.

In the table, the *P* values designated with a dagger (†) are from one-sample paired *t* tests. The first *P* (0.05) shows a significant change in quality of life in the treatment group during the study; the second *P* value (0.16) shows no significant change in the control group. However, this analysis does not permit inferences about differences *between* the groups, and it would be wrong to conclude that there was a significant effect of the treatment.

The *P* values designated with a (*) represent the *appropriate* two-sample *t* test results. The first two *P* values (0.87 and 0.64) are two-sample unpaired *t* tests that show no statistically significant between-group differences in the initial or final measurements for quality of life. The last *P* value (0.17) is a two-sample paired *t* test; it is closer to 0.05 than the *P* value for the end of study values (0.64) because the paired mean differences have smaller standard deviations. However, the mean quality of life improvement of 1.3 points in the treatment group was not significantly different from the mean improvement of 0.9 points in the placebo group. Thus, the correct conclusion is that the study did not find the treatment to be effective.

TABLE 6F CORRECT (AND INCORRECT) WAYS TO ANALYZE PAIRED DATA

	QUALITY OF LIFE, AS MEAN ± SD		
TIME OF MEASUREMENT	TREATMENT (*N* = 100)	CONTROL (*N* = 100)	*P* VALUE
Baseline	7.0 ± 4.5	7.1 ± 4.4	0.87*
End of study	8.3 ± 4.7	8.0 ± 4.6	0.64*
Difference (end – baseline)	1.3 ± 2.1	0.9 ± 2.0	0.17*
P value	0.05†	0.16†	

*Comparing treatment with control.

†Comparing difference with zero.

APPENDIX 6G
Exercises for Chapter 6. Estimating Sample Size and Power: Applications and Examples

1. Review exercise 1 of Chapter 5. Determine how many cases of stomach cancer would be required for the study. What if the investigator wanted a power of 0.90? Or a level of statistical significance of 0.01? Extra credit: Suppose the investigator had access to only 60 cases. What could she do?

2. Muscle strength declines with advancing age. Preliminary evidence suggests that part of this loss of muscle strength might be due to progressive deficiency of dehydroepiandrosterone (DHEA). Investigators plan a randomized trial to administer DHEA or an identical placebo for 6 months to elderly participants and then measure muscle strength. Previous studies have reported a mean grip strength in elderly persons of 20 kg with a standard deviation of 8 kg. Assuming alpha (two-sided) = 0.05 and beta = 0.10, how many participants would be required to demonstrate a 10% or greater difference between strength in the treated and placebo groups? How many participants would be needed if beta = 0.20?

3. In exercise 2, sample size calculations indicated more participants were needed than can be enrolled. A colleague points out that elderly people have great differences in grip strength. This accounts for much of the variability in the strength measured after treatment and might be obscuring the treatment effect. She suggests that you measure strength at baseline and again after treatment, using the change in strength as the outcome variable. A small pilot study shows that the standard deviation of the change in strength during a 6-month period is only 2 kg. How many participants would be required to detect the same effect size (2 kg), per group, using this design, assuming alpha (two-sided) = 0.05 and beta = 0.10?

4. An investigator suspects that left-handedness is more common in dyslexic than in non-dyslexic third graders. Previous studies indicated that about 10% of people are left-handed and that dyslexia is uncommon. A case-control study is planned that will select all the dyslexic students in a school district as cases, with an equal number of nondyslexic students randomly selected as controls. What sample size would be required to show that the odds ratio for dyslexia is 2.0 among left-handed students compared with right-handed students? Assume alpha (two-sided) = 0.05 and beta = 0.20.

5. An investigator seeks to determine the mean IQ of medical students in her institution, with a 99% CI of ±3 points. A small pilot study suggests that IQ scores among medical students range from about 110 to 150. Approximately what sample size is needed?

CHAPTER 7

Addressing Ethical Issues

Bernard Lo and Deborah G. Grady

Research with human participants raises ethical concerns because people accept inconvenience and risks to advance scientific knowledge to benefit others. The public, who participate in and help fund clinical research, needs to trust that research follows high ethical standards.

In this chapter, we begin with the history of research oversight and then review ethical principles and federal regulations guiding research with human participants, especially requirements for **institutional review board** (IRB) approval and **informed consent**. We finally turn to issues of **scientific misconduct**, authorship, and **conflicts of interest**, as well as ethical concerns in specific types of research.

■ HISTORY OF REGULATIONS ON CLINICAL RESEARCH

Current regulations and guidelines for clinical research have developed in response to abuses, including "research" by Nazi physicians during World War II, research in the United States on prisoners, residents of long-term care facilities and other vulnerable populations, and the Tuskegee study (Case 7.1).

Case 7.1 The Tuskegee Study

The U.S. Department of Health and Human Services started the Tuskegee study in 1932 to determine the long-term effects of untreated syphilis (1). The men enrolled in the study were impoverished, poorly educated Black men in rural Alabama who received meals, some basic medical care, and burial insurance. Researchers falsely told the men that they were receiving treatment for syphilis, for example misrepresenting lumbar punctures done for research purposes as "special free treatments." When antibiotics for syphilis became available during World War II and were later recommended as a public health measure, researchers took steps to keep those enrolled in the study from receiving treatment. The results of the study were published widely, and it took persistent efforts from whistleblowers to end it. In 1974, in response to the Tuskegee study, the federal government issued regulations on human subjects research, which required informed consent from participants and review by IRBs. In 1997, President Bill Clinton apologized formally for the Tuskegee study.

■ ETHICAL PRINCIPLES

Four ethical principles, which had been violated in the Tuskegee study and others, were articulated to guide research with human participants (2). First, the principle of **respect for persons** recognizes that everyone has the right to make her own decisions about research participation, including providing informed consent and being free to discontinue participation at any time. Persons who do not have decision-making capacity, such as children and adults with advanced dementia, may participate in research if a surrogate gives permission and the participant does not object.

Second, the principle of **beneficence** requires that the scientific knowledge to be gained from the study must outweigh the inconvenience and risk experienced by research participants and that risks be minimized. Risks include both physical harm from research interventions and also psychosocial harm, such as breaches of confidentiality, stigma, and discrimination. The risks of participating in a study can be reduced, for example, by screening potential participants to exclude those likely to suffer harm, monitoring participants for adverse effects, making sure that study staff are trained and certified, and ensuring confidentiality. Beneficence can be difficult to assess, especially because risks apply only to the small group of study participants, whereas the potential benefits apply to a much larger number of patients with a specific disease or even to society in general. Phase 1 drug trials are good examples of this tension. In these trials, new drugs are often tested in a small group of healthy persons to determine whether the drugs cause harms such as liver, kidney, or blood abnormalities. In this situation, participants may contribute to identifying an effective treatment but may suffer risks with no possibility of benefit.

Third, the principle of **justice** requires that the benefits and burdens of research be distributed fairly. Disadvantaged and vulnerable populations, such as people with low income, limited education, poor access to health care, or impaired decision-making capacity, should not be chosen as participants if other populations would also be suitable to address the research questions. Studying vulnerable groups primarily because of easy access, cooperation, and follow-up takes unfair advantage of them.

Justice also requires equitable access to the potential benefits of research. Because clinical research may provide access to new therapies, participation should be available regardless of income, insurance, or education. Children, women, and members of ethnic minorities have been underrepresented in clinical research, resulting in a weak evidence base and potentially suboptimal care for these groups. National Institutes of Health (NIH)–funded clinical researchers must have adequate representation of children, women, and members of ethnic minorities in studies, unless there are good reasons why these groups might be underrepresented.

Finally, the Tuskegee study violated the principle of **truth-telling** because the investigators lied to the participants about the real purpose of the study and withheld information about the treatment of syphilis even after penicillin was known to be effective. Truth-telling does not mean merely avoiding outright lies: It also requires that investigators provide relevant information, explain potential risks, and be honest about any possible benefits or risks of participation.

■ FEDERAL REGULATIONS FOR RESEARCH ON HUMAN SUBJECTS

Federal regulations apply to all federally funded research as well as to research that will be submitted to the U.S. Food and Drug Administration (FDA) in support of a new drug or device application (3). In addition, most universities require that research on human participants conducted by affiliated faculty and staff comply with core regulations regarding informed consent and IRB review, including research funded privately or conducted off-site. Although the federal regulations refer to human "subjects," the term "participants" is preferred, because it recognizes that people can be involved in a research study, rather than just being subjects to be experimented on or used as sources of data.

Several definitions in these federal regulations are important to understand:

- **Research** is "systematic investigation designed to develop or contribute to generalizable knowledge." Unproven clinical care that is directed toward benefiting an individual patient—not toward publication—is not considered research. Some clinical quality improvement projects might be treated as research, although most meet criteria for exemption, which we discuss later.
- **Human subjects** are living individuals about whom an investigator obtains either "data through interaction with the individual" or "identifiable private information."

- **Private information** comprises information that a person can reasonably expect is not being observed or recorded and will not be made public (eg, a medical record).
- **Information is identifiable** if "the identity of the subject is or may be readily ascertained by the investigator."
- **Coded research data are not identifiable** if the key that links data collected previously to participants is destroyed before the analysis begins or if the investigators cannot access it.

Institutional Review Board Approval

Federal regulations require that research with human participants be approved by an IRB, sometimes called an independent ethics committee, ethical review board, or research ethics board. An IRB reviews proposals to ensure that the research is ethical and that the welfare and rights of research participants are protected. The IRB has the authority to approve, disapprove, or require modifications of research proposals. IRBs are overseen by the Office for Human Research Protections within the Department of Health and Human Services. Most institutions require IRB oversight of all human participant research, even if it is not federally funded. Although most IRB members are researchers, IRBs must also include community members and persons knowledgeable about legal and ethical issues concerning research.

When approving a research study, the IRB must determine that (3):

- Risks to participants are minimized.
- Risks are reasonable in relation to anticipated benefits and the importance of the knowledge that is expected to result.
- Selection of participants is equitable.
- Informed consent will be obtained from participants or their legally authorized representatives.
- Confidentiality is adequately maintained.

Most universities, medical centers, and hospitals have their own IRBs that implement federal regulations using their own forms, procedures, and guidelines; there is no appeal to a higher body. Many universities also have established relationships with commercial IRBs, which are nonacademic, independent companies that provide IRB services.

For multi-institutional research projects, federal regulations require sites in the United States to rely on approval by a single IRB (sometimes called the "IRB of record" or "central IRB"). This requirement aims to avoid duplicative reviews that can cause delays in cooperative research. Site IRBs need to communicate local information to the central IRB, such as relevant state laws and regulations and institutional policies regarding conflicts of interest and consent form language.

IRBs and federal regulations have been criticized for placing undue emphasis on consent forms rather than the consent process and for failing to adequately scrutinize the design and scientific merit of the research study (4, 5). Although IRBs need to review protocol revisions and monitor adverse events, they typically do not check to determine whether the study itself is carried out in accordance with the approved protocol. Many IRBs lack the resources and expertise to fulfill their mission of protecting research participants. For these reasons, federal regulations and IRB approval should be regarded as a minimal ethical standard for research. Ultimately, the judgment and character of the investigator are the most essential elements for assuring that a study is ethically acceptable.

Exceptions to Full IRB Review

Most research using surveys and interviews, as well as secondary analyses of de-identified existing records and specimens may be **exempted from IRB review** (Table 7.1). The ethical justification for such exemptions is that the research involves low risk, almost all people would consent to such research, and obtaining consent from each participant would make such studies prohibitively expensive or difficult. Many IRBs, however, require researchers to submit some information about the project to verify that it qualifies for exemption.

TABLE 7.1 RESEARCH THAT IS EXEMPT FROM FEDERAL RESEARCH REGULATIONS

1. Surveys, interviews, or observations of public behavior unless:
   - Participants can be readily identified, *and*
   - Disclosure of participants' responses could place them at risk of legal liability or damage their reputation, financial standing, or employability. For example, questionnaires on such issues as drug addiction, depression, HIV risk behaviors, or illegal immigration are not exempt.
2. Studies of existing records, data, or specimens, provided that data are:
   - Publicly available (eg, data sets released by state and federal agencies), *or*
   - Recorded by the investigator in such a manner that the identity of participants cannot be readily ascertained, for example, because the investigator cannot obtain the key to the code linking data and participant identities.
3. Research on normal educational practices.

An IRB may also allow certain minimal risk research to undergo **expedited review** by a single IRB member rather than the full committee (Table 7.2). The Office for Human Research Protections website lists the types of research eligible for expedited review (6). The concept of **minimal risk** to participants is important in federal regulations, as indicated in Table 7.2. Minimal risk is defined as risk that is "ordinarily encountered in daily life or during the performance of routine physical or psychological tests." Both the magnitude and probability of risk must be considered by the IRB.

Informed and Voluntary Consent

Investigators must obtain voluntary informed consent from research participants. Informed consent is the process of telling potential research participants about the key elements of a research study, what their participation will involve, the potential risks and benefits of the study and alternatives to participation, and then obtaining their agreement.

Disclosure of Information to Participants

The federal regulations require that the informed consent process include several topics, including:

- **The nature of the research study.** The prospective participant should be told explicitly that research is being conducted, what its purpose is, who is in charge of the research project, and what kind of people are being recruited as participants. The specific study hypothesis need not be stated.

TABLE 7.2 RESEARCH THAT MAY UNDERGO EXPEDITED IRB REVIEW

1. Certain minimal risk research procedures, including:
   - Collection of specimens through venipuncture, saliva or sputum collection, or skin or mucosal swabs.
   - Collection of specimens through noninvasive procedures employed routinely in clinical practice, such as electrocardiograms and magnetic resonance imaging. X-rays, which expose participants to radiation, require full IRB review.
   - Research involving data, records, or specimens collected for clinical purposes.
   - Research using surveys or interviews that is not exempt from IRB review.
2. Minor changes in approved research protocols.
3. Renewal of IRB approval for studies that are complete except for data analysis or accessing follow-up data from procedures that participants would undergo in routine clinical care.

- **The procedures of the study.** Participants need to know what they will be asked to do in the research project. On a practical level, they should be told how much time will be required and how often visits or contacts will be required. Procedures that are not standard clinical care should be identified. If the study involves blinding or randomization, these concepts should be explained in terms the participant can understand. In interview or questionnaire research, participants should be informed of the topics to be addressed.
- **The potential risks and benefits of the study and the alternatives to participating in the study.** Medical, psychosocial, and economic risks and benefits should be described in lay terms. Potential participants also need to be told the alternatives to participation; for example, whether the treatment in a clinical trial is also available outside the study.

Concerns have been voiced that the information provided to participants often understates the risks—and overstates the benefits of the trial—and fails to discuss its aims (7). For example, research on new drugs or procedures is sometimes described as offering benefits to participants. However, most new interventions, despite encouraging preliminary results, show no significant advantages over standard therapy. Many participants substantially overestimate the potential personal benefit of the trial (7), a phenomenon called "therapeutic misconception." Investigators should make clear that it is not known whether the study drug or intervention is more effective than standard therapy and that promising drugs sometimes cause serious harms.

Consent Forms

Written, signed, and witnessed consent forms are generally required to document that the process of informed consent—discussions between an investigator and the participant—has occurred. The consent form needs to contain the required information discussed in the previous section. Alternatively, a short form may be used, which states that the required elements of informed consent have been presented orally. If the short form is used, there must be a witness to the oral presentation, who must also sign it.

IRBs usually have template consent forms that they prefer investigators to use; these forms may require more information than is required by federal regulations.

Participants' Understanding of Disclosed Information

Research participants commonly have serious misunderstandings about the goals of research and the benefits of the study. In discussions and consent forms, researchers should avoid technical jargon and complicated sentences. Investigators should adopt strategies to increase comprehension by participants, including extended discussion with study participants; simpler, shorter, more understandable consent forms, using a question-and-answer format; and checking that participants understand key features of the study (8).

The Voluntary Nature of Consent

Ethically valid consent must be voluntary as well as informed. Researchers must minimize the possibility of coercion or **undue influence**, such as excessive payments to participants and enrolling prisoners or the investigator's students as research participants. Undue influence is problematic if it leads participants to discount the risks of a research project or undermines their ability to decline to participate. Declining to participate in a study must not compromise participants' medical care, and they must be free to withdraw from the project at any time; these assurances must be documented on the consent form.

Exceptions to Informed Consent

Some scientifically important studies would be difficult or impossible to carry out if informed consent were required from each participant.

Research With Leftover De-Identified Specimens and Data

Case 7.2 Research With Neonatal Blood Specimens

Shortly after birth, infants have a heel stick to collect blood onto filter paper to screen for genetic diseases. In most states, parental permission is not required for this mandated screening; hence, the specimens represent the entire population of newborns. Specimens left over after clinical screening have been valuable for research on genetic causes of birth defects and preterm birth, environmental exposures during pregnancy, and gene-environment interactions (9).

Informed consent and IRB review are not required to use de-identified specimens in research (Table 7.1), but many IRBs still require investigators to notify them of such research. When original research is submitted for publication, many journals require authors to declare that an IRB approved the protocol or determined that IRB review was not needed.

Waiver of Informed Consent

Some valuable research projects require identified information and specimens. Such studies do not qualify for exemption from IRB review but may qualify for a waiver of informed consent.

Case 7.2 Research With Neonatal Blood Specimens (*Continued*)

A research team would like to use identified neonatal blood specimens to study the association between maternal environmental exposures to selected chemicals, as determined in neonatal blood samples, and low birth weight, prematurity, and perinatal deaths. Researchers can link identified specimens to birth certificates, death certificates, and hospital records (9). Because of the large number of children who need to be studied to achieve adequate power to detect associations, it would not be feasible to obtain permission from parents or guardians.

Under federal regulations, IRBs may grant waivers of informed consent if all of the conditions in Table 7.3 apply. For example, most IRBs would waive consent for a study of maternal environmental exposures and low birth weight.

TABLE 7.3 RESEARCH THAT MAY RECEIVE A WAIVER OF INFORMED CONSENT

1. The research involves no more than minimal risk to the participants, *and* the waiver or alteration will not adversely affect the rights and welfare of the participants, *and* the research could not practicably be carried out without the waiver.
2. For research involving identifiable information or biospecimens, the research could not practicably be carried out without the use of identifiable information or specimens.
3. Whenever appropriate, the participants will be provided with additional pertinent information after participation. This provision allows some research involving deception, for example, when disclosing the purpose of the research during the consent process would undermine study validity.

Rationale for Exceptions to Informed Consent

Some scientifically important research presents such low risks that consent would be burdensome while doing little to protect research participants. Every patient has benefited from knowledge obtained from research that used existing medical records and specimens. Fairness in the sense of reciprocity suggests that people who receive such benefits should be willing to participate in similar very low-risk research to benefit others.

Objections to Exceptions to Informed Consent

Even though the federal regulations permit de-identified neonatal blood specimens to be used for research without parental permission, there is significant public opposition.

Case 7.2 Research With Neonatal Blood Specimens (*Continued*)

Parents in several states have objected to the storage of neonatal blood specimens for unspecified research without their permission or the opportunity to withdraw from research, bringing lawsuits in two states. The plaintiffs did not contest the collection of blood for neonatal screening but objected that de-identification of the specimens failed to address their concerns about loss of privacy and parental autonomy.

Several states now require consent for research using neonatal specimens collected in state screening programs. Thus, what is legally permitted in federal research regulations might not be permitted in some states, particularly for research regarded as sensitive.

Participants Who Lack Decision-Making Capacity

When participants are not capable of giving informed consent, permission to participate in the study should be obtained from the participant's parent or guardian in the case of young children and the legally authorized representative in the case of adults. Also, the protocol should be subjected to additional scrutiny to ensure that the research question could not be studied among participants who are capable of giving consent.

Minimizing Risks

Researchers need to anticipate and minimize the risks that might occur in research projects, for instance, by identifying and excluding persons who are very susceptible to adverse events, monitoring for adverse events, and substituting less invasive measurements. An important aspect of minimizing risk is maintaining participants' confidentiality.

Confidentiality

Breaches of confidentiality might cause stigma or discrimination, particularly if the research addresses sensitive topics such as sexual attitudes or practices, use of alcohol or drugs, illegal conduct, and psychiatric illness. Breaches of confidentiality might also put study participants at financial risk if personal identifiers are not protected. Strategies for protecting confidentiality include coding research data, protecting or destroying the key that identifies participants, limiting personnel who have access to identifiers, and having strong data security protections.

However, investigators should not make unqualified promises of confidentiality. Confidentiality may be overridden if research records are audited or subpoenaed or if conditions are identified that must be reported legally, such as child abuse, certain infectious diseases, and serious threats of violence. In projects where such reporting can be foreseen, the protocol should specify how field staff should respond, and participants should be informed of these plans.

Certificates of confidentiality provide legal protection to research participants. These certificates prohibit disclosure of individually identifiable data to anyone not associated with the research (including by subpoena or court order), except when the participant consents to disclosure (10). Certificates of confidentiality are issued by federal agencies automatically upon approving or funding a project. When research is not federally funded, researchers may still apply to NIH for a certificate at https://grants.nih.gov/policy/humansubjects/coc/coc-nih-funded.htm.

The HIPAA Health Privacy Rule

The federal Health Privacy Rule (commonly known as HIPAA, after the **Health Insurance Portability and Accountability Act**) protects individually identifiable information collected in the process of routine health care, billing, or administration, which is termed protected health information (PHI). Under the Privacy Rule, individuals must sign an authorization for the use of PHI in a research project (11). This HIPAA authorization form is in addition to the informed consent form required by the IRB. For example, in addition to consent to be in a randomized trial, participants need to sign a separate authorization allowing their data or biologic materials to be placed in a databank for future research. Authorization is not required if data are not identifiable and in certain other situations. Researchers should contact their IRB with questions about the Privacy Rule and how it differs from the Federal Regulations on the Protection of Human Subjects.

Protections for Vulnerable Research Participants

Vulnerable research participants are those who might be at greater risk for being used in ethically inappropriate ways in research. Federal regulations define all children and prisoners as vulnerable. These regulations focus on protecting vulnerable participants by restricting them from risky research. However, such restrictions limit the evidence on the efficacy and safety of interventions in the care of these groups. Furthermore, other persons not mentioned in the regulations may be vulnerable in some research projects. An alternative framework based on the **reason for vulnerability** has many advantages (12). Vulnerable research participants may be unable to protect their own interests because they have difficulty understanding the risks and benefits of research or are subject to undue influence or coercion. Vulnerabilities can often be ameliorated by enhancing the consent process to promote more informed and voluntary decisions about research participation. For example, patient advocates, relatives, or friends can help a participant understand the nature of the research, its risks and benefits, and her right to decline. Identifying different types of vulnerability allows researchers to adopt safeguards tailored to the specific vulnerability and thereby allow participants to enroll in research that strengthens the evidence base for clinical care.

Participants who are ill may be vulnerable in another sense: They are at greater risk for adverse medical events. This vulnerability can be addressed by conducting pilot studies of the intervention, excluding participants at the highest risk, and close monitoring for adverse events throughout the study.

Research with Children

Children are vulnerable in research because they cannot give informed consent for themselves but face risks in research participation. In addition, young children may be more susceptible to certain harms, such as exposures that affect neurodevelopment. Investigators must obtain the permission of the parents *and* the assent of the child if developmentally appropriate. According to Subpart D of the federal regulations, research with children involving more than minimal risk is permissible only if:

- It offers the prospect of direct benefit to the child *or*
- The increase over minimal risk is minor, and the research is likely to yield "generalizable knowledge of vital importance about the child's disorder or condition."

Researchers can minimize vulnerability of children who are capable of forming their own opinion by seeking their assent to research separately from parental permission for research, presenting information about the research that is understandable to them, and being aware of family dynamics and cultural expectations that make it difficult for a child to voice disagreement (13).

Research with Pregnant Women

Interventional research with pregnant women presents benefits and risks to both the woman and her fetus. Pregnant women are not defined as vulnerable research participants *per se*, but Subpart B of the federal regulations, which is aimed at protecting the fetus, may also impact pregnant women. Generally, pregnant women can be involved in research only if the purpose of the research is to address health risks in the mother or fetus *and* risk to the fetus is minimal. If the purpose of the research is to benefit the fetus, consent of both the pregnant woman and the father is required, except when the father is unavailable or incompetent or the pregnancy resulted from rape or incest (3).

Historically, pregnant women have been excluded from most clinical trials. These exclusions have narrowed the evidence base for the clinical care of pregnant women and how medicines affect the fetus. Moreover, the regulations have perpetuated the misconception that pregnant women cannot make informed decisions for themselves and their fetus. Researchers and sponsors should strive to include pregnant women in trials of treatments for serious conditions for which no treatments are known to be safe and effective during pregnancy. Information about possible fetal abnormalities needs to be presented to the IRB.

Research with Prisoners

Prisoners are vulnerable in research because they might not feel free to refuse to participate in research and might be influenced by cash payments, breaks from prison routine, or parole considerations. Subpart C of the federal regulations limits the types of research that are permitted with prisoners using federal funding and requires stricter IRB review, as well as approval by the Department of Health and Human Services. However, many institutions require the same strict IRB review for any research with prisoners. In recent years, to improve the evidence base, advocates have pressed for the inclusion of prisoners in clinical trials for promising new therapies, such as for HIV infection and hepatitis C.

Research on Persons Who Have Difficulty Understanding the Risks and Benefits of Research

There are many common causes of vulnerability that federal regulations do not address, including impaired decision-making capacity, low educational level, and lack of health literacy and numeracy. For example, persons with low literacy or with impaired memory can be protected through consent processes that present information orally and in small segments, check participant comprehension, and include family members or advocates to encourage questions and provide support.

Power Differences

Persons who reside in institutions, such as nursing homes, might feel pressure to participate in research and to defer to persons who control their daily routine. Residents might not understand that they may decline to participate in research without retaliation by authorities or jeopardy to other aspects of their everyday lives.

If the investigator in the research project is also a potential participant's treating physician, that person might hesitate to decline to participate, fearing that the physician would then be less interested in her care. This can be mitigated by having someone other than the treating physician obtain informed consent and ensuring that the physician does not know whether the patient participated. Similarly, students and trainees might feel pressured to enroll in research conducted by their instructors or superiors. To counteract this, IRBs can require that investigators recruit participants who are not their students or trainees and prohibit them from knowing who does not participate.

Social and Economic Disadvantages

Persons with low socioeconomic status or poor access to health care might join a research study to obtain payment or medical care, even if they would regard the risks as unacceptable if they had a higher income. Participants with poor education or low health literacy might fail to comprehend information about the study or be more susceptible to influence by other people.

Case 7.3 Research with Nursing Home Residents in a Low-Income Country

During the COVID-19 pandemic, researchers might have planned a randomized, placebo-controlled trial of a COVID-vaccine that had received emergency use authorization by the United States and other countries but was not available in a low-income country where the researchers had ongoing collaborations. At the time of the study, the safety and efficacy of authorized COVID-vaccines have not been studied in nursing home residents over 75 years of age—a group at very high risk for COVID infection and death. The trial sponsor was the vaccine manufacturer. The findings would have direct benefits for the care of patients such as those in the study.

At the time, vaccine guidelines from the Centers for Disease Control and Prevention (CDC) placed residents of skilled nursing facilities at the highest priority for COVID vaccination. Critics would have argued that it would be unethical to conduct a trial in which an intervention recommended by public health guidelines was withheld from the control group.

Case 7.3 Research with Nursing Home Residents in a Low-Income Country (*Continued*)

The study sponsor and principal investigator might have proposed to carry out the study in a low-income country that had very little access to vaccine during the duration of the study. If the vaccine proved safe and effective, participants in the placebo arm would receive active vaccine, as per CDC recommendations, at the conclusion of the study.

Historically, low-income countries have been the sites of clinical trials of interventions that would not be available there even after they were shown to be effective and safe. Early in the HIV epidemic, placebo-controlled trials of new antivirals were carried out in developing countries. These trials would have been unethical in developed countries, where effective antiretrovirals were available for use in the control group. It is now considered unethical to carry out such trials if patients in the developing country will not have posttrial access to therapies found to be effective (14, 15).

Today, using a placebo control in a trial of a new intervention in low-income countries when there are standard-of-care treatments in well-resourced countries is considered ethical only if there are strong justifications for this study design, if the results of the trial will provide benefit to persons in the host country, and if there are credible (not just aspirational) plans for posttrial access in the host country.

In Case 7.3, participants were vulnerable in several ways that may have limited their ability to give voluntary and informed consent:

- Living in a low-income country, they had little access to the vaccine outside of a trial and may have thus believed that there was no alternative to entering a research study to obtain the benefits of the vaccine (16).
- Nursing home residents with impaired cognition, low education, or low health literacy may be incapable of informed consent.
- Residents in institutional settings such as nursing homes have their autonomy restricted in many ways (such as determining who has access to their room, scheduling of meals and housecleaning, etc.) that may make them more vulnerable to coercion.

The principle of justice requires fair distribution of the burdens and benefits of research. It is unfair, and could be perceived as exploitative, for residents of low-income countries to bear the risks and inconveniences of research that is considered unethical in the researchers' home country.

Researchers and the IRBs overseeing such studies can provide additional protection to these vulnerable participants in the following ways:

- There must be IRB review both in the country where the research is to be carried out and in the country of the study sponsor and investigators. The IRBs should include advocates for persons in nursing homes, and IRB(s) in the United States should also include individuals familiar with the culture of the country and the challenges of carrying out research there.
- The consent process must ensure that disclosed information is understandable to potential participants. This requires translation of documents into the languages of the participants, an assessment of research concepts that are culturally unfamiliar in the host country, vetting of the consent process by patient advocates, and pretesting in the host country to ensure that there is not undue influence due to power dynamics that are not apparent to foreign investigators. The IRB might require consent monitors from trusted community-based organizations in the host country to observe consent discussions.
- It would be preferable ethically to enroll only participants who are able to give informed and voluntary consent for themselves, unless the host country has robust protections for nursing home residents in research.
- Finally, the sponsor and the host country government should agree before the trial to provide fair access to an effective vaccine (if one is found) after the trial. The agreement might include, for example, doses of free vaccine to other nursing home residents in the country, as well as additional doses of vaccine at the manufacturer's cost. In negotiations over posttrial access, the host country government might want to consult with international organizations such as the World Health Organization, global vaccine advocates, global philanthropies, and a community advisory board.

■ RESPONSIBILITIES OF INVESTIGATORS

Scientific Misconduct

The federal Office for Research Integrity defines **research misconduct** as fabrication, falsification, and plagiarism (17).

- **Fabrication** is making up results and recording or reporting them.
- **Falsification** is manipulating research data, materials, equipment, or procedures or changing or omitting data or results so that the research record misrepresents the actual findings.
- **Plagiarism** is appropriating another person's ideas, results, or words without giving appropriate credit.

According to this definition, misconduct must be intentional (in the sense that the investigators were aware that their conduct was wrong) or reckless (aware that what they were doing had a substantial risk but disregarded it). Research misconduct excludes honest error and legitimate scientific differences of opinion. The federal definition does not address other unethical actions, such as publishing the same material more than once (double publication), refusal to share research materials, sloppy research and statistical methodology, and sexual harassment; research institutions should deal with them under other policies. The following case is a recent example of research misconduct that seriously harmed research participants.

Case 7.4 Genome-Based Prediction Model of Response to Cancer Therapy

A young investigator developed several gene-expression-based tests of tumor specimens to predict cancer patients' responses to chemotherapy. These findings were published in high-impact journals, and the tests were used in NIH-sponsored clinical trials. Biostatisticians at another university were unable to reproduce his findings. They identified several serious errors in his publications, including reversal of labels for sensitive and resistant tumors, incorrect gene lists due to data entry errors, duplicate use of some test data samples, and failure to lock down the algorithm before its performance was evaluated. The investigator did not address these errors even after they were published, and the NIH was unable to reproduce key results.

Because the validity of the tests could not be reproduced, the NIH terminated three randomized clinical trials using these predictive models. Eventually, 14 articles reporting the predictive tests were retracted. After the investigator was found to have falsified his curriculum vitae, he resigned his faculty position. The federal Office for Research Integrity found that he had committed research misconduct by falsifying research data in published papers and a federal grant application (18).

In other highly publicized cases, researchers intentionally fabricated or altered data in alleging a link between measles-mumps-rubella vaccine and childhood autism (19) and in claiming to derive a human stem cell line using somatic cell nuclear transplantation (20, 21). Such misconduct undermines public and physician trust in research and threatens public funding for research.

When research misconduct is alleged, both the federal funding agency and the investigator's institution have the responsibility to carry out a fair and timely investigation (22). During such an investigation, both whistleblowers and accused scientists have rights that must be respected. Whistleblowers need to be protected from retaliation, and accused scientists need to be told the charges and given an opportunity to respond. Punishment for proven research misconduct may include suspension of a grant; debarment from future grants; loss of academic position; and other administrative, academic, criminal, or civil sanctions.

Authorship

To merit authorship (22), researchers must:

- **Make substantial contributions to study conception and design, or data analysis and interpretation, and**

- Make substantial contributions to drafting or revising the manuscript, and
- Give final approval of the manuscript before submission for publication.

Guest authorship and ghost authorship are unethical. **Guest authors** (or honorary authors) are listed as authors despite having made only trivial contributions to a research manuscript, abstract, or other publication, for example, by providing name recognition, access to participants, reagents, laboratory assistance, or funding. It is not appropriate for someone to become an author after the study is completed, the data analyzed, and the first draft written. **Ghost authors**, on the other hand, make substantial contributions to a publication but are *not* listed as authors. They are generally employees of pharmaceutical companies or medical writing companies. Omission of ghost writers misleads readers into underestimating a company's role in the manuscript. According to one study, 25% of original research articles in high-impact general journals have guest authors, and 12% have ghost authors (23).

Disagreements arise commonly regarding who should be an author or the order of authors. These issues are best discussed explicitly and decided before a manuscript is drafted. Changes in authorship should be negotiated if decisions are made to shift responsibilities for the work. Suggestions have been made for carrying out such negotiations diplomatically (24). Because there are no criteria to determine the position of authors, some journals describe the contributions of each author in the published article.

Conflicts of Interest

A researcher's primary interests should be providing valid answers to important scientific questions and protecting the safety of participants. **Conflicts of interest** arise when researchers have other interests that might lead to bias in the research, impair its objectivity, or undermine public trust in research (25, 26).

Types of Conflicts of Interest

- **Financial conflicts of interest.** Studies of new drugs, devices, and tests are commonly funded by industry. The ethical concern is that financial arrangements might lead to bias in the design and conduct of a study, overinterpretation of positive results, or failure to publish negative results (25). If investigators hold patents on the study intervention, or equity in the company making the drug or device under study, they might reap large financial rewards if the treatment is shown to be effective. Finally, receipt of consulting fees, honoraria, or in-kind gifts might bias an investigator's judgment in favor of the company's product.
- **Professional conflicts of interest.** Nonfinancial incentives, such as professional reputation and intellectual commitment to an idea, may cause bias in favor of a preconceived result.

Responding to Conflicting Interests

All conflicts of interest should be disclosed, and some have such great potential for biasing research results that they should be managed or avoided.

- **Reduce the likelihood of bias.** In well-designed clinical trials, several standard precautions help keep competing interests in check. Investigators can be blinded to the intervention a participant is receiving to prevent bias in assessing outcomes. An independent Data and Safety Monitoring Board (see Chapter 11), whose members have no conflict of interest, can review interim data and terminate the study if there is convincing evidence of benefit or harm. The peer-review process for grants, abstracts, and manuscripts also helps reduce bias.
- **Separate conflicting roles.** Ideally, researchers with strong personal financial incentives or intellectual commitments should be excluded from key roles in planning a study, analyzing the data, or interpreting the results; others without such relationships should fill those roles. This would exclude, for example, the patent holder of the study intervention from serving

as principal investigator. In reality, however, drug and device manufacturers are commonly responsible for key roles in clinical trials they sponsor.

- **Control of analysis and publications.** In research funded by a pharmaceutical company, academic investigators who are first or senior authors need to ensure that the research contract gives them control over the primary data and statistical analysis, and the freedom to publish findings, whether or not the investigational drug is found to be effective (27). The investigator has an ethical obligation to take responsibility for all aspects of the research. The sponsor may review the manuscripts, make suggestions, and ensure that patent applications have been filed before the article is submitted to a journal. However, the sponsor should not have the power to veto or censor publication or to insist on specific language in the manuscript.
- **Disclose conflicting interests.** The NIH, other funding and federal agencies, local IRBs, scientific meetings, and medical journals require disclosure of conflicts of interest when grants, abstracts, or papers are submitted. Pharmaceutical companies are also required to publicly disclose payments to individual physicians in the United States on the website https://openpaymentsdata.cms.gov/. Although disclosure alone is often an inadequate response to serious conflicts of interest, it might deter investigators from ethically problematic practices, and it allows editors, reviewers, and readers of journal articles to assess the potential for undue influence.
- **Manage conflicts of interest.** If a particular study presents significant conflicts of interest, the research institution, funding agency, or IRB may require additional safeguards, such as closer monitoring of the informed consent process or modification of the conflicted investigator's role.
- **Prohibit certain situations.** To prevent conflicts of interest, funders or academic institutions might prohibit the patent holder on an intervention or an officer of the company manufacturing the intervention from serving as principal investigator in a clinical trial.

■ ETHICAL ISSUES SPECIFIC TO CERTAIN TYPES OF RESEARCH

Randomized Clinical Trials

Although randomized clinical trials are the most rigorous design for evaluating interventions, they present two unique ethical concerns: researchers carry out interventions on participants, and who receives which intervention is determined by chance. One ethical justification for assigning study interventions randomly is that they are in **equipoise**, a concept that seems clear intuitively but is challenging to define (28). Equipoise does not require an exact balance among the study arms, but there should be genuine uncertainty or controversy over which arm of the trial is superior, so that participants will not be harmed significantly if they allow their care to be determined by randomization rather than by their personal physician.

Participants in a clinical trial receive an intervention whose adverse effects are often unknown. Thus, trials require careful monitoring to make sure that participants are not being harmed. For most trials, this includes establishing an independent Data and Safety Monitoring Board that reviews study data intermittently and that has the authority to recommend stopping the trial if there is statistically and clinically significant harm associated with the intervention (see Chapter 11).

Interventions for control groups may also raise ethical concerns. If there is a standard of effective care for a condition, the control group should receive it. However, placebo controls may be justified in short-term trials that do not have serious risks to participants, such as studies of mild, self-limited pain. Participants need to be informed of effective interventions that are available outside the research study.

It is also unethical to continue a clinical trial if there is compelling evidence that the treatment is either effective or harmful or if the trial will not answer the research question because of low enrollment, high dropout, or an inadequate rate of outcomes. The periodic analysis of interim data by an independent Data and Safety Monitoring Board can determine whether a trial should be terminated prematurely for these reasons (29). Such interim analyses should not be carried out by the researchers themselves, because unblinding investigators to interim findings can lead to bias if the study continues, and investigators often have conflicting interests about whether to continue or stop a study. Procedures for examining interim data and statistical stopping rules should be specified before enrolling participants.

Clinical trials in developing countries present additional ethical dilemmas, as in Case 7.3.

Research on Previously Collected Specimens and Data

Biobanks of blood and tissue specimens allow future studies to be carried out without the collection of additional samples. Although research on previously collected specimens and data offers no physical risks to participants, there might be ethical concerns. Consent for unspecified future studies is problematic because no one can anticipate what kind of research might be carried out later. Furthermore, participants might object to specific future use of data and biospecimens, even if their identity cannot be readily ascertained. If breaches of confidentiality occur, such as through reidentification of genomic sequences, they might lead to stigma and discrimination. Groups participating in research might be harmed even if individual participants are not, as in Case 7.5.

Case 7.5 Research with Specimens Previously Collected for Research

Investigators at the University of Arizona studied genetic markers associated with diabetes in the Havasupai Native American tribe, who are at high risk for developing the disease. Although the consent form stated that specimens could be used to study behavioral or medical disorders, communication with the tribe and consent discussions with participants focused on diabetes. Later, the specimens were used for studies of the genetic basis of schizophrenia and ancestral migration patterns. The tribe claimed these studies were outside the scope of the original consent. Moreover, the studies of schizophrenia were stigmatizing, and the evolutionary genetics study contradicted the tribe's origin story. The tribe sued the University of Arizona for $50 million and won a settlement of $700,000. The University apologized and returned the remaining genetic samples (30).

Currently, research can be carried out without consent on biologic specimens that have already been collected if the identity of the participants cannot be ascertained readily. However, it has been suggested that patients should be asked to consent prospectively for secondary research carried out on biospecimens collected for clinical care but no longer needed for that purpose, such as leftover blood, biopsies, or surgical specimens (31).

When new biologic specimens are collected for research, consent forms should allow participants to agree to or refuse certain broad categories of future research using the specimens. For example, participants might allow their specimens to be used:

- For all future research that is approved by an IRB and scientific review panel; *or*
- Only for research on specific conditions; or
- Only in the current research study, not in future studies.

Participants should also know whether identifiable data and specimens will be shared with other researchers. Furthermore, participants should understand that research discoveries from the specimens might be patented and developed into commercial products that could have monetary value.

Research Using Artificial Intelligence and Big Data

Using artificial intelligence (AI), computers carry out tasks typically done by humans. Machine learning is a type of AI that automatically learns and improves its performance without further programming. Nonclinical examples include protocols for facial recognition, suggesting additional purchases, screening job applicants, and assessing creditworthiness. These techniques hold promise to improve clinical care and health care administration, such as diagnosing skin cancer and eye diseases and reading radiology images. However, machine learning algorithms are difficult to understand due to the "black box" nature of the process, and reliance on underlying data without clinical validation might result in erroneous, limited, or biased protocols. Outside of clinical medicine, bias is common in widely used AI algorithms because of unrepresentative derivation and validation data.

Case 7.6 Machine Learning Algorithm to Predict High-Cost Patients

A researcher develops a machine learning algorithm to predict which patients experience adverse health care outcomes, using de-identified data from about 50,000 patients' electronic health records. The goal is to target care management programs to high-risk patients to improve their outcomes. As the outcome variable, the researcher chooses future health care costs. A successful algorithm might allow the health care organization to improve quality of care for high-risk patients or to save money by avoiding hospital readmissions, postacute care, and other expensive care (32).

On average, Black patients have lower health care costs than Whites (except for emergency visits and dialysis), most likely because they have less access to health care. Based on these data, AI algorithms that target high-cost patients for care management may offer such programs preferentially to White patients over sicker Black patients (32). Such bias violates the principle of justice by denying access to beneficial care to patients with greater need. However, if the outcome for the algorithm is changed to health status, defined as the number of active chronic illnesses, the percentage of Black patients offered the program would be doubled, because they have more—and more severe—chronic medical conditions than do Whites. Moreover, the percentage of total costs incurred (and thus potentially saved) among patients identified by the algorithm increases. Hence the choice of the outcome variable can lead both to bias and reduced effectiveness of the algorithm.

Researchers developing and testing predictive AI algorithms can reduce bias by employing training and validation data sets that are representative of the target population to which the algorithm will be applied and ensuring that the training set does not include historical cases in which decisions were biased. For example, AI algorithms for diagnosis of skin cancer should include in the training data set cases in Blacks and Asians, which tend to present differently than cases in Whites. Algorithms to predict coronary artery disease need to ensure that they do not yield biased results in women and Blacks because appropriate tests available in the data set were not ordered. Furthermore, the algorithm should be tested in diverse populations, in which it should achieve equitable performance (33). There are consensus guidelines for designing clinical trial protocols using AI interventions (34).

Trials Using Sensors and Mobile Health Devices

Smartphone apps and wearable sensors make it possible to collect a wide range of health-relevant data, including heart rate and rhythm, blood glucose levels, physical activity, and voice and speech patterns. These technologies—collectively called mobile health—allow passive collection of health information and have been employed in conditions such as arrhythmia, hypertension, diabetes, Parkinson's disease, and depression. Mobile health may offer the opportunity to identify risk factors for disease, track natural history, and support randomized trials with mobile health predictors or outcomes. However, most mobile health devices and application are inaccurate (or have not been tested for accuracy) (35), and populations that use these devices regularly may be highly selected.

The following case involving research using electronic sensors in a low-income country demonstrates some related ethical issues.

Case 7.7 Malaria Research Using Digital Sensors

A malaria researcher proposes a descriptive study of adherence to insecticide-treated bednets in a low-income country with a high incidence of malaria (36). These bednets are a standard public health intervention, but their actual use is poorly studied. Sensors can provide more accurate measurements of adherence than self-report of use of bednets. First-generation sensors detect simply whether the bednet is deployed or not. Second-generation sensors, which have video recording and proximity sensors, can also detect whether someone is under the bednet and identify that person. Knowing which uninfected children, who are at highest risk, are under bednets would help plan more effective preventive interventions.

Although this proposed study addresses a major global health problem, it raises several ethical issues. First, monitors raise privacy and confidentiality concerns, particularly for persons sleeping in the bed who did not give consent to be studied or even know that research was being carried out. Their privacy will be violated, and breaches of confidentiality may cause them harm, for example if there is an extramarital sexual relationship. Stigma of marital infidelity may be greater for women than for men in the local culture. The stakes for confidentiality are high if the research team plans to hire research assistants from the area where the research will be carried out. This policy facilitates enrollment in the study and provides tangible benefits to the villages that are the study sites. However, it also increases the likelihood that the research assistants will know the study participants.

Before implementing a study such as Case 7.7, researchers should assess the acceptability of digital sensors, particularly video sensors, through pilot studies, community advisory boards, and community-based participatory research methods (36, 37).

■ OTHER ISSUES

Payment to Research Participants

Participants in clinical research deserve payment for their time and effort, as well as reimbursement for out-of-pocket expenses such as transportation and childcare. Practically speaking, compensation might also be needed to enroll and retain participants. A common practice is to offer higher payment for studies that are very inconvenient or risky. However, incentives also raise ethical concerns about undue inducement and justice. If participants are paid more to participate in riskier research, persons of lower socioeconomic status might undertake risks against their better judgment. To avoid undue influence, it has been suggested that participants be compensated only for actual expenses and time at a local hourly rate for unskilled labor (38).

Clinical Impact of Research

Early in their careers, researchers may be motivated to publish articles to establish their professional stature. However, stature is earned on the basis of the importance of publications, not just their quantity. It is unethical to use research resources and to put participants at risk without addressing questions that will improve patients' health and quality of life, to use a weak study design, or conduct a poor quality study that cannot answer the research question.

■ SUMMARY

1. Investigators must assure that their projects observe the ethical principles of respect for persons, beneficence, justice, and truth-telling.
2. Investigators must assure that research meets the requirements of applicable federal regulations, the key features being informed consent from participants and IRB review. During the informed consent process, investigators must explain to potential participants the nature of the project and the risks, potential benefits, and alternatives. Investigators must assure the confidentiality of participant information, observing the HIPAA Health Privacy Rule.
3. Vulnerable populations, such as children, prisoners, and people with cognitive deficits or social disadvantage, require additional protections.
4. Investigators must have ethical integrity. They must not commit scientific misconduct, which regulations define as fabrication, falsification, or plagiarism. Investigators need to disclose and appropriately manage conflicts of interest. Investigators should follow criteria for appropriate authorship by listing themselves as an author on a manuscript only if they made substantial intellectual contributions and by ensuring that all persons who contributed substantially to a manuscript are listed as authors.
5. In certain types of research, additional ethical issues must be addressed. In randomized trials, the intervention arms must be in equipoise, control groups must receive appropriate interventions, and the trial must not be continued once it has been demonstrated that one arm is more effective or harmful. When research is carried out on previously collected specimens and data, special attention needs to be given to confidentiality. In research conducted in low- and middle-income countries, justice requires particular attention.

REFERENCES

1. Jones JH, King NMP. Bad blood thirty years later: a Q&A with James H. Jones. *J Law Med Ethics*. 2012;40(4):867-872.
2. The National Commission for the Protection of Human Subjects of Biomedical and Behavioral Research. The Belmont Report. Ethical Principles and Guidelines for the Protection of Human Subjects of Research [Internet]. HHS.gov. 1979 [cited 2021 Feb 12]. https://www.hhs.gov/ohrp/regulations-and-policy/belmont-report/read-the-belmont-report/index.html.
3. Department of Health and Human Services. *Federal Policy for the Protection of Human Subjects*. 45 CPR 46 [Internet]. Electronic Code of Federal Regulations (eCFR). 2017 [cited 2021 Feb 12]. https://www.ecfr.gov/.
4. Lo B, Barnes M. Federal research regulations for the 21st century. *N Engl J Med*. 2016;374(13):1205-1207.
5. Emanuel EJ, Menikoff J. Reforming the regulations governing research with human subjects. *N Engl J Med*. 2011;365:1145-1150.
6. Office of Human Research Protections. *Expedited Review Procedures Guidance* (2003) [Internet]. HHS.gov. 2003 [cited 2021 Feb 12]. https://www.hhs.gov/ohrp/regulations-and-policy/guidance/guidance-on-expedited-review-procedures/index.html.
7. Joffe S, Mack JW. Deliberation and the life cycle of informed consent. *Hastings Cent Rep*. 2014;44(1):33-35.
8. Nishimura A, Carey J, Erwin PJ, Tilburt JC, Murad MH, McCormick JB. Improving understanding in the research informed consent process: a systematic review of 54 interventions tested in randomized control trials. *BMC Med Ethics*. 2013;14(1):28.
9. Institute of Medicine. *Challenges and Opportunities in Using Residual Newborn Screening Samples for Translational Research: Workshop Summary* [Internet]. 2010 [cited 2021 Mar 4]. https://www.nap.edu/catalog/12981/challenges-and-opportunities-in-using-residual-newborn-screening-samples-for-translational-research.
10. Wolf LE, Beskow LM. New and improved? 21st century cures act revisions to certificates of confidentiality. *Am J Law Med*. 2018;44(2-3):343-358.
11. Nass SJ, Levit LA, Gostin LO, editors. *Beyond the HIPAA Privacy Rule: Enhancing Privacy, Improving Health Through Research [Internet]*. National Academies Press (US); 2009 [cited 2021 Feb 12]. http://www.ncbi.nlm.nih.gov/books/NBK9578/.

12. Gordon BG. Vulnerability in research: basic ethical concepts and general approach to review. *Ochsner J.* 2020;20(1):34-38.

13. Weisleder P. Helping them decide: a scoping review of interventions used to help minors understand the concept and process of assent. *Front Pediatr.* 2020;8:25.

14. HIV Prevention Trials Network. *Updated Ethics Guidance for HIV Prevention Research* [Internet]. 2020 [cited 2021 Jan 31]. https://www.hptn.org/news-and-events/announcements/updated-ethics-guidance-hiv-prevention-research.

15. *The Ethics of Research in Developing Countries* [Internet]. The Nuffield Council on Bioethics. 2002 [cited 2021 Jan 31]. https://www.nuffieldbioethics.org/topics/research-ethics/research-in-developing-countries.

16. Ndebele P. The Declaration of Helsinki, 50 years later. *JAMA.* 2013;310(20):2145-2146.

17. Office of Research Integrity. *Definition of Research Misconduct | ORI—The Office of Research Integrity* [Internet] [cited 2021 Feb 12]. https://ori.hhs.gov/definition-misconduct.

18. Institute of Medicine. *Evolution of Translational Omics: Lessons Learned and the Path Forward* [Internet]. 2012 [cited 2020 Dec 28]. https://www.nap.edu/catalog/13297/evolution-of-translational-omics-lessons-learned-and-the-path-forward. (See Appendix B).

19. Godlee F, Smith J, Marcovitch H. Wakefield's article linking MMR vaccine and autism was fraudulent. *BMJ.* 2011;342:c7452.

20. Chong S, Normile D. How young Korean researchers helped unearth a scandal. *Science.* 2006;311(5757):22-25.

21. Chong S. Investigations document still more problems for stem cell researchers. *Science.* 2006;311(5762):754-755.

22. Mello MM, Brennan TA. Due process in investigations of research misconduct. *N Engl J Med.* 2003;349(13):1280-1286.

23. Wislar JS, Flanagin A, Fontanarosa PB, Deangelis CD. Honorary and ghost authorship in high impact biomedical journals: a cross sectional survey. *BMJ.* 2011;343:d6128.

24. Browner WS. Authorship. In: *Publishing and Presenting Clinical Research.* 3rd ed. Wolters Kluwer; 2013.

25. Lo B, Field M, editors. *Conflict of Interest in Medical Research, Education, and Practice* [Internet]. 2009 [cited 2021 Feb 13]. https://www.nap.edu/catalog/12598/conflict-of-interest-in-medical-research-education-and-practice.

26. Fineberg HV. Conflict of interest: why does it matter? *JAMA.* 2017;317(17):1717-1718.

27. DeAngelis CD, Fontanarosa PB. Ensuring integrity in industry-sponsored research: primum non nocere, revisited. *JAMA.* 2010;303(12):1196-1198.

28. Joffe S, Miller FG. Equipoise: asking the right questions for clinical trial design. *Nat Rev Clin Oncol.* 2012;9(4):230-235.

29. Ellenberg SS, Fleming TR, DeMets DL. *Data Monitoring Committees in Clinical Trials: A Practical Perspective.* 2nd ed. Wiley; 2019:496.

30. Mello MM, Wolf LE. The Havasupai Indian tribe case—lessons for research involving stored biologic samples. *N Engl J Med.* 2010;363(3):204-207.

31. Wolinetz CD, Collins FS. Recognition of research participants' need for autonomy: remembering the legacy of Henrietta Lacks. *JAMA [Internet].* 2020 [cited 2020 Nov 6];324:1027-1028. https://jamanetwork.com/journals/jama/fullarticle/2769506.

32. Obermeyer Z, Powers B, Vogeli C, Mullainathan S. Dissecting racial bias in an algorithm used to manage the health of populations. *Science.* 2019;366(6464):447-453.

33. Zou J, Schiebinger L. AI can be sexist and racist—it's time to make it fair. *Nature.* 2018;559(7714):324-326.

34. Rivera SC, Liu X, Chan A-W, et al. Guidelines for clinical trial protocols for interventions involving artificial intelligence: the SPIRIT-AI Extension. *BMJ [Internet].* 2020 [cited 2020 Dec 27];370. https://www.ncbi.nlm.nih.gov/pmc/articles/PMC7490785/.

35. Freeman K, Dinnes J, Chuchu N, et al. Algorithm based smartphone apps to assess risk of skin cancer in adults: systematic review of diagnostic accuracy studies. *BMJ [Internet].* 2020 [cited 2021 Feb 13];368. https://www.ncbi.nlm.nih.gov/pmc/articles/PMC7190019/.

36. Krezanoski P, Haberer J. Objective monitoring of mosquito bednet usage and the ethical challenge of respecting study bystanders' privacy. *Clin Trials Lond Engl.* 2019;16(5):466-468.

37. Fairchild AL. Objective monitoring of mosquito bednet usage and the ethical challenge of privacy revelations about study bystanders: ethical analysis. *Clin Trials Lond Engl.* 2019;16(5):469-472.

38. Gelinas L, Largent EA, Cohen IG, Kornetsky S, Bierer BE, Lynch HF. A framework for ethical payment to research participants. *N Engl J Med [Internet].* 2018 [cited 2021 Feb 13]. https://www.nejm.org/doi/10.1056/NEJMsb1710591.

APPENDIX 7A
Exercises for Chapter 7. Addressing Ethical Issues

1. The research question is to identify genes that are associated with an increased risk of developing Type II diabetes mellitus. The investigator finds that frozen blood samples and clinical data are available from a completed prospective cohort study on risk factors for coronary artery disease. That study collected baseline data on diet, exercise, clinical characteristics, and measurements of cholesterol and hemoglobin A1c levels. Follow-up data are available on coronary endpoints and the development of diabetes. The proposed study will carry out DNA sequencing on participants; no new blood samples are required.
   a. Can the proposed study be done under the original informed consent that was obtained for the cohort study?
   b. If the original informed consent did not provide permission for the proposed study, how can the proposed study be done?
   c. When designing a study that will collect blood samples, how can investigators plan to allow future studies to use their data and samples?
2. The investigator plans a phase III randomized controlled trial of a new cancer drug that has shown promise in treating advanced colon cancer. To reduce sample size, she would like to carry out a placebo-controlled trial rather than compare it to current therapy.
   a. What are the ethical concerns about a placebo control in this situation?
   b. Is it possible to carry out a placebo-controlled study in an ethically acceptable manner?
3. The investigator plans a study to prepare for a future HIV vaccine trial. The goals of the study are to determine if it is possible to recruit a cohort of participants who have a high HIV seroconversion rate despite state-of-the-art HIV prevention counseling, and if the follow-up rate in the cohort will be sufficiently high to carry out a vaccine trial. Participants will be persons at increased risk for HIV infection, including injection drug users, persons who trade sex for money, and persons with multiple sexual partners. Most participants will have low literacy and poor health literacy. The study will be an observational cohort study, following participants for 2 years to determine seroconversion and follow-up rates.
   a. What do the federal regulations require to be disclosed to participants as part of informed consent?
   b. What steps can be taken to ensure that consent is truly informed in this context?
   c. What is the investigator's responsibility during this observational study to reduce the risk of HIV infection in these high-risk participants?

Study Designs

CHAPTER 8

Designing Cross-Sectional and Cohort Studies

Thomas B. Newman, Warren S. Browner, and Steven R. Cummings

Observational studies have two primary purposes: **descriptive**, examining the distributions of variables in a population, and **analytic**, examining associations among them. In this chapter, we present two basic observational designs, which are categorized according to the time frame for making the measurements.

In a **cross-sectional study**, the investigator makes all of his measurements on a single occasion or within a short time. He draws a sample from the population and looks at distributions of variables within that sample, sometimes designating them as predictors or outcomes based on biologic plausibility, historical information, and his research hypotheses. For example, if he is interested in studying the relationship between bodyweight and blood pressure, he could measure these variables at a single clinic visit for each study participant and examine whether participants with higher bodyweights were more likely to have hypertension.

In a **cohort study**, measurements take place over a period of time in a group of participants who have been identified at the beginning of the study (the "cohort"). The defining characteristic of cohort studies is that this group is assembled at the outset and is followed **longitudinally** (over time). Just as in a cross-sectional study there is no structural difference between predictors and outcomes, in a cohort study there is no structural difference between a predictor of particular interest (often an exposure or treatment) and other predictors of outcome (often called covariates). For example, the investigator could measure egg consumption and covariates (such as other dietary habits, age, and tobacco smoking) on a cohort of study participants and then follow them to determine the relationship between egg consumption and the **incidence** of cardiovascular disease; the same study could also quantify the effects of the covariates (1). In this chapter, we discuss **prospective** and **retrospective cohort** designs, as well as **multiple-cohort** designs. We also address the importance of optimizing cohort retention during follow-up and basic approaches to statistical analysis.

■ CROSS-SECTIONAL STUDIES

Basic Design

In a cross-sectional study, all the measurements are made at about the same time, with no follow-up period (Figure 8.1). Cross-sectional designs are well suited to the goal of describing variables and their distribution patterns. In the National Health and Nutrition Examination Survey (NHANES-I), for example, a sample designed to represent the entire US population aged 1 to 74 was interviewed and examined from 1971 to 1975. This cross-sectional study was a major source of information about the health and habits of the US population in the year it was carried out, providing estimates of such things as the prevalence of smoking in various demographic groups. The NHANES I was followed by NHANES II (1976 to 1980), Hispanic HANES (1982 to 1984), and NHANES III (1988 to 1994); since 1999, NHANES surveys (revised every

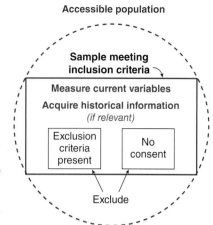

Accessible population

Sample meeting
inclusion criteria

Measure current variables

Acquire historical information
(if relevant)

Exclusion
criteria
present

No
consent

Exclude

■ **FIGURE 8.1 Cross-sectional study**. In a cross-sectional study, the steps are to:
• Sample participants meeting inclusion criteria from the accessible population,
• Exclude those with exclusion criteria or who do not consent, and
• Measure current values of predictor and outcome variables, often supplemented by historical information.

2 years) have been carried out continuously (2). All NHANES data sets and data collection forms are available for public use from the Centers for Disease Control (CDC; www.cdc.gov/nchs/nhanes.htm).

Cross-sectional studies can be used for examining associations, although the choice of which variables to label as predictors and which as outcomes depends on the cause-and-effect hypotheses of the investigator rather than on the study design. This choice is easy for constitutional factors such as age, race, and sex assigned at birth; these cannot be altered by other variables and are therefore always predictors. For other variables, however, the choice can go either way. For example, in NHANES III there was a cross-sectional association between childhood obesity and hours spent watching television (3). Whether to label obesity or television-watching as the predictor and the other as the outcome depends on the causal hypothesis of the investigator.

Unlike cohort studies, which have a longitudinal time dimension and can be used to estimate **incidence** (the proportion who *develop* a disease or condition over time), cross-sectional studies provide information only about **prevalence**, the proportion who *have* a disease or condition at one point in time (Table 8.1). Cross-sectional studies of clinical populations (eg, emergency department patients with abdominal pain) are helpful to clinicians, who must estimate the likelihood that the patient in front of them has a particular disease (eg, appendicitis); the greater the prevalence, the greater the "prior probability" of the disease (Chapter 12). Cross-sectional studies are also useful to health planners who want to know how many people have certain diseases so that they can allocate enough resources to care for them. When analyzing cross-sectional

TABLE 8.1 DIFFERENCE BETWEEN INCIDENCE AND PREVALENCE

TYPE OF STUDY	STATISTIC	DEFINITION
Cross-sectional	Prevalence	Number of people who HAVE a disease or condition at a given point in time
		Number of people at risk
Cohort	Cumulative incidence or incidence proportion	Number of people who GET or GOT a disease over a given point of time
		Number of people at risk
Cohort	Incidence rate	Number of people who GET or GOT a disease
		Number of people at risk × time period at risk

Example 8.1 Cross-Sectional Study

Sargent et al. (4) sought to determine whether exposure to movies in which the actors smoked is associated with smoking initiation. The steps in performing the study were to:

1. Define selection criteria and recruit the population sample. The investigators did a random-digit-dial survey of 6522 US children aged 10 to 14 years.
2. Measure the predictor and outcome variables. They quantified smoking in 532 popular movies and for each participant asked which of a randomly selected subset of 50 movies they had seen. Participants were also asked about a variety of covariates such as age, race, gender, parental smoking and education, sensation-seeking (eg, "I like to do dangerous things"), and self-esteem (eg, "I wish I were someone else"). The outcome variable was whether the child had ever tried smoking a cigarette.

The prevalence of ever having tried smoking varied from 2% in the lowest quartile of movie smoking exposure to 22% in the highest quartile. After adjusting for age and other confounders, these differences were statistically significant; the authors estimated that 38% of smoking initiation was attributable to exposure to movies in which the actors smoked. Subsequent studies in multiple other countries have confirmed the importance of smoking in movies as a contributor to smoking initiation among adolescents (5-7).

studies, the prevalence of the outcome can be compared in those with and without an exposure, yielding the *prevalence ratio* of the outcome, the cross-sectional equivalent of the **risk ratio**.

Sometimes cross-sectional studies describe the prevalence of ever having been exposed to something or ever having had a disease or condition. But, of course, the older a person is, the more opportunity they will have had to be exposed or to get a disease. Therefore, age (or anything else associated with greater opportunity to be exposed, such as duration of employment when studying a work-related exposure) needs to be accounted for when studying associations between these types of "ever having" variables. This is illustrated in Example 8.1, in which the prevalence of ever having tried smoking was studied in a cross-sectional study of children with differing levels of exposure to movies in which the actors smoked. Of course, children who had seen more movies were also older and therefore had more opportunity to have tried smoking, so it was important to adjust for age in multivariable analyses (see Chapter 10).

Strengths and Weaknesses of Cross-Sectional Studies

A major advantage of cross-sectional studies is that there is no waiting for the outcome to occur. This makes them fast and inexpensive and avoids the problem of loss to follow-up. Another advantage is that a cross-sectional study can be included as the first step in a cohort study or clinical trial at little or no added cost. The results define the demographic and clinical characteristics of the study group at baseline, allow for exclusion of those who already have the outcome from subsequent longitudinal studies, and can sometimes reveal cross-sectional associations of interest. Cross-sectional studies are also useful for studies of diagnostic tests, in which patients already have the disease of interest and the focus is on the accuracy of tests to diagnose it (Chapter 13).

Cross-sectional designs are the best approach to studying associations between characteristics that influence each other within short periods. For instance, the association between patterns of sleep and tests of cognition is best studied by measurements taken on the same day (8).

However, as previously noted, it's often difficult to establish causal relationships from cross-sectional data. Because cross-sectional studies measure only prevalence, rather than incidence, it is important to be cautious when drawing inferences about the causes, prognosis, or natural history of a disease. That's because a factor that is associated with prevalence of disease may be a cause of the disease—but could also just be associated with *duration* of the disease, by affecting either the likelihood of mortality or the likelihood of disease resolution.[1] For example, the prevalence of chronic kidney disease is affected not only by its incidence, but also by survival once it has occurred. Given the observation that obesity is associated with greater survival among dialysis patients (9), a cross-sectional study of the predictors of prevalent chronic kidney failure would overestimate the association between obesity and chronic kidney failure incidence.

Serial Surveys

Occasionally, investigators perform **serial cross-sectional surveys** in the same population, say, every 5 years. This design can be used to draw inferences about changing patterns over time, as is done with the previously described NHANES. Sometimes, such surveys can reveal dramatic changes in prevalence over a relatively short period. For example, McMillen et al. (10), using annual cross-sectional surveys of representative samples of US adults, reported that the prevalence of electronic cigarette use increased from 0% to 14.2% of young adults (18 to 24 years) between 2010 and 2013.

Serial surveys have a longitudinal time frame, but they are not the same as a cohort study, because a new sample is drawn each time. As a result, changes within individuals cannot be assessed, and findings may be influenced by people entering or leaving the population (and, thus, the samples) due to births, deaths, and migration.

■ COHORT STUDIES

Cohort was the Roman term for a group of soldiers that marched together. In clinical research, a cohort is a group of participants, specified at the outset and followed over time.

Prospective Versus Retrospective Studies

Cohort studies are often classified as either *prospective* or *retrospective* (literally, looking forward or looking backward), but definitions of these terms vary (11), and there is not a sharp dichotomy (Examples 8.2 and 8.3): cohort studies can look forward at some variables and backward at others ("*ambidirectional* cohort studies") (12). Indeed, the terms are best applied to aspects of a study, rather than being all-or-nothing phenomena. Studies with many prospective features are less subject to bias, but they also tend to be more difficult and expensive, because the investigator must assemble and follow a cohort of participants, sometimes over many years. Thus, they may be impractical for new investigators. New investigators can often take advantage of prospective studies by using data or specimens from ongoing or completed cohort studies (Chapter 16).

In its purest form, a prospective cohort study involves **identifying a group of participants at risk of the outcome to be studied** (eg, by excluding those who already have the outcome or who no longer have the organ in which it occurs), **defining and measuring predictors at baseline and then following the participants,** using a strict ascertainment protocol, **for the new occurrence of or change in that outcome.** For example, blood cadmium levels and other predictors could be measured in 3000 participants free of peripheral neuropathy at baseline. They could then be followed at regular intervals for the development of peripheral neuropathy by measurement of touch, pain, and vibration sensation in the feet.

Several prospective features of a study can increase its validity (Table 8.2), most notably those that ensure that the occurrence and measurement of the outcome (eg, peripheral neuropathy) cannot affect the measurement of the predictor (eg, cadmium level). In addition, making

---

[1]The prevalence of a disease is, in fact, the product of its incidence and (average) duration: $P = I \times D$.

Example 8.2 Example of a (Mostly) Prospective Cohort Study

The classic Nurses' Health Studies (NHS) have examined the **epidemiology** of common diseases in women since the original study, which began enrollment in 1976. (Beginning in 2015, NHS-3 extended recruitment to include male nurses.) (13)

In 2020, Wang et al. reported on the association between menstrual cycle regularity and the risk of death before 70 years in the Nurses' Health Study II (NHS-II). The steps in performing the study were to:

1. **Define selection criteria and assemble the cohort.** The NHS-II began in 1989 with the enrollment of 116,429 female US registered nurses aged 25 to 42 years from 14 states.
2. **Measure predictor variables, including potential confounders.** NHS-II was focused particularly on oral contraceptives and other reproductive risk factors for disease. At baseline in 1989, participants were asked to recall characteristics of their menstrual cycles when they were 14 to 17 and 18 to 22 years old. In 1993, the women (then 29 to 46 years old) were asked about their current menstrual cycles. Values of other covariates in 1993 were taken as baseline measurements.
3. **Follow up the cohort and measure outcomes.** Mortality was ascertained from state vital statistics records, periodic searches of the national death index, or by reports from next of kin or the postal authorities.

The investigators found that women who reported that their usual cycle length was 40 days or more were more likely to die before age 70 years compared with women whose usual cycle length was 26 to 31 days (adjusted hazard ratios 1.34 [95% CI, 1.06 to 1.69] for long cycle length at ages 18 to 22 years and 1.40 [95% CI, 1.17 to 1.68] for long cycle length at 29 to 46 years). Adjusting for potential confounding factors did not change the result.

Comment: The measurement of menstrual cycle characteristics at age 14 to 17 and 18 to 22 years was based on participants' recall at the time of recruitment and so in that sense was *retrospective*. On the other hand, the measurement of current menstrual cycles was *prospective*. Given that the outcome was total mortality before age 70 years, there is little risk of bias in its measurement, and its occurrence could not have affected the measurement of exposures.

Example 8.3 Example of a (Mostly) Retrospective Cohort Study

Antithrombotic ("blood thinning") therapy can improve outcomes from acute ischemic stroke if given within a few hours of symptom onset. Man et al. (14) studied the association between "door-to-needle time" (the time it took from hospital arrival to deliver tissue plasminogen activator (tPA) therapy to the patient) and 1-year mortality among Medicare patients. The steps were as follows:

1. **Identify a suitable existing cohort.** The investigators studied 61,426 Medicare beneficiaries ≥65 years old who were seen at hospitals participating in the Get With the Guidelines (GTWG)-Stroke quality-improvement program and who received tPA within 4.5 hours of symptom onset.
2. **Collect exposure data and covariates.** Trained hospital personnel collected data on door-to-needle time and other clinical predictors of outcome as part of the Get With the Guidelines (GWTG)-Stroke quality-improvement program. The authors obtained data on hospital-level characteristics from the American Hospital Association database.

3. **Ascertain outcomes.** To obtain data on deaths and hospital admissions in the following year, the investigators linked GWTH-Stroke records to Medicare claims files by "matching on a series of indirect identifiers," including admission and discharge dates, hospital, and the patient's sex and date of birth.

Using the Cox proportional hazards model to adjust for baseline covariates, the investigators found a dose-response relationship between door-to-needle time and all-cause mortality, with an adjusted hazard ratio of 1.04 (95% CI, 1.02 to 1.05) per 15-minute increase in door-to-needle time. (The Cox model is logarithmic; thus, the estimated effect of a 1-hour increase in door-to-needle time would be to increase the risk of death by a factor of 1.04 for each 15 minutes of that hour, or $1.04^4 = 1.17$.) However, shorter door-to-needle times were also associated with a wide variety of the measured baseline patient and hospital characteristics.

Comment: The inference that the association is causal thus depends on the assumption that the statistical model adequately adjusted for all of these differences and that there were no significant differences in unmeasured characteristics related to mortality (Chapter 10). The main exposure variable in this study, door-to-needle time, was carefully measured in the participants as part of the GWTG-Stroke quality-improvement project. If door-to-needle time had been measured by the research team rather than hospital quality-improvement staff, and/or if the patients had provided consent to be in the study, it seems likely that the investigators would have called this study a prospective cohort study rather than a retrospective cohort study.

TABLE 8.2 ADVANTAGES AND DISADVANTAGES OF FEATURES OF COHORT STUDIES THAT MAKE THEM MORE PROSPECTIVE

FEATURE	ADVANTAGES (+) AND DISADVANTAGES (−)
Investigators recruit eligible participants into the cohort	+ Specification of enrollment criteria and control over recruitment eligibility
	− Expense of recruitment, data and specimen collection, etc.
Investigators check for the outcome at baseline and exclude anyone who has already had it	+ Avoids having outcome precede (or even cause) the exposure
	− Baseline physical measurement of endpoints might be expensive
	− Time and expense of screening more people for enrollment than qualify for the study
Investigators measure exposures and covariates, rather than relying on previous measurements	+ Allows investigators to maximize accuracy and precision of measurements
	+ Allows investigators to minimize missing data on exposure and covariates
	− Time and expense to make these measurements
Exposures measured before outcomes occur	+ Prevents the outcome from affecting measurement of exposure
Investigators measure outcomes as they occur or at the end of follow-up, rather than relying on measurements of outcome that have already occurred	+ Prevents the outcome from affecting measurement of exposure
	+ Allows greater control over ascertainment of outcomes
	+ May reduce missing data on outcome
	− Time consuming (must wait for outcomes to occur) and expensive

measurements of predictor and outcome variables prospectively gives the investigator much more control over the *quality* of the measurements. For example, cadmium levels are best measured in whole blood collected in special metal-free tubes, whereas a retrospective study might have stored only serum and plasma in regular tubes. Similarly, in a prospective study, participants could be examined by a neurologist biannually for 10 years using a standardized instrument to ascertain whether peripheral neuropathy had developed, whereas a retrospective study might rely on diagnoses of peripheral neuropathy in the electronic medical record. You can see why the prospective study would be of higher quality but would be much more costly and take much longer to complete.

To make matters more complicated, nearly all prospective studies also measure predictors that started or occurred before the study began, for example, by asking participants about a prior history of binge drinking. Although that predictor was measured retrospectively (looking backward), because this measurement occurred at the onset of the study, neither knowledge nor occurrence of the outcome (eg, neuropathy) could have affected its occurrence or measurement.

Moreover, data from prospective studies are often used to answer research questions that the investigators had not considered when the study began. For example, in the Study of Osteoporotic Fractures, we studied whether low bone density was associated with an increase in the risk of stroke (15). Although bone density was measured at baseline using a strict protocol, strokes were not originally adjudicated as outcomes. They needed to be validated subsequently by a review of medical records, which were obtained only in those women who reported being hospitalized for a stroke. This was a less rigorous method of stroke ascertainment than if all participants had undergone regular neurologic evaluations and a standard evaluation for stroke in the event of any sudden neurologic symptoms.

Finally, even case-control studies (Chapter 9)—in which the outcomes occur before the study begins, so they are usually thought of as retrospective—may have prospective features. For example, the investigators can create a rigorous case definition and enroll cases meeting that definition as they occur. Similarly, predictors (eg, from previous driving records) may have been measured before the outcomes occurred. This approach increases validity because it prevents the outcome from affecting the predictor or its measurement.

When determining the "prospectiveness" of a study, it isn't always obvious when a study *begins*. In this context, what matters most is when the study's key predictors and outcomes occur, and if and when the investigator starts to measure them rigorously. For example, an ongoing cohort study might add a new measurement (say, performance on a balance test) at the second follow-up visit. Subsequently, an investigator might study whether self-reported insomnia at baseline affects balance. However, unless insomnia was of major interest as a predictor when the baseline data were collected, it may not have been measured rigorously. In addition, the absence of information about balance at baseline means that there will be uncertainty whether insomnia preceded any difficulty with balance.

Range of Complexity of Cohort Studies

Cohort studies can range from simple to complex (Table 8.3). The simplest cohort studies measure predictors only at baseline, have a short enough follow-up period that loss to follow-up is not a concern, and simply compare the cumulative incidence (risk) of the outcome between people with different values of predictor variables at the end of the study (Figure 8.2). For example, in a study of predictors of survival to hospital discharge in the early months of the COVID-19 pandemic (16), the outcome was known on all participants and the time course was short, so this design was suitable.

The next level of complexity takes follow-up time into account and measures outcomes as they occur, but still measures exposures only at entry into the cohort (Figure 8.3). These studies can account for differential follow-up time and loss to follow-up, as commonly occurs when studies last for more than a few months or when participants are hard to reach. They do this by considering not just the number of people at risk, but also the time they were at risk; the

TABLE 8.3 FEATURES OF SIMPLE VERSUS MORE COMPLEX COHORT STUDIES

LEVEL OF COMPLEXITY	MEASUREMENT OF EXPOSURE AND COVARIATES	MEASUREMENT OF OUTCOMES	DEALING WITH LOSS TO FOLLOW-UP	MEASURE OF INCIDENCE	MEASURES OF ASSOCIATION	MULTIVARIABLE ANALYSIS
Simple	At baseline only	At end of study	Must be minimal for study to be valid; sensitivity analyses	Cumulative incidence; incidence proportion (eg, cases per 100 at risk)	Risk ratio, odds ratio	Logistic regression
Moderate	At baseline only	As they occur or as determined periodically	Participants are censored when lost to follow-up (f/u); sensitivity analyses	Incidence rate (eg, cases per 100 person-years at risk)	Incidence rate ratio or hazard ratio	Poisson or Cox regression
Complex	At baseline with periodic updating; exposure and covariate levels may change over time, but covariates are not affected by the exposure of interest	As they occur or as determined periodically	Patients are censored when lost to f/u; sensitivity analyses	Incidence rate (eg, cases per 100 person-years at risk)	Hazard ratio	Cox model with time-dependent covariates
Most complex	At baseline with periodic updating; exposure and covariate levels may change over time, and covariates may be affected by exposure of interest	As they occur or as determined periodically	Patients are censored when lost to f/u; sensitivity analyses	Incidence rate (eg, cases per 100 person-years at risk)	Hazard ratio	Advanced (and difficult) methods such as marginal structural models. Consider a simpler design!

product of these two is the **person-time** at risk. Analyses of such studies compare **rates**, which have person-time at risk in the denominator, rather than risks, which have only people at risk in the denominator (see Section "Approach to Analyzing Cohort Studies"). These studies must account for **censoring** of participants—meaning incomplete knowledge about their outcome—because some participants will be lost to follow-up or because the study may end before they have had the outcome.

When measurements of predictors are periodically updated (Figure 8.4), the analysis becomes more complicated (and less intuitive) because a simple comparison between exposed and unexposed persons is no longer possible: The same person can contribute person-time at different levels of exposure during different time periods of the study. For example, a participant might start doing crossword puzzles (the exposure of interest) halfway through the study. Thus, analyses tend to compare the risk of events in exposed versus unexposed *person-time*, rather than in exposed and unexposed *people*. This can be especially challenging if the effects of exposure are

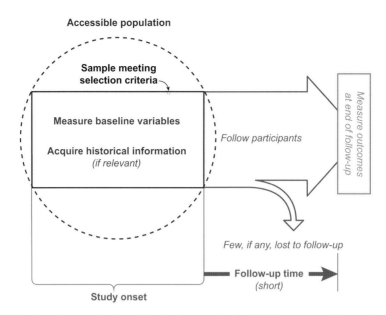

■ **FIGURE 8.2 Simple cohort study**. In a simple cohort study, the initial steps are similar to those for a cross-sectional study (Figure 8.1). Then the steps are to:
• Follow all participants for a specified period and
• Identify participants who developed the outcome (or repeat the measurement of outcome variable) at the end of the period.

delayed, and thus the past history of the exposure is also relevant. Furthermore, if outcomes are being measured as they occur, but predictors are being updated only periodically, it is possible that the values of predictors at the time the outcome occurred are different from what they were when they were last measured. This is illustrated poignantly in an unfortunate example from the Nurses' Health Study (NHS), Example 8.4.

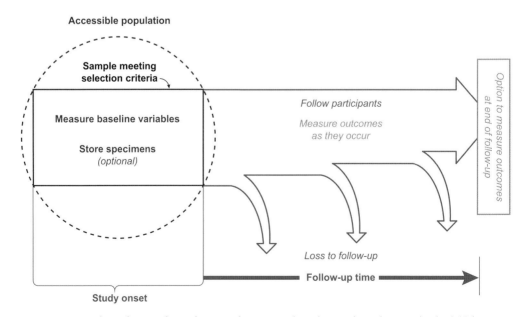

• **FIGURE 8.3 Moderately complex cohort study**. In a moderately complex cohort study, the initial steps are similar to those for a simple cohort study (Figure 8.2), except that investigators:
• Follow all participants until they develop the outcome, are lost to follow-up or the study ends; and
• Keep track of when each of these events occurs.

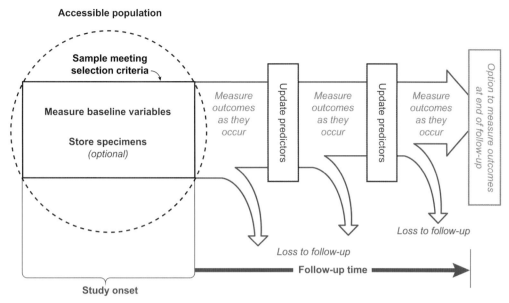

■ **FIGURE 8.4 Complex cohort study**. In a complex cohort study, the steps are similar to those for a moderately complex cohort study (Figure 8.3), except that the investigators:
• Make repeated measurements to update predictor variables; and
• May analyze the data taking into account the most recent values as well as past values of predictor variables.

Example 8.4 A Costly Error from Studying Prevalent Use and Trying Too Hard To Be "Prospective"

One of the great failures of 20th century epidemiology was the promotion of postmenopausal hormone therapy to increase longevity. Multiple observational studies had found that women who reported taking these hormones had lower rates of heart disease, including the Nurses' Health Study, which reported in the New England Journal of Medicine that women who took estrogen with progestin had an adjusted relative risk of 0.39 (95% CI: 0.19 to 0.78) for major coronary heart disease (17).

What went wrong: The study compared *prevalent users* of hormones to nonusers, which is problematic for reasons discussed in the section "Cohort Studies of Treatments or Interventions" (p. 128). But there was also an error in determining timing of exposure that led to cardiovascular events in the first year or two after starting hormone treatment being counted as if they had occurred in women not exposed to hormones!

This happened because exposure to hormone therapy was based on the questionnaires returned by the study participants and *only updated every 2 years*. A woman who indicated that she had not been taking hormones in 1980 but had started taking them in 1981 was counted as a nonuser until she returned the 1982 questionnaire, when (if she was still taking hormones) her time would start to be counted as a user. If she had had a coronary event during that first year on hormones, it would have been counted as an event in a nonuser, even though the hormones may have caused it!

This **misclassification** of exposure was intentional. As described in Table 8.2, one of the features of a study that make it more prospective is if the measurement of the exposure precedes the outcome. If women had a coronary event before reporting the hormone use that preceded it, the study would not have been as prospective. The authors wrote, "*To maintain the prospective nature of the study*, hormone use (including duration) during each 2-year period was established from women's reports *at the start of the period*; thus, we probably underestimate duration of use by an average of 1 year" (18).

What the investigators did not realize—until it was suggested by randomized trials—was that hormone use seems to increase coronary events primarily in the first year or two. When the NHS was analyzed more like a series of target trials, in which hormone therapy *initiators* were compared with *noninitiators*, this early adverse effect became apparent (19).

Finally, if one is studying the effect of an exposure (perhaps to a treatment, like a statin drug) that is both caused by a covariate, such as a high level of low-density lipoprotein (LDL)-cholesterol, and alters the level of that covariate (as statin drugs reduce LDL-cholesterol levels), the design and interpretation of cohort studies are most complex. The advanced methods needed to analyze the data from these studies make them unappealing for most investigators and reports of their results opaque and unconvincing to most readers.

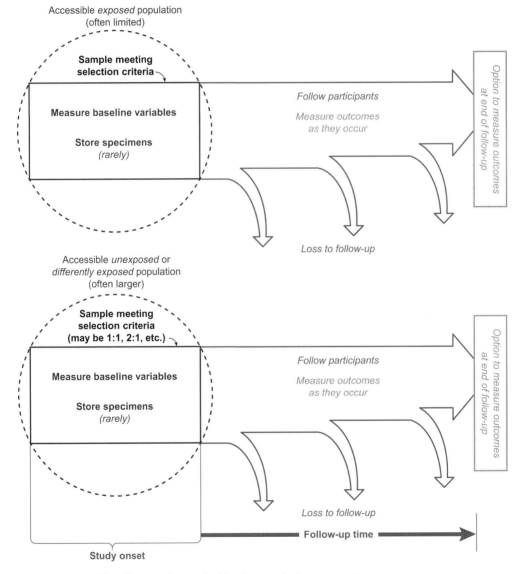

■ **FIGURE 8.5 Double-cohort study**. In a double-cohort study the steps are to:
• Select two cohorts from populations with different levels of the exposure (main predictor), but otherwise meeting the same inclusion and exclusion criteria;
• Measure other predictors at baseline; and
• Measure outcome variables as they occur or at the end of follow-up.

Double-Cohort Studies, Multiple-Cohort Studies, and External Controls

A **double-cohort study** involves two separate cohorts of participants with different levels of exposure. They may be sampled from different populations, as in Figure 8.5, or (preferably) from the same population, in which case the double-cohort study is called **nested**. The investigator may choose equal-sized cohorts or (especially if the number of some exposed participants is limited) increase power by sampling a larger number from the other (eg, unexposed) population, for example, with a 2:1 or 3:1 ratio of unexposed to exposed. (A similar strategy, involving oversampling of controls relative to cases, was illustrated in Chapter 6.) Sometimes, the comparison cohort is selected by matching on values of some variables (eg, age and sex) in the exposed cohort. Such matching is more often done in case-control studies, as discussed in Chapters 9 and 10.

After defining exposed and unexposed cohorts, the investigator measures baseline levels of other covariates, follows the cohorts, and assesses outcomes either as they occur, at the end of follow-up, or at specified time intervals after exposure. Because the level of exposure defines the follow-up groups, these studies are generally simple or only moderately complex; there is usually no need to make repeated measures of covariates.

The use of two different samples of participants in a double-cohort design should not be confused with the use of two samples in the case-control design (Chapter 9). In a double-cohort study, the two groups of participants are chosen on the basis of the level of the exposure, whereas

Example 8.5 Example of a Nested Double-Cohort Study

There are concerns that azithromycin, an antibiotic commonly prescribed to outpatients, might increase the risk of sudden cardiac death. No such concern has been reported for amoxicillin, another antibiotic commonly prescribed to outpatients. To investigate this risk of azithromycin, Zaroff et al. (20):

1. **Identified a cohort from which to draw their participants:** Patients enrolled in one of two large health plans (Kaiser Permanente of Northern or Southern California) with electronic medical records of encounters and prescriptions from January 1, 1998, to December 31, 2014.
2. **Defined exposure groups:** The authors identified outpatient prescriptions for either azithromycin ($N=$ ~1.7 million) or amoxicillin ($N=$ ~6.1 million) among patients who had been enrolled in the health plan with prescription benefit coverage for at least 12 months before their prescription date. They excluded anyone who had serious underlying medical conditions prior to the prescription date. Multiple demographic and clinical potential confounding variables (Chapter 10) were obtained from the electronic medical record as well.
3. **Defined and measured outcomes in the two exposure groups:** The primary outcomes were cardiovascular death 0 to 5 days and 6 to 10 days from the prescription. These were obtained from diagnosis codes on death certificates, with cardiovascular deaths and a random sample of noncardiovascular deaths adjudicated by a panel of cardiologists.

The authors found that those who had received azithromycin had significantly higher risk of cardiovascular death within 5 days (adjusted hazard ratio 1.82; 95% CI, 1.23 to 2.67), but not at 6 to 10 days. However, they cautioned that the causality of this association was unclear, particularly because they found a similar association with noncardiovascular mortality (adjusted hazard ratio 2.17; 95% CI, 1.44 to 3.26).

Comment: The retrospective design allowed the authors to capture rare events from a large population over a 16-year period, providing adequate power to test their hypothesis. The exposures and outcomes are likely to have been measured accurately.

in a case-control study the two groups are chosen on the basis of the presence or absence of an outcome. (Unfortunately, sometimes the exposed and unexposed groups in these studies are mislabeled as "cases" and "controls," and the study is erroneously referred to as a "case-control study.")

Multiple-cohort studies are similar to double-cohort studies but include more than two cohorts, either to allow the same exposed cohort to be compared with two or more unexposed cohorts or to allow more than one exposed cohort to be compared with a single unexposed cohort. For example, in the Jaundice and Infant Feeding (JIFee) study, the investigators compared a single unexposed cohort (randomly selected from the birth cohorts from which the exposed cohorts arose) with two different exposed cohorts, one that had high bilirubin levels and the other that had been readmitted to the hospital for dehydration (Example 8.6).

In a variation on the multiple-cohort design, the outcome rate in one or more exposed cohorts can be compared with the outcome rate from *external controls*, obtained from census, **registry**, or vital statistics data. For example, several studies have examined suicide rates of male and female physicians and found female physician suicide rates higher and male physician suicide rates lower than those of the general female and male populations (23).

Cohort Studies of Treatments or Interventions

Although the fundamental structure of cohort studies is the same regardless of whether the exposure being studied is a risk factor or a treatment for disease, there are enough differences to warrant this separate section about cohort studies of disease treatments and a separate tool for evaluating the risk of bias in such studies (24).

One difference is that unlike most risk factors for disease, disease treatments can—and generally should—be studied with randomized trials. Because cohort studies, particularly retrospective cohort studies, may be more ethical or feasible than randomized trials, they still have a role in evaluating treatments, but it should usually be a secondary one.

Example 8.6 (Nested) Multiple-Cohort Design

To determine whether substantial neonatal jaundice or dehydration has subtle adverse effects on neurodevelopment, investigators from UCSF and Kaiser Permanente of Northern California (KPNC) (21, 22) undertook a triple-cohort study. The steps in performing the study were to:

1. **Identify cohorts with different exposures.** The investigators used electronic databases to identify term and near-term newborns who were born between 1995 and 1998 at KPNC hospitals ($N = 106,627$) and:
   a. had a maximum total serum bilirubin level of ≥25 mg/dL ($N = 147$), or
   b. were readmitted for dehydration with a serum sodium of ≥150 mEq/L or weight loss of $\geq12\%$ from birth ($N = 197$), or
   c. were randomly selected from the birth cohort ($N = 428$; no exposed participants were sampled)
2. **Apply exclusion criteria.** Because this step required review of paper charts and contacting primary care providers, it could not be done until cohorts had been sampled. (Seven participants with hyperbilirubinemia, 15 with dehydration, and 9 controls were excluded.)
3. **Collect outcome data.** The investigators used electronic databases to search for diagnoses of neurologic disorders and did full neurodevelopmental examinations at the age of 5 for consenting participants (blinded to which of the three cohorts the participant belonged to).

Neither hyperbilirubinemia nor dehydration was associated with subtle adverse outcomes.

When designing cohort studies of treatments, it is helpful to have the cohort study emulate as closely as possible a randomized trial (called the "target trial" by Hernán and Robins) (25) that would have been designed to answer the research question (24). For example, what would be the inclusion and exclusion criteria for such a trial? If there are people who would have been excluded from the target trial because randomization to either one treatment arm or the other would be unethical, those people probably do not belong in a cohort study of that treatment. Similarly, in a randomized trial, the starting point for follow-up is generally clear: It is the date of randomization. In complex cohort studies of treatments, this is not so clear. Among participants who begin taking a medication, exposed follow-up time can begin at the time they fill their first prescription. But when does follow-up time begin for those who do not begin taking a medication?

It is helpful if there is a triggering event that can act as a starting point that would make one eligible for a target trial. For example, if some patients are started on medication after a seizure and others are not, the seizure could be the starting point for follow-up in both treated and untreated people; one could imagine a target trial for which people would become eligible after a seizure. Similarly, a triggering event could be a second high hemoglobin A1c level in people with diabetes or a second high blood pressure reading in people with hypertension, each of which could be an inclusion criterion for a target trial comparing medication changes among people whose disease is not well controlled with a single medicine.

Once the timing of eligibility for the target trial has been established, as described previously, events that happen subsequently should not be used to alter the defined exposure groups, just as participants randomized to treatment need to be analyzed according to their randomization group. ("Once randomized, always analyzed"; see Chapter 11.) For example, a study of the effect of antibiotics on length of hospital stay in patients hospitalized with asthma (initially) allowed people in the exposed group to have been started on antibiotics *after* the day of admission (which would have been the randomization date in a target trial) and required that they be treated with antibiotics for at least 2 days. If patients started on antibiotics were discharged before they had been treated for 2 days, they were not included in the antibiotic group (26). The investigators reported that treatment with antibiotics was associated with a 1-day longer median length of stay. When the possible bias introduced by their study design was pointed out (27) and they redid their analysis, counting only antibiotics started on day 1 and not requiring a minimum duration of antibiotic treatment in the exposed group, the difference in median length of stay disappeared (28).

The bias that resulted from patients in the exposed group not being susceptible to discharge until after receiving 2 days of antibiotics is called **immortal time bias** (27, 29, 30), because the bias was initially described in studies in which exposed participants were given credit for surviving time periods during which the design of the study made it impossible for them to die (31). The target trial framework can help identify and prevent immortal time bias and "other self-inflicted injuries in observational studies" (32).

What about people who are already receiving the treatment (eg, taking the medication) at the onset of the study? So-called **prevalent users** are problematic to study for several reasons (33-36). First, people who are adherent to prescribed medication will be overrepresented among prevalent users: Those who started medication and stopped for whatever reason before the study began will not be counted as users. This is a problem because people who take prescribed medication have more favorable outcomes, even when that medication is a placebo and investigators control for other salutary factors (37, 38)! This is not a small effect: The pooled odds ratio for mortality among good adherers to *placebo* in a meta-analysis was 0.56 (95% CI, 0.43 to 0.74) (37). Thus, comparing prevalent users with nonusers will tend to make any medication (including placebo!) look beneficial.

Second, participants may be more likely to receive a treatment for a variety of uncommonly measured reasons, such as an interest in prevention or a close relationship with a clinician. These factors could influence physicians' prescription of the treatment and also affect the risk of the outcome, leading to a "healthy user" effect. For example, in cohort studies, women who are prescribed drug treatments for osteoporosis appear to have 25% to 60% lower overall mortality than comparable untreated women, but no such benefit is observed in large, randomized placebo-controlled trials (39).

Third, including prevalent users will miss early adverse effects from starting a medication. This is important when adverse effects (including deaths) occur early. For example, it appears that women taking hormone replacement therapy have higher rates of cardiovascular disease mainly in the first year after starting that therapy (19, 40).

Fourth, studying prevalent users complicates control of confounding (Chapter 10), because the values of confounding variables may already have been affected by the treatment when the study begins. We alluded to this problem in the discussion of Table 8.2, when we used the example of an investigation into the efficacy of a statin drug in a study with multiple measurements of LDL-cholesterol. Similar considerations would apply to controlling for viral load in a study of prevalent antiretroviral drug users and to controlling for bone density in a study of drugs for osteoporosis. In each case, the baseline value of the confounding variable may have already been affected by the treatment, so some of the benefit of the treatment could be hidden by controlling for the confounder.

Finally, it is not possible to map a study that compares prevalent users and nonusers to a target trial. If someone is not yet taking a medication, one could imagine a target trial that would compare those who start medication with those who do not; this trial would inform the decision whether to start medication. For those who are already taking medication, one could imagine a target trial that would compare those who continue the medication with those who stop it; this would inform the decision whether to stop medication. But there is no target trial that would compare the effect of *being on* medication to not being on it.

Strengths and Weaknesses of Cohort Studies

A major strength of the cohort design is that, unlike cross-sectional designs, it allows the calculation of incidence—the rate or proportion who develop a condition over time (Table 8.1). The longitudinal approach can also be used to examine changes in continuous outcomes, such as blood pressure, over time. Measuring levels of the predictor before the outcome occurs establishes the time sequence of the variables, which strengthens the process of inferring the causal basis of an association.

All cohort studies share the general weakness of observational studies (relative to clinical trials), namely that causal inference is challenging, and interpretation is often muddied by the influences of confounding variables (Chapter 10). Two additional weaknesses of prospective cohort studies are their expense and their inefficiency for studying rare outcomes. Even diseases we think of as relatively common, such as lung cancer, happen at such a low rate in any given year that large numbers of people must be followed for long periods to observe enough outcomes to produce meaningful results. Cohort designs are more efficient for dichotomous outcomes that are more common and immediate, and for continuous outcomes.

Although they are prone to several biases in studying the efficacy and safety of treatments, cohort studies may be the only feasible way to estimate the efficacy of some treatments. For example, when the condition is rare or there is strong belief in the efficacy of a treatment for a condition that has few or no other treatment options, it may be impossible to conduct a randomized blinded trial with sufficient sample size.

Some argue that analyzing the effect of treatments in observational studies that include people who would not have been eligible for clinical trials provides better "real world" evidence about the effectiveness and safety of treatment. Such studies might discover adverse effects, particularly in older patients with other medical conditions that could not have been found in clinical trials. However, favorable reports of effectiveness in "real world" cohort studies are prone to the many biases described previously and must be considered with skepticism.

Retrospective cohort studies have many of the strengths of prospective cohort studies, and they have the advantage of being much less costly and time consuming. The participants are already assembled, baseline measurements have already been made, and the follow-up period has already taken place. The main disadvantages are the limited control the investigator has over the approach to sampling and follow-up of the population, and over the nature and the quality of the measurements. The existing data may be incomplete, inaccurate, or measured in ways that are not ideal for answering the research question.

The double- or multiple-cohort design may be the only feasible approach for studying rare exposures to potential occupational and environmental hazards. Using data from a census or registry as the external control group has the additional advantage of being population based and economical. Otherwise, the strengths of this design are similar to those of other cohort studies. A concern with multiple-cohort studies is that when participants with different exposures are sampled from separate populations, there is a greater risk of **selection bias** because the cohorts may differ in important ways (besides the exposure variable) that influence the outcomes. Although some of these differences, such as age and race, can be matched or used to adjust the findings statistically, other differences in the two underlying populations (eg, geographic location) may make exposed and unexposed groups not comparable. This is why **nested multicohort studies**, in which both exposed and unexposed cohorts are drawn from the same population, are more desirable, as was done in the azithromycin/amoxicillin study (Example 8.5) and the JIFee study (Example 8.6). If ascertainment of outcomes is difficult or expensive, and the exposure is rare, a nested double- or multiple-cohort study can be much more efficient than studying the entire cohort.

Tools to assess the risk of bias have been proposed for both cohort studies of exposures (41) and of interventions (24). Investigators planning a cohort study can review these tools to make sure they address at least any easily remedied threats to validity in the design stage of the study.

Approach to Analyzing Cohort Studies

Measures of Outcome Frequency

Risks, **odds**, and **rates** are estimates of the frequency of a dichotomous outcome in participants who have been followed for a certain period. These three measures are closely related, sharing the same numerator—the number of participants who develop the dichotomous outcome. Implicit in these three measures is the concept of being *at risk*, which means that the participant did not already have the outcome of interest at the beginning of the study. In a prospective study of the predictors of angina, a woman who had angina at baseline would not be at risk, because she already had the outcome of interest. The observed *risk* of an outcome is just the number of people in whom the outcome occurred divided by the number at risk. The observed *odds* of an outcome are the number in whom the outcome occurred divided by the number in whom it did not occur; odds are also risk/(1 − risk).

In many cohort studies, **loss to follow-up**, deaths, or other events that preclude ascertainment of the outcome may occur. To account for this, the investigator must measure the amount of **person-time** each participant contributes, from entry into the cohort until she either develops the outcome of interest or is **censored** due to loss to follow-up or death. In any group (say those exposed), the **incidence rate** is the number of outcomes divided by the sum of that group's person-time at risk.

Consider a study of 1000 people who were followed for 2 years to see who developed lung cancer and among whom 50 new cases occurred each year. Risk, odds, and rate are shown in Table 8.4.

Of the three measures, risk is the easiest to understand because of its everyday familiarity—the risk of getting lung cancer in 2 years was 100 out of a thousand (10%). Odds are harder to grasp intuitively—the odds of getting lung cancer were 100 to 900, or 0.111. For rare outcomes, the odds are quantitatively similar to risk; the 10% risk in the current example is at about the upper limit of when the risk and odds are similar. The rate of the outcome takes into account that those who had the outcome in the first year were no longer at risk in the second and therefore should not be included in the denominator for year 2. Thus, the *rate* of the outcome in the second year (50 cases/~925 person-years) was a little higher than in the first.

TABLE 8.4 SIMPLIFIED CALCULATION OF RISK, ODDS, AND RATE FOR A STUDY OF 1000 PEOPLE FOLLOWED FOR 2 YEARS WITH 50 NEW CASES PER YEAR.

STATISTIC	FORMULA	CALCULATION
Risk	N who develop outcome/N at risk	100/1000 = 0.10 (or 10%)
Odds	N who develop outcome/N who do not develop the outcome	100/900 = 0.111
Rate	N who develop the outcome/Person-time at risk[a]	100/1900 person-years = 5.3% per year or 5.3 per 100 person-years

[a]The denominator is approximately the number of person-years at risk in the first year (there were 1000 participants at the beginning and 950 at the end, so about 975) plus the number at risk in the second year (950 at the beginning and 900 at the end, so about 925) = 1900 person-years. Note that in this example the rate is increasing slightly over time because the number of cases per year is constant, whereas the number of people at risk is decreasing.

Some outcomes can occur more than once in the same person, such as repeated episodes of the same disease (eg, strep throat) or outcomes that reflect exacerbations of disease, such as admissions to the hospital for heart failure. If most of the participants have 0 or 1 outcome, little is lost and some simplicity is gained by making a dichotomous variable for 0 versus ≥1 episode. On the other hand, if many participants have multiple outcomes, the average count of outcomes per person or average counts divided by person-time at risk can be calculated.[2]

Measures of Association

In studies comparing two groups, the **risk difference** is just that: The difference in risk between groups, customarily expressed as the risk in the exposed group minus the risk in the unexposed group. If the exposure prevents, rather than causing the outcome (perhaps because it is a treatment), the risk difference will be negative, in which case its absolute value is called the **absolute risk reduction**.

The quotient of the risks in the two groups, again customarily expressed as the risk in the exposed divided by the risk in the unexposed, is the **risk ratio** or **relative risk (RR)**. The **odds ratio (OR)**, the ratio of the odds of the outcome in the exposed to the odds in the unexposed, is similar to the risk ratio *when the outcome is rare*. However, because (especially when outcomes are common) odds tend to be confusing, odds ratios are best avoided in the analysis of cohort studies. The exception to this guidance is when a multivariable method called **logistic regression** is used, because that method quantifies associations using odds ratios.[3]

As is true of the risk ratio, the **rate ratio** can be estimated as the quotient of rates in people who do and do not have a particular risk factor. The **Cox proportional hazard model** provides a method for multivariable analysis of data of this form (sometimes called "time to event" data); it allows estimation of **hazard ratios**, which are similar to rate ratios and commonly used as the measure of association in **cohort studies**.

Maximizing Follow-Up

Follow-up of the entire cohort is important, and prospective studies should take several steps to achieve this goal (Table 8.5). Good relationships between investigators, study staff, and participants, and positive and engaging experiences at study visits are essential to complete follow-up; study participants often look forward to contacts with staff or the study. These relationships can be strengthened by such things as newsletters that include personal profiles, recipes, or other news that reinforces attachment to the study.

---

[2]It is important not to mix the person-time from different people together if some people have more than one outcome event, because multiple outcomes on the same person are not independent. If that last sentence expresses anything unfamiliar to you, it would be a good idea to consult with a statistician.

[3]Odds ratios are often used in analyses of cross-sectional and case-control studies (Chapter 9), in which situation they may be ratios of prevalence odds rather than incidence odds.

TABLE 8.5 STRATEGIES FOR MINIMIZING LOSS TO FOLLOW-UP

During Enrollment

1. Build relationships between study staff and participants
   - Make the baseline and follow-up visits interesting, enjoyable, and engaging.
2. Exclude those likely to be lost:
   - Planning to move
   - Uncertainty about willingness to return
   - Ill health or fatal disease unrelated to research question
3. Obtain information to allow future tracking:
   - Address, telephone number (mobile phone numbers are particularly useful), and email address of participant
   - Social Security/Medicare number and permission to use these for future outcome tracking
   - Name, address, telephone number, and email address of close friends or relatives who do not live with the participant
   - Name, address, telephone number, and email address of physician(s)

During Follow-up

1. Periodic contact with participants to collect information, provide results, and be supportive:
   - By telephone: may require calls during weekends and evenings
   - By mail: repeated mailings by email or with stamped, self-addressed return cards
   - Newsletters, birthday cards, token gifts
   - Provide results of tests that may be taken during follow-up, if it would not influence outcomes.
2. For those who are not reached by phone or mail:
   - Contact friends, relatives, or physicians.
   - Request forwarding addresses from postal service.
   - Seek address through other public sources, such as telephone directories and the internet, and (if permission initially obtained) a credit bureau search.
   - For participants receiving Medicare, collect data about hospital discharges from the Social Security Administration.
   - Determine vital status from the state health department or National Death Index.

At All Times

1. Treat study participants with appreciation, kindness, and respect, helping them to understand the research question so they will want to join as partners in making the study successful.

For studies that require in-person measurements, participants who plan to move out of reach during the study should be excluded at the outset. The investigator should collect information early on that can help to find participants who move or die. This information would include the address, telephone number, and email address of the participant, her personal physician, and close friends or relatives who do not live in the same house. Mobile telephone numbers and personal email addresses are particularly helpful, because they often remain unchanged when participants, friends, or family move or change jobs. If feasible, obtaining the participant's social security number will help in determining the vital status of those lost to follow-up and obtaining hospital discharge information from the Social Security Administration for participants who receive Medicare. Periodic contact with the participants at least once or twice a year helps in keeping track of them and may improve the timeliness and accuracy of recording the outcomes of interest. Finding participants for follow-up assessments sometimes requires persistent and repeated efforts by mail, email, telephone, or even house calls.

Despite investigators' best efforts, follow-up in most studies is less than 100%. In that case, **sensitivity analyses** can examine whether the conclusions from the study are sensitive to assumptions about the outcomes of those lost to follow-up—such as by redoing analyses assuming none of the exposed and all of the unexposed who were lost to follow-up had the outcome or vice versa. If the study's conclusions are not sensitive to assumptions about the outcomes of those lost to follow-up, the study will be more convincing.

■ SUMMARY

1. In a **cross-sectional study**, the variables are all measured at a single point in time, with no structural distinction between predictors and outcomes. Cross-sectional studies yield weaker evidence for causality than cohort studies because the predictor variable is not shown to precede the outcome.

2. Cross-sectional studies are valuable for providing descriptive information about **prevalence** and have the advantage of avoiding the time, expense, and dropout problems of a follow-up design; they are often useful as the **first step of a cohort study** or experiment and can be linked in independently sampled serial surveys to reveal population changes over time.

3. In **cohort studies**, a group of participants identified at the outset is **followed over time** to describe the incidence or natural history of a condition and to discover predictors (risk factors) for various outcomes.

4. Cohort studies are typically divided into prospective and retrospective cohort studies, but these terms are used inconsistently; it is important to specify how and when the exposure and outcome variables will be measured to fully capture the risk of bias.

5. **Prospective cohort studies** generally begin at the outset of follow-up and may require large numbers of participants to be recruited and followed for long periods. They provide greater control over measurements but are often time consuming and expensive.

6. This disadvantage can sometimes be overcome by identifying a **retrospective cohort** in which measurements of predictor variables and outcomes have already occurred, although this provides less control over measurements.

7. The **multiple-cohort design**, which compares the incidence of outcomes in cohorts that differ in the nature or level of the exposure, is useful for studying the effects of rare and occupational exposures. A nested retrospective multiple-cohort design can be a good design for studying the effects of rare exposures within a population.

8. The risk of bias in **cohort studies of treatments** or interventions can be reduced by modeling them on a target trial, the randomized trial of the treatment you would do if it were feasible.

9. **Risks, odds, and rates** are three ways to estimate the frequency of a dichotomous outcome during follow-up. Among these, incidence rates, which take into account **person-time** at risk, are the basis for modern approaches to calculating multivariable hazard ratios using Cox proportional hazard models.

10. The strengths of a cohort design can be undermined by **incomplete follow-up**. Losses can be minimized by excluding people at the outset who may not be available for follow-up, by collecting baseline information that facilitates tracking and by staying in touch with all participants regularly.

REFERENCES

1. Drouin-Chartier JP, Chen S, Li Y, et al. Egg consumption and risk of cardiovascular disease: three large prospective US cohort studies, systematic review, and updated meta-analysis. *BMJ.* 2020;368:m513.

2. Centers for Disease Control NCHS. *National Health and Nutrition Examination Survey (NHANES): History 2020* [cited 2020 Dec 15]. https://www.cdc.gov/nchs/nhanes/history.htm.

3. Andersen RE, Crespo CJ, Bartlett SJ, Cheskin LJ, Pratt M. Relationship of physical activity and television watching with body weight and level of fatness among children: results from the Third National Health and Nutrition Examination Survey. *JAMA.* 1998;279(12):938-942.

4. Sargent JD, Beach ML, Adachi-Mejia AM, et al. Exposure to movie smoking: its relation to smoking initiation among US adolescents. *Pediatrics.* 2005;116(5):1183-1191.

5. Morgenstern M, Sargent JD, Engels R, et al. Smoking in movies and adolescent smoking initiation: longitudinal study in six European countries. *Am J Prev Med.* 2013;44(4):339-344.

6. Dal Cin S, Stoolmiller M, Sargent JD. Exposure to smoking in movies and smoking initiation among black youth. *Am J Prev Med.* 2013;44(4):345-350.

7. Mejia R, Perez A, Pena L, et al. Smoking in movies and adolescent smoking initiation: a longitudinal study among Argentinian adolescents. *J Pediatr.* 2017;180:222-228.

8. Blackwell T, Yaffe K, Ancoli-Israel S, et al. Association of sleep characteristics and cognition in older community-dwelling men: the MrOS sleep study. *Sleep.* 2011;34(10):1347-1356.

9. Kalantar-Zadeh K, Abbott KC, Salahudeen AK, Kilpatrick RD, Horwich TB. Survival advantages of obesity in dialysis patients. *Am J Clin Nutr.* 2005;81(3):543-554.

10. McMillen RC, Gottlieb MA, Shaefer RM, Winickoff JP, Klein JD. Trends in electronic cigarette use among U.S. adults: use is increasing in both smokers and nonsmokers. *Nicotine Tob Res.* 2015;17(10):1195-1202.

11. Vandenbroucke JP. Prospective or retrospective: what's in a name? *BMJ.* 1991;302(6771):249-250.

12. Rothman KJ, Greenland S, Lash TL. *Modern Epidemiology.* 3rd ed. Wolters Kluwer Health/Lippincott Williams & Wilkins; 2008:758.

13. Bao Y, Bertoia ML, Lenart EB, et al. Origin, methods, and evolution of the three nurses' health studies. *Am J Public Health.* 2016;106(9):1573-1581.

14. Man S, Xian Y, Holmes DN, et al. Association between thrombolytic door-to-needle time and 1-year mortality and readmission in patients with acute ischemic stroke. *JAMA.* 2020;323(21):2170-2184.

15. Browner WS, Pressman AR, Nevitt MC, Cauley JA, Cummings SR. Association between low bone density and stroke in elderly women: the study of osteoporotic fractures. *Stroke.* 1993;24(7):940-946.

16. Evans DS, Kim KM, Jiang X, Jacobson J, Browner W, Cummings SR. Prediction of in-hospital mortality among adults with COVID-19 infection. *medRxiv.* 2021.

17. Grodstein F, Stampfer MJ, Manson JE, et al. Postmenopausal estrogen and progestin use and the risk of cardiovascular disease. *N Engl J Med.* 1996;335(7):453-461.

18. Grodstein F, Manson JE, Colditz GA, Willett WC, Speizer FE, Stampfer MJ. A prospective, observational study of postmenopausal hormone therapy and primary prevention of cardiovascular disease. *Ann Intern Med.* 2000;133(12):933-941.

19. Hernán MA, Alonso A, Logan R, et al. Observational studies analyzed like randomized experiments: an application to postmenopausal hormone therapy and coronary heart disease. *Epidemiology.* 2008;19(6):766-779.

20. Zaroff JG, Cheetham TC, Palmetto N, et al. Association of azithromycin use with cardiovascular mortality. *JAMA Netw Open.* 2020;3(6):e208199.

21. Newman TB, Liljestrand P, Jeremy RJ, et al. Outcomes among newborns with total serum bilirubin levels of 25 mg per deciliter or more. *N Engl J Med.* 2006;354(18):1889-1900.

22. Escobar GJ, Liljestrand P, Hudes ES, et al. Five-year neurodevelopmental outcome of neonatal dehydration. *J Pediatr.* 2007;151(2):127-133, 133 e1.

23. Duarte D, El-Hagrassy MM, Couto TCE, Gurgel W, Fregni F, Correa H. Male and female physician suicidality: a systematic review and meta-analysis. *JAMA Psychiatry.* 2020;77(6):587-597.

24. Sterne JA, Hernán MA, Reeves BC, et al. ROBINS-I: a tool for assessing risk of bias in non-randomised studies of interventions. *BMJ.* 2016;355:i4919.

25. Hernán MA, Robins JM. Using big data to emulate a target trial when a randomized trial is not available. *Am J Epidemiol.* 2016;183(8):758-764.

26. Stefan MS, Shieh MS, Spitzer KA, et al. Association of antibiotic treatment with outcomes in patients hospitalized for an asthma exacerbation treated with systemic corticosteroids. *JAMA Intern Med.* 2019;179(3):333-339 [original version, subsequently retracted].

27. Newman TB. Possible immortal time bias in study of antibiotic treatment and outcomes in patients hospitalized for asthma. *JAMA Intern Med.* 2021;181(4):568-569.

28. Stefan MS, Shieh M-S, Spitzer KA, et al. Association of antibiotic treatment with outcomes in patients hospitalized for an asthma exacerbation treated with systemic corticosteroids. *JAMA Intern Med.* 2019;179(3):333-339 [replaced version of retracted article].

29. Newman T, Kohn M. *Evidence-Based Diagnosis: An Introduction to Clinical Epidemiology.* 2nd ed. Cambridge University Press; 2020:231-243.

30. Newman TB. Antibiotic treatment for inpatient asthma exacerbations: what have we learned? *JAMA Intern Med.* 2021;181(4):427-428.

31. Suissa S. Immortal time bias in pharmaco-epidemiology. *Am J Epidemiol.* 2008;167(4):492-499.

32. Hernán MA, Sauer BC, Hernandez-Diaz S, Platt R, Shrier I. Specifying a target trial prevents immortal time bias and other self-inflicted injuries in observational analyses. *J Clin Epidemiol.* 2016;79:70-75.

33. Vandenbroucke J, Pearce N. Point: incident exposures, prevalent exposures, and causal inference: does limiting studies to persons who are followed from first exposure onward damage epidemiology? *Am J Epidemiol.* 2015;182(10):826-833.

34. Hernán MA. Counterpoint: epidemiology to guide decision-making: moving away from practice-free research. *Am J Epidemiol.* 2015;182(10):834-839.

35. Vandenbroucke J, Pearce N. Vandenbroucke and Pearce respond to "incident and prevalent exposures and causal inference". *Am J Epidemiol.* 2015;182(10):846-847.

36. Ray WA. Evaluating medication effects outside of clinical trials: new-user designs. *Am J Epidemiol.* 2003;158(9):915-920.

37. Simpson SH, Eurich DT, Majumdar SR, et al. A meta-analysis of the association between adherence to drug therapy and mortality. *BMJ*. 2006;333(7557):15.

38. Avins AL, Pressman A, Ackerson L, Rudd P, Neuhaus J, Vittinghoff E. Placebo adherence and its association with morbidity and mortality in the studies of left ventricular dysfunction. *J Gen Intern Med*. 2010;25(12):1275-1281.

39. Cummings SR, Lui LY, Eastell R, Allen IE. Association between drug treatments for patients with osteoporosis and overall mortality rates: a meta-analysis. *JAMA Intern Med*. 2019;179(11):1491-1500.

40. Hulley S, Grady D, Bush T, et al. Randomized trial of estrogen plus progestin for secondary prevention of coronary heart disease in postmenopausal women. Heart and Estrogen/progestin Replacement Study (HERS) Research Group. *JAMA*. 1998;280(7):605-613.

41. Bero L, Chartres N, Diong J, et al. The risk of bias in observational studies of exposures (ROBINS-E) tool: concerns arising from application to observational studies of exposures. *Syst Rev*. 2018;7(1):242.

APPENDIX 8A
Exercises for Chapter 8. Designing Cross-sectional and Cohort Studies

1. The research question is: "Do low vitamin B_{12} levels cause hip fractures in the elderly?"
   a. Briefly outline a way to address this research question using a prospective cohort study design.
   b. An alternative approach would be to take a sample from a geriatric clinic and compare vitamin B_{12} levels in those with a previous hip fracture to levels in (all) those who did not have a previous hip fracture. Compared with this cross-sectional approach, list at least one advantage and one disadvantage of a prospective cohort design.
   c. Could this research question be addressed as a retrospective cohort study? If so, how would this affect these advantages or disadvantages?
2. Sung et al. (1) examined the association between the frequency of urinary incontinence and depressive symptoms among 338 overweight or obese women at least 30 years old when they first enrolled in the PRIDE (Program to Reduce Incontinence by Diet and Exercise) clinical trial. They found that women with depressive symptoms ($N = 101$) reported a greater number of episodes of incontinence per week than women without depressive symptoms (28 vs 23; $P = 0.005$).
   a. What kind of study design was this?
   b. One possible explanation is that depression increases the frequency of urinary incontinence. What are some other explanations for this association, and how might changes in the study design help you sort them out?

REFERENCE

1. Sung VW, West DS, Hernandez AL. Association between urinary incontinence and depressive symptoms in overweight and obese women. *Am J Obstet Gynecol*. 2009;200(5):557.e1-557.e5.

CHAPTER 9

Designing Case-Control Studies

Thomas B. Newman and Warren S. Browner

In Chapter 8 we introduced cohort studies, in which the investigators follow a sample of participants over time to estimate the incidence of an outcome among people who were exposed (or not exposed) to various risk factors. In contrast, in a **case-control study** the investigator starts with a sample of people who have already had the outcome (the **cases**) and a sample without that outcome (the **controls**) and looks backward, measuring previous exposures in both groups to find differences that might explain why the cases developed the outcome and the controls did not.

For example, a case-control study might involve assembling a group of cases of ocular melanoma and a sample of healthy controls, after which data are gathered from each group about previous exposure to arc welding to estimate how that exposure affects that disease's risk (1). The case-control design is relatively inexpensive and particularly well suited to studying rare diseases and disease outbreaks.

This chapter also presents several variations on the case-control design. A **nested case-control** design compares incident cases that occur within a defined cohort with controls sampled from the remaining cohort. The nested case-cohort design allows a random sample of the *entire* cohort (including cases) to serve as the control group, often for several different sets of cases. Using an **incidence-density case-control** design allows investigators to take into account changes in risk factors over time and loss to follow-up. **Case-crossover** studies allow cases to serve as their own controls. The chapter ends with advice on choosing among the observational study designs discussed in Chapter 8 and this chapter.

■ CASE-CONTROL STUDY BASICS

Because most diseases are relatively uncommon, both cohort and cross-sectional studies of general population samples are expensive designs, requiring thousands of participants to identify risk factors for a rare disease like ocular melanoma. Although a **case series** of patients with the disease can identify an obvious risk factor (such as injection drug use for AIDS) using prior knowledge of the prevalence of the risk factor in the general population, for most risk factors it is necessary to assemble a reference group so that exposure to the risk factor in the cases can be compared with exposure in the controls.

In most of the ways described in Chapter 8, case-control studies are **retrospective**. The investigator identifies one group of people with the disease and another without it and then looks backward in both groups to measure predictors that predated the development of the disease (Figure 9.1). However, all the outcomes need not have occurred at the time the investigator begins the study. For example, for investigation of disease outbreaks, a team of epidemiologists may be dispatched to identify the cause of the outbreak while cases are still occurring. They may create a case definition and enroll new cases and controls prospectively as the cases occur, until the cause of the outbreak is identified (Example 9.1).

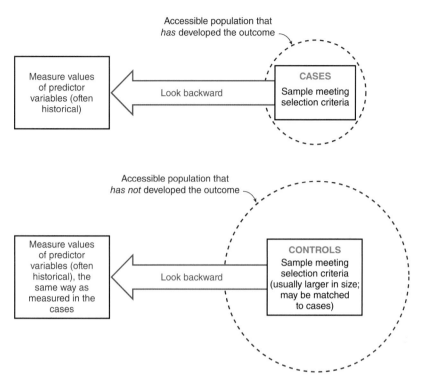

Accessible population that
has developed the outcome

Measure values
of predictor
variables (often
historical)

Look backward

CASES
Sample meeting
selection criteria

Accessible population that
has not developed the outcome

Measure values
of predictor
variables (often
historical), the
same way as
measured in the
cases

Look backward

CONTROLS
Sample meeting
selection criteria
(usually larger in size;
may be matched
to cases)

■ **FIGURE 9.1 Case-control study.** In a case-control study, the steps are to:

• Define selection criteria and recruit one sample from a population of cases and a second sample from a population of controls.
• Measure current values of relevant variables, often supplemented by historical information.

Case-control studies are the "house red" on the research design wine list: more modest and a little riskier than the other selections, but much less expensive and sometimes surprisingly good. The design of a case-control study is challenging because of the increased opportunities for bias, but there are many examples of well-designed case-control studies that have yielded

Example 9.1 Case-Control Study of a Disease Outbreak

A 2018 multistate outbreak of Hepatitis A in Australia triggered an investigation by public health authorities (2). *Cases* had Hepatitis A genotype IB identified between April 13 and June 8, 2018. *Controls* had other reportable infectious diseases (like salmonellosis, campylobacteriosis, or cryptosporidiosis). The controls came from the same or a neighboring local government area as the cases and were frequency matched by age group (0 to 14, 15 to 39, ≥40 years) in a 2:1 ratio to the cases. (This means that for each age group they selected 2 controls in that age group for each case; see Chapter 10.) Both cases and controls were questioned about potential exposures during the period prior to their illness.

The authors found the exposure most strongly associated with case status was consumption of frozen pomegranate arils (9 of 13 cases compared with 1 of 21 controls, odds ratio (OR) = 45.0, 95% CI: 3.8 to 2065; see Appendix 9A). Subsequent investigation identified Hepatitis A virus in two packages of frozen pomegranate arils from an Egyptian manufacturer whose products had been linked to a 2012 Hepatitis A outbreak in British Columbia (3). This outbreak led the Australian Department of Agriculture and Water Resources to begin inspection and testing of all future consignments from that manufacturer.

important results. These include the links between maternal diethylstilbestrol use and vaginal cancer in daughters (a classic study that provided a definitive conclusion based on just seven cases!) (4), and between prone sleeping position and sudden infant death syndrome (5), a simple result that has saved thousands of lives (6).

Case-control studies cannot yield estimates of the incidence or prevalence of a disease because the proportion of study participants who have the disease is determined by how many cases and how many controls the investigator chooses to sample, rather than by their frequencies in the population. Case-control studies do provide descriptive information on the characteristics of the cases and, more important, an estimate of the strength of the association between each predictor variable and the outcome. These estimates are in the form of **odds ratios**, which approximate the **risk ratio** if the **risk** of the outcome in both exposed and unexposed participants is relatively low (about 10% or less; see Appendix 9B).

Case-control studies began as epidemiologic studies to identify risk factors for diseases. For this reason, and because it makes the discussion easier to follow, we generally refer to "cases" as those with the disease and often refer to the exposures being compared between cases and controls as "risk factors." However, the case-control design can also be used to look at other uncommon outcomes, such as death among those with a usually nonfatal disease. In addition, for some studies the exposure of interest may be hypothesized to protect against the disease rather than being a risk factor, as in case-control studies of vaccine or treatment effectiveness. In that case, investigators may seek to show that the risk of the outcome is lower in the exposed group (ie, that the odds ratio is <1).

Strengths of Case-Control Studies

Efficiency for Rare Outcomes

One of the major strengths of case-control studies is their rapid yield of information from relatively few participants. Consider a study of the effect of circumcision on subsequent carcinoma of the penis. This cancer is very rare in circumcised men but also rare in uncircumcised men, whose lifetime cumulative incidence is about 0.16% (7). To do a cohort study with a reasonable chance (80%) of detecting whether circumcision increases the risk of penile cancer 50-fold would require following more than 6000 men for decades (assuming about half were circumcised). A randomized clinical trial of circumcision at birth would require the same sample size, but the cases would occur at a median of 67 years after entry into the study—it would take two or three generations of investigators to follow the participants!

Now consider a case-control study of the same question. For the same chance of detecting the same relative risk, only 16 cases and 16 controls would be required. Of course, one still needs to find a representative 16 cases; the rarer the disease, the more effort that may be required to find them. This topic is discussed in the Weaknesses section. Nonetheless, for diseases that are rare or that have long latent periods between exposure and disease, case-control studies are not only far more efficient than other designs, they are often the only feasible option.

Usefulness for Generating Hypotheses

The retrospective approach of case-control studies and their ability to examine many predictor variables makes them useful for generating hypotheses about the causes of a new outbreak of disease. Although outbreaks are usually due to infectious diseases (as in Example 9.1), this is not always the case. For example, a case-control study of an epidemic of deaths from acute renal failure in Haitian children (8) found an odds ratio of 53 for ingestion of locally manufactured acetaminophen syrup. Further investigation revealed that the renal failure was due to poisoning by a contaminant, diethylene glycol, a problem that, unfortunately, continues to occur (9, 10).

Weaknesses of Case-Control Studies

Case-control studies have great strengths but also major disadvantages. First, only one outcome can be studied (the presence or absence of the disease that was the criterion for drawing the two samples), whereas cohort and cross-sectional studies (and clinical trials) can study several outcomes. Second, as mentioned, the information available in case-control studies is limited: there is no direct way to estimate the incidence or prevalence of the disease unless the investigator also knows the population and time period from which the cases arose. But the biggest weakness of case-control studies is their susceptibility to bias, which comes chiefly from two sources: the separate selection of the cases and controls and the retrospective measurement of the predictor variables. These two problems and strategies for dealing with them are the topic of the next two sections.

Selection Bias and How to Avoid It

Finding and sampling the cases The sampling in a case-control study begins with the cases. Ideally, the sample of cases would include everyone in a defined population who developed the disease under study, or a random selection from those cases. An immediate problem comes up, however: How do we know who has developed the disease and who has not? In cross-sectional and cohort studies, the disease is ascertained systematically in all the study participants, but in case-control studies the cases must be sampled from patients in whom the disease has already been diagnosed and who are available for study. This sample may not be representative of all patients who develop the disease because those who are undiagnosed, misdiagnosed, unavailable for study, or dead are unlikely to be included (Figure 9.2).

In general, selection bias matters when the sample of cases is unrepresentative with respect to the risk factor being studied. Diseases that almost always require hospitalization and are straightforward to diagnose and confirm, such as hip fracture and traumatic amputation, can be sampled safely from diagnosed and accessible cases, at least in populations with good access to medical care. Similarly, in nested case-control studies (discussed later in this chapter), in which the cases come from a defined cohort, if the participants are followed for a sufficiently long time and the disease is almost always eventually diagnosed, cases can approximate the population with newly occurring disease.

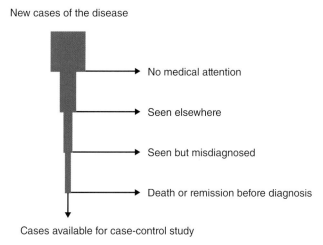

FIGURE 9.2 Some reasons why the cases in a case-control study may not be representative of all new cases of the disease.

On the other hand, conditions that do not always come to medical attention are more difficult to study with case-control studies because of the selection that precedes diagnosis. For example, some studies have raised concerns that vasectomy might increase prostate cancer risk (11). However, the diagnosis of prostate cancer may depend on screening so that cases may over-represent men who have received medical care (especially from urologists), such as those who have had a vasectomy. Indeed, prostate cancer *screening* is more common among men who have had a vasectomy (12).

Sampling the controls Although it is important to think about these issues, the selection of cases is often limited to the accessible sources of participants. The sample of cases may not be entirely representative, but it may be all that the investigator has to work with. The difficult decisions faced by an investigator designing a case-control study then relate to the more open-ended task of selecting appropriate controls. The general goal is to sample controls from the population who would have become a case in the study if they had developed the disease. Three strategies for sampling controls follow:

- Clinic-, hospital-, or registry-based controls. The most convenient source of controls for a case-control study is often the same clinic or hospital at which the cases were seen, or the same registry to which the cases were reported, simply because these are the people to whom the investigators have easy access. **Clinic-** or **hospital-based controls** may also partially compensate for the possible **selection bias** caused by obtaining cases from a clinic or hospital, because they are people who would likely have sought care at that facility if they had been cases. Similarly, in Example 9.1, the investigators of the Hepatitis A outbreak had ready access to contact information for people who had been diagnosed with other reportable infectious diseases and presumably also would have been reported as cases if they had had Hepatitis A.

  However, selection of an unrepresentative sample of controls to compensate for an unrepresentative sample of cases can be problematic. If the risk factor of interest causes a medical problem for which the controls seek care, the prevalence of that risk factor in the control group will be falsely high, diminishing or reversing the association between the risk factor and the outcome. For example, if the investigators in the Hepatitis A study had been interested in exposures related to general food and water safety, a control group made up of people diagnosed with salmonellosis, campylobacteriosis, or cryptosporidiosis would be problematic; those with poor food hygiene would be overrepresented. Similarly, in a case-control study linking proximity to oil and gas wells to hematologic cancers in children and young adults (13), the investigators used children and young adults reported to their registry with nonhematologic cancers as controls. If the chemicals found near oil and gas wells caused any of these other types of cancer, the association with hematologic cancers would be underestimated.

  Because controls with diseases other than the one under study may have conditions caused by the risk factor(s) being studied, these types of controls can produce misleading findings. Thus, it is essential to consider whether the convenience of such controls is worth the possible threat to the validity of the study.

- Using population-based samples of cases and controls. Because of the rapid increase in the use of disease registries and digital clinical and administrative data in geographic populations and within health plans, population-based case-control studies are now feasible for many diseases. Cases obtained from such registries and databases are generally representative of the patient population with the disease in the area or health plan, thus simplifying the choice of a control group, which can be a representative sample of "noncases" from the population or database covered by the registry.

  When registries or other databases are available, population-based case-control studies are the most desirable design. As a disease registry approaches completeness and the population it covers approaches stability (no migration in or out), a population-based case-control study approaches a case-control study that is nested within a cohort study or clinical trial, assuming that the controls can be identified and enrolled. Those latter tasks are relatively straightforward when the population has been enumerated and medical records are available to investigators.

It's important to recognize, however, that even in a well-integrated health system, the filtering process leading to the identification of cases shown in Figure 9.2 may affect different segments of the population differently. Thus, bias can be introduced any time participants need to access the health care system to be diagnosed and/or need to be contacted and to consent to be included in a study because some people (say, those who do not speak English or who have lower levels of trust in the scientific establishment) may be less likely to be included.

• **Using two or more control groups.** Because selection of a control group can be so tricky, particularly when the cases may not be a representative sample of those with disease, it is sometimes advisable to use two or more control groups selected in different ways. For example, in a case-control study to estimate the effectiveness of oral cholera vaccine, investigators from Haiti compared vaccination histories of cholera cases with those of two different sets of controls (14). A "test-negative" control group had presented with watery diarrhea to the same cholera treatment centers as the cases but had negative tests for cholera. A second "community" control group had no diarrhea; these controls (up to four per case) were matched to cholera cases by age group, time, and neighborhood. The effectiveness estimates for self-reported receipt of 2 doses of the oral cholera vaccine were reassuringly similar for the two control groups (73% and 74%).

Unfortunately, sometimes the biases associated with different strategies for selecting controls may cause the results using different control groups to conflict with one another, thereby revealing the inherent fragility of the case-control design for the research question at hand. When this happens, the investigator should seek additional information to try to determine the magnitude of potential biases from each of the control groups (Chapter 10). For example, if the concern is that clinic-based controls might have excess exposure to the risk factor of interest (say smoking) because it contributed to them seeking medical attention for other problems (say fatigue), the investigator could see how much the prevalence of the risk factor in the control group varies by the reason for their clinic visit. In any case, it is better to have inconsistent results and conclude that the answer is not known than to have just one control group and draw the wrong conclusion.

Any of these strategies may also include **matching**, a simple method of ensuring that cases and controls are comparable with respect to major factors that are or may be related to the disease but not the major exposure of concern. Because many risk factors and diseases are related to age, sex, and geographic location, for example, the study results may be more convincing if the cases and controls are comparable with regard to these variables. One approach to achieving this comparability is to choose controls that match the cases on age, sex, and some measure of location. However, matching does have potential disadvantages, particularly if modifiable predictors such as income or serum cholesterol level are matched. The reasons for this and the alternatives that are often preferable to matching are discussed in Chapter 10.

Differential Measurement Bias and How to Avoid It

The second major weakness of case-control studies is the increased risk of bias due to **measurement error**. This is caused by the retrospective approach to measuring the exposures, whether it is done by the investigators, treating clinicians (as reflected by entries in the medical record), or the cases and controls themselves, who may be asked to recall exposures that happened years before. Unfortunately, people's memories for past exposures are imperfect. If they are similarly imperfect in cases and controls, the problem is called **nondifferential misclassification** of the exposure, which makes it more difficult to find associations. (In epidemiologic terms, the odds ratio is biased toward 1.) Of greater concern, however, is that being diagnosed with a disease may lead cases to remember or report their exposures differently from controls; this **differential misclassification** of exposure, called **recall bias**, has unpredictable effects on associations measured in a study.

For example, widespread publicity about the relationship between sun exposure and malignant melanoma might lead cases diagnosed with that cancer to recall their history of sun exposure differently from controls. Cockburn et al. (15) found some evidence of this in a clever study of twins discordant for melanoma: The matched odds ratio for sunbathing as a child was 2.2 (95% CI: 1.0 to 4.7) when the twin with melanoma was asked which twin had sunbathed more as a child, but only 0.8 (95% CI: 0.4 to 1.8) when the co-twin without melanoma was asked the same question. However, for some other questions, such as which twin tanned or burned more easily, there was no evidence of recall bias.

Recall bias cannot occur in a cohort study because the participants are asked about exposures before the disease has been diagnosed. A case-control study of malignant melanoma nested within a cohort with sun exposure data collected years earlier provided a direct test of recall bias: the investigators compared self-reported sun exposure in cases and controls both before and after the case was diagnosed with melanoma (16). The investigators found some inaccuracies in recollections of exposure in both cases and controls but little evidence of recall bias. Thus, while it is important to consider the possibility of recall bias, it is not inevitable (17).

In addition to the strategies set out in Chapter 4 for controlling bias in measurements (standardizing the operational definitions of variables, choosing objective approaches, supplementing key variables with data from several sources, etc.), here are two specific strategies for avoiding bias in measuring exposures in case-control studies:

- **Use data recorded before the outcome occurred.** For example, in the previously cited case-control study of oral cholera vaccine effectiveness (14), actual vaccination records were used in addition to self-reported vaccination status. However, this excellent strategy is limited to the extent that recorded information about the risk factor of interest is available and reliable. In the cholera vaccine trial, verified vaccination histories were available for only about half of those reporting vaccination (both cases and controls).
- **Use blinding.** The general approach to blinding was discussed in Chapter 4, but there are some issues that are specific to designing interviews in case-control studies. In theory, both observers and study participants could be blinded to the case-control status of each participant and to the risk factor being studied; thus, four types of blinding are possible (Table 9.1).

Ideally, neither the study participants nor the observers should know who is a case and who is a control. In practice, this is often difficult. The participants know whether they are sick or well, so they can be blinded to case-control status only if controls are also ill with diseases that

TABLE 9.1 APPROACHES TO BLINDING IN A CASE-CONTROL STUDY

PEOPLE BLINDED	BLINDING CASE-CONTROL STATUS	BLINDING RISK FACTOR MEASUREMENT
Study participants	Possible if both cases and controls have diseases that could plausibly be related to the risk factor	Include "dummy" risk factors and be suspicious if they differ between cases and controls
		May not work if the risk factor for the disease has already been publicized
Observers	Possible if cases are not externally distinguishable from controls, but subtle signs and statements volunteered by the participants may make it difficult	Possible if the interviewer is not the investigator, but may be difficult to maintain

they believe might be related to the risk factors being studied. Efforts to blind interviewers are hampered by the obvious nature of some diseases (an interviewer can hardly help noticing if someone is jaundiced or has had a laryngectomy) and by the clues that interviewers may discern in the participant's responses.

Blinding to specific risk factors being studied is usually easier than blinding to case-control status. Case-control studies are often the first step in investigating an illness, so there may not be just one risk factor of particular interest. Thus, the study participants and the interviewer can be kept in the dark about the study hypotheses by including "dummy" questions about plausible risk factors not associated with the disease. For example, in a study of honey consumption as a risk factor for infant botulism, equally detailed questions about yogurt and bananas could be included in the interview. This type of blinding does not prevent differential bias but allows an estimate of whether it is a problem: If the cases report more exposure to honey but no increase in the other foods, then differential measurement bias is less likely. This strategy would not work if an association between eating honey and infant botulism had been widely publicized, or if some of the dummy risk factors turned out to be real ones.

Blinding the observer to the case-control status of the study participant is a particularly good strategy for laboratory measurements such as blood tests and x-rays. Blinding under these circumstances is easy and should always be done, simply by having someone other than the individual who will make the measurement apply a coded identification label to each specimen (or patient). The importance of blinding was illustrated by 15 case-control studies comparing measurements of bone mass between hip fracture patients and controls; much larger differences were found in the studies that used unblinded measurements than in the blinded studies (18).

■ NESTED CASE-CONTROL, INCIDENCE-DENSITY NESTED CASE-CONTROL, AND CASE-COHORT STUDIES

A **nested case-control** design has a case-control study "nested" within a defined cohort (Figure 9.3). The cohort may already have been defined by the investigator as part of a formal cohort study, often including banking of specimens, images, and so on, to be analyzed in the future after outcomes occur. Alternatively, the investigator can design a nested case-control study *de novo*, in a cohort that is not already defined, in which case describing the cohort will be the first step.

The investigator begins by identifying a cohort at risk for the outcome that is large enough to yield sufficient numbers of cases to answer the research question and that provides the ability to measure the exposure variable, either because specimens have been banked or medical records with exposure information are available. As described in Chapter 8, definition of the cohort will include the specific inclusion and exclusion criteria that define a population at risk. In addition, the *date of entry* into the cohort must be clear for each participant. This could be a fixed date (eg, everyone meeting inclusion criteria who was enrolled in a health plan on January 1, 2021), or it could be a variable date on which a period at risk begins (eg, the date of enrollment in a cohort study or the date of first myocardial infarction in a study of risk factors for recurrent myocardial infarction).

The investigator next describes the criteria that define the occurrence of the outcome of interest, which will be after the date of entry into the cohort and before the end of the defined follow-up period. If the outcome is rare, follow-up close to complete, and a single measurement of the exposure at baseline sufficient, then this process is simple. The investigator identifies all the individuals in the cohort who developed the outcome by the end of follow-up (the cases) and then selects a random sample of the participants who were also part of the cohort but did not develop the outcome (the controls). The investigator then measures the predictor variables for cases and controls and compares levels of the risk factor in cases to the levels in the sample of controls.

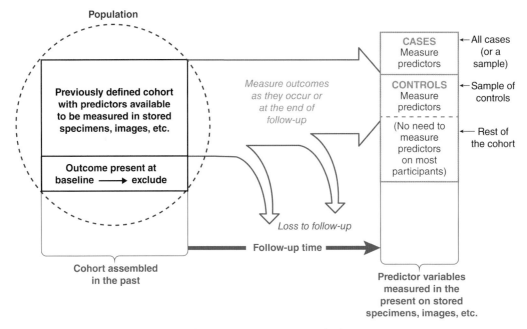

■ **FIGURE 9.3 Nested case-control study.** A nested case-control study. The steps are to:

- Identify a cohort from the population with previously stored specimens, images, and other data.
- Measure the outcome variable that distinguishes cases from controls.
- Measures predictor variables in specimens, images, and other data stored since the cohort was formed, as well as other variables, in all the cases and in a sample of the controls.

If follow-up is *variable* or *incomplete*, or the exposure of interest *changes over time*, a single measurement of exposure at entry into the cohort in the cases and a random sample of controls will not be sufficient. In that situation, it is better to design an **incidence-density** nested case-control study and sample the controls from **risk sets**. A risk set is defined for each case as it occurs to include the members of the cohort who were followed the same length of time as the case but had not yet become cases (Figure 9.4). As is true of any other form of matching of controls to cases, this matching on follow-up time needs to be accounted for in the analysis.

For example, if entry in the cohort was a fixed date (eg, January 1, 2018), the controls for a case diagnosed on July 1, 2019, would be sampled from among the risk set of participants who had not yet developed the outcome as of July 1, 2019. If the date of entry into the cohort was variable, controls for a case diagnosed 18 months after entry would be sampled from the risk set of those who had not yet become a case after 18 months of follow-up. Depending on the research hypothesis about the timing and duration of exposure required to cause the disease, values of the exposure at entry, average values, or values at some fixed point (eg, 3 months) before the case was diagnosed could be compared between cases and controls.

This sampling according to risk sets introduces the possibility that someone may be selected as a control for a case that occurs early in follow-up and later become a case himself, perhaps even after his value for the exposure variable changes. In effect, what this design does (with the help of appropriate statistical analysis) is consider chunks of person-time at risk, using values of predictor variables in that time period (and sometimes a previous period, so-called **lagged variables**) to predict occurrence of cases in that chunk of person-time, with the boundaries of each time chunk defined by the occurrence of the cases. This is called an incidence-density design (Example 9.2).

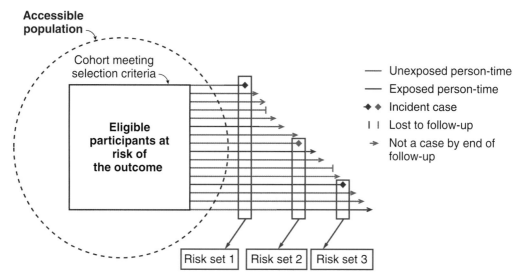

■ **FIGURE 9.4 Incidence-density nested case-control study.** An incidence-density nested case-control study can be either prospective or retrospective. For the prospective version, the steps are to:

- Define selection criteria and recruit a cohort from the population.
- Define the date of entry for each member of the cohort to align follow-up times.
- Store specimens, images, etc., for later analysis.
- Follow the cohort to identify cases and the date they were diagnosed.
- Sample one or more controls for each case from "risk sets," defined as members of the cohort who have been followed for the same amount of time as the case and who have not become a case, died, or been lost to follow-up at the time the case was diagnosed.
- Measure predictor variables in specimens, images, etc., stored since baseline, as well as other current variables, on cases and matched controls.
- For retrospective incidence-density case-control studies, the first four steps will already have been done.

Example 9.2 A Nested Incidence-Density Case-Control Study of Opiate Overdose Deaths in Italy

Opiate overdose is a leading cause of death in high-income countries. Treatment with opiate agonists (such as methadone) may reduce the risk. Because treatment among substance users varies over time as they go in and out of treatment, investigators from Italy, Australia, and the United Kingdom used an incidence-density nested case-control design to efficiently quantify the benefit of opiate agonists and other treatments (19). The steps were to:

1. **Identify the cohort and time period at risk.** This case-control study was nested within the VEdeTTE cohort, for which the investigators recruited heroin users from public treatment centers in Italy from 1998 to 1999. They ascertained mortality on 4444 participants from two Italian regions from September 1998 through December 31, 2005.
2. **Identify the cases, including dates of occurrence.** Study staff blinded to the case/control status of the participants retrieved vital status from clinical records. There were 316 deaths during the follow-up period, of which 95 were coded as due to overdose.
3. **Sample controls from "risk sets" matched to each case.** For each fatal overdose case, the investigators randomly selected four controls who were still alive on the date of the case's death (called the *index date* for controls), matched on region, age (±5 years), and sex. Controls could be matched with multiple cases, and cases were eligible to be selected as controls for cases who died before them.

4. **Measure predictors in the cases and controls.** The investigators (blinded to case/control status) retrieved information about drug treatment type from clinical records for the 2 months before the date of death for cases and before the index date for controls. For those out of treatment for the 2 months before that date, they retrieved information on types and dates of last treatments. The incidence-density case-control design allowed them to retrieve this information on a much smaller number of people and over a much more limited period than if they had done a cohort study.

The investigators (appropriately) used conditional logistic regression to analyze the data. They found that opiate agonist treatment was associated with a >90% reduction in the odds of mortality (OR = 0.09, 95% CI: 0.03 to 0.24); adjustment for homelessness, HIV-positivity, alcohol use, legal problems, and overdose reported at baseline did not change the result (adjusted OR = 0.08, 95% CI: 0.03 to 0.23).

A nested **case-cohort** design is similar to the nested case-control design except that, instead of selecting controls who did not develop the outcome of interest, the investigator selects a random sample of all the members of the cohort, regardless of outcomes. A few people who are part of that random cohort sample may have developed the outcome(s); that number is small when the outcome is uncommon. An advantage of the case-cohort design is that a single random sample of the cohort can provide the controls for several different outcomes, as illustrated in Example 9.3. In addition, the random sample of the cohort provides information on the overall prevalence of risk factors in the cohort.

Example 9.3 Plasma ACE2 and Risk of Death or Cardiometabolic Diseases: A Nested Case-Cohort Study

Circulating levels of angiotensin-converting enzyme 2 (ACE2) might serve as a marker of dysregulation of the renin-angiotensin system. Investigators primarily from the Population Health Research Institute, in Hamilton, Ontario, Canada, studied how well plasma ACE2 levels predicted several adverse health outcomes (20). The basic steps in performing the study were to:

1. **Identify a cohort.** The investigators used the Prospective Urban Rural Epidemiology (PURE) study, a cohort study of individuals 35 to 70 years old at baseline from 27 low-, middle-, and high-income countries. The PURE study included a biobanking initiative with baseline blood samples stored at −165 °C on a subset of the participants from 14 countries. Participants were eligible if they had stored analyzable samples and belonged to the major self-reported ethnicity in the residing country (eg, European ancestry in Sweden). The samples were collected in 2005 to 2006, and the median follow-up time was 9.4 years.
2. **Identify the cases.** The outcome events for the study (cases) were incident death (N = 1985), myocardial infarction (N = 882), stroke (N = 663), heart failure (N = 264), and diabetes (N=1715). These events had already been ascertained as part of the PURE study.
3. **Sample the cohort.** The investigators selected a random sample ("subcohort") of 5084 of the 55,246 PURE participants with analyzable samples. Of note, people were *not* excluded from this subcohort if they had one of the outcome events under study. Thus, this was a case-cohort rather than a nested case-control study.

4. **Measure predictors in the cases and the sample of the cohort.** The investigators measured levels of ACE2 on biobank specimens and analyzed previously collected data on traditional cardiovascular risk factors, such as sex, body mass index, cigarette smoking, and blood pressure.

The investigators found that ACE2 was a strong predictor of all of the outcomes studied, with hazard ratios of 1.21 to 1.44 per standard deviation increase (21) in ACE2 level after adjustment for traditional cardiovascular risk factors. ACE2 levels were stronger predictors than clinical risk factors, including smoking, diabetes, blood pressure, lipid levels, and body mass index.

Strengths

Nested case-control and case-cohort studies are especially useful for costly measurements on serum and other specimens or images that have been archived at the beginning of the study and preserved for later analysis. Making expensive measurements on all the cases and a sample of the controls is much less costly than making the measurements on the entire cohort.

When those making measurements are blinded, these designs preserve the advantages of cohort studies that result from collecting predictor variables before the outcomes have occurred. In addition, these designs avoid the potential biases of conventional case-control studies that cannot make measurements on fatal cases and that draw cases and controls from different populations.

Weaknesses

These designs share certain disadvantages of other observational designs: the possibilities that observed associations are due to the effect of unmeasured or imprecisely measured confounding variables and that baseline measurements may be affected by silent preclinical disease ("effect-cause" rather than cause-effect; see Chapter 10).

Other Considerations

Nested case-control and case-cohort designs have been used less often than they should be. An investigator planning large prospective studies should consider preserving biologic samples (eg, banks of frozen sera) or storing images or records that are expensive to analyze for subsequent nested case-control analyses. He should ensure that the conditions of storage will preserve substances of interest for many years. It may also be useful to collect new samples or information during the follow-up period, which can be most efficiently used in subsequent incidence-density case-control studies.

■ CASE-CROSSOVER STUDIES

The **case-crossover** design is a variant of the case-control design that is useful for studying the short-term effects of intermittent exposures. These retrospective studies begin with a group of cases who have had the outcome of interest. However, unlike traditional case-control studies, in which the exposures of the cases are compared with exposures of a group of controls, in case-crossover studies each case serves as his own control. Exposures of the cases at the time (or right before) the outcome occurred are compared with exposures of those same cases at one or more other points in time.

For example, McEvoy et al. studied cases who were injured in car crashes and who owned or used a mobile phone (22). Using phone company records, they compared mobile phone usage in the 10 minutes before the crash with usage when the cases were driving at the same time of day

24 hours, 72 hours, and 7 days before the crash. They found that mobile phone usage was about four times more likely in the 10 minutes before a crash than in the comparison time periods.

The analysis of a case-crossover study is similar to that of a matched case-control study, except that the control exposures are exposures of the case at different time periods, rather than exposures of the matched controls. This is illustrated in Appendix 9A, scenario number 3. Case-crossover designs have been used in large populations to study time-varying exposures such as levels of particulate air pollution; associations have been found with hospital admissions (23) and total mortality in older adults (24), out-of-hospital cardiac arrest (25), and even infant mortality (26).

■ CHOOSING AMONG OBSERVATIONAL DESIGNS

The pros and cons of the main observational designs presented in the last two chapters are summarized in Table 9.2. We have already described these issues in detail and will make only one final point here. Among all these designs, none is best and none is worst; each has its place and purpose, depending on the research question and the circumstances.

TABLE 9.2 ADVANTAGES AND DISADVANTAGES OF THE MAJOR OBSERVATIONAL DESIGNS

DESIGN	ADVANTAGES	DISADVANTAGES[a]
	Cross-sectional	
	Relatively short duration	Does not establish sequence of events
	A good first step for a cohort study or clinical trial	Not feasible for rare predictors or rare outcomes
	Yields prevalence of multiple predictors and outcomes	Does not yield incidence
	Cohort Designs	
All	Establishes sequence of events	Often requires large sample sizes
	Multiple predictors and outcomes	Less feasible for rare outcomes
	Number of outcome events grows over time	
	Yields incidence, relative risk, excess risk	
Prospective cohort	More control over participant selection and measurements	Follow-up can be lengthy
	Avoids bias in measuring predictors	Often expensive
Retrospective cohort	Follow-up is in the past	Less control over participant selection and measurements
	Relatively inexpensive	
Multiple cohort	Useful when distinct cohorts have different or rare exposures	Bias and confounding from sampling distinct populations
	Case-Control	
	Useful for rare outcomes	Bias and confounding from sampling two populations
	Short duration, small sample size	Differential measurement bias
	Relatively inexpensive	Limited to one outcome variable
		Sequence of events may be unclear
		Does not yield prevalence, incidence, or excess risk unless nested within a cohort

TABLE 9.2 ADVANTAGES AND DISADVANTAGES OF THE MAJOR OBSERVATIONAL DESIGNS (*continued*)

DESIGN	ADVANTAGES	DISADVANTAGES[a]
	Hybrid Designs	
Nested case-control	Advantages of a retrospective cohort design, and less costly if measurement of predictors is expensive	Measurements of risk factors subject to bias if not previously measured or based on banked specimens or images stored previously; usually requires a pre-existing defined cohort
Incidence-density nested case-control	Allows investigators to analyze risk relationships taking into account changes over time in risk factor levels and loss to follow-up	Requires measurements of risk factor levels and incidence of cases over time during follow-up; usually requires a pre-existing defined cohort
Nested case-cohort	Same as nested case-control and can use a single control group for multiple case-control studies with different outcomes	Same as nested case-control
Case-crossover	Cases serve as their own controls, reducing random error and confounding	Requires that the exposure have only immediate, short-term effects

[a]All these observational designs have the disadvantage (compared with randomized trials) of being susceptible to the influence of confounding variables—see Chapter 10.

■ SUMMARY

1. In a **case-control study**, the prevalence of a risk factor in a **sample of cases** who have the outcome of interest is compared with the prevalence in a **sample of controls** who do not. This design, in which people with and without the disease are sampled separately, is relatively **inexpensive** and uniquely **efficient for studying rare diseases**.

2. One problem with case-control studies is their susceptibility to **selection bias**. Three approaches to reducing selection bias are (a) to sample controls and cases in the same (admittedly unrepresentative) way; (b) to do a population-based study; and (c) to use several control groups, sampled in different ways. Any of these strategies can also include matching the cases and controls on variables like age, sex, and location.

3. The other major problem with case-control studies is their retrospective design, which makes them susceptible to **measurement bias**, affecting cases and controls differentially. Such bias can be reduced by **using measurements** of the predictor **made prior to the outcome** and by **blinding** the participants and research staff.

4. The best way to avoid both selection and measurement bias is to design a **nested case-control study** in which **random samples of cases and controls** are drawn from a larger cohort study. In addition to controlling both of these biases, expensive measurements on serum, images, and so on, can be made at the end of the study on a relatively small number of study participants.

5. The **incidence-density case-control** design allows investigators to efficiently analyze risk relationships, taking into account changes over time in risk factor levels and in the availability of follow-up.

6. The **nested case-cohort design** uses a random sample of the entire cohort in place of the noncases; this can serve as a control group for studying more than one outcome and provides direct information on the overall prevalence of risk factors in the cohort.

7. **Case-crossover studies** are a variation on the matched case-control design in which observations at two or more points in time allow each case to serve as his own control.

REFERENCES

1. Guenel P, Laforest L, Cyr D, et al. Occupational risk factors, ultraviolet radiation, and ocular melanoma: a case-control study in France. *Cancer Causes Control*. 2001;12(5):451-459.

2. Franklin N, Camphor H, Wright R, Stafford R, Glasgow K, Sheppeard V. Outbreak of hepatitis A genotype IB in Australia associated with imported frozen pomegranate arils. *Epidemiol Infect*. 2019;147:e74.

3. Swinkels HM, Kuo M, Embree G, et al. Hepatitis A outbreak in British Columbia, Canada: the roles of established surveillance, consumer loyalty cards and collaboration, February to May 2012. *Euro Surveill*. 2014;19(18):20792.

4. Herbst AL, Ulfelder H, Poskanzer DC. Adenocarcinoma of the vagina. Association of maternal stilbestrol therapy with tumor appearance in young women. *N Engl J Med*. 1971;284(15):878-881.

5. Beal SM, Finch CF. An overview of retrospective case-control studies investigating the relationship between prone sleeping position and SIDS. *J Paediatr Child Health*. 1991;27(6):334-339.

6. Mitchell EA, Blair PS. SIDS prevention: 3000 lives saved but we can do better. *N Z Med J*. 2012;125(1359):50-57.

7. Kochen M, McCurdy S. Circumcision and the risk of cancer of the penis. A life-table analysis. *Am J Dis Child*. 1980;134(5):484-486.

8. O'Brien KL, Selanikio JD, Hecdivert C, et al. Epidemic of pediatric deaths from acute renal failure caused by diethylene glycol poisoning. Acute Renal Failure Investigation Team. *JAMA*. 1998;279(15):1175-1180.

9. Fatal poisoning among young children from diethylene glycol-contaminated acetaminophen—Nigeria, 2008–2009. *MMWR Morb Mortal Wkly Rep*. 2009;58(48):1345-1347.

10. Llamas M. Drug Makers Warned for Potential Diethylene Glycol Toxin Contamination: Drugwatch.com; 2020 [updated April 20, 2020]. https://www.drugwatch.com/news/2020/04/20/diethylene-glycol-toxin-contamination/

11. Nutt M, Reed Z, Kohler TS. Vasectomy and prostate cancer risk: a historical synopsis of undulating false causality. *Res Rep Urol*. 2016;8:85-93.

12. Shang Y, Han G, Li J, et al. Vasectomy and prostate cancer risk: a meta-analysis of cohort studies. *Sci Rep*. 2015;5:9920.

13. McKenzie LM, Allshouse WB, Byers TE, Bedrick EJ, Serdar B, Adgate JL. Childhood hematologic cancer and residential proximity to oil and gas development. *PLoS One*. 2017;12(2):e0170423.

14. Franke MF, Jerome JG, Matias WR, et al. Comparison of two control groups for estimation of oral cholera vaccine effectiveness using a case-control study design. *Vaccine*. 2017;35(43):5819-5827.

15. Cockburn M, Hamilton A, Mack T. Recall bias in self-reported melanoma risk factors. *Am J Epidemiol*. 2001;153(10):1021-1026.

16. Parr CL, Hjartaker A, Laake P, Lund E, Veierod MB. Recall bias in melanoma risk factors and measurement error effects: a nested case-control study within the Norwegian Women and Cancer Study. *Am J Epidemiol*. 2009;169(3):257-266.

17. Gefeller O. Invited commentary: recall bias in melanoma—much ado about almost nothing? *Am J Epidemiol*. 2009;169(3):267-270; discussion 71-72.

18. Cummings SR. Are patients with hip fractures more osteoporotic? Review of the evidence. *Am J Med*. 1985;78(3):487-494.

19. Faggiano F, Mathis F, Diecidue R, et al. Opioid overdose risk during and after drug treatment for heroin dependence: an incidence density case-control study nested in the VEdeTTE cohort. *Drug Alcohol Rev*. 2021;40(2):281-286.

20. Narula S, Yusuf S, Chong M, et al. Plasma ACE2 and risk of death or cardiometabolic diseases: a case-cohort analysis. *Lancet*. 2020;396(10256):968-976.

21. Newman TB, Browner WS. In defense of standardized regression coefficients. *Epidemiology*. 1991;2(5):383-386.

22. McEvoy SP, Stevenson MR, McCartt AT, et al. Role of mobile phones in motor vehicle crashes resulting in hospital attendance: a case-crossover study. *BMJ*. 2005;331(7514):428.

23. Wei Y, Wang Y, Di Q, et al. Short term exposure to fine particulate matter and hospital admission risks and costs in the Medicare population: time stratified, case crossover study. *BMJ*. 2019;367:l6258.

24. Di Q, Dai L, Wang Y, et al. Association of short-term exposure to air pollution with mortality in older adults. *JAMA*. 2017;318(24):2446-2456.

25. Kojima S, Michikawa T, Matsui K, et al. Association of fine particulate matter exposure with bystander-witnessed out-of-hospital cardiac arrest of cardiac origin in Japan. *JAMA Netw Open*. 2020;3(4):e203043.

26. Scheers H, Mwalili SM, Faes C, Fierens F, Nemery B, Nawrot TS. Does air pollution trigger infant mortality in Western Europe? A case-crossover study. *Environ Health Perspect*. 2011;119(7):1017-1022.

APPENDIX 9A
Calculation of Odds Ratios for Case-Control Studies

CASE-CONTROL STUDY

Example 9.1 was an investigation of an outbreak of Hepatitis A. The authors reported that 9 of 13 cases, compared with only 1 of 21 controls, reported having eaten frozen pomegranate arils. Table 9A.1 shows these results. The odds ratio is the **odds** of exposure in the cases (a/c) divided by the odds of exposure in the controls (b/d), which is mathematically equivalent to ad/bc.

The odds ratio provides a good estimate of the risk ratio when the disease is rare ($<\sim$10%), as Hepatitis A was in this example. Thus, this study suggests that people who ate the contaminated frozen pomegranate arils were about 45 times more likely to get Hepatitis A than those who did not.

TABLE 9A.1 CALCULATION OF THE ODDS RATIO IN EXAMPLE 9.1

PREDICTOR VARIABLE: ATE FROZEN POMEGRANATE ARILS	OUTCOME VARIABLE: DIAGNOSIS OF HEPATITIS A	
	YES	NO
Yes	9(*a*)	1(*b*)
No	4(*c*)	20(*d*)
Total	13	21

$$\text{Relative risk} \approx \text{Odds ratio} = \frac{a/c}{b/d} = \frac{ad}{bc} = \frac{9 \times 20}{4 \times 1} = 45$$

MATCHED CASE-CONTROL STUDY

To illustrate the similarity between analysis of a matched case-control study and a case-crossover study, we will use the same example for both. The research question is whether mobile telephone use increases the risk of car crashes among mobile telephone owners. A traditional matched case-control study might consider self-reported frequency of using a mobile telephone while driving as the risk factor. Then the cases would be people who had been in crashes, and they could be compared with controls who had not been in crashes, matched by age, sex, and mobile telephone prefix to the cases. The cases and controls would then be asked whether they ever use a mobile telephone while driving. (To simplify, for this example, we dichotomize the exposure and consider people as either "users" or "nonusers" of mobile telephones while driving.) We then classify each case/control pair according to whether both are users, neither is a user, or the case was a user but not the control, or the control was a user but not the case. If we had 300 pairs, the results might look like this:

TABLE 9A.2 EXAMPLE OF A HYPOTHETICAL PAIR-MATCHED CASE-CONTROL STUDY OF (HABITUAL) CELL PHONE USE DURING DRIVING AS A RISK FACTOR FOR CRASH INJURIES

MATCHED CONTROLS	CASES (WITH CRASH INJURIES)		
	USER	NONUSER	TOTAL
User	110	40	150
Nonuser	90	60	150
Total	200	100	300

Table 9A.2 shows that there were 90 pairs where the case used a mobile phone while driving, but not the matched control, and 40 pairs where the matched control but not the case was a "user." Note that this 2 × 2 table is different from the 2 × 2 table from the Hepatitis A study in Table 9A.1, in which each cell in the table is the number of people in that cell. In the 2 × 2 table for a *matched* case-control study, the number in each cell is the number of *pairs* of participants in that cell; the total N in Table 9A.2 is therefore 600 (300 cases and 300 controls).

The odds ratio for such a table is simply the ratio of the number of pairs in which the case was exposed and the control was not to the number of pairs in which the control was exposed and the case was not ("discordant pairs"). Note that the case-control pairs that share the same exposure level ("concordant pairs") contribute no information about the association between exposure and outcome. In Table 9A.2 the OR = 90/40 = 2.25. Because crashes are rare, the odds ratio approximates the risk ratio, so the study result (if real) would suggest that users of mobile phones had more than double the risk of being in a crash.

CASE-CROSSOVER STUDY

Now consider the case-crossover study of the same question. Data from the study by McEvoy et al. (22) are shown in the following table.

TABLE 9A.3 CALCULATION OF THE ODDS RATIO FROM A CASE-CROSSOVER STUDY OF RECENT CELL PHONE USE AS A RISK FACTOR FOR CRASH INJURIES

SEVEN DAYS BEFORE CRASH	CRASH TIME PERIOD		
	DRIVER USING PHONE	NOT USING	TOTAL
Driver using phone	5	6	11
Not using	27	288	315
Total	32	294	326

For the case-crossover study (22), each cell in Table 9A.3 is a number of cases, not a number of pairs, but *each cell represents two time periods* for that one case: the period just before the crash and a comparison period 7 days before. Therefore, the 5 in the upper left cell means there were 5 drivers involved in crashes who were using a mobile phone just before they crashed and also using a mobile phone during the comparison period 7 days before, whereas the 27 just below the 5 indicates that there were 27 drivers involved in crashes who were using a phone just before crashing but *not* using a phone during the comparison period 7 days before.

Similarly, there were 6 drivers involved in crashes who were not using their phone at the time of the crash but were using them in the comparison period 7 days before. The odds ratio is the ratio of the numbers of discordant time periods, in this example 27/6 = 4.5, meaning that driving during periods of mobile phone use was associated with a 4.5-fold higher risk of a crash than driving during periods when not using a mobile phone.

APPENDIX 9B
When and Why the Odds Ratio Approximates the Risk Ratio

A two-by-two table can be used to represent the association between an exposure and a disease, as follows:

	DISEASE	NO DISEASE
Exposure present	a	b
Exposure absent	c	d

■ WHAT ARE RISKS AND ODDS?

The risk of a disease is the number of people who develop that disease divided by the number of people at risk (ie, $a/(a+b)$ in the exposed, and $c/(c+d)$ in the unexposed). The odds of a disease are the number of people who develop that disease divided by the number of people who do not develop it (ie, either a/b or c/d).

■ THERE ARE TWO WAYS TO CALCULATE AN ODDS RATIO— BUT ONLY ONE ODDS RATIO

The first way (let's call it OR_1), which is used in cohort studies and clinical trials, divides the odds of the disease in those who are exposed by the odds of the disease in those who are unexposed. This is simply $OR_1 = (a/b) \div (c/d) = ad/bc$. The second way ($OR_2$), which is used in case-control studies, divides the odds of the exposure in those with the disease (cases) by the odds of the exposure in those without the disease (controls). This is simply $OR_2 = (a/c) \div (b/d) = ad/cb$.

These two approaches and formulas give the same value, because $ad/cb = ad/bc$. There is only one odds ratio ($OR_2 = OR_1$).

■ ODDS AND RISK—AND THE ODDS RATIO AND RISK RATIO— ARE SIMILAR WHEN A DISEASE IS RARE

When a disease is rare in both the exposed and the unexposed, most people don't develop the disease, so the number of people at risk is similar to the number of people who don't develop the disease. Thus, the odds of a rare disease and the risk of a rare disease are similar.

So when a disease is rare, the odds ratio (OR_1) comparing the odds of the disease in the exposed and in the unexposed, and the risk ratio (RR) comparing the risks of the disease in the exposed and in the unexposed, are also similar ($OR_1 \approx RR$). That in turn means that the odds ratio (OR_2) comparing the odds of exposure in those with the disease (the cases) and those without the disease (the controls), which can be estimated in case-control studies, must also be similar to the risk ratio ($OR_2 = OR_1 \approx RR$).

APPENDIX 9C
Exercises for Chapter 9. Designing Case-Control Studies

1. In Exercise 1c of Chapter 8, you designed a retrospective cohort study of low vitamin B_{12} levels as a risk factor for hip fractures. Describe how you could use the same cohort to answer the research question more efficiently using a case-control study.

2. The research question is: "How much does a family history of ovarian cancer increase the risk of ovarian cancer?" The investigator plans a case-control study to answer this question.

   a. What would be a good way to pick the cases?

   b. Given your answer to part a, how should he pick the controls?

   c. Comment on potential sources of bias in the sampling of cases and controls and the direction in which they might bias the results.

   d. How would he measure "family history of ovarian cancer" as the predictor variable of interest? Comment on the sources of bias in this measurement.

   e. What measure of association would he use, and what test of statistical significance?

   f. Do you think the case-control method is an appropriate approach to this research question? Discuss the advantages and disadvantages of the case-control design relative to other possibilities for this research question.

3. The researcher wants to investigate the relationship between playing video games with car racing and the risk of being involved in a real car crash (as the driver).

   a. Assume the exposure of interest is long-term effects of habitual use of these video games. How would he select cases and controls and measure the exposure for a case-control study of this question?

   b. Now imagine the exposure of interest is whether use of such games in the hour immediately preceding driving increases short-term risk. What is a design for studies of short-term effects of intermittent exposures? Lay out how such a study would be carried out for this research question.

CHAPTER 10

Estimating Causal Effects Using Observational Studies

Thomas B. Newman and Warren S. Browner

Most observational studies are designed to estimate the **causal effect** of an exposure on an outcome, for example, the effect of eating red meat on the risk of colon cancer. (Exceptions are observational studies whose goal is **prediction**, such as studies of diagnostic and prognostic tests, discussed in Chapter 13.) As introduced in Chapter 1, this process begins by drawing inferences from measured variables in the study sample to phenomena of interest in the target population. But so far these inferences have been only about **associations** in the target population. Additional effort is needed to estimate causal effects, which are of greater interest than associations because they can provide insights into the underlying pathophysiology of a disease, identify ways to prevent its occurrence, and even suggest potential treatments.

■ COUNTERFACTUAL FRAMEWORK FOR UNDERSTANDING CAUSALITY

To understand causal effects, we can do a thought experiment that compares the risk of an outcome (eg, colon cancer) in the target population if everyone were exposed (the entire target population ate red meat) with the risk in that same population if no one were exposed (nobody ate red meat).[1] Of course, in the real world, everyone either is or is not exposed, so there's no way to know what would happen in these so called **counterfactual** worlds—in which many of the exposures are "counter to the facts." Causal effects are best estimated by studies that allow an investigator to estimate and compare what the counterfactual outcomes would have been under these counterfactual exposures (Figure 10.1).

The simplest way to do this is a randomized trial, as discussed in detail in the next chapter. For now, we'll just focus on how a trial is used to estimate counterfactual outcomes. First, we need to enroll people for whom the causal effect would be of interest, that is, those who, at least theoretically, could have either exposure level. For example, if there were people who (perhaps for religious, ethical, or medical reasons) would or could not eat red meat under any circumstances, we would want to exclude them from the trial. The same is true for those who would insist on eating red meat.

Then, by allocating the remaining participants to the exposure at random, we create similar ("exchangeable" in epidemiologic parlance) groups, one of which is exposed (assigned to eat red meat, in this example) and the other unexposed (assigned to not eat red meat). Because randomization has made the groups exchangeable, the colon cancer rate in the red meat group can be used to estimate what would have happened to the no red meat group if they had eaten red meat. Moreover, the outcomes in the no red meat group can be used to estimate what would have happened in the meat-eating group if they had abstained from red meat. Thus, the between-group difference in observed risks in a randomized trial (if there is good adherence to

---

[1]We are keeping this discussion simple by making both the predictor and outcome dichotomous. The same principles apply to estimating causal effects generally.

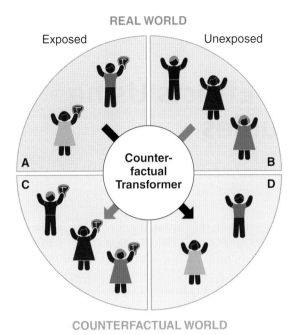

REAL WORLD

Exposed   Unexposed

A

Counter-factual Transformer

B

C

D

COUNTERFACTUAL WORLD

■ **FIGURE 10.1 Thought experiment to understand causal effects in terms of counterfactual worlds.** In the real world, the effects of an exposure (eg, eating red meat, symbolized by over-sized T-bone steaks in the figure) are estimated by comparing outcomes (eg, colon cancer) in people who eat red meat (Quadrant A) with the outcomes in (different) people who do not eat red meat (Quadrant B), trying to control for other differences between them (eg, in the figure more women do not eat red meat). In the thought experiment there is a counterfactual transformer that creates people in the counterfactual world who are identical to people in the real world but with opposite exposures. We could determine the causal effect of red meat on colon cancer from the difference in colon cancer rates between a world in which everyone ate red meat (Quadrants A and C) and an otherwise identical world in which no one ate red meat (Quadrants B and D).

treatment assignment) provides a valid estimate of the causal effect. Enhancing causal inference in observational studies usually involves emulating a randomized trial of the research question as much as possible.

■ WHY AN ASSOCIATION IN AN OBSERVATIONAL STUDY MIGHT DIFFER FROM THE CAUSAL EFFECT

Trying to emulate a randomized trial with an observational study in which exposures are not under the control of the investigator can, however, be challenging. Consider again the question of whether eating red meat causes colon cancer. An observational study of this topic is relevant because colon cancer is the second-leading cause of cancer mortality in the United States (1), because for some people compassion for mammals and the proven adverse environmental effects of producing red meat (especially from ruminants like cattle and sheep) (2) are not sufficient motivation to change their diets, and because a trial randomizing people to eat or not eat red meat and then following them long enough to observe colon cancer outcomes would be extremely impractical. Let's treat red meat exposure as a dichotomous (yes/no) variable and assume an observational study finds that red meat eaters had about twice the risk of developing colon cancer compared with those who did not eat red meat.

One possibility—presumably the one most important to the investigator—is that eating red meat doubles the risk of colon cancer. Before reaching this conclusion, however, we must consider four reasons (Table 10.1) why this might not be correct: chance, **bias**, **confounding**, and **effect-cause**.[2] Obtaining an accurate estimate of the causal effect of eating red meat on colon cancer requires reducing the influence of distortions due to these four possibilities.

---

[2]Some epidemiologists consider confounding to be a type of bias because, like all biases, it distorts a study's estimate of the parameter (ie, a measure of the causal effect) being estimated. We prefer to consider confounding separately, because the other types of bias cause the association in the study to differ from the true association in the target population and thus will be problematic whether or not the goal is to estimate causal effects. Confounding, on the other hand, is a problem only when the goal is to estimate causal effects: it causes the *association* in the target population to differ from the *causal* effect.

TABLE 10.1 FOUR REASONS FOR DISTORTIONS OF ESTIMATED CAUSAL EFFECTS IN A STUDY OF RED MEAT INTAKE AS A CAUSE OF COLORECTAL CANCER

REASON FOR DISTORTION	DOES THE STUDY ESTIMATE REFLECT THE ASSOCIATION IN THE TARGET POPULATION?	WHAT IS REALLY GOING ON IN THE POPULATION?	CAUSAL MODEL
1. Chance	No	Association is distorted by random error.	Eating red meat CRC (no connecting arrow)
2. Bias	No	Association is distorted by systematic error.	Example: selection bias in a hospital-based case-control study (see text) Eating red meat ↓ CVD ↘ [Hospitalization] CRC ↗
3. Effect-cause	Yes	Colon cancer causes people to eat more red meat.	CRC ↓ Anemia ↓ Eating red meat
4. Confounding	Yes	A third factor causes both red meat intake and colon cancer.	Male gender ↙ ↘ Eating red meat ⟶ CRC

CVD, cardiovascular disease; CRC, colorectal cancer.

If chance or bias were the explanation, those who ate red meat would have twice the risk of colon cancer in the study—even though that association does not exist in the population. Rather, the apparent doubling in risk would be attributable to bad luck or to a problem with how the study was designed, executed, or interpreted.

The other two alternatives—effect-cause and confounding—are true biologic phenomena so that the association in the sample may reflect the association in the population. However, that association may not be (entirely) a causal effect of the exposure. In one situation, the association is attributable to effect-cause: having colon cancer causes people to eat more red meat, perhaps because they crave it as a result of anemia from intestinal blood loss. (This is just cause and effect in reverse and is primarily a concern with retrospective studies.) The final possibility, confounding, occurs when a third factor, such as male gender identity (hereafter just "male gender"), causes both red meat intake and colon cancer.

In the remainder of the chapter, we will review strategies for estimating and minimizing the distortion caused by these four errors when estimating a causal effect in an observational study. These strategies can be used while designing a study or when analyzing its results. Although this book emphasizes research design, understanding the analytic options can influence the choice of design, so we will discuss both topics.

◼ MINIMIZING ERRORS DUE TO CHANCE

Suppose that there is no association between red meat intake and colon cancer among members of the target population, 50% of whom eat red meat. If we were to randomly sample 20 cases with colon cancer and 20 controls, we would expect that about 10 people in each group (50% of 20) would eat red meat. However, *by chance alone*, we might enroll 14 red meat eaters among the 20 cases of colon cancer but only 6 in the 20 controls. If that happened, we would observe a spurious—yet statistically significant—association between red meat intake and colon cancer in our study (odds ratio = 5.4; 95% confidence interval, 1.2 to 26; $P = 0.03$).

Chance is sometimes called **random error**, because it has no underlying explanation. When an association attributable to random error is statistically significant, it's known as a **type I error** (Chapter 5). Strategies for reducing random error are available in both the design and the analysis phases of research (Table 10.2). *Design strategies*, such as increasing the **precision** of measurements and increasing the **sample size**, are discussed in Chapters 4 and 6, respectively. The *analysis strategy* of calculating *P* **values** helps the investigator quantify the magnitude of the observed association in comparison with what might have occurred by chance alone. For example, a *P* value of 0.03 (as in the previous paragraph) means that an association at least that strong could occur about 3% of the time by chance when there is no association in the target population.

Even more useful than *P* values, **confidence intervals** show the possible values for parameters describing an association (risk ratios, odds ratios, etc.) that fall within the range of random error estimated in the study. Confidence intervals are especially helpful for results that are not statistically significant, because they show whether a large and important effect might have been missed by chance (3, 4).

TABLE 10.2 MINIMIZING DISTORTIONS IN THE ESTIMATE OF CAUSAL EFFECTS BY GETTING THE ESTIMATE OF THE ASSOCIATION IN THE TARGET POPULATION CORRECT

REASON FOR DISTORTION	DESIGN PHASE (HOW TO PREVENT THE DISTORTION)	ANALYSIS PHASE (HOW TO EVALUATE THE DISTORTION)
Chance (due to random error)	Increase sample size and other strategies to increase precision (Chapters 4 and 6).	Calculate *P* values and confidence intervals, and interpret them in the context of prior evidence (Chapters 5 and 11).
Bias (due to systematic error)	Carefully consider the potential consequences of each difference between the research question and the study plan (Figure 10.2); alter the study plan if necessary.	Check consistency with other studies (especially those using different designs).
	Do not use variables affected by the exposure of interest as inclusion criteria or matching variables.	Do not control for variables affected by your predictor variable.
	Employ blinding and other strategies to minimize differences in measurement accuracy and precision between exposure groups.	Look for systematic differences in means or standard deviations between observers, centers, etc.
	Collect additional data that will allow assessment of the extent of possible biases (falsification tests), for example, outcomes not expected to be associated with exposure and vice versa.	Analyze additional data (falsification tests) to see if there is evidence suggesting that the potential biases have occurred.

■ MINIMIZING ERRORS DUE TO BIAS

There are many kinds of bias—also called systematic error—and dealing with them is a major topic of this book. Along with the specific strategies described in Chapters 3, 4, 8, and 9, we now add a general approach to reducing the likelihood of bias.

As was discussed in Chapter 1, there are almost always differences between the original research question and the one that is answered by the study. Those differences reflect the compromises that were made for the study to be feasible as well as mistakes in the design or execution of the study. Bias occurs when those differences cause the estimates provided by the study to differ systematically from what they were trying to estimate. As described in Chapter 9, the two main categories of bias are **selection bias** (also called sampling bias) and **measurement bias**. Strategies for minimizing bias are available in both the design and analysis phases of research (Table 10.2).

Design Phase

Begin by writing the research question next to the study plan, as in Figure 10.2. Then think through the following three concerns as they pertain to the research question:

1. Do the samples of study participants (eg, cases and controls, or exposed and unexposed participants) represent the population(s) of interest?
2. Do the measurements of the exposure variables represent the predictors of interest?
3. Do the measurements of the outcome variables represent the outcomes of interest?

For each question answered "no" or "maybe not," consider whether the bias applies similarly to one or both groups studied (eg, cases and controls, or exposed and unexposed participants) and whether the bias is likely to be large enough to affect the answer to the research question.

To illustrate this with our red meat and colon cancer example, consider a hospital-based case-control study in which the controls are sampled from patients hospitalized for diseases other than colon cancer. If many of these patients have cardiovascular illnesses that were caused by meat intake, the sample of controls will not represent the target population from which the

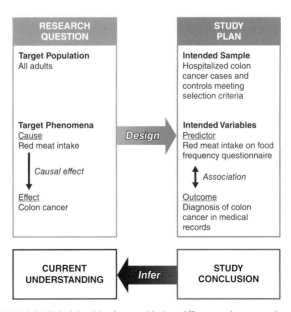

■ **FIGURE 10.2** Minimizing bias by considering differences between the research question and the study plan.

colon cancer cases arose: There will be an excess of carnivores in the control group, resulting in an association between red meat and colon cancer that is lower than the one in the population. The study might even find that eating red meat protects against colon cancer. This would be an example of selection bias.[3]

Measurement bias is also a potential problem for our study. For example, what if we were doing our study using an existing data set and measurement of red meat intake was based on a 24-hour food frequency questionnaire? A participant's 24-hour recall might differ from his actual intake of red meat that day or his usual past or future meat intake by chance alone (we happened to sample a day when he ate chicken nuggets) or due to systematic error, such as a general tendency for people to underreport behaviors believed to be less healthy.

Measurement bias can also affect how a study's outcome is ascertained. Most cohort studies estimate the incidence of the outcome as a proportion or rate, whose numerator is the number of new occurrences of the outcome during follow-up. To get it right, care must be taken to make sure that ascertainment of the outcome is applied uniformly across exposure groups, for example, by blinding those adjudicating whether a participant developed the outcome to exposure status. The denominator for incidence is either the population at risk (for a cumulative incidence) or person-time at risk (for the incidence rate). These denominators can be tricky, especially for exposures measured more than once during the follow-up period. As discussed in Chapter 8, designing an observational study to emulate a "target trial" can help avoid immortal time bias and other errors resulting from counting people as having been at risk when they were not or vice versa (5-7).

The next step is to think about possible strategies for preventing each potential bias, such as selecting more than one control group in a case-control study (Chapter 9) or the strategies for reducing measurement bias described in Chapter 4. In each case, judgments are required about the likelihood of bias and how easily it could be prevented with changes in the study plan. If the bias is easily preventable, revise the study plan and ask the three questions again. If the bias is not easily preventable, decide whether the study is still worth doing by judging the likelihood of the potential bias and the degree to which it will distort the association you are trying to estimate.

Potential biases may either be unavoidable or costly to prevent, or there may be uncertainty as to the extent to which they will be a problem. In either situation, the investigator should consider designing the study to collect additional data that will allow an assessment of the seriousness of the biases. These are called **falsification tests**, and it is important that they be prespecified by being included in the study design (8).

For example, in the case-control twin study of malignant melanoma and sun exposure described in Chapter 9, investigators concerned about the possibility of recall bias asked both twins which one had sunbathed more as a child. They found that the twins with melanoma reported greater sun exposure than the control twins, who reported that their sun exposures had been similar to those of the case twin. It is not possible to know which twin was correct, but the difference in their answers suggests that there was a problem with recall of childhood sun exposure.[4]

If the investigator is concerned that a 24-hour food frequency questionnaire does not accurately reflect usual red meat intake, he could use a more detailed (but time-consuming) 7-day food diary on a subset of the cases and controls to determine its agreement with the 24-hour food frequency questionnaire. Similarly, if he is concerned that rather than causing colon cancer, red meat increases survival among colon cancer patients (which could lead to red meat eaters being overrepresented in a sample of colon cancer survivors), a case-control study could

---

[3]We'll revisit this example when we discuss collider stratification bias and directed acyclic graphs in Appendix 10A.
[4]We don't know whether this was *recall bias*, which typically leads cases to overestimate exposures compared with controls, or just imperfect recall, a type of measurement error that affects both cases and controls similarly.

identify colon cancer patients who died and interview their surviving partners about their previous dietary habits.

Analysis Phase

Once the data have been collected, the goal shifts from minimizing bias to assessing its likely severity. The first step is to analyze data that have been collected for the prespecified falsification tests. For example, an investigator anticipating imperfect recall of red meat intake may have included questions about how sure the cases and controls are of their answers. The association between red meat and colon cancer could then be examined after stratifying on certainty about red meat intake, to see whether the association is stronger among those more certain of their exposure history.

The investigator can also look at the results of other studies. If the conclusions are consistent, the association is less likely to be attributable to bias. This is especially true if the other studies have used different designs and are thus unlikely to share the same biases. The decision on how vigorously to pursue additional information and how best to discuss these issues in reporting the study are matters of judgment, for which it is helpful to seek advice from colleagues.

■ GETTING THE DIRECTION RIGHT: EFFECT-CAUSE

Chance and bias are reasons why the estimate of the association between the measured variables in your sample may not reflect the true association between the phenomena of interest in the target population. But even if your estimate of the association is valid, it may not represent the causal effect.

One possibility is that the cart has come before the horse—the outcome has caused the predictor (Table 10.3). Effect-cause is often a problem in cross-sectional and case-control studies: Does a sedentary lifestyle cause obesity, or vice versa? Effect-cause can also be a problem in case-crossover studies. For example, in the study of mobile phone use and motor vehicle accidents described in Chapter 9 (9), it was important to know the exact timing of the calls and the car crash, because a car crash could cause the driver to make a mobile phone call to report the crash, rather than the crash having been caused by an inattentive driver.

Effect-cause is less commonly a problem in cohort studies of disease causation because risk factor measurements can be made among participants who do not yet have the disease. Even in cohort studies, however, effect-cause is possible if the disease has a long latent period and those with subclinical disease cannot be identified at baseline. For example, Type 2 diabetes is associated with subsequent risk of pancreatic cancer. Some of this association may well be effect-cause, because pancreatic cancer could affect the pancreatic islet cells that secrete insulin,

TABLE 10.3 STRATEGIES FOR GETTING THE DIRECTION OF CAUSALITY RIGHT IN OBSERVATIONAL STUDIES

DESIGN PHASE	ANALYSIS PHASE
• Do a longitudinal study to discover which came first • Obtain data on the historic sequence of the variables • (Ultimate solution: do a randomized trial)	• Consider biologic plausibility • Compare the strength of the association immediately after the exposure to the predictor with the strength later • Consider findings of other studies with different designs

thus causing diabetes. Consistent with effect-cause, the risk of pancreatic cancer is highest just after diabetes is diagnosed (10). The association diminishes with the duration of diabetes, but some excess risk of pancreatic cancer persists even 4 years or more after the onset of diabetes (10-12) suggesting that at least some of the relationship may be cause-effect.

This example illustrates a general approach to ruling out effect-cause: looking for a diminution in the association with increasing time between the presumed cause and its effect. Of course, for short-term exposures with rapid effects, causal effect will also diminish over time, so this strategy works best for chronic exposures, for which the cumulative exposure increases over time (as with diabetes), so that an increase, rather than a decrease, in the association over time would be expected if there was a cause-effect relationship.

A second approach is to assess the biologic plausibility of effect-cause versus cause-effect. In this example, effect-cause was plausible because pancreatic cancer could damage the pancreas, but the observation that having diabetes for more than 10 years is associated with an increased risk of a variety of other cancers as well as pancreatic cancer (12) increases the biologic plausibility of diabetes causing pancreatic cancer.

■ CONFOUNDING

The other reason why the association in the population might differ from the causal effect is confounding. As noted previously, this occurs when a third factor, such as a male gender, causes both red meat intake and colon cancer.[5] This is a plausible concern for male gender because eating red meat is tied with some men's notion of masculinity (13) and men have higher age-specific incidence of colon cancer (14). If this is the case, then the association between red meat intake and colon cancer in the target population might not entirely represent a causal effect. Appendix 10B gives a numeric example of how confounding by gender could be partly responsible for the association between red meat and colon cancer.

What if eating red meat altered the intestinal microbiome, which then caused colon cancer? (15). In that case, the microbiome is called a **mediator** of the causal effect of eating red meat on colon cancer and not a confounder. In general, the strategies for coping with confounders described later in this chapter should not be used for factors that lie along the causal path between a predictor and an outcome (ie, mediators).

Aside from bias, confounding is often the only likely alternative explanation to cause-effect and the most important one to try to rule out. It is also the most challenging; much of the rest of this chapter is devoted to strategies for coping with confounders. It is worth noting, however, that all these strategies involve judgments and that no amount of epidemiologic or statistical sophistication can substitute for understanding the underlying biology.

■ COPING WITH CONFOUNDERS IN THE DESIGN PHASE

Most strategies for coping with confounding variables require that an investigator measure them, so it is helpful to begin by listing the variables (such as age and gender) that may cause (or share a cause with) the exposure and also cause the outcome. The investigator must then choose among design and analysis strategies for controlling for the influence of these potential confounding variables.

---

[5]We have simplified a bit here. The confounder need not cause the exposure if it *shares a common cause* with the exposure. For example, colon cancer screening does not cause people to eat less red meat, but it might share a common cause (health consciousness) with red meat intake. This could be true if people who are more health conscious are more adherent to colon cancer screening and also less likely to eat red meat. In this example, it would be important to control for colon cancer screening to prevent it from confounding the effect of red meat on colon cancer incidence. A more rigorous understanding of confounding (and mediation) depends on directed acyclic graphs (DAGs, Appendix 10A).

TABLE 10.4 DESIGN-PHASE STRATEGIES FOR COPING WITH CONFOUNDERS

STRATEGY	ADVANTAGES	DISADVANTAGES
Specification	• Easily understood • Focuses the sample of participants for the research question at hand	• Limits generalizability and sample size
Matching	• Can eliminate influence of strong constitutional confounders like age and gender • Can eliminate the influence of confounders that are difficult to measure • Can increase precision by balancing the number of cases and controls in each stratum • May be a sampling convenience, making it easier to select the controls in a case-control study	• May be time-consuming and expensive; may be less efficient than increasing the number of participants • Decision to match must be made at outset of study and has an irreversible effect on analysis • Requires early decision about which variables are predictors and which are confounders • Eliminates the option of studying matched variables as predictors or as mediating variables • Requires dropping cases that cannot be matched • Creates the danger of overmatching (ie, matching on a factor that is not a confounder, thereby reducing power) • Only feasible for case-control and multiple-cohort studies
"Opportunistic" study designs	• Can provide great strength of causal inference • May be a lower cost and elegant alternative to a randomized trial	• Only possible in select circumstances where predictor variable is randomly or virtually randomly assigned or there is an instrumental variable

The first two design-phase strategies (Table 10.4), **specification** and **matching**, involve changes in the sampling scheme. Cases and controls (in a case-control study) or exposed and unexposed participants (in a cohort study) can be sampled in such a way that they have comparable values of the confounding variable. This removes the confounder as an explanation for any association that is observed between predictor and outcome. A third design-phase strategy, using **opportunistic study designs**, is only applicable to selected research questions for which the right conditions exist. However, when applicable, these designs can resemble randomized trials in their ability to reduce or eliminate confounding not only by measured variables but by unmeasured variables as well.

Specification

The simplest strategy is to use an inclusion criterion that specifies a value of the potential confounding variable and excludes everyone with a different value, a process called specification. For example, one way to prevent confounding by gender is to specify that only women be included in the study. If an association were then observed between red meat and colon cancer, it could not be due to confounding by gender.

Specification is an effective strategy, but, as with all restrictions in the sampling scheme, it has disadvantages. First, even if red meat does not cause colon cancer in women, it may do so in men or gender-nonbinary people. This phenomenon—an effect of red meat on colon cancer that differs by gender—is called **effect modification**; see the section on this topic under Other

Pitfalls in Quantifying Causal Effects and Appendix 10B. Thus, specification limits the generalizability of information available from a study, in this instance compromising our ability to generalize to those who do not identify as female. A second disadvantage is that specification will necessarily reduce the sample size. These disadvantages can become serious if specification is used to control too many confounders or to control them too narrowly. For example, sample size and generalizability would be major problems if a study were restricted to lower-income, nonsmoking, 70- to 74-year-old women.

Matching

Matching is used to control for confounding in the design phase[6] by selecting cases and controls (or exposed and unexposed) who have the same or similar ("matching") values of the confounding variable(s). Matching and specification both prevent confounding by allowing comparison only of cases and controls who share similar levels of the confounder. Matching differs from specification, however, in that participants at all levels of the confounder can be studied.

Matching is often done individually (**pairwise matching**). To control for age and gender in a study of red meat consumption and colon cancer, for example, each case (someone with colon cancer) could be individually matched to one or more controls of the same gender and age group (eg, women 55-59 years old). The red meat intake of each case would then be compared with that of the matched control(s).

An alternative approach, called frequency matching, is based on the number of cases and controls in each subgroup of interest. For example, frequency matching by age and gender would include the same number of controls as cases in each subgroup (or the appropriate multiple, as appropriate). If the study called for two controls per case and there were 20 cases who were 55- to 59-year-old women, the investigators would select 40 controls who were 55- to 59-year-old women to match to them. The case-control study of hepatitis A (Example 9.1) used frequency matching in broad age groups.

Matching is most commonly used in **case-control studies**, but it can also be used with **multiple-cohort designs**. For example, to investigate the effects of service in the 1990-1991 Gulf War on subsequent fertility in male veterans, Maconochie et al. (16) compared men deployed to the Gulf region during the war with men who were not deployed but who were frequency-matched by service, age, fitness to be deployed, serving status, and rank. They found a higher risk of reported infertility and a longer time to their partner's conception in the Gulf War veterans.

Advantages of Matching

- Matching is an effective way to **prevent confounding by constitutional factors** such as age and gender that are strong determinants of outcome, not susceptible to intervention, and unlikely to be intermediaries on a causal path.
- Matching can be used to **control confounders that cannot be measured** and controlled in any other way. For example, matching siblings (or, better yet, twins) with one another can control for a whole range of genetic and familial factors that would be impossible to measure. Matching for clinical site in a multicenter study can control for unspecified differences among the populations or staff who are dispersed geographically.
- Matching may **increase the precision** of comparisons between groups (and therefore the power of the study to find a real association) by **balancing the number** of cases and controls at each level of the confounder. This may be important if the available number of cases is limited or if the cost of studying the participants is high. However, the effect of matching

---

[6]Matching is generally a design phase strategy, but, as will be discussed later, it may also be used with propensity scores in the analysis phase.

on precision is modest and not always favorable (see **overmatching**, below). In general, the desire to enhance precision is a less important reason to match than the need to control confounding.

- Finally, matching may be used as a **sampling convenience**, to narrow down an otherwise impossibly large number of potential controls. For example, in a study of marijuana use as a risk factor for testicular germ cell tumors (17), investigators asked cases (men with testicular tumors) to suggest friends of similar age without tumors to be in the control group. This convenience, however, also runs the risk of overmatching.

Disadvantages of Matching

- Matching often requires additional **time and expense**. In case-control studies, for example, the more matching criteria there are, the larger the pool of controls that must be searched to match each case. The possible increase in statistical power from matching must therefore be weighed against the increase in power that might be obtained at the same expense by enrolling more cases.

- When matching is used as a sampling strategy, the decision to match must be made at the beginning of the study. It is therefore **irreversible**. This precludes further analysis of the effect of the matched variables on the outcome. It also can create a serious error if the matching variable is not a constitutional variable like age or gender but an intermediary in the causal path between the predictor and the outcome. For example, consider a case-control study of the effect of parental smoking during pregnancy on the risk of sudden infant death syndrome. If the investigator matched on the infant's gestational age at birth, he would miss any harmful effects of maternal smoking mediated through an increase in the risk of prematurity. Although the same error can occur with the analysis phase strategies, matching builds the error into the study in a way that cannot be undone; with the analysis phase strategies, the error can be avoided by altering the analysis.

- Correct analysis of pair-matched data requires special analytic techniques (matched analyses) that compare each participant only with his match(es) and not with other participants who have differing levels of confounders. This means **cases for whom a match cannot be found must be excluded**. In the study of marijuana use and germ cell tumors, for example, 39 of the 187 cases did not provide a friend control and had to be excluded (17). The use of unmatched analytic techniques on matched data can lead to incorrect results (generally biased toward no effect) because the assumption that the groups are sampled independently is violated.[7]

- A final disadvantage of matching is the possibility of **overmatching**, which occurs when the matching variable is associated with the exposure but turns out not to be a confounder because it is not associated with the outcome. Overmatching can reduce the power of a case-control study because it makes the cases and controls more similar. Indeed, in a pairwise matched study, the analysis discards "concordant" case-control sets (those that share the same level of exposure) because they are uninformative: what matters is the number of discordant sets in which the case, but not the control, has the exposure—and vice versa (Appendix 9A). In the marijuana and germ cell tumor study, for example, use of friend controls may have reduced the power by increasing the **concordance** in exposures between cases and their matched controls: the cases and their friends might tend to have similar patterns of marijuana use.

---

[7]Frequency-matched cohort data can be analyzed with multivariable methods without taking the matching into account as long as the matching variables are included as covariates.

Opportunistic Studies

Occasionally, there are opportunities to control for confounding variables in the design phase even without measuring them; we call these "opportunistic" designs because they utilize unusual opportunities to control confounding. What all these studies have in common is something that provides an **opportunity to estimate counterfactual outcomes**, namely, what would have happened to those who were exposed if they had not been exposed and vice versa.

Natural Experiments

A particularly opportunistic design is a **natural experiment**, in which participants are either exposed or not exposed to a particular risk factor through a ("quasi-random") process that, in effect, acts randomly (18). For example, Lofgren et al. (19) studied the effects of discontinuity of in-hospital care by taking advantage of the fact that patients admitted after 5:00 PM to their institution were alternately assigned to senior residents who either maintained care of the patients or transferred them to another team the following morning. They found that patients whose care was transferred had 38% more laboratory tests ordered ($P = 0.01$) and 2-day longer median length of stay ($P = 0.06$) than those kept on the same team. In this case, the outcomes of patients that stayed on the same team are used to estimate the counterfactual outcomes of those who had been transferred (ie, what would have happened to those who were transferred if they had not been transferred).

Similarly, Bell and Redelmeier (20) studied the effects of nursing staffing by comparing outcomes for emergency department patients with selected diagnoses admitted on weekends to those admitted on weekdays. They found higher mortality on weekends from all three conditions (ruptured abdominal aortic aneurysm, acute epiglottitis, and pulmonary embolism) that they predicted would be affected by reduced weekend staffing ratios. So, in this study, the patients admitted on weekdays provided the estimate for the counterfactual outcomes of those admitted on weekends for the same conditions. The authors also prespecified a falsification test: they found no increase in weekend mortality for patients hospitalized emergently for conditions they hypothesized would not be susceptible to staffing differences.

Mendelian Randomization

As genetic differences underlying exposures or (especially) susceptibility to specific exposures are elucidated, the opportunity for studies using **Mendelian randomization** (21) may arise. This opportunity works because, for common genetic polymorphisms, the allele a person receives is determined at random within families (and, to a less certain extent, within populations with similar ancestry)[8] and is therefore not linked to most confounding variables. If alleles associated with greater exposure to a risk factor are also associated independently with the disease thought to be caused by that risk factor, it can provide convincing evidence of causality. For example, the CHRNA5 gene codes for a subunit of a receptor for nicotine; the rs16969968 allele for that gene is associated with more severe nicotine addiction, which manifests as heavier smoking (22) and more trouble quitting (23). This allele is also independently associated with a variety of smoking-related diseases, such as lung cancer (23, 24), chronic obstructive pulmonary disease (25), and low birth weight (26).

Mendelian randomization can also be used more qualitatively to study *susceptibility* to exposures. For example, a proposed mechanism for at least some of the association between red meat intake and colon cancer is that heterocyclic aromatic amines produced from high-temperature cooking of red meat are converted to carcinogens in the body (27). This is facilitated by the action of N-acetyltransferase 2 (NAT-2) whose genetically determined activity can be used to classify people as rapid, intermediate, or slow acetylators. Several studies (27, 28) have found

---

[8]Mendelian randomization in studies that involve populations rather than families is susceptible to a type of confounding called *population stratification*, in which differences in ancestry affect both the genotype and disease being studied. This is most likely when diverse populations are studied, and, therefore, the ancestry of cases and controls may differ.

stronger associations between red meat intake and colon cancer among rapid acetylators, consistent not only with a causal association between red meat and colon cancer but also with this proposed mechanism.

Mendelian randomization does have some limitations. Genetic variants may explain only a small proportion of the variation in the level of or susceptibility to a risk factor. In addition, genetic variants may affect multiple biologic pathways, which can affect the outcome in ways other than through the exposure of interest. Finally, Mendelian exposures generally begin to occur at birth and may have different biologic meaning compared with exposures encountered later in life.

Instrumental Variables

Natural experiments and Mendelian randomization are closely related to a more general approach to enhancing causal inference in observational studies, the use of **instrumental variables** (29, 30). These are variables associated with the exposure of interest, but not independently associated with the outcome. Whether someone is admitted on a weekend, for example, is associated with staffing levels but was thought not to be otherwise associated with mortality risk (for the diagnoses studied), so admission on a weekend can be considered an instrumental variable.

Instrumental variable analyses differ from natural experiments in that they involve explicit measurement of the exposure of interest at different levels of the instrument (eg, number of nurses per 100 patients on weekdays and weekends) and then attempt to quantify the effects of that exposure (rather than just the instrument) on outcome. So, in this example, they would estimate the number of additional deaths that might be prevented by increasing staffing by 3 nurses per 100 patients.

One common type of instrument in clinical research is the frequency of use of specific treatments or diagnostic tests, which may differ among providers, hospitals, or regions. For example, cerebral aneurysms can be treated with clipping (a neurosurgical procedure) or coiling (an interventional radiology procedure in which a coil of wire is placed in the aneurysm). Belekis et al. (31) reported that the proportion of Medicare beneficiaries with unruptured cerebral aneurysms treated with coiling rather than clipping varied dramatically across 306 hospital referral regions, from 35% for Modesto, CA, to 99% for Tacoma, WA. Using the regional proportion of coiling as an instrument to compare the outcomes of the two procedures, they found that mortality was similar but that clipping led to substantially longer hospital stays and a much greater likelihood of discharge to a rehabilitation facility.

Regression Discontinuity Designs

In a randomized trial, the exposure is randomly assigned by the investigator. In an instrumental variable study, it is determined by an external factor not otherwise associated with outcome. In a **regression discontinuity** study, exposure is determined by whether an underlying continuous variable (called the "running variable") is above a threshold that leads to the exposure.

For example, Bor et al. (32) studied the effect of early versus delayed treatment of HIV with antiretroviral therapy. Simply comparing mortality rates in patients who were treated early with antiretrovirals to those who were treated later is susceptible to confounding if, for example, sicker patients are more likely to be treated early. The investigators used data from a large South African cohort in which patients first qualified for antiretroviral treatment when their CD4 cell count (the running variable) fell below 200 cells/μL. Including only patients with CD4 counts between 50 and 350 cells/μL, they found that patients whose CD4 count was just below 200 cells/μL had a hazard ratio for total mortality of 0.65 (95% CI: 0.45 to 0.94) compared with those just above, strongly suggesting that early treatment was highly beneficial.

The ability to use a regression discontinuity design depends on the existence of continuous running variable that either completely determines ("*sharp*" regression discontinuity) or strongly influences ("*fuzzy*" regression discontinuity) the exposure of interest. Examples of running variables (33) include age (which may determine eligibility for programs or legality of activities that may affect health), clinical measures like CD4 count, birth weight, blood lead levels, and systolic blood pressure, all of which can trigger interventions if above or below some threshold, and calendar time commonly divided into before/after changes in policies or incidents, discussed in the next section.

The regression discontinuity design provides one of the strongest alternatives to randomized trials for estimating causal effects and is probably underutilized in clinical research (34). The main assumption is that the only thing affecting outcome that differs on opposite sides of the threshold is the exposure of interest. This assumption gets more likely as the discontinuity sharpens and the sample gets larger so that comparisons between people in very narrow ranges on either side of the threshold can be sufficiently precise. When sample size is more limited and people farther from the threshold need to be included to estimate counterfactual outcomes, investigators can *model* the relationship between the running variable and the outcome separately on each side of the threshold and use the difference between these two models (one approaching from below and one from above) to estimate the causal effect at the threshold.

Interrupted Time Series Designs

Time is a common running variable for regression discontinuity designs: something happens, such as a new policy or program being introduced, and investigators wish to make before/after comparisons, that is, to use the person-time before the defining event to estimate what would have happened if the event had not occurred. These are called **interrupted time series designs** (see also Chapter 12). Changes in outcome over time are modeled before and after the threshold event (eg, as a linear increase or decrease over time) and the model estimates from the before- and after-models are compared at the event time. These designs can express an effect as either a change in the intercept at the time of the threshold event or a change in the slope of the line or both. For example, an intervention might accelerate the rate of decline of a postoperative infection rate that was already declining.

However, time is a particularly challenging running variable, because things outside the control of the investigator may change at about the same time as the event or intervention being studied. For example, the Health in Pregnancy program provided an unconditional cash transfer of GBP 190 at 25 weeks' gestation for pregnant women in the United Kingdom, beginning with those with a due date on or after April 6, 2009 (35). Investigators compared birth outcomes in Scotland before and after the program took effect and found an odds ratio of 1.84 (95% CI: 1.22 to 2.78) for neonatal death during the intervention period. They hypothesized that this unexpected (and profoundly disappointing) result may have been caused by the 2009 swine flu outbreak or the global financial crisis.

Difference in Differences Designs

An alternative approach to using only the period before an event or intervention in a single population to estimate counterfactual outcomes is to have a comparison population during the same time that was not exposed to the event or intervention. This other population can provide an estimate of how the outcome would have changed over time in the exposed population in the absence of exposure. For example, if the swine flu or global financial crisis were responsible for the increase in neonatal mortality in Scotland in 2009, perhaps the increase would have been even worse if not for the cash transfers. Having a comparison population with similar exposure to swine flu, the global financial crisis, and other events during the study period—but that did not receive the cash transfers—would allow the testing of this hypothesis: the before-after difference in neonatal mortality and other outcomes in those exposed to the intervention could be compared with the difference in those not exposed, hence the name "**difference in differences.**" The more closely the time trends of the outcome in the comparison population tracked with those in the study population before the intervention, the more reasonable it is to use the comparison population to estimate the counterfactual outcomes of the treated or exposed group after the intervention.

■ COPING WITH CONFOUNDERS IN THE ANALYSIS PHASE

The design-phase strategies of specification and matching require decisions at the outset of the study as to which variables are confounders, and the investigators cannot subsequently estimate the effects of those confounders on an outcome. By contrast, analysis phase strategies keep the investigator's options open, so that he can change his mind about which variables to control for at the time of analysis.

Sometimes, there are several predictor variables, each of which may act as a confounder to the others. For example, although red meat intake, lack of exercise, and smoking are associated with colon cancer, they are also associated with each other. The goal is often to estimate the causal effects of many predictor variables at the same time. In this section, we discuss analytic methods for assessing the **independent** causal effects of predictor variables in observational studies. These methods are summarized in Table 10.5.[9]

Stratification

Like specification and matching, **stratification** ensures that only cases and controls (or exposed and unexposed participants) with similar levels of a potential confounding variable are compared. It involves segregating the participants into *strata* (subgroups) according to the level of a potential confounder and then examining the relationship between the predictor and the outcome separately in each stratum. Stratification is illustrated in Appendix 10B. By considering men and women separately ("stratifying on gender"), the confounding effects of gender on the association between red meat intake and colon cancer can be controlled.

Appendix 10B also illustrates **interaction (effect modification)**,[10] in which stratification reveals that the association between predictor and outcome varies with the level of a third variable (ie, the effect of the predictor on the outcome is modified by that third factor). Interaction introduces additional complexity, because a single measure of association can no longer summarize the relationship between predictor and outcome. By chance alone, the estimates of association in different strata will rarely be precisely the same, and it is only when the estimates vary markedly or the study is very large that effect modification will be statistically significant. Examining many subgroups increases the likelihood of at least one interaction being statistically significant due to chance. In any case, it is prudent to see if the apparent interaction can be replicated in another population. Biologic plausibility, or the lack thereof, may also contribute to the interpretation. The issue of interaction also arises for subgroup analyses of clinical trials (Chapter 11).

Stratification has the advantage of *flexibility*: by performing several stratified analyses, the investigator can decide which variables appear to be confounders and ignore the remainder. This can be done by combining knowledge about the likely directions of causal relationships

---

[9]Similar questions arise in studies of medical tests (Chapter 13), but in those situations the goal is not to determine a causal effect but whether the test being studied adds substantial predictive power to information already available when the test was done.

[10]Although the terms "effect modification" and "interaction" are often used interchangeably (including by us), there is a subtle difference between them. Effect modification means that the estimate of association (eg, a risk ratio) between cause X and effect Y differs by levels of a third variable C. If the reason for this is that C is also a cause of Y, then we say there is interaction. But effect modification can exist even if C is not a cause of Y. For example, if the risk ratio for red meat and colon cancer were different in men and women because both red meat intake and male gender caused colon cancer, we would say there was an interaction. But there might be effect modification by another variable caused by gender that was *not* a cause of colon cancer, for example being talked over at meetings or having one's ideas ignored until repeated by someone of the opposite gender. For a more detailed explanation, see VanderWeele (36).

TABLE 10.5 ANALYSIS PHASE STRATEGIES FOR COPING WITH CONFOUNDERS

STRATEGY	ADVANTAGES	DISADVANTAGES
Stratification	• Easily understood • Flexible and reversible; can choose which variables to stratify upon after data collection	• Number of strata limited by sample size needed for each stratum • Few covariables can be considered • Few strata per covariable lead to incomplete control of confounding • Relevant covariables must have been accurately measured
Statistical modeling (using a model for outcome)	• Multiple confounders can be controlled simultaneously • Information in continuous variables can be fully used • Flexible and reversible	Model may not fit: • Incomplete control of confounding (if model does not fit confounder-outcome relationship) • Inaccurate estimates of strength of effect (if model does not fit predictor-outcome relationship) • Results may be hard to understand. (Many people do not readily comprehend the meaning of a regression coefficient.) • Relevant covariables must have been accurately measured
Propensity scores (statistical modeling using a model for exposure)	• Multiple confounders can be controlled simultaneously • Information in continuous variables can be fully used • Enhances the ability to control for confounding when the exposure is more common than the outcome • Especially useful for studying *treatments* because the determinants of treatments are often better understood than determinants of outcome • If a stratified or matched analysis is used, does not require model assumptions • Flexible and reversible • Lack of overlap of propensity scores can highlight subgroups in whom control of confounding is difficult or impossible	• Results may be hard to understand • Relevant covariables must have been accurately measured • Only one exposure at a time can be evaluated • Exposure must be dichotomous • Add a layer of opacity and offer more opportunities for "P-hacking" • Seem to be imbued with magical "confounding-correcting" properties by some investigators, reviewers, and readers

(encoded in a directed acyclic graph [DAG], see Appendix 10A) with analyses determining whether the results of stratified analyses differ substantially from those of unstratified analyses (see Appendix 10B). Stratification also has the advantage of being *reversible*: No choices need to be made at the beginning of the study that might later be regretted.

The principal disadvantage of stratified analysis is the limited number of variables that can be controlled simultaneously. The more variables there are and the more strata there are for each variable, the smaller the sample size in each stratum—like dicing an onion. For example, possible confounders in the red meat and colon cancer study might include age, body mass index, fiber intake, colon cancer screening frequency, and cigarette smoking. To stratify on these five variables—with only three strata for each—would require $3^5 = 243$ strata! With this many strata, the sample sizes in each stratum may be small, and there will be many strata with no cases or no controls, which cannot be used at all.

To maintain enough participants in each stratum, a variable is often divided into broader strata. When the strata are too broad, however, the confounder may not be adequately controlled. For example, if the preceding study stratified age using only two strata (eg, <50 and ≥50 years), some residual confounding would still be possible if within each age stratum those eating red meat were older or younger and therefore at different levels of risk of colon cancer.

Multivariable Modeling

Multivariable statistical models adjust for confounders by **modeling** the nature of the associations among the variables to isolate the effects of predictor variables and confounders. For example, a study of the effect of lead levels on the intelligence quotient (IQ) in children might examine parental education as a potential confounder. Statistical modeling might model the relationship between parents' years of schooling and the child's IQ as a straight line, in which each year of parent education is associated with a fixed increase in child IQ. The IQs of children with different lead levels could then be adjusted to remove the effect of parental education using the approach described in Appendix 10C.

Often, an investigator wants to adjust simultaneously for several potential confounders—such as age, gender, race/ethnicity, and education. This requires using multivariable modeling techniques, such as multivariable linear or logistic regression, or Cox proportional hazards analysis. These techniques have another advantage: They enable the use of all the information in continuous variables. It is easy, for example, to adjust for a parent's education level in 1-year intervals, rather than stratifying it into just a few categories. In addition, **interaction terms** can be used to model effect modification among the variables.

There are, however, disadvantages of multivariable modeling. Most important, **the model may not fit**. Computerized statistical packages have made these models so accessible that the investigator may not stop to consider whether their use is appropriate for the predictor and outcome variables in the study. Taking the example in Appendix 10C, the investigator should examine whether the relationship between the parents' years of schooling and the child's IQ is actually linear. If the pattern is very different (eg, the slope of the line decreases and eventually becomes negative with increasing education), then attempts to adjust IQ for parental education using a linear model will be imperfect, and the estimate of the causal effect of lead will be incorrect.

Second, with the exception of linear models with dichotomous predictors, for which coefficients simply represent the expected difference between means, **the resulting statistics are often difficult to understand**. Both odds ratios (produced by logistic regression) and hazard ratios (produced by the Cox model) are harder to understand and explain than risk ratios or risk differences. When predictor variables are continuous, the coefficients depend on the units of measurement, adding to the possibilities for misinterpretation. Interpretability is particularly a problem if transformations of variables (eg, parental education squared) or interaction terms are used. Investigators should spend the necessary time with a statistician (or take the necessary courses) to make sure they can explain the meaning of coefficients or other highly derived statistics they plan to report. As a safety precaution, it is a good idea to always start with simple, stratified analyses and to seek help understanding what is going on if more complicated analyses yield substantially different results.

Propensity Scores

Propensity scores can be particularly useful for observational studies of the efficacy of a treatment, policy, or other intervention. The major threat to validity in such studies is **confounding**

by indication—the problem that patients for whom a treatment is indicated (and prescribed) are often at higher risk, or otherwise different, from those who do not get the treatment (37). Recall that in order to be a confounder, a variable must cause or have a common cause with both the predictor and the outcome. Instead of adjusting for all factors that predict *outcome*, use of propensity scores involves creating a multivariable model to predict receipt of the *treatment*. Each participant can then be assigned a predicted probability of treatment—a "propensity score." This single score can be used as the only confounding variable in a stratified (eg, in quintiles of propensity score) or multivariable analysis.

Alternatively, participants who did and did not receive the treatment can be *matched* by propensity score and outcomes compared between matched pairs. Unlike the use of matching as a design-phase (sampling) strategy, propensity matching resembles other analysis phase strategies in being reversible. However, the analysis must exclude participants who cannot be matched (ie, those for whom there is no one with a similar propensity score but the opposite exposure). This happens most often for participants with propensity scores close to 0 or 1, who have a very low or very high propensity to be exposed; thus, there will be few people with that score and the opposite exposure. Although this reduces sample size, it may also be advantageous, because calculating propensity scores identified a problem—the lack of comparability among unmatchable participants—that might not have been apparent with other analytic methods. The unmatched people in a propensity analysis resemble those who would meet the exclusion criteria in a clinical trial: people in whom either the treatment is contraindicated or so nearly mandatory that it would be unethical to randomize them to the alternative. It is difficult to estimate the causal effects of the exposure in such people, but those effects are usually not of much interest clinically.

Analyses using propensity scores have several advantages. The number of potential confounding variables that can be modeled as predictors of an intervention is usually greater than the number of variables that can be modeled as predictors of an outcome, because the number of people treated is generally much greater than the number who develop the outcome (2310 compared with 276 in the Example 10.1). Another reason that more confounders can be included is that there is no danger of "overfitting" the propensity model—interaction and quadratic terms and multiple indicator variables can all be included. That said, variables known to have no association with the outcome should be excluded.[11] Finally, investigators are usually more confident in identifying the determinants of treatment than the determinants of outcome, because the treatment decisions were made by clinicians on the basis of a limited number of patient characteristics. It is easier to ask a clinician why a person got treated than to ask a deity (or find one to ask!) why a person got a disease.

Of course, as with other multivariable techniques, the use of propensity scores still requires potential confounding variables to be identified and measured. A limitation of this technique

Example 10.1 Example of a Propensity Analysis

Gum et al. (38) studied 6174 consecutive adults who underwent stress echocardiography, 2310 of whom (37%) were taking aspirin and 276 of whom died in the 3.1-year follow-up period. In unadjusted analyses, aspirin use was not associated with mortality (4.5% in both groups). However, when 1351 patients who had received aspirin were matched to 1351 patients who had the same propensity to receive aspirin but who did not, mortality was 47% lower in those who were treated ($P = 0.002$).

---

[11]Variables associated with exposure but not otherwise with outcome are called instruments. The reason not to include them in propensity scores is that their inclusion is not necessary to control confounding. However, including them diminishes the overlap in propensity scores between the exposed and unexposed, and it is only in areas of overlap that the causal effect can be estimated.

is that it does not provide information about the relationship between any of the confounding variables and outcome—the only result is for the chosen predictor (usually, a treatment). However, because this is an analysis phase strategy, it does not preclude also doing more traditional multivariable analyses.

This brings up a final problem with propensity scores: they add a layer of opacity and manipulability to the analysis. Because there are many ways to both create the propensity scores and include them in the analysis, there is greater potential to do the analysis several ways and selectively publish or emphasize the analyses that give results most appealing to the investigator, a process called "P-hacking" (39). This problem is compounded, in our experience, by the tendency of some investigators and readers to imbue these scores with almost magical ability to control for confounding simply because they may have been created from hundreds of predictor variables. But, as will be discussed in Chapter 16, data quantity is a poor substitute for data quality: garbage in, garbage out.

■ OTHER PITFALLS IN QUANTIFYING CAUSAL EFFECTS

Conditioning on a Shared Effect (Collider Stratification Bias)

One of the most important insights from using directed acyclic graphs (DAGs; Appendix 10A) is the concept of a **collider**: a variable that is a common effect of two causes. (In a DAG, it is a variable that has two arrows pointing into it.) If we stratify ("condition") on such a variable, it can lead to a tricky kind of bias. Rather than diving right into a complicated explanation, we will first give a few examples of how it might occur and then try to explain it.

Consider a study of people who have lost at least 15 pounds in the previous year. An investigator finds that those who have been dieting have a lower risk of cancer than those who have not been dieting. Do you think dieting prevents cancer?

If you stop and think, you'll probably answer no, because cancer also causes weight loss. You can imagine that if someone loses weight for no apparent reason it is much more likely to signify a cancer than if someone loses weight while dieting. *As a result, among people who have lost weight*, if the weight loss was not caused by dieting, it is more likely to have been caused by something more ominous. Because weight loss has arrows from both cancer and dieting pointing into it, it is a collider. The investigators created an inverse association between dieting and cancer by **conditioning** on (restricting attention to) a collider (weight loss, which is caused by both dieting and cancer; Figure 10.3 Panel A).

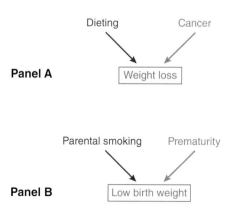

■ FIGURE 10.3 Directed acyclic graphs showing collider examples in text.
By convention, a box around a variable means it has been conditioned on.

Here's another example. Among low-birth-weight babies, those whose mothers smoked during pregnancy were less likely to be born prematurely than those whose mothers did not smoke. Should we encourage more mothers to smoke during pregnancy? Definitely not! The reason for this observation is that smoking causes low birth weight, but so do other things, especially prematurity. So, *among low-birth-weight babies*, if the low birth weight was not caused by smoking, it is more likely to have been caused by prematurity. The investigators created an inverse association between smoking and prematurity by conditioning on (restricting attention to) a collider (low birth weight, which is caused by both smoking and prematurity; Figure 10.3 Panel B).[12]

The possibility of collider stratification bias elucidates an important difference between traditional, population-based epidemiology and clinical epidemiology. Because clinical epidemiology studies often include only patients with a particular disease or symptom, they are limited in their ability to study causes of that disease or symptom—a representative sample of those not affected would be required. For example, Newman et al. (40) studied predictors of urinary tract infections (UTI) among babies <3 months old with fevers. A factor associated with reduced risk of UTI was if the baby had sick family members. It is unlikely that having, say, an older sibling with a cold prevents UTIs. Rather, fever, which was an inclusion criterion for the study, is a shared effect of colds and of UTI. Thus, anything that made a baby more likely to have a cold made him less likely to have a UTI.

Clinical populations are fine for studying diagnostic tests and efficacy of treatments. But it is risky to try to study causes of diseases using only clinical rather than population-based samples.

Effect Modification and Interaction

Effect modification (interaction) is just what it sounds like: one variable modifying the effect of another. For example, if we were measuring the causal effect of red meat intake on colon cancer using the risk ratio, effect modification by gender would mean that the risk ratios would be different in men and women (Appendix 10B).

Effect modification depends on the scale used to quantify the effects of an exposure. Unless the exposure has no effect on outcome, if there is no effect modification on the multiplicative scale (which uses risk ratios, hazard ratios, or odds ratios to quantify effects), there will be effect modification on the additive scale (which uses risk and rate differences) and vice versa. This is illustrated in Example 10.2.

Whether to quantify an association on the multiplicative or additive scale (or both) depends on the investigator's model for how the exposure causes (or prevents) disease and how the results of the study will be used. Many exposures (both favorable and unfavorable) fit the multiplicative model reasonably well, and risk ratios and other multiplicative measures provide stronger evidence for causality the farther they are from 1. On the other hand, risk differences are more important for clinical and public health decision making (Example 10.2).

Underestimation of Causal Effects

Although confounding is often thought of as inflating risk ratios, making exposures seem to be stronger risk factors than they are, it can also lead to attenuation of real associations. This type of confounding, in which the effects of a beneficial factor are hidden by its association with a cause of the outcome, is sometimes called **suppression** (41). It is a common problem for observational studies of treatments, because **treatments** are often indicated in those at higher risk of a bad outcome. The result, noted earlier, is that a beneficial treatment can appear to be useless (as aspirin did in Example 10.1) or even harmful until the confounding by indication is controlled.

---

[12]In both examples, the common causes of the collider were positively associated with it. In such situations, conditioning on the collider tends to create inverse associations between the common causes. But if one of the arrows pointing into the collider is from a factor that *decreases* risk, conditioning on the collider will tend to create positive associations between the common causes.

Example 10.2 Numerical Illustration of Additive versus Multiplicative Interactions

Consider two risk factors for fatal car crashes—drinking and texting—and assume that we can divide drivers into those who habitually text and drive, drink and drive, do both, or do neither. The following partially filled in 2 × 2 table shows hypothetical crash fatality rates per 100,000 per year:

CRASH FATALITIES PER 100K/YEAR	NO TEXTING	TEXTING
No Drinking	10	30
Drinking	40	?

What number would we expect in the "?" cell if there were no interaction? We asked three transportation safety researchers.

Additive Ada: I can see that texting adds 20 to the rate per 100,000/year in the No Drinking group, so if there's no interaction, I should add 20 to 40 in the drinking group to get 60 in the Drinking Texting group. Alternatively, it looks like drinking adds 30 to the risk in those who do not text, so I can add 30 to the 30 in the Texting-No Drinking group and I get 60 again! I did this two ways and got 60 both times, so I must be right!

CRASH RATES PER 100K/YEAR		
ADA'S TABLE	NO TEXTING	TEXTING
No Drinking	10	30
Drinking	40	60

Multiplicative Mia: I can see that texting multiplies the rate of crashes per 100,000 by 3 in the No Drinking group, so if there's no interaction, I should multiply 40 by 3 in the drinking group and get 120 in the Drinking Texting group. Alternatively, it looks like drinking quadruples the risk in those who do not text, so I can multiply 30 by 4 in the Texting-No Drinking group and I get 120 again! I did this two ways, and got the same answer both times, so I must be right!

CRASH RATES PER 100K/YEAR		
MIA'S TABLE	NO TEXTING	TEXTING
No Drinking	10	30
Drinking	40	120

Sophisticated Sophie: Ada and Mia, you are both right! Under the additive model, the risk *differences* are maintained (ie, an additional 20 crashes per 100,000 per year from texting and an additional 30 crashes per 100,000 per year from drinking alcohol), but the risk ratios are not. In contrast, under the multiplicative model, the risk *ratios* are maintained (ie, 3 times as many crashes from texting and 4 times as many from drinking alcohol), but the risk differences are not.

This is why when talking or writing about interactions, it is important to specify whether your model is additive or multiplicative.

Because clinical and public health decisions should generally be based on additive models, additive interactions are arguably more relevant. For example, if Mia's table was based on actual data, some people might say, "There was no interaction, so the effect of texting is the same among drinkers and nondrinkers." But, in fact, the effect of texting is 4 times as big in drinkers: If we could eliminate texting in drinkers, we could prevent 80 crashes per 100,000 per year, compared with only 20 per 100,000 per year if we eliminated texting among non-drinkers! So, it is important to remember that anytime someone finds an effect with no multiplicative interactions, it means there will be additive interactions, and they may be important.

■ CHOOSING A STRATEGY

What general guidelines can be offered for deciding whether to cope with confounders during the design or analysis phases and how best to do it? The use of *specification* to control confounding is most appropriate for situations in which the investigator is chiefly interested in specific subgroups of the population; this is just a special form of the general process of establishing criteria for selecting the study participants (Chapter 3). However, for studies in which causal inference is the goal, there's the additional caution to avoid inclusion criteria that could be caused by predictor variables you wish to study (ie, avoid conditioning on a shared effect).

An important decision to make in the design phase of the study is whether to *match*. Matching is most appropriate for case-control studies and fixed constitutional factors such as age and sex. Matching may also be helpful when the sample size is small compared with the number of strata necessary to control for known confounders and when the confounders are more easily matched than measured. However, because matching can permanently compromise the investigator's ability to observe real associations, it should be used sparingly, particularly for variables that may be in the causal chain. In many situations, the analysis phase strategies (stratification, modeling, and propensity scores) are just as good for controlling confounding and have the advantage of being *reversible*—they allow the investigator to add or subtract covariates to explore different causal models.

Although not available for all research questions, it is always worth considering the possibility of an *opportunistic* study design. If you don't stop and consider (and ask your colleagues about) these studies, you might miss a great opportunity to do one.

The final decision to *stratify, model,* or use *propensity scores* need not be made until after the data are collected; in many cases, the investigator may wish to do all the above. However, it is important during study design to consider which factors may later be used in multivariable models in order to know which variables to measure. In addition, because different analysis phase strategies for controlling confounding do not always yield the same results, it is best to specify a primary analysis plan in advance. This may help investigators resist the temptation to select the analysis strategy that provides the most desired results.

■ EVIDENCE FAVORING CAUSALITY

The approach to enhancing causal inference has largely been a negative one thus far—how to rule out the four rival explanations in Table 10.1. A complementary strategy is to seek characteristics of associations that provide positive evidence for causality, the most important of which are the consistency and strength of the association, the presence of a dose-response relationship, and biologic plausibility.

When the results are **consistent** in studies of various designs, it is less likely that chance or bias is the cause of an association. Real associations that represent effect-cause or confounding, however, will also be consistently observed. In that case, consistency across multiple investigators, study designs, and methods for controlling for confounding can strengthen the evidence for causality.

The **strength** of the association is also important. For one thing, stronger associations give more significant *P* values and confidence intervals farther from no effect, making chance a less likely explanation. Stronger associations also provide better evidence for causality by reducing the likelihood of confounding. Associations due to confounding are indirect (ie, via the confounder) and are therefore generally weaker than direct cause-effect associations.

A **dose-response** relationship provides positive evidence for causality. The association between cigarette smoking and lung cancer is an example: Moderate smokers have higher rates of cancer than do nonsmokers, and heavy smokers have even higher rates. Whenever possible, predictor variables should be measured continuously or in several categories so that any dose-response relationship that is present can be observed. Once again, however, a dose-response relationship can be observed with effect-cause associations or with confounding.

Finally, **biologic plausibility** is an important consideration for drawing causal inference—if a causal mechanism that makes sense biologically can be proposed, evidence for causality is enhanced, whereas associations that do not make sense given our current understanding of biology are less likely to represent cause-effect. For example, in the study of marijuana use as a risk factor for germ cell tumors, use of marijuana less than once a day was associated with lower risk than no use (17). It is hard to explain this biologically. It is important not to overemphasize biologic plausibility, however. Investigators seem to be able to come up with a plausible mechanism for virtually any association, and some associations originally dismissed as biologically implausible, such as a bacterial etiology for peptic ulcer disease, have turned out to be real.

■ SUMMARY

1. The goal of many studies is to estimate **causal effects**. The association observed in a population may differ from the causal effect for four reasons: **chance, bias, effect-cause, and confounding**.
2. The role of **chance** (random error) can be minimized by designing a study with adequate sample size and precision to reduce the influence of random error. Once the study is completed, potential random error can be estimated from the width of the 95% confidence interval and the consistency of the results with previous evidence.
3. **Bias** (systematic error) arises from differences between the population and phenomena addressed by the research question and the actual participants and measurements in the study. Bias can be minimized by basing design decisions on a judgment as to whether these differences will lead to a wrong answer to the research question and can be assessed by prespecifying falsification tests.
4. **Effect-cause** is made less likely by designing a study that permits assessment of temporal sequence and by considering biologic plausibility.
5. **Confounding** may be present when a third variable is a cause of (or shares a common cause with) the predictor of interest and is a cause of the outcome. It can be made less likely by the following strategies, all of which require potential confounders to be anticipated and measured accurately:
    a. **Specification** or **matching** in the design phase, which alters the sampling strategy to ensure that only groups with similar levels of the confounder are compared. These strategies should be used judiciously because they can irreversibly limit the information available from the study.
    b. Analysis phase strategies that accomplish the same goal and preserve options for investigating causal paths:
       • **Stratification**, which in addition to controlling for confounding can reveal effect modification, in which the magnitude of the predictor-outcome association depends on a third variable.
       • **Multivariable modeling**, which can permit the effects of many predictor variables to be controlled simultaneously.
       • **Propensity scores**, which are especially useful for addressing confounding by indication in observational studies of the efficacy of treatments and other interventions.
6. Investigators should be on the lookout for opportunistic observational designs, including **natural experiments, Mendelian randomization**, and other **instrumental variable** and **regression discontinuity** designs that offer a strength of causal inference that can approach that of a randomized clinical trial. Causal inference with **interrupted time series designs** can be enhanced if there is a comparison group not exposed to the change being studied; in that case a **difference in differences** can be calculated.

7. Investigators should avoid **conditioning on shared effects** in the design phase by not selecting participants based on covariates that might be caused by the predictor and should avoid it in the analysis phase by not controlling for these covariates.
8. Causal inference can be enhanced by positive evidence, notably the consistency and strength of the association, the presence of a dose-response relationship, and biologic plausibility.

REFERENCES

1. National Cancer Institute Surveillance, Epidemiology, and End Results Program. *Cancer stat facts: common cancer sites.* Published 2020. https://seer.cancer.gov/statfacts/html/common.html.
2. Tilman D, Clark M. Global diets link environmental sustainability and human health. *Nature.* 2014;515(7528):518-522.
3. Bacchetti P. Current sample size conventions: flaws, harms, and alternatives. *BMC Med.* 2010;8:17.
4. Newman T, Kohn M. *Evidence-Based Diagnosis: An Introduction to Clinical Epidemiology.* 2nd ed. Cambridge University Press; 2020:292-295.
5. Hernan MA, Sauer BC, Hernandez-Diaz S, Platt R, Shrier I. Specifying a target trial prevents immortal time bias and other self-inflicted injuries in observational analyses. *J Clin Epidemiol.* 2016;79:70-75.
6. Newman TB. Antibiotic treatment for inpatient asthma exacerbations: what have we learned? *JAMA Intern Med.* 2021;181(4):427-428.
7. Newman TB. Possible immortal time bias in study of antibiotic treatment and outcomes in patients hospitalized for asthma. *JAMA Intern Med.* 2021;181(4):568-569.
8. Prasad V, Jena AB. Prespecified falsification end points: can they validate true observational associations? *JAMA.* 2013;309(3):241-242.
9. McEvoy SP, Stevenson MR, McCartt AT, et al. Role of mobile phones in motor vehicle crashes resulting in hospital attendance: a case-crossover study. *BMJ.* 2005;331(7514):428.
10. Magruder JT, Elahi D, Andersen DK. Diabetes and pancreatic cancer: chicken or egg? *Pancreas.* 2011;40(3):339-351.
11. Huxley R, Ansary-Moghaddam A, de Gonzalez Berrington A, Barzi F, Woodward M. Type-II diabetes and pancreatic cancer: a meta-analysis of 36 studies. *Br J Cancer.* 2005;92(11):2076-2083.
12. Bosetti C, Rosato V, Polesel J, et al. Diabetes mellitus and cancer risk in a network of case-control studies. *Nutr Cancer.* 2012;64(5):643-651.
13. Love HJ, Sulikowski D. Of meat and men: sex differences in implicit and explicit attitudes toward meat. *Front Psychol.* 2018;9:559.
14. Abotchie PN, Vernon SW, Du XL. Gender differences in colorectal cancer incidence in the United States, 1975-2006. *J Womens Health (Larchmt).* 2012;21(4):393-400.
15. Song M, Chan AT, Sun J. Influence of the gut microbiome, diet, and environment on risk of colorectal cancer. *Gastroenterology.* 2020;158(2):322-340.
16. Maconochie N, Doyle P, Carson C. Infertility among male UK veterans of the 1990-1 Gulf war: reproductive cohort study. *BMJ.* 2004;329(7459):196-201.
17. Trabert B, Sigurdson AJ, Sweeney AM, Strom SS, McGlynn KA. Marijuana use and testicular germ cell tumors. *Cancer.* 2011;117(4):848-853.
18. Bor J. Capitalizing on natural experiments to improve our understanding of population health. *Am J Public Health.* 2016;106(8):1388-1389.
19. Lofgren RP, Gottlieb D, Williams RA, Rich EC. Post-call transfer of resident responsibility: its effect on patient care [see comments]. *J Gen Intern Med.* 1990;5(6):501-505.
20. Bell CM, Redelmeier DA. Mortality among patients admitted to hospitals on weekends as compared with weekdays. *N Engl J Med.* 2001;345(9):663-668.
21. Davey Smith G, Ebrahim S. 'Mendelian randomization': can genetic epidemiology contribute to understanding environmental determinants of disease? *Int J Epidemiol.* 2003;32(1):1-22.
22. Ware JJ, van den Bree MB, Munafo MR. Association of the CHRNA5-A3-B4 gene cluster with heaviness of smoking: a meta-analysis. *Nicotine Tob Res.* 2011;13(12):1167-1175.
23. Chen LS, Hung RJ, Baker T, et al. CHRNA5 risk variant predicts delayed smoking cessation and earlier lung cancer diagnosis-a meta-analysis. *J Natl Cancer Inst.* 2015;107(5):djv100.
24. Zhou W, Zhu W, Tong X, et al. CHRNA5 rs16969968 polymorphism is associated with lung cancer risk: a meta-analysis. *Clin Respir J.* 2020;14(6):505-513.
25. Pillai SG, Ge D, Zhu G, et al. A genome-wide association study in chronic obstructive pulmonary disease (COPD): identification of two major susceptibility loci. *PLoS Genet.* 2009;5(3):e1000421.
26. Yang Q, Millard LAC, Davey Smith G. Proxy gene-by-environment Mendelian randomization study confirms a causal effect of maternal smoking on offspring birthweight, but little evidence of long-term influences on offspring health. *Int J Epidemiol.* 2020;49(4):1207-1218.

27. Doaei S, Hajiesmaeil M, Aminifard A, Mosavi-Jarrahi SA, Akbari ME, Gholamalizadeh M. Effects of gene polymorphisms of metabolic enzymes on the association between red and processed meat consumption and the development of colon cancer; a literature review. *J Nutr Sci.* 2018;7:e26.
28. Wang H, Iwasaki M, Haiman CA, et al. Interaction between red meat intake and NAT2 genotype in increasing the risk of colorectal cancer in Japanese and African Americans. *PLoS One.* 2015;10(12):e0144955.
29. Greenland S. An introduction to instrumental variables for epidemiologists. *Int J Epidemiol.* 2000;29(6):1102.
30. Rassen JA, Schneeweiss S, Glynn RJ, Mittleman MA, Brookhart MA. Instrumental variable analysis for estimation of treatment effects with dichotomous outcomes. *Am J Epidemiol.* 2009;169(3):273-284.
31. Bekelis K, Gottlieb DJ, Su Y, et al. Comparison of clipping and coiling in elderly patients with unruptured cerebral aneurysms. *J Neurosurg.* 2017;126(3):811-818.
32. Bor J, Moscoe E, Mutevedzi P, Newell ML, Barnighausen T. Regression discontinuity designs in epidemiology: causal inference without randomized trials. *Epidemiology.* 2014;25(5):729-737.
33. Hilton Boon M, Craig P, Thomson H, Campbell M, Moore L. Regression discontinuity designs in health: a systematic review. *Epidemiology.* 2021;32(1):87-93.
34. Moscoe E, Bor J, Barnighausen T. Regression discontinuity designs are underutilized in medicine, epidemiology, and public health: a review of current and best practice. *J Clin Epidemiol.* 2015;68(2):122-133.
35. Leyland AH, Ouedraogo S, Nam J, et al. *Evaluation of Health in Pregnancy grants in Scotland: A Natural Experiment Using Routine Data.* Public Health Research; 2017.
36. VanderWeele T. On the distinction between interaction and effect modification. *Epidemiology.* 2009;20(6): 863-871.
37. Braitman LE, Rosenbaum PR. Rare outcomes, common treatments: analytic strategies using propensity scores. *Ann Intern Med.* 2002;137(8):693-695.
38. Gum PA, Thamilarasan M, Watanabe J, Blackstone EH, Lauer MS. Aspirin use and all-cause mortality among patients being evaluated for known or suspected coronary artery disease: a propensity analysis. *JAMA.* 2001;286(10):1187-1194.
39. Bruns SB, Ioannidis JP. p-Curve and p-hacking in observational research. *PLoS One.* 2016;11(2):e0149144.
40. Newman TB, Bernzweig JA, Takayama JI, Finch SA, Wasserman RC, Pantell RH. Urine testing and urinary tract infections in febrile infants seen in office settings: the Pediatric Research in Office Settings' Febrile Infant Study. *Arch Pediatr Adolesc Med.* 2002;156(1):44-54.
41. Katz MH. *Multivariable Analysis: A Practical Guide for Clinicians.* 2nd ed. Cambridge University Press; 2006:xv, 192 p.

APPENDIX 10A
Using Directed Acyclic Graphs (DAGs) to Represent Associations Among Variables

Using observational data to model the associations among variables has been enhanced through the use of **directed acyclic graphs** (abbreviated **DAGs**, rhymes with rags). DAGs are a schematic representation of how an investigator believes the variables in his study are related to one another. The mathematical principles that underlie DAGs enable the estimation of causal effects.

DAGs use unidirectional arrows to indicate the causal direction between two variables. Thus A → B indicates that the investigator believes that predictor A causes outcome B; for example, that excessive alcohol consumption causes hip fractures. DAGs are so named because they involve a network of variables connected by directed arrows that are acyclic (they can't contain a loop) and represented graphically.

Although DAGs can get complicated, connecting 10 or more variables, they are relatively easy to understand when there are only three variables: a predictor that you believe causes an outcome and a third variable that may be related to the other two variables. For example, an investigator studying whether low vitamin D levels cause hip fractures might be concerned about the confounding effects of outdoor exercise, which increases vitamin D levels and also improves strength and balance. Of course, the investigator is likely to also be interested in many other factors, such as a history of falls, nutritional status, and place of residence. Still, the basic approach is straightforward. After creating the causal model (ie, drawing the DAG), the investigator must decide which, if any, variables affect the way study participants should be selected and which variables—beyond the predictor and outcome—need to be measured so they can be included in statistical models when the data are analyzed.

As we did in Chapter 1 when introducing clinical research, we will begin by discussing the anatomy of DAGs, illustrating and naming the different forms they can take. Then we will cover their physiology—how using DAGs can help with causal inference and choosing a sample.

■ EXAMPLES OF DAGS

When investigating whether a predictor causes an outcome, there are only eight ways (Figures 10A.1 to 10A.8) that a third variable can be associated with them. We will review all eight possibilities, always putting the predictor variable in purple text (since the words predictor and purple start with a p) and the outcome variable in ocher. Pay close attention, however, to the position of—and the blue arrows connected to—the third variable (in teal). *These differ, sometimes subtly, in each example.* We have followed the convention of having the connecting arrows point in the purported causal direction and, to the extent possible, from up to down and/or from left to right.

■ DAGS THAT DO NOT CONNECT ALL THREE VARIABLES

Two of these examples (Figures 10A.1 and 10A.2) occur when the third variable causes the predictor but not the outcome or the outcome but not the predictor. In both these DAGs, the third variable is not relevant to the question of whether the predictor causes the outcome.

For example, suppose you are studying whether a predictor (a history of severe head trauma) causes the outcome of Parkinson's disease (Figure 10A.1). A third variable (failure to wear a bike helmet when riding) causes the predictor (thus the arrow from wearing a bike helmet to head trauma). But because you do not believe that wearing (or not wearing) a bike helmet directly causes Parkinson's disease, there is no arrow between them. Thus, you would not have to be concerned about how wearing a bike helmet affects the causal effect of the predictor (head trauma) on the outcome (Parkinson's disease).

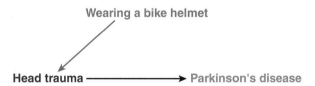

■ **FIGURE 10A.1** An example of an association that does not connect all three variables; the history of wearing a bike helmet need not be considered to estimate the causal effect of head trauma on Parkinson's disease. Note this is the DAG for an instrumental variable analysis, with wearing a bike helmet as the instrument.

Let's now consider a study of whether having type A blood increased the risk of being hospitalized with COVID-19 (Figure 10A.2). Men were at increased risk of COVID-19 hospitalization (thus, there is an arrow from male sex to COVID-19 admission in Figure 10A.3), but sex has no association with—and thus no arrow to—blood type A, which is equally frequent in both sexes. Therefore, there is no need to be concerned about whether male sex might be responsible for the causal effect of blood group A on COVID-19 admission. (That said, including sex in an analytic model might improve the *precision* of the estimated effect of blood type on admission; it might also be useful when seeing whether sex modifies that effect.)

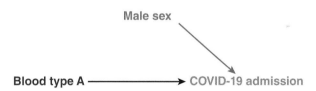

■ **FIGURE 10A.2** An example of an association that does not connect all three variables; male sex cannot be responsible for an association between blood type A and COVID-19 admission.

Next, there are two examples where a third variable is caused by the predictor but has no connection with the outcome (Figure 10A.3) or where it is caused by the outcome but has no connection with the predictor (Figure 10A.4).

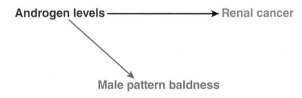

■ **FIGURE 10A.3** An example of an association that does not connect all three variables; male-pattern baldness would not influence the causal effect of androgen levels on renal cancer.

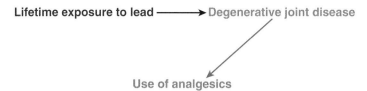

■ **FIGURE 10A.4** An example of an association that does not connect all three variables; use of analgesics would not change the estimated causal effect of lead exposure on joint disease.

Suppose you are interested in determining whether elevated androgen levels in men are a cause of renal cancer and are concerned about the possible effects of male-pattern baldness. Although men with higher androgen levels may be more susceptible to male-pattern baldness, there is no reason to think that baldness causes renal cancer. So you would not need to account for its effects or even ask about it (Figure 10A.3).

In another situation, the third variable (say, using analgesics) is caused by the outcome (degenerative joint disease), but not by the predictor (exposure to lead), except insofar as lead exposure causes joint disease (Figure 10A.4). Again, there would be no need to account for analgesic use when studying the association between lead exposure and joint disease.

■ DAGS THAT CONNECT ALL THREE VARIABLES

There are four ways that a third variable can be connected to both the predictor and the outcome (Figures 10A.5 to 10A.8). These require additional attention because the investigator must decide whether to include that variable when analyzing the data—and sometimes even when choosing the study's selection criteria, as will be discussed later in the sections called "Using DAGs to make inferences about causality" and "DAGs and sampling."

DAG Showing Mediation

Of the four, **mediation** is easiest to understand (Figure 10A.5). It occurs when a predictor (say, serum LDL cholesterol level) causes another factor (carotid artery stenosis), which in turn causes the outcome (stroke). It's called mediation because some of or all the effects of LDL cholesterol on stroke may be mediated through carotid stenosis.

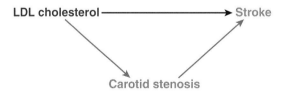

■ **FIGURE 10A.5** An example of mediation. Some of the causal effect of LDL cholesterol level on stroke may be mediated through its effects on carotid stenosis.

DAG Showing Shared Effects

The next DAG (Figure 10A.6) represents the phenomenon of a **shared effect**; the point (node) where the arrows meet is often called a **collider**. This happens when the predictor and the outcome both cause a third variable. Consider a study of whether low-calorie diets cause gastric carcinoma. Both low-calorie diets and gastric carcinoma cause weight loss, which is thus a shared effect.

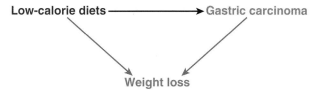

■ **FIGURE 10A.6** An example of a shared effect. Stratifying on weight loss may bias the estimate of the causal effect of low-calorie diets on gastric carcinoma.

Shared effects can be problematic: When a collider is used as an inclusion criterion, or included in a statistical model, it can cause bias and even make true causal associations disappear. In this example, a study that enrolled only patients with weight loss would create an inverse association between low-calorie diets and gastric carcinoma, because having one negates the need to have the other to explain the weight loss. This could make low-calorie diets appear protective against gastric carcinoma or mask a true-positive association between them.

DAG Showing Confounding

The best-known DAG (Figure 10A.7) illustrates **confounding**, which occurs when the third factor causes both the predictor and the outcome. For example, if you are interested in determining whether marijuana smoking causes lung cancer, tobacco smoking is a potential confounder, since it causes lung cancer and increases the likelihood of marijuana smoking.

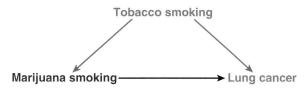

■ **FIGURE 10A.7** An example of confounding. Tobacco smoking could contribute to an association between marijuana smoking and lung cancer.

If the effect of marijuana smoking on lung cancer is accounted for entirely by tobacco smoking, adjusting for it in an analytic model will remove the effect of marijuana smoking on lung cancer. There can also be partial confounding, in which **adjustment** reduces the effect. There is even reverse confounding (called **suppression**), in which adjustment for the confounder makes an association stronger (see the section on "Underestimation of Causal Effects").

A "DAG" That Isn't One

The final situation occurs when the causal diagram includes a cycle (Figure 10A.8), meaning that a predictor (obesity) causes the outcome (osteoarthritis), which in turn causes a third factor (sedentary lifestyle), which then affects the predictor (obesity).

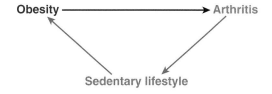

■ **FIGURE 10A.8** An example of a cyclic graph, to which the principles underlying DAGs do not apply.

This situation is not actually a DAG, because it's not acyclic—and thus the rules for DAGs don't work. There are special methods to deal with situations like this, such as making repeated measurements of the variables over time to untangle "the chicken and egg" problem of which variable is the cause and which the effect.

■ USING DAGS TO MAKE INFERENCES ABOUT CAUSALITY

Once you've drawn your DAG and determined which of these situations apply, you next must decide what, if anything, to do about the third variable or set of variables. The answer will depend on which situations are represented.

A DAG guides how to design your study and analyze your data to estimate the causal effect of the predictor on the outcome. Think of the arrows in a DAG as pipes (or paths) through which causal information flows from one variable to another. Pipes allow information to flow, no matter which way the arrows point, so they are generally referred to as being "open."

There is one important exception: when arrows from two different variables point into the same variable, the path between those two variables is said to be "closed" (eg, in Figure 10A.6, the path from low-calorie diet through weight loss to gastric carcinoma is closed). To remember this rule, think of arrows that point at one another as getting in each other's way. As you gain experience using DAGs, you will get better at identifying which paths are open and which are closed—and why it matters. Publicly available software (eg, daggity.net) can help.

What variables should be included in models when planning your data analysis? (Including a variable in an analytic model is the same as adjusting for it; this process is sometimes called conditioning on that variable.) To start, you want to include the *direct* path from the predictor to the outcome (Predictor → Outcome): After all, that's the causal effect you're trying to estimate. So, you always include the predictor and the outcome in your models.

But you don't want there to be "causal flow" along paths that involve shared effects or confounding (Table 10A.1). Fortunately, there's a way to prevent this from happening, namely, by using an important rule about DAGs: **Adjusting for a variable along an open path closes that path, whereas adjusting for a variable that has closed a path opens it.** Specifically, you will want to close every confounding path by including a variable in such a path in the adjustment model. In contrast, you will want to leave a shared effect path alone: it's already closed, and you do not want to open it.

TABLE 10A.1 GUIDANCE ABOUT LEAVING A PATH OPEN OR CLOSING IT

SITUATION	EXAMPLE	CURRENT STATE OF PATH THROUGH BLUE ARROWS	DESIRED STATE OF PATH THROUGH BLUE ARROWS	ACTION	QUESTION ANSWERED BY THAT ACTION
Mediation	LDL → Stroke → Carotid stenosis	Open	Leave the path open	Leave carotid stenosis out of the model to determine *total* effect of LDL cholesterol	What is the causal effect of LDL cholesterol on stroke risk, *including* its effects on carotid stenosis?
Mediation	LDL → Stroke → Carotid stenosis	Open	Close the path	Adjust for carotid stenosis in model to determine *direct* effect of LDL cholesterol[a]	What is the causal effect of LDL cholesterol on stroke risk, *aside from* its effects on carotid stenosis?

TABLE 10A.1 GUIDANCE ABOUT LEAVING A PATH OPEN OR CLOSING IT (*continued*)

SITUATION	EXAMPLE	CURRENT STATE OF PATH THROUGH BLUE ARROWS	DESIRED STATE OF PATH THROUGH BLUE ARROWS	ACTION	QUESTION ANSWERED BY THAT ACTION
Confounding	Tobacco smoking → Marijuana smoking → Lung cancer	Open	Close the path	Adjust for tobacco smoking in model	What is the causal effect of marijuana smoking on lung cancer, accounting for the effects of tobacco smoking?
Shared effect	Low-cal diet → Gastric cancer → Weight loss	Closed	Leave the path closed	Leave weight loss out of model	What is the causal effect of low-calorie diets on gastric cancer?

^aAnalyses involving mediation sometimes introduce a subtle complication. If there are confounders of the mediator-outcome relationship (eg, hypertension could confound the association between carotid stenosis and stroke), including the mediator can open a path that was previously closed (because the mediator was "pointed to" by both the confounder and the predictor). This is not a problem if you include the confounder in the model, thus reclosing the path.

LDL, serum low-density lipoprotein cholesterol level.

You have a choice with paths that involve mediators. If you want to determine the *total* effect of the predictor on the outcome, don't include the mediator in the analytic model. If you want to determine the *direct* effect of the predictor (the part that isn't a result of its effects on the mediator), then include the mediator—and confounders of the mediator-outcome association—in the model.

■ DAGS AND SAMPLING

DAGs can also clarify whether the sampling scheme for a study causes selection bias. For example, at one time it was controversial whether women taking postmenopausal hormone replacement therapy (HRT) were more likely to develop endometrial cancer (36). The question facing investigators was what to do about postmenopausal uterine bleeding, which is both a consequence of HRT and a symptom of endometrial cancer.

Restricting the sample to just patients who had (or didn't have) postmenopausal bleeding introduces that symptom as a shared effect (Figure 10A.9). Both variables (use of HRT, endometrial cancer) increase the risk of bleeding, so a study among just those with (or without) postmenopausal bleeding will likely give an erroneous result. This problem can occur when the predictor and the outcome both affect the likelihood that a participant will be included in the study.

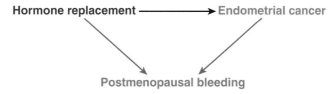

■ **FIGURE 10A.9** An example of a shared effect (the collider is postmenopausal bleeding), which can bias the estimate of the causal effect of postmenopausal hormone replacement therapy on endometrial cancer if it influenced who was studied or if it was included (inappropriately) in an analytic model.

■ SHARING A CAUSE

Earlier in the chapter, we noted that to be a confounder, a variable must cause—*or have a common cause with*—the exposure of interest and also cause the outcome. We will now illustrate the meaning of "have a common cause with" by using a DAG.

Consider a study of whether eating red meat causes colon cancer. Is screening for colon cancer a confounder? Although cancer screening is causally related to the outcome—most cases of colorectal cancer are detected by screening, and some might even go undetected without screening—it presumably does not cause someone to eat (or not eat) red meat. However, cancer screening shares a common cause with (not) eating red meat, namely, following a "healthy lifestyle." Thus, there is a confounding path—from eating red meat through healthy lifestyle through cancer screening to colorectal cancer—that needs to be closed. Although it may not be possible to measure healthy lifestyle per se, the path can be closed by adjusting for cancer screening (Figure 10A.10).

This example illustrates another point about DAGs. The arrow connecting two variables—though its direction should *always* point from the cause to the effect—can represent either an increase or a decrease in the likelihood of that effect. In this example, a healthy lifestyle is thought to reduce the likelihood of eating red meat. Sometimes, a + sign alongside an arrow is used to indicate that the investigator believes a cause increases the likelihood of an effect; a − sign indicates that the cause decreases that likelihood.

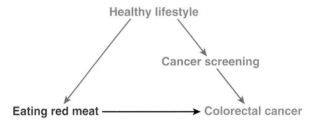

■ **FIGURE 10A.10 An example of a common cause (healthy lifestyle), which can lead to confounding of the association between eating red meat and colorectal cancer, because the path (eating red meat → healthy lifestyle → cancer screening → colorectal cancer) is open.** The path can be closed by including cancer screening in the analytic model.

■ AN EXAMPLE TO DEMONSTRATE THESE PRINCIPLES

All of this is pretty abstract stuff that can confuse even experienced epidemiologists. Let's do an example by returning to the question of whether red meat consumption increases the risk of developing colorectal cancer, perhaps through its effects on the intestinal microbiome. Suppose you have access to the electronic health records of many thousands of patients who received a nutritional assessment as part of a health maintenance program that also included a colonoscopy at baseline and at recommended intervals thereafter. (By including only those who have had colonoscopies, you closed the path, discussed in the previous example, from eating red meat through healthy lifestyle through cancer screening to colorectal cancer.) There are now more than 20 years of follow-up since that initial assessment was made. Moreover, blood and even stool samples from participants have been stored in a deep freeze.

You plan to do a retrospective cohort study, including everyone who had a normal colonoscopy at baseline. The predictor variable will be the dietician's baseline assessment of the patient's weekly red meat consumption, and the outcome variable will be the subsequent diagnosis of colorectal cancer. You will abstract data on baseline dietary fiber consumption and intercurrent fecal occult blood testing (FOBT) (as well as other covariates that we will ignore). In a nested case-control study, you will compare the fecal microbiome in cases of colorectal cancer and a sample of those who did not develop cancer, as well as look at various genetic polymorphisms that have been associated with gastrointestinal cancers.

Recall that you want to see whether eating red meat causes colorectal cancer. So, the first analysis you would do at the end of the study would be to see if participants who ate more red meat were, indeed, at a greater risk of developing colorectal cancer. However, you will also need to decide how to account for other variables—such as polymorphisms in cancer genes and dietary fiber consumption—that may be responsible for a noncausal association between eating red meat and developing colon cancer. We will begin by discussing these other variables separately; they are all portrayed in a single DAG (Figure 10A.11).

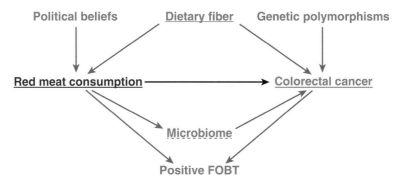

■ **FIGURE 10A.11 An example of a DAG including several relationships.** Only variables that are underlined should be included in analytic models to estimate the causal effect of eating red meat on colorectal cancer. Political beliefs and genetic polymorphisms are not associated with both the predictor (red meat consumption) and the outcome (colorectal cancer) and need not be included in the model, though including genetic polymorphisms that have strong associations with colorectal cancer would likely improve the model's precision. Dietary fiber is a confounder in this DAG and should be included to close an open path. The specific components of the microbiome are mediators: the dotted underlining indicates that the investigator must decide whether to include them. A positive fecal occult blood test (FOBT) is a shared effect and should not be included in the analytic model to avoid opening a closed path.

Variables not Causally Associated with Both Eating Red Meat and Colorectal Cancer

Polymorphisms in cancer genes, although likely to affect the risk of cancer, are unlikely to be associated with someone's dietary choices and thus need not be included when estimating the causal effect of red meat consumption on cancer. (To be sure, it would be easy to do an analysis to verify that the polymorphisms were not related to diet.) However, if polymorphisms did have a strong association with colorectal cancer, including them in an analytic model would enhance precision; it would also allow one to look for interactions among them, eating red meat, and colorectal cancer.

Similarly, although **political views** (assuming you had measured them!) may be related to eating red meat, they are not likely to affect a patient's risk of developing colorectal cancer; again, that assumption would be easy to test.

Variables Associated with Both Red Meat Consumption and Colorectal Cancer

Components of the microbiome. The research question suggested an explanation for why diet might affect cancer risk, namely, through its effects on components of the intestinal microbiome (say, increases in the proportions of *Bacteroides fragilis* or *Fusobacterium nucleatum* organisms), which are thus potential mediators. Analyses could determine whether and how information about the microbiome affects the association between red meat consumption and colorectal cancer. The decision about whether to include microbiologic data in an adjustment model depends on whether you want to determine the total effect of eating red meat on colorectal cancer or just the effect mediated (or not) through the microbiome.

Dietary fiber consumption, on the other hand, is a potential confounder. Patients who eat lots of dietary fiber (such as vegans and vegetarians) are less likely to eat red meat; they may also be at lower risk of developing colorectal cancer for that or other reasons. This confounding path needs to be closed by including fiber in the model. (Note that it is also possible that high levels of red meat consumption cause a reduction in dietary fiber; thus, the arrow could go in the other direction. In that situation, including dietary fiber in an analytic model would enable the determination of the direct effect of red meat consumption on colorectal cancer.)

Fecal occult blood testing (FOBT) is a shared effect: both consumption of red meat and the development of cancer cause can lead to positive tests (and subsequent additional workups). This path is already closed (the arrows collide at FOBT), and you do not want to open it, so FOBT results should *not* be included in the model.

■ LIMITATIONS OF DAGS

Using DAGs isn't a perfect solution to problems in causal inference. Although the diagrams are often simple to draw, determining the underlying causal models can be challenging: Not every 3-way relationship is straightforward, let alone 4-, 5-, and 10-way relationships. Sometimes, the direction of an arrow may not be obvious, or it's not clear whether two variables should be connected. Or it may seem that an arrow should be bidirectional: Does depression cause lack of exercise, or vice versa? We've already seen an example in which the connection among variables appears to be circular (obesity causes arthritis, which causes lack of exercise, which causes obesity, etc.).

As additional variables are considered, keeping track of the paths—and determining the connections among variables—gets even more complex. Indeed, drawing a DAG can help to identify which variables are *not* related to one another and therefore don't need to be accounted for! Finally, another limitation is that there isn't a straightforward way to represent or address interaction and effect modification with DAGs.

The good news is that it is not necessary to specify exactly what the *final* DAG will look like at the time a study is designed, although it is essential to ensure that potential colliders do not affect the sampling plan to avoid conditioning on a shared effect. Although the final DAG can wait until it's time to make causal inferences as results are analyzed, it is important to *measure* variables that you believe are likely to appear in causal models, even if there is uncertainty about their eventual roles.

APPENDIX 10B
Hypothetical Examples to Demonstrate Confounding and Effect Modification

The entries in these tables are numbers of participants in an imaginary case-control study of eating red meat as a risk factor for colorectal cancer (CRC). CRC + indicates a case of colorectal cancer; CRC – indicates a control. Red meat + indicates that the case or control ate red meat; red meat – indicates that the case or control did not eat red meat. Some numbers are in color to help you see where they came from.

Panel 1. Left: If we look at the entire group of study participants, the association between eating red meat and CRC has an odds ratio of 2.25. Right: the DAG guiding our analysis.

BOTH MEN AND WOMEN			
	CRC +	CRC –	Total
Red meat +	90	60	150
Red meat –	60	90	150
Total	150	150	300

$$OR = \frac{90 \times 90}{60 \times 60} = 2.25$$

Panel 2. However, based on our DAG, this could be partly due to **confounding**, as shown by the tables stratified by gender:

MEN			
	CRC +	CRC –	Total
Red meat +	78	42	120
Red meat –	32	28	60
Total	110	70	180

WOMEN			
	CRC +	CRC –	Total
Red meat +	12	18	30
Red meat –	28	62	90
Total	40	80	120

$$OR = \frac{78 \times 28}{32 \times 42} = 1.63$$

$$OR = \frac{12 \times 62}{28 \times 18} = 1.48$$

The stratum-specific odds ratios are quite a bit lower than 2.25: 1.63 in men and 1.48 in women. We can see that gender was associated with both CRC (73% [110 of 150] of the CRC cases were men, compared with only 47% [70 of 150] of the controls) and eating red meat (67% [120 of 180] of men but only 25% [30 of 120] of women ate red meat). In this example, stratifying by gender reduced but did not eliminate the association between red meat and CRC.

Panel 3. Effect Modification

The association between red meat and CRC in Panel 1 would be modified by gender (**effect modification**) if the association between red meat intake and CRC differed (appreciably) in men and women. Of course, small differences in stratum-specific effect measures, such as those

191

shown in Panel 2, are to be expected. In the following tables, the interaction is dramatic: the overall OR of 2.25 in Panel 1 results from an OR of 4.70 in men and only 0.73 in women:

MEN	CRC +	CRC −	Total
Red meat +	78	42	**120**
Red meat −	17	43	**60**
Total	**95**	**85**	**180**

WOMEN	CRC +	CRC −	Total
Red meat +	12	18	**30**
Red meat −	43	47	**90**
Total	**55**	**65**	**120**

$$OR = \frac{78 \times 43}{17 \times 42} = 4.70$$

$$OR = \frac{12 \times 47}{43 \times 18} = 0.73$$

When effect modification is present, the odds ratios in different strata are different and should be reported separately.

Of course, when data are from actual research, rather than being made up, the numbers are likely not to be clear cut. In that case, it is helpful to combine knowledge from outside the study with tests of statistical significance to judge whether the amount of apparent confounding or effect modification observed is plausibly explained by chance variation in the data.

APPENDIX 10C
Simplified Example of Modeling

Suppose that a study finds two major predictors of the IQ of children: the parental education level and the child's blood lead level. Consider the following hypothetical data on children with normal and high lead levels:

	AVERAGE YEARS OF PARENTAL EDUCATION	AVERAGE IQ OF CHILD
High lead level	10.0	95
Normal lead level	12.0	110

Note that the parental education level is also associated with the child's blood lead level. The question is "Is the difference in IQ between children with normal and high lead levels more than can be accounted for on the basis of the difference in parental education?" To answer this question we look at how much difference in IQ the difference in parental education levels would be expected to produce. We do this by plotting parental educational level versus IQ in the children with normal lead levels (Figure 10C.1).[13]

The diagonal dashed line in Figure 10C.1 shows the relationship between the child's IQ and parental education in children with normal lead levels; there is an increase in the child's IQ of 5 points for every 2 years of parental education. Therefore, we can adjust the IQ of the normal lead group to account for the difference in mean parental education by sliding down the line from point A to point A′. (Because the group with normal lead levels had 2 more years

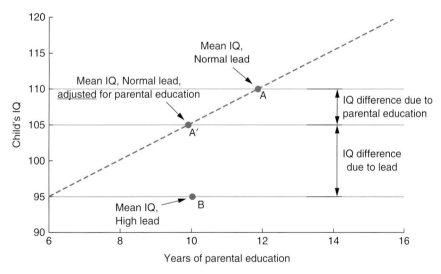

■ **FIGURE 10C.1** Hypothetical graph of child's IQ as a linear function (dashed line) of years of parental education.

---

[13]This description of analysis of covariance (ANCOVA) is simplified. Actually, parental education is plotted against the child's IQ in both the normal and the high lead groups, and the single slope that fits both plots the best is used. The model for this form of adjustment, therefore, assumes linear relationships between parental education and IQ in both groups, and that the slopes of the lines in the two groups are the same. Other more complicated "regression adjustment" models allow slopes (and intercepts) to differ between groups.

of parental education on the average, we adjust their IQs downward by 5 points to make them comparable in mean parental education to the high lead group.) This still leaves a 10-point difference in IQ between points A and B, suggesting that lead has an independent effect on IQ of this magnitude. Therefore, of the 15-point difference in IQ of children with low and high lead levels, 5 points can be accounted for by their parents' different education levels, and the remaining 10 are attributable to the lead exposure.

APPENDIX 10D
Exercises for Chapter 10. Estimating Causal Effects Using Observational Studies

1. The investigator undertakes a case-control study to address the research question: "Does eating more fruits and vegetables reduce the risk of coronary heart disease (CHD)?" Suppose that her study finds an odds ratio of 0.6 for those with fruit and vegetable intake above the median.
    a. What are some possible reasons why this observed lower risk of CHD in those with higher fruit and vegetable intake may not represent the causal effect? Give special attention to the possibility that the association between eating fruits and vegetables and CHD may be confounded by exercise (if people who eat more fruits and vegetables also exercise more, and this is a cause of their lower CHD rates).
    b. What approaches could you use to cope with exercise as a possible confounder, and what are the advantages and disadvantages of each plan?
2. A study by the PROS (Pediatric Research in Office Settings) network of pediatricians found that among young infants (<3 months) brought to their pediatricians for fever, uncircumcised boys had about 10 times the risk of urinary tract infection, compared with circumcised boys (39), an association that has been seen in numerous studies. Interestingly, uncircumcised boys in that study appeared to have a *lower* risk of ear infections (risk ratio = 0.77; $P = 0.08$). Explain how including only babies with fever in this study could introduce an association between circumcision and ear infections that is not present in the general population of young infants.
3. In Exercise 2 of Chapter 2, we asked you to suggest studies to address the question of whether acetaminophen causes asthma. A proposed mechanism for this association is acetaminophen-induced depletion of glutathione, which protects the lungs from oxidative injury that might contribute to asthma. Describe briefly how you could take advantage of variation in maternal antioxidant genotypes to enhance the inference that an association between maternal acetaminophen use and asthma in the offspring is causal.

CHAPTER 11

Designing Randomized Blinded Trials

Steven R. Cummings, Deborah G. Grady, and Alison J. Huang

In a clinical trial, the investigator applies an **intervention** and observes its effect on one or more outcomes. The major advantage of a trial over an observational study is the ability to demonstrate causality if the trial involves **randomization** and **blinding**. Randomly assigning the intervention minimizes the influence of **confounding variables**, and blinding minimizes the possibility that its apparent effects result from the **placebo effect**, the differential use of other **cointerventions**, or biased reporting or ascertainment of the outcomes.

This chapter focuses on designing a randomized, blinded trial: choosing the intervention and **control** conditions, defining and measuring outcomes and adverse events, selecting participants, and determining approaches to randomization and blinding. We also address issues related to conducting clinical trials and analyzing the results and the value of **pilot studies**. In the next chapter, we will address alternative trial designs.

■ SELECTING THE INTERVENTION AND CONTROL CONDITIONS

The "classic" randomized trial involves participants who are randomly assigned either to receive the intervention to be tested or to a control, which can be an inactive placebo or a different treatment. Optimally, these assignments are blinded, such that the investigators, participants, and study staff do not know whether a participant is assigned to the intervention or the comparison group. The investigator administers the active and control interventions, follows the participant over time, and compares the outcomes between the groups (Figure 11.1). The words "parallel group" are sometimes appended to the description of this design; they indicate that the intervention and control groups are enrolled and followed concurrently.

Choice of Intervention

Choosing the intervention is the critical first step in designing a clinical trial. All types of interventions, including drugs, behavioral programs, and surgical procedures, raise similar considerations, including the method of delivery, dose or intensity, and frequency and duration of administration. Several goals in choosing the intervention must be balanced: **efficacy** and safety, acceptability to participants, and ease of implementation.

The efficacy of the intervention—how well it treats the condition of interest—is the paramount consideration in designing trials of interventions to treat severe illnesses or to reduce high risks of disability or death. In these situations, it is best to choose the highest tolerable dose, frequency, and duration of treatment. For conditions with less severe consequences—and especially for preventive interventions in healthy people—investigators must place greater weight on safety: if efficacious, the intervention will prevent or ameliorate the condition in only *some* people, whereas *everyone* receiving it will be at risk of the adverse effects.

Sometimes, an investigator may decide to compare more than one dose or duration of an intervention with a control group. This is sometimes a reasonable choice but will require a larger trial.

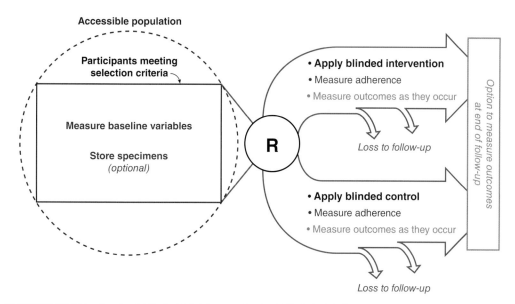

■ **FIGURE 11.1 Randomized blinded trial**. In a randomized blinded trial, the steps are to
- Select a sample of participants from the accessible population in whom the intervention is warranted and safe.
- Measure baseline predictor variables and, if appropriate, the baseline level of the outcome variable.
- Consider the options of making additional measurements and storing specimens for later analysis.
- Randomly assign (represented by the letter R) the blinded intervention and control condition (eg, placebo).
- Follow the participants over time, minimize loss to follow-up, and assess adherence with the intervention and control.
- Measure the outcome variables as they occur or at the end of follow-up.

Occasionally, it may be best to design an intervention so that the dose of active drug or behavioral treatment can be titrated to optimize efficacy. To maintain blinding, corresponding changes should also be made in the "dose" of the placebo among participants in the control group.

Trials to test single interventions are much easier to plan and implement than those testing a combination of interventions. The most important disadvantage of testing a combination of interventions, such as exercise and diet, is that the result cannot provide clear conclusions about any one element of the intervention. The Women's Health Initiative, for example, compared a combination of postmenopausal estrogen and progestin therapy versus placebo, finding an increased risk of several outcomes, including breast cancer; however, it was unclear whether the effect was due to the estrogen or the progestin (1).

The investigator should consider how receptive participants will be to the intervention, whether it can be blinded, and its applicability to clinical practice. Participants are more likely to enroll in trials and more likely to be adherent to trial interventions that are not burdensome. Complicated interventions with components that are difficult to standardize, such as multifaceted counseling to change behavior, may not be feasible to incorporate in general practice because they are difficult to replicate, time consuming, or costly. As a result, such interventions are less likely to have public health impact even if a trial proves that they are efficacious.

Choice of Control

The best control group is "treated" in a way that can be blinded, which for medications generally requires a placebo or alternate drug that is indistinguishable from the trial medication. This strategy compensates for any placebo effect of the active intervention (ie, through suggestion or expectation) so that any difference in outcomes between study groups can be ascribed to a specific effect of the intervention. However, it can be difficult or impossible to construct a blinded control for interventions such as education, behavioral training, or medical procedures.

In some trials, it may be appropriate to ask participants to avoid other treatments during the trial that might influence the outcome. For example, in a study of a new treatment for osteoporosis, participants should not take other drugs for that condition. But it is often not possible to withhold such treatments: a trial of a drug to reduce the risk of myocardial infarction in persons with known coronary heart disease (CHD) cannot prohibit or discourage participants from taking treatments, such as statins, that are indicated clinically. One solution is to give standard (or usual) care to all participants in the trial, supplemented by the study treatment in the intervention group and placebo in the control group. This approach tests the most relevant clinical question—whether the new intervention improves the outcome when added to standard care—but it will reduce the overall event rate, thus increasing the required sample size.

Cointerventions

Cointerventions are treatments or behaviors other than the study intervention that change the risk of developing the outcome of interest. They are particularly problematic if they are more likely to occur in the one group than the other. For example, in a trial of strength training to improve motor function among patients with Parkinson's disease, participants in the control group may begin to walk more to compensate for not receiving the intervention. When the use of an efficacious cointervention, such as exercise, differs between the treatment and control groups, the results of the study will be biased.

Blinding can minimize differences in cointerventions between groups, as discussed later in this chapter. If blinding is not possible, the protocol must include plans to obtain data, such as periodic objective measurements of exercise, to allow statistical adjustment for differences between the groups in the use of such cointerventions. However, measuring cointerventions may be difficult, and adjusting for such *postrandomization* differences should be viewed as a secondary or explanatory analysis because it violates the **intention-to-treat** principle discussed later in this chapter.

■ CHOOSING OUTCOME MEASUREMENTS

Selection and definition of the specific outcomes of the trial influence many other design components, as well as the cost and feasibility of the trial. Trials often include several end points to increase the richness of the results and the possibilities for secondary analyses. However, there should always be one primary outcome that reflects the main question, guides calculation of the sample size, and sets the priority for efforts to implement the study. Secondary end points should be considered only if the size and duration of the trial provide sufficient statistical power for a meaningful result.

Changes in the risk of clinical outcomes (such as strokes and fractures) or in participants' health, function, and quality of life provide the best evidence about the value of an intervention. But many clinical outcomes, such as new-onset dementia, are uncommon, and trials to find efficacious treatments must be large, long, and expensive. As noted in Chapter 6, outcomes measured as continuous variables, such as the change in cognitive function measured with a standard instrument, can be studied with fewer participants than dichotomous outcomes.

Biomarkers are intermediate measurements, typically measured in biologic samples, that are associated with a clinical outcome. For example, a reduction in an elevated white blood cell count is associated with successful treatment of pneumonia. However, biomarkers can be considered surrogate markers for the clinical outcome *only* to the extent that treatment-induced changes in the marker consistently predicted effects on the clinical outcome in previous trials of treatments of the same type (2). For example, treatment-related changes in bone density of the femoral neck predict how well a treatment reduces the risk of fractures, because bone density is a major determinant of bone strength and predictor of fracture risk, and a meta-analysis of previous trials showed that improvement in femoral neck bone density predicted a reduction in hip and nonspine fractures (3). Few **intermediate markers** satisfy these conditions. Even biomarkers that predict clinical outcomes may be misleading as end points of trials (2, 4, 5). For example, greater levels of high-density lipoprotein (HDL) cholesterol and lower levels of low-density lipoprotein (LDL) cholesterol predict a decreased risk of cardiovascular disease and death. However, a clinical trial found that torcetrapib, despite having very favorable effects on both HDL- and LDL-cholesterol levels, *increased* the risk of both total mortality and cardiovascular events (6).

Number of Outcome Variables

It is often desirable to have several outcome variables that measure different aspects of the phenomena of interest. That said, having many secondary outcomes complicates the conduct of the trial and increases its cost.

For example, in a trial of adults hospitalized with COVID-19 infection who were randomized to treatment with hydroxychloroquine or placebo, the primary outcome was clinical status 14 days after randomization. This allowed the investigator to determine the sample size and duration of the study, while avoiding the problems of interpreting tests of **multiple hypotheses**. The investigators also measured 12 secondary outcomes, such as time to recovery and adverse events. When investigators found no benefit for the primary outcome or any of the secondary outcomes, they were able to draw a more definitive conclusion that the treatment was not efficacious (7).

Composite Outcomes

Some trials use outcomes that include several related events, such as myocardial infarction, coronary revascularization procedures, and stroke. This may be reasonable if each outcome is important clinically and affected similarly by the intervention. If so, a **composite outcome** provides greater power than a single outcome because there will be more events. But composite outcomes that include events that have different biologic mechanisms or frequency can result in misleading findings. For example, if coronary revascularization occurs much more commonly than the other components, it will dominate the composite outcome—and an intervention that appears to lower the risk of "cardiovascular events" may in reality only reduce the risk of revascularization. Furthermore, a treatment may have different biologic effects, say, on coronary revascularization and hemorrhagic stroke, so that a reduction in "cardiovascular events" may not mean that treatment is beneficial for both.

Adverse Events

The investigator should also ascertain the occurrence of **adverse events** that may result from the intervention or from other aspects of the trial, such as coronary angiograms to assess the progression of atherosclerosis. Revealing whether the beneficial effects of an intervention outweigh the adverse ones is a major goal of most clinical trials, even those that test seemingly innocuous interventions like a health education program or cancer screening test. Adverse events may range from minor symptoms, such as upper respiratory tract infections, to serious and even fatal complications, such as reactivated tuberculosis. Because the sample size requirements for detecting rare adverse events, such as renal failure, are large, most trials will not have adequate power to detect an increased risk of these outcomes. They are discovered (if at all) by analyses of large medical databases or case reports after an intervention is in widespread clinical use.

In the early stages of testing a new intervention—when its potential adverse events are unclear—investigators should ask open-ended questions about whether any adverse events have occurred. In addition, specific queries should be designed to discover important adverse events that are anticipated because of previous research or clinical experience.

Adverse events should be categorized for analysis. Standard dictionaries—like MedDRA (www.ich.org/products/meddra.html) and SNOMED (https://www.nlm.nih.gov/research/umls/)—group adverse events in several ways, such as by symptom, diagnosis, and organ system. Adverse events are also often classified by the likelihood they are related to the study intervention and by their severity; serious adverse events are defined as those that are fatal or life-threatening, that require or extend hospitalization or medical treatment, or that lead to disability, permanent damage, or birth defects (www.fda.gov/Safety/MedWatch/HowToReport/ ucm053087.htm). Certain disease areas, such as cancer, have established methods for classifying adverse events (http://ctep.cancer.gov/protocolDevelopment/electronic_applications/ctc. htm). Serious adverse events that may be related to trial interventions or that are unexpected should be reported promptly to the institutional review board (IRB) and the sponsor of the trial. When data from a trial are used to apply for regulatory approval of a new drug, the trial design must satisfy regulatory expectations for reporting adverse events (http://www.fda.gov/Drugs/ InformationOnDrugs/ucm135151.htm).

■ SELECTING THE PARTICIPANTS

Chapter 3 discussed how to specify **selection criteria** defining a target population that is appropriate to the research question, how to design an efficient and scientific approach to selecting participants, and how to recruit them. Here we cover issues that are especially relevant to clinical trials.

Selection Criteria for Clinical Trials

A trial must enroll and follow enough participants who have a sufficient risk of the primary outcome to have adequate power to find an important effect of the intervention (Chapter 5). Selection criteria should balance the need to include those most likely to benefit from the intervention against the goals of recruiting the desired sample size and maximizing the generalizability of the study findings. For example, if the outcome of interest is an uncommon event, such as new-onset breast cancer, it is usually necessary to recruit high-risk participants to reduce the sample size and follow-up time to feasible levels. However, narrowing the **inclusion criteria** to high-risk women limits the generalizability of the results and makes it more difficult to recruit enough participants.

To plan the sample size, the investigator must estimate the risk of the primary outcome, or rate of change in the end point, that would have occurred among potential participants without the intervention. This estimate can be based on data from vital statistics or longitudinal observational studies. For example, expected rates of mortality from pancreatic cancer can be estimated from registry data. The investigator should keep in mind, however, that volunteers who qualify for and agree to enter clinical trials are healthier than average people with disease; thus, event rates among trial participants are often lower than in the target population and rates of change in an end point may be different. It may be preferable to estimate the risk of the primary outcome from the results in the untreated group in studies that had inclusion criteria similar to those in the planned trial.

Although probability samples of the target population confer advantages in observational studies, this type of sampling is generally not feasible or necessary for randomized trials. Inclusion of participants with diverse characteristics will increase the confidence that the results of a trial apply broadly, so long as there are sufficient numbers of important groups, such as women and ethnic minorities, to determine that the effects are consistent. However, unless there are biologic or genetic differences between populations that influence the effect of an intervention, it is generally true that results of a trial conducted in a convenience sample (eg, women with CHD who respond to advertisements) will be similar to results obtained in probability samples of eligible people (all women with CHD). Occasionally, the effects of an intervention depend on other covariates, like age or sex/gender; this is termed **effect modification** (Chapter 10).

Stratified sampling of participants by a characteristic, like being at least 80 years of age, that may influence the effect of the intervention or its generalizability ensures that a specified number of participants with that characteristic are enrolled. Recruitment to the stratum can be closed when the

TABLE 11.1 REASONS FOR EXCLUDING PEOPLE FROM A CLINICAL TRIAL

REASON	EXAMPLE: LOW-DOSE METHOTREXATE (MTX) FOR THE PREVENTION OF ATHEROSCLEROTIC EVENTS (8)
1. A study treatment may be harmful.	
• Unacceptable risk of harm if assigned to active treatment.	History of alcohol abuse, unwilling to limit consumption to <4 drinks per week. (There is an adverse interaction between MTX and alcohol.)
• Unacceptable risk of harm if assigned to control.	Patient needs to take a medication that alters folate metabolism.
2. Active treatment is unlikely to be efficacious.	
• At low risk for the outcome.	Young adult with very low risk for coronary heart disease.
• Has a type of disease that is not likely to respond to treatment.	Within a short time period (<60 days) of a prior myocardial infarction or procedure, when recurrent events are more likely.
• Taking a treatment that is likely to interact adversely with the intervention.	Requires treatment with corticosteroid therapy or other immunosuppressive treatment.
3. Unlikely to adhere to the intervention.	Poor adherence during the initial MTX run-in period.
4. Unlikely to complete follow-up.	Plans to move before trial ends and will not be available for final outcome measures.
	Life expectancy <3 years (not enough time for follow-up for the outcome).
5. Practical problems with participating in the protocol.	Impaired cognitive function that prevents accurate answers to questions.

goal has been reached. However, this strategy may have limited value if the trial is not designed with enough power to test that the effect differs significantly in that subgroup when compared with other participants.

Exclusion criteria should be parsimonious, because unnecessary exclusions make it more difficult to recruit the needed number of participants, diminish the generalizability of the results, and increase the complexity and cost of recruitment. That said, there are several reasons for excluding people from a clinical trial (Table 11.1).

Potential participants should be excluded if the active or control intervention may be unsafe for them. For example, persons with advanced renal disease are usually excluded from trials of medications that are excreted by the kidneys, and persons with severe depression should not be entered into a placebo-controlled trial of a new antidepressant. Persons in whom the active intervention is unlikely to be efficacious should also be excluded, as well as those who are unlikely to be adherent to the intervention or unlikely to complete follow-up. Occasionally, practical issues justify exclusion, such as impaired mental status or language barriers that make it difficult for a participant to follow instructions. However, investigators should weigh potential exclusion criteria that apply to many people (eg, diabetes or upper age limits) as these may have a large impact on the feasibility and costs of recruitment as well as the generalizability of the results.

Determine an Adequate Sample Size and Plan the Recruitment Accordingly

Trials that are not designed to include enough participants to detect important effects are arguably wasteful and unethical, as they may produce misleading conclusions. Estimating the sample size is therefore one of the most important early parts of planning a trial. The process should recognize that outcome rates in clinical trials are usually lower than estimated due to healthy volunteer bias. In addition, recruitment for a trial is often more difficult than for an observational study, because participants must be willing to be randomized to a placebo or "experimental" treatment and comply with the intervention. For these reasons, the investigator should plan to recruit from a large accessible population of eligible people and have enough resources to enroll the desired number of participants when—as often happens—the barriers to doing so turn out to be greater than expected.

■ MEASURING BASELINE VARIABLES

Describe the Participants

In addition to collecting robust contact information about participants, investigators should collect information on risk factors for the outcome and other characteristics that may affect the efficacy and risk of the intervention. These measurements also provide a way to check the comparability of the randomized study groups at baseline and to assess the generalizability of the findings. The goal is to make sure that differences in baseline characteristics do not exceed what might be expected from the play of chance, thus suggesting a technical error or bias in carrying out the randomization. In small trials that are prone to sizable maldistributions of baseline characteristics across randomized groups by chance alone, measurement of important predictors of the outcome may allow statistical adjustment for such maldistributions. Measuring predictors of the outcome also allows the investigator to examine whether the intervention's effect differs in various subgroups (effect modification, Chapter 10).

Measure the Baseline Value of the Outcome Variable

If outcomes are defined as a change in a variable, that variable must be measured at the beginning of the study in the same way that it will be measured at its end. In studies that have a continuous outcome variable (eg, pain severity score), the best measure is almost always the change in that variable during the study. This approach usually provides more power than comparing values at the end of the trial. In studies that have a dichotomous outcome (eg, incidence of lung cancer), it is often essential to demonstrate—using clinical history, examination, and diagnostic testing—that the outcome was not present at the trial outset.

Additional Measurements

Although baseline measurements have many uses, the design of a randomized trial does not require that *any* be measured, because randomization minimizes the problem of confounding by factors that are present at the outset. Adding measurements enables the investigators to answer additional questions, but making more measurements adds complexity and expense. In a randomized trial that has a limited budget, time and money may be better spent on vital aspects of the study, such as the adequacy of the sample size, the success of randomization and blinding, and the completeness of adherence and follow-up.

Bank Specimens

If participants provide blood, tissue samples, or other biologic specimens at baseline, then storage of these samples will allow subsequent measurement of changes caused by the treatment, markers that predict the outcome, and factors such as genotype that might identify people who respond well or poorly to the treatment. Stored specimens can also be a rich resource to study other research questions not related to the main outcome.

■ RANDOMIZING AND BLINDING

A key step in any trial involves assigning the participants randomly to two (or more) groups. In the simplest design, one group receives an active intervention and the other receives an inactive placebo or alternative intervention. Randomization ensures that baseline characteristics that could confound an observed association—even those that are unknown or unmeasured—will be distributed equally, except for chance variation, among the randomized groups. Blinding is important to minimize differential placebo effects, maintain the comparability of the study groups during the trial, and ensure unbiased outcome ascertainment.

Randomization

It is important that each participant complete screening evaluations, be found eligible for inclusion, and give consent to enter the study before randomization. Participants are then assigned to the study groups randomly.

Simple trials use a computer algorithm to generate treatment assignments. Randomization can be performed at the research site or by a research pharmacy that dispenses active treatment or control. Most multicenter trials use a central facility that the clinical site contacts when an eligible participant is ready to be randomized. Occasionally, when computerized randomization is not feasible, simple trials may enclose treatment assignment in opaque envelopes that are opened at the time of enrollment. Randomization must be tamperproof because investigators might find themselves under pressure to influence the randomization process (eg, for an individual who seems particularly suitable for the active treatment group in a placebo-controlled trial).

Consider Special Randomization Techniques

Typically, participants are assigned randomly in equal proportions to each intervention group. Trials of small-to-moderate size will have a small gain in power if special randomization procedures are used to balance the number of participants in each group (**blocked randomization**) and the distribution of baseline variables that predict the outcome (**stratified blocked randomization**).

Blocked randomization is used in blinded trials to ensure that the number of participants is distributed equally among the study groups, with "blocks" of predetermined size. For example, if the block size is six, randomization proceeds normally within each block of six until three persons have been randomized to one of the groups, after which participants are assigned to the other group until the block of six is completed. This means that in a study of 30 participants, exactly 15 will be assigned to each group; in a study of 33 participants, the disproportion could be no greater than 18:15. Blocked randomization with a fixed block size is less suitable for nonblinded studies because the intervention assignment of the participants at the end of each block could be anticipated and manipulated. This problem can be minimized by varying the size of the blocks randomly (ranging, eg, from blocks of four to eight) according to a schedule that is not known to the investigator.

Stratified blocked randomization ensures that an important predictor of the outcome is more evenly distributed between the study groups than chance alone would dictate. In a trial of the effect of an exercise intervention to prevent development of diabetes, obesity is such a strong predictor of outcome that it may be best to ensure that similar numbers of people who are obese are assigned to each group. This can be achieved by carrying out blocked randomization separately by "strata"—those with and without obesity. Stratified blocked randomization can slightly enhance the power of a small trial by reducing the variation in outcome due to chance disproportions in important baseline predictors. It is of little benefit in large trials because random assignment ensures nearly even distribution of baseline variables.

An important limitation of stratified blocked randomization is that only a few (up to two or three) baseline variables can be balanced by this technique. This limitation can be addressed by adaptive randomization, which uses a "biased coin" to alter the probability of assigning each new participant. Using this approach, a participant with a high risk score (based on any number of baseline prognostic variables) would be slightly more likely to be randomized to the study group that had a lower average risk. This method requires an interactive computerized system that recomputes the probabilities with each randomization.

Usually, the best decision is to assign equal numbers of participants to each study group, as this maximizes power for any given total sample size. However, the attenuation in power of even a 2:1 disproportion is modest (9), and unequal allocation of participants to treatment and control groups may sometimes be appropriate (10):

- Increasing the proportion of those assigned to the active treatment can make a trial more attractive to potential participants, such as those who would like the greater chance of receiving active treatment if they enroll.
- Increasing the proportion in the active treatment group can augment the sample size for exploration of mediating variables in that group, as with the Program to Reduce Incontinence with Diet and Exercise Trial, in which two-thirds of overweight or obese participants were randomized to the intensive behavioral weight loss group (11).
- Decreasing the proportion receiving an intervention can make the trial affordable when the intervention is very expensive, as in the Women's Health Initiative low-fat diet trial (12).
- Increasing the proportion assigned to a group serving as the control for several active intervention groups will increase the power of each comparison by increasing the precision of the control group estimate, as in the Coronary Drug Project trial (13).

Randomization of matched pairs is another strategy for balancing baseline confounding variables. It requires selecting pairs of participants who are matched on important characteristics like age and sex, then randomly assigning one member of each pair to each study group. However, this approach complicates enrollment, because an eligible participant must wait for randomization until a suitable match has been identified. In addition, matching is not necessary in large trials in which random assignment balances the groups. However, an attractive version of this design can be used when the circumstances permit a contrast of active and control intervention effects in two parts of the same individual. For example, some Asians have a genetic predisposition to facial flushing from drinking alcohol. A trial in Asian participants who suffered from the flushing syndrome randomly assigned application of a gel of brimonidine (an alpha-adrenergic receptor agonist) or placebo to one or the other cheek (14). By comparing changes across cheeks in the same individual, the study demonstrated that the active gel reduced redness after the participants drank alcohol.

Blinding

Blinding the assessment of the outcome is important when it could be influenced by knowledge of the intervention assignment. Whenever possible, the study investigators, participants, staff interacting with participants, persons obtaining measurements, and those ascertaining and adjudicating outcomes should not know the assignment. When it is not possible to blind everyone, it is particularly important to blind participants and the personnel who make the outcome determinations. Blinding minimizes differential placebo effects and cointerventions, and biased ascertainment and adjudication of outcomes, especially those that are subjective, like self-reported symptoms. For example, in a trial of a new intervention to reduce fatigue, if participants know their treatment status, their perceptions of fatigue may be influenced by their belief in the intervention's potential to improve their energy levels (placebo effect). Those who adjudicate reported outcomes must also be blinded. For example, if the outcome of a trial is myocardial infarction, investigators may collect data on symptoms, ECG findings, and cardiac enzyme levels. Experts blinded to the intervention group then use these data and specific definitions to adjudicate whether a myocardial infarction occurred.

Results of the Canadian Cooperative Multiple Sclerosis trial illustrate the importance of blinding for unbiased outcome adjudication (15). Persons with multiple sclerosis were randomly assigned to plasma exchange with or without cyclophosphamide and prednisone, or sham plasma exchange and placebo medications. At the end of the trial, the severity of multiple sclerosis was assessed using a structured examination by neurologists blinded to treatment assignment and again by neurologists who were unblinded. Therapy was not efficacious based on the assessment of the blinded neurologists but was efficacious based on the assessment of the unblinded neurologists. The unblinded neurologists were not trying to bias the outcome of the trial, but there is a strong human desire to see patients improve after treatment, especially if the treatment is painful or potentially harmful. Blinding minimizes such biased outcome adjudication.

Biased assessment or reporting of outcomes may be less likely if the trial has "hard" outcomes such as death or automated measurements, like blood glucose levels. However, most other outcomes, such as cause of death, disease diagnosis, physical measurements, questionnaire scales, and self-reported conditions, are susceptible to biased ascertainment and adjudication.

It is often a good idea at the end of a trial to assess whether the participants and investigators were aware of the treatment assignment by asking them to guess about it. The proportion of participants guessing that they were assigned to the active intervention should be similar in both groups. If this is not the case, then the published discussion of the findings should include an assessment of the potential biases that unblinding may have caused.

What to Do When Blinding Is Difficult or Impossible

Blinding is not always possible, such as when an exercise intervention is compared with a control group that receives a pamphlet. Surgical interventions can be challenging to blind because it may seem unethical to perform sham surgery in the control group. However, invasive procedures such as surgery are always associated with some risk, so it is important to determine if the procedures are efficacious before they are recommended to the public. Surgery is also likely to influence participants' use of cointerventions and perceptions of their health, so unblinded surgical trials are susceptible to differential use of cointerventions as well as biased outcome reporting. For example, a patient undergoing coronary angioplasty and stenting may expect his symptoms of chest pain to improve. However, a trial that randomized patients with symptomatic coronary artery disease to angioplasty or an identical sham procedure (without treating the arterial lesion) showed no difference in patient-reported symptoms (16). In this case, the need for rigorous evidence about the efficacy of this very common treatment outweighed the risk to participants in the control group. Similar considerations apply to many behavioral interventions, in which a sham intervention omits the key aspects of the therapy and instead just engages participants in nondirected therapy.

If intervention assignment cannot be blinded, the investigator should ensure that individuals who adjudicate the outcomes are blinded and take active steps to limit the use of cointerventions. For example, an investigator testing the effect of a yoga program for relief of back pain could instruct both yoga and control participants to refrain from starting new treatments for back pain until the trial has ended. Also, study staff who collect information on the severity of pain should not also provide the yoga training, because they are likely to remember which participants were in the active treatment group.

Even if the nature of the intervention makes it impossible to blind participants, it may be possible to promote **equipoise** between groups and minimize differential expectations about intervention effects, which will in turn minimize differential placebo effects and use of cointerventions or biased reporting of outcomes. For example, in the case of a trial of a yoga intervention for back pain, the control intervention could be a physical activity program that required a similar amount of time and attention from participants. This would avoid between-group differences in the level of engagement. The control may also offer other plausible benefits for participants' health, which will enable the investigators to recruit and retain participants who may expect something in return for their investment of time in the study.

■ PILOT STUDIES

Sometimes it is valuable to conduct a small study to collect information for planning a larger clinical trial, to determine, say, the best approaches to recruiting participants and the time required for clinical visits. Pilot studies are not suited to estimating the efficacy of the intended intervention because their small size leaves them prone to imprecise estimates. Appendix 11A describes the uses of pilot studies.

■ CLINICAL TRIALS EMBEDDED IN HEALTH CARE

Most trials are conducted in a clinical setting, with in-person visits, measurements, and data collection. However, several other settings can support randomized trials. For example, it is now possible to use electronic health record systems to introduce interventions and to collect data while health care is being delivered. These "embedded" trials most often study quality improvement for clinical processes. Some of these trials are classic randomized, blinded trials, while others have **before-after** or **interrupted time series designs** (Chapter 12).

■ TRIALS FOR REGULATORY APPROVAL OF NEW INTERVENTIONS

Many trials are done to test the efficacy and safety of new treatments before approval for marketing by the U.S. Food and Drug Administration (FDA) or another regulatory body. Trials are also done to determine whether drugs that have FDA approval for one condition might be efficacious for the treatment or prevention of other conditions. The design and conduct of these trials are the same as for other trials, but regulatory requirements must be considered.

The FDA publishes guidelines on how such trials should be conducted. Investigators and staff conducting trials with the goal of obtaining FDA approval of a new medication or device should seek specific training on general guidelines, called **Good Clinical Practice**. In addition, the FDA provides specific guidance for studies of certain outcomes. For example, studies designed to obtain FDA approval of treatments for hot flashes in menopausal women must currently include participants with at least 7 hot flashes per day or 50 per week. FDA guidelines are updated regularly; similar guidelines are available from international regulatory agencies.

Trials for regulatory approval of new treatments are described by phase, which refers to an orderly progression in the testing of a new treatment, beginning with **preclinical studies** in animals, human cell cultures, or tissues; initial unblinded, uncontrolled treatment of a few human volunteers to test safety (**Phase I**); then small randomized or time series trials that test the effect of a range of doses on adverse effects and biomarkers or clinical outcomes (**Phase II**); then randomized trials large enough to test the hypothesis that the treatment improves the targeted condition (such as blood pressure) or reduces the risk of disease (such as stroke) with acceptable safety (**Phase III**) (Table 11.2). The FDA usually defines the end points for Phase III trials that are required to obtain approval to market a new drug. **Phase IV** refers to large studies that may be randomized trials but are often observational studies conducted after a drug is approved to assess the rate of serious side effects when the drug is used in large populations or to test additional uses of the drug.

TABLE 11.2 STAGES IN TESTING NEW THERAPIES

Preclinical	Studies in cell cultures, tissues, and animals
Phase I	Unblinded, uncontrolled studies in a few volunteers to test safety
Phase II	Relatively small randomized or time series trials to test tolerability and different intensity or dose of the intervention on biomarkers or clinical outcomes
Phase III	Relatively large randomized blinded trials to test conclusively the effect of the therapy on clinical outcomes and adverse events
Phase IV	Large trials or observational studies conducted after the therapy has been approved by the FDA to assess the rate of uncommon serious side effects and suggest additional therapeutic uses

FDA, U.S. Food and Drug Administration.

■ CONDUCTING A CLINICAL TRIAL

Follow-up and Adherence to the Protocol

In order for a trial to achieve its goal of determining the effects of an intervention, the study participants must adhere to the protocol and provide follow-up data. As a result, investigators planning a trial must think carefully about procedures to maximize adherence and follow-up to ensure that the trial does not end up with underpowered or biased findings (Table 11.3).

TABLE 11.3 MAXIMIZING FOLLOW-UP AND ADHERENCE TO THE PROTOCOL

PRINCIPLE	EXAMPLE
Choose participants who are likely to be adherent to the intervention and protocol.	Require completion of two or more visits before randomization
	Exclude those who are nonadherent in a prerandomization run-in period.
	Exclude those who are likely to move or be noncompliant.
Make the intervention simple.	Use a single tablet once a day if possible.
Make study visits convenient and enjoyable.	Establish good interpersonal relationships with participants.
	Collect information by phone, e-mail, or electronic remote device.
	Consider collecting measurements and providing treatment at home instead of clinic visits.
	Make clinic visits available in the evening or on weekends.
	Have sufficient and well-organized staff to prevent waiting.
	Provide reimbursement for travel and parking.
Make study measurements painless and interesting.	Prefer noninvasive tests.
	Provide test results of interest to participants with counseling or referrals, if appropriate.
Encourage participants to continue in the trial.	Never discontinue follow-up for protocol violations, adverse events, or stopping the intervention.
	Send newsletters and e-mail messages.
	Emphasize the importance of adherence and follow-up.
	Send participants birthday and holiday cards.
Find participants who are lost to follow-up.	Ask close contacts of participants.
	Use a tracking service.

The effect of an active intervention is reduced to the degree that participants do not receive it. When possible, the investigator should design the study intervention so that it is easy to apply and well-tolerated. Drugs that can be taken in a single daily dose, or less often, are the easiest to remember and therefore preferable. Behavioral interventions that require hours of practice by participants are likely to have lower levels of adherence. The protocol should include provisions that will enhance adherence to interventions, such as instructing participants to take the study pill at a standard point in their morning routine, giving them pill containers labeled with the day of the week, or sending reminders to their cell phones. In the case of a behavioral intervention, this may include reinforcements or incentives for attending training sessions.

There is also a need to consider how to measure adherence to the intervention, using approaches like self-report, pill counts, pill containers with sensors that record when the container is opened, intervention practice diaries or logs, and serum or urinary metabolite levels that correlate with use of an intervention. This information can identify participants who are not complying, so that approaches to improving adherence can be instituted and the investigator can interpret the findings of the study appropriately.

Adherence to study visits and measurements can be enhanced by discussing what is involved in the study before consent is obtained, by scheduling the visits at convenient times when there is enough staff to prevent waiting, by calling or e-mailing the participant the day before each visit, and by reimbursing travel, parking, and other out-of-pocket costs. As discussed in the next section, conducting assessments from participants' homes may improve adherence by removing the barriers and inconvenience of visits to clinical sites (17). It is important to make participants feel appreciated. Participants often say that their personal relationship with the research staff is one of the most important reasons that they continue to attend study visits and adhere to treatments.

Failure to follow participants and measure the outcome of interest can result in biased results, diminished credibility of the findings, and decreased statistical power. For example, a trial of nasal calcitonin spray to reduce the risk of osteoporotic fractures reported that treatment reduced fracture risk by 36% (18). However, about 60% of those randomized were lost to follow-up, and it was not known if fractures had occurred in these participants. Because the overall number of fractures was small, even a few fractures in the participants lost to follow-up could have altered the findings of the trial and this uncertainty diminished the credibility of the study findings (19).

Even if participants violate the protocol or discontinue the trial intervention, they should be followed so that their outcomes can be used in intention-to-treat analyses (see Section "Analyzing the Results" later in this chapter). In many trials, participants who violate the protocol (by enrolling in another study, missing visits, or discontinuing the intervention) are removed from follow-up; this can result in biased or uninterpretable results. Consider, for example, a study medication that causes a side effect, which results in its frequent discontinuation. If participants who discontinue study medication are not followed, this can bias the findings if the side effect is associated with the main outcome or with a serious adverse event.

At the outset of the study, participants should be informed of the importance of follow-up and investigators should record the name(s) of, and contact information for, one or two family members or close acquaintances who will always know where the participant lives. In addition to enhancing the investigator's ability to assess vital status, the ability to contact participants by phone or e-mail may provide access to proxy outcome measures from those who refuse to come for a visit at the end.

Two design aspects that are specific to trials—screening visits before randomization and a run-in period—may improve adherence and follow-up. Asking participants to attend one or two screening visits before randomization may exclude participants who find that they cannot complete such visits. The trick here is to set the hurdle for entry into the trial high enough to exclude those who will later be nonadherent, but not so high as to exclude participants who will turn out to have satisfactory adherence.

A run-in period may be useful for increasing the proportion of study participants who adhere to the intervention and follow-up procedures. During the baseline period, all participants are placed on placebo. A specified time later (usually a few weeks), only those who have complied with the intervention (eg, taken at least 80% of the assigned placebo) are randomized. Excluding nonadherent participants before randomization in this fashion may increase the power of the study and permit a better estimate of the full effects of intervention. However, a run-in period delays entry into the trial, the proportion of excluded participants is generally small, and participants randomized to the active drug may notice a change in their medication following randomization, contributing to unblinding. It is also not clear that a placebo run-in is more effective in increasing adherence than the requirement that participants complete one or more screening visits before randomization. In the absence of a specific reason to suspect that adherence in the study will be poor, it is not necessary to include a run-in period.

A variant approach uses the active drug during the run-in period. In addition to increasing adherence among those who enroll, an active run-in can select participants who tolerate and respond to the intervention: The absence of adverse events, or the presence of a desired effect of treatment on a biomarker associated with the outcome, can be used as criteria for randomization. For example, in a placebo-controlled trial testing the effect of continuous nitroglycerin treatment on hot flushes, the investigators used an active run-in period and excluded women who stopped nitroglycerin due to headache (20). This approach maximizes power by increasing the proportion of the intervention group that tolerated the drug and were likely to be adherent. However, the findings of trials using this strategy will not be generalizable to those who were excluded.

Using an active run-in may also underestimate the rate of adverse events, as occurred in a trial of the effect of carvedilol on mortality in 1094 patients with congestive heart failure. During the 2-week active run-in period, 17 people had worsening congestive heart failure and 7 died (21). These people were not randomized in the trial, and these adverse events of drug treatment were not included as outcomes.

Clinical Trials Outside of Traditional Clinical Sites

Some trials, sometimes called "virtual trials," "remote trials," or "disseminated trials," are performed at least in part outside of clinical sites, for example, by enrolling participants online and conducting the trial from home (17). This is commonly done for trials of online behavioral interventions, such as weight reduction programs. However, trials of drugs and supplements can also be done without clinical sites, or with fewer visits to sites, using online informed consent and assessments of eligibility, delivery, and administration of treatments to participants at home, obtaining biologic specimens by phlebotomists in homes or local laboratories, and assessment of outcomes by self-report and by medical records. A trial that does not have bricks-and-mortar clinical sites may be able to recruit participants without geographic limitations and at any time of day, potentially reaching many more people than trials based in sites. When functions of a trial are done without the help of research staff in clinical sites, protocols must be simple, and the systems for enrollment and follow-up must be designed to be intuitive and done with little or no assistance.

Monitoring Clinical Trials

Even if investigators believe that the procedures in a trial pose no undue risks and do not deprive participants of well-established benefits, this may change over the course of a trial. New data from other studies may change the perceived benefit-to-risk ratio, or even answer the research question posed by the trial. Although it is desirable to have more than one study that provides evidence about a given research question, if definitive evidence for either benefit or harm becomes available during a trial, it may be unethical to continue it.

Early trends within a trial may also suggest that the intervention is more harmful or beneficial than expected. Challenges in recruitment, adherence, or outcomes assessment may decrease the likelihood that a trial will be able to provide a definitive answer to its study question. Investigators must ensure that participants are neither exposed inappropriately to a harmful intervention, denied a beneficial intervention, nor continued in a trial if the research question is unlikely to be answered. Each of these three considerations must be monitored during a trial to see if it should be stopped early.

- **Stopping for harm.** The most pressing reason to monitor clinical trials is to make sure that the intervention does not turn out unexpectedly to be harmful. If harm is judged to outweigh benefits, the trial should be stopped.
- **Stopping for benefit.** If an intervention is more efficacious than was estimated when the trial was designed, statistically significant benefit can be observed early in the trial. When clear benefit has been proved, it may be unethical to continue the trial and delay offering the intervention to participants on placebo and to others who could benefit.
- **Stopping for futility.** If there is a very low probability that enrolling additional participants will change the answer to the research question, it may be unethical to continue a trial. If a clinical trial is scheduled to last 5 years, for example, but after 4 years there is little difference in the rate of outcome events in the intervention and control groups, the "conditional power" (the likelihood of rejecting the null hypothesis in the remaining time, given the results thus far) becomes very small and stopping the trial should be considered. Sometimes trials are stopped early if investigators are unable to recruit or retain enough participants and maintain sufficient adherence to treatment to provide adequate power to answer the research question.

Appendix 11B provides examples of trials that were stopped early.

Most clinical trials should include an **interim monitoring** plan; indeed, some organizations that fund trials, such as the National Institutes of Health (NIH), may require such monitoring. In small trials with interventions likely to be safe, the trial investigators might monitor safety themselves or appoint a single independent data and safety monitor. In large trials and those in which adverse events of the intervention are unknown or potentially dangerous, interim monitoring is generally performed by a committee, usually known as the Data and Safety Monitoring Board (DSMB), consisting of experts in the disease or condition under study, biostatisticians, clinical trialists, ethicists, and sometimes a representative of the patient group being studied. These experts are not involved in the trial and should have no personal or financial interest in its continuation. DSMB guidelines and procedures should be detailed in writing before the trial begins.

The interim monitoring plan for a trial may include a plan for scheduled, periodic interim assessments of the effects of interventions on the primary outcome and on safety to detect early evidence of benefit, harm, or futility. This interim plan should use statistical techniques that compensate for multiple looks at the findings. There are many statistical methods for monitoring the interim results of a trial. Analyzing the results of a trial repeatedly ("multiple peeks") is a form of **multiple hypothesis testing** and increases the probability of a **type I error**. For example, if a significance level (alpha) of 0.05 is used for each interim test and the results of a trial are analyzed four times during the trial and again at the end, the probability of making a type I error is increased from 5% to about 14% (22). To address this issue, statistical methods for interim monitoring generally decrease the alpha for each interim test so that the overall alpha is close to 0.05.

Stopping a trial should always be a careful decision that balances ethical responsibility to the participants and the advancement of scientific knowledge. Trends in the apparent interim effects of interventions should be evaluated for consistency over time and across subgroups. It may be preferable to modify a trial, such as by extending follow-up or discontinuing a lower risk subgroup (in which outcomes are unlikely), rather than terminating it completely. Whenever a trial is stopped early, the chance to provide more conclusive results will be lost, particularly about adverse events that may occur with longer term use. Early termination can also have a negative impact on the credibility of the findings and the ability to answer important secondary questions (Appendix 11B).

Bayesian trials take a different approach to monitoring. Rather than testing for statistical significance at designated points, they update the likely efficacy of treatment continuously as data accrue (Appendix 12A). Thus, there are no stopping rules based on *P* values.

Analyzing the Results: Intention-to-Treat, Per-Protocol, and As-Treated Analyses

Statistical analysis of the primary hypothesis of a clinical trial involves comparing outcomes in those assigned to the intervention group with those assigned to the control group. This approach is known by the rubrics "once randomized, always analyzed" and "**intention-to-treat analysis**," because **participants are compared based on the group to which they were randomized, even if they never received the intervention or control.** Results can only be analyzed by intention-to-treat if follow-up measures are completed regardless of whether participants adhere to intervention, so investigators must collect outcomes data for participants even if they discontinue an intervention early or adhere to it poorly.

An intention-to-treat analysis preserves the key benefit of randomization, namely, that the groups being compared will have similar distributions of potential confounding variables. This helps to ensure that the intervention itself—rather than any baseline differences, measured or unmeasured, in the participants—is the only causal explanation for any observed differences in outcomes between the groups (see Section "Counterfactual Framework for Understanding Causality" in Chapter 10). Potential confounding of the causal relationship between the intervention and the outcome, such as by race/ethnicity and sex, can only arise if they are maldistributed by chance, which is unusual, especially in large clinical trials.

In an intention-to-treat analysis, participants who **cross over**—those assigned to the active intervention group who do not get or adhere to the intervention, as well as those assigned to the control group who end up getting the active intervention—are analyzed according to their randomized group assignment (how participants were intended to be treated). An intention-to-treat analysis may underestimate the full effect of the intervention, but it guards against confounding.

By contrast, a "**per-protocol**" analysis includes only participants who adhered to the protocol. This is defined in various ways, but often includes only participants in both groups who adhered to the assigned study intervention, completed a certain proportion of visits or measurements, and had no other protocol violations. (Participants who did not follow the protocol are excluded from a per-protocol analysis.) Another approach is an "**as-treated**" analysis in which participants who received the intervention or the control are analyzed according to the treatment received—even if they had been assigned randomly to the other group. (In this situation, participants who did not receive either the intervention or the control are excluded.) These analyses seem reasonable because participants can only be affected by an intervention they receive. However, participants who adhere to the study treatment and protocol almost always differ in important ways from those who do not—and those differences can confound the causal relationship between the intervention and the outcome.

In an intention-to-treat approach, participants who do not receive the assigned intervention are included in the estimate of the effects of that intervention. Therefore, substantial discontinuation or crossover between treatments will cause an intention-to-treat analysis to underestimate the magnitude of the effect of treatment. For this reason, trials are often evaluated with both intention-to-treat and per-protocol analyses. If the results of an intention-to-treat and a per-protocol analysis differ, the intention-to-treat results should be used for estimates of efficacy because they preserve the value of randomization. In addition, unlike a per-protocol analysis, an intention-to-treat analysis can only bias the estimated effect of the intervention in the conservative direction (favoring the null hypothesis). However, **for estimates of harm, as-treated or per-protocol analyses provide the most cautious estimates: An intervention can only cause harm in someone who receives it.**

Consider a randomized trial comparing two options for treatment of hip fractures in the elderly: internal fixation (using screws to put the hip back together) and hip replacement (with an artificial hip) (23). In the trial, 5 of the 229 patients randomized to hip replacement were treated with screws instead, because they were thought to be too sick for hip replacement, a longer and riskier operation (Figure 11.2).

Figure 11.3 shows the three options for how to analyze the patients who do not receive their assigned treatment. In the **intention-to-treat analysis** (Panel A), randomization is preserved, and the patients are analyzed according to their assigned group. As discussed earlier, this preserves the randomization but can lead to bias toward no difference between groups. In **the as-treated analysis**, the patients are analyzed according to the treatment received (Panel B). You can see that the as-treated analysis is particularly unfair to the screw group, because that group now includes some of the highest risk patients who had been randomized to receive hip replacement. Finally, even the **per-protocol analysis** (Panel C) is unfair to the screw group, because it eliminates those high-risk patients from the hip replacement group but keeps them in the screw group.

Of course, in other clinical situations, crossover might happen in both directions—or the patients crossing over might be at lower, rather than higher, risk. But the basic principle remains: Because those who cross over from their assigned treatment are not a random sample, analyzing them according to the treatment they received—or excluding them from analysis—will likely lead to bias.

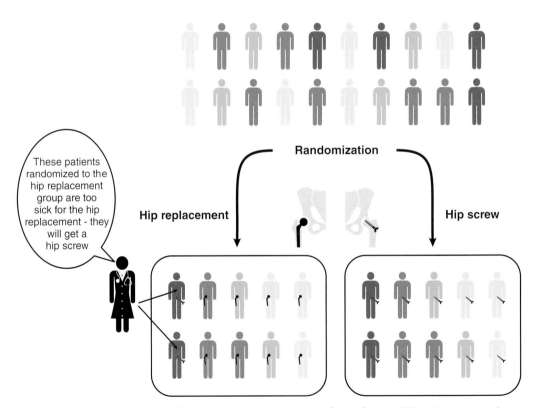

■ **FIGURE 11.2** A randomized trial of hip replacement versus hip screw for hip fracture (23). Patients are not always treated according to the group to which they were randomized. This is especially problematic if those not treated according to the protocol differ in some way, such as being sicker (darker red color), as in the figure. Note: Right hips are shown receiving replacements and left hips receiving screws to make them easier to tell apart. (Illustration by Martina Steurer. From Newman TB and Kohn MA: *Evidence-Based Diagnosis, An Introduction to Clinical Epidemiology, 2nd edition (2020)* reprinted with permission from Cambridge University Press.)

A

Intention to treat
All patients are analyzed according to the randomization group, regardless of the treatment received.

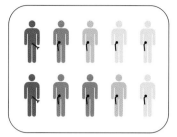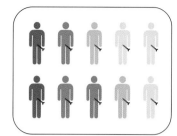

B

As treated
Patients are analyzed according to the treatment received.

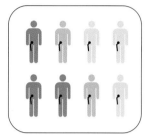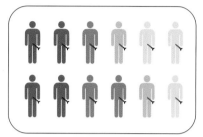

C

Per protocol
Only patients treated according to the study protocol are analyzed.

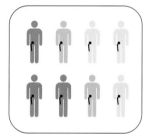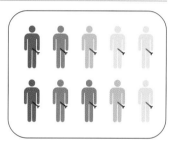

■ **FIGURE 11.3 A-C** Three ways of analyzing a randomized trial with imperfect adherence to assigned treatment. (Illustration by Martina Steurer. From Newman TB and Kohn MA: *Evidence-Based Diagnosis, An Introduction to Clinical Epidemiology, 2nd edition* (*2020*) reprinted with permission from Cambridge University Press.)

Subgroup Analyses

Subgroup analyses compare the intervention and control groups in various subsets of the participants, such as by sex. The main reason for doing these analyses is to look for effect modification ("interaction"), for example, whether the effects of the studied treatment differ in men and women. These analyses have a mixed reputation because they are easy to misuse and can lead to wrong conclusions. With proper caution, however, they can provide useful information and expand the inferences that can be drawn from a clinical trial.

To preserve the value of randomization, subgroups should be defined by measurements made before the interventions are applied. For example, in a trial that found that denosumab decreased the overall risk of nonvertebral fracture by 20%, a preplanned subgroup analysis revealed that the treatment was efficacious (a 35% reduction in fracture risk) among women with low bone density at baseline, but not in women with higher bone density ($P = 0.02$ for effect modification) (24). Subgroup analyses based on *postrandomization* factors, such as adherence to randomized treatment, do not preserve the value of randomization and often produce misleading results.

However, even if they are based on *prerandomization* factors, subgroup analyses can be problematic. First, subgroup comparisons involve fewer participants than the main trial, so investigators should avoid claiming that a drug "was not efficacious" in a subgroup when the finding might reflect insufficient power to find an important difference. Second, investigators often examine results in many subgroups, increasing the likelihood of finding a different effect of the intervention in one subgroup by chance. To address this issue, planned subgroup analyses should be defined before the trial begins, and the number of subgroups analyzed should be reported (25). Claims about different responses in subgroups should be supported by evidence that there is a statistically significant difference in the effect of treatment by the subgroup characteristic, and a separate study should confirm the effect modification before it is considered established.

■ SUMMARY

1. A randomized blinded trial, designed and carried out properly, provides the most definitive causal inference for evidence-based medicine and practice guidelines.
2. The choice and dose of intervention is a difficult decision that balances judgments about efficacy and safety. Other considerations include relevance to clinical practice, suitability for blinding, and whether to use a combination of drugs.
3. When possible, the comparison group should be a placebo control or alternate medication that allows participants, investigators, and study staff to be blinded.
4. Clinically relevant outcomes such as pain, quality of life, occurrence of cancer, and death are the most meaningful outcomes of trials. Intermediary outcomes, such as change in bone density, are valid surrogate markers for clinical outcomes to the degree that treatment-induced changes in the marker predict changes in the clinical outcome.
5. Measuring more than one outcome variable can be helpful but combining them into a composite outcome requires careful consideration. A single primary outcome should be specified to test the main hypothesis.
6. All clinical trials should include measures of potential adverse effects of the intervention, including open-ended measures, with procedures to ensure that serious adverse events are reported promptly to IRBs and sponsors.
7. Study participants should be likely to have the most benefit and the least harm from treatment, and to adhere to treatment and follow-up protocols. Choosing participants at high risk of the outcome will decrease the necessary sample size but may make recruitment more difficult and decrease the generalizability of the findings.
8. Baseline variables should describe participants' characteristics and measure risk factors for (and baseline values of) the outcome to enable later examination of the effects of the intervention in selected subgroups. Consider storing biologic specimens for later analyses.
9. Randomization minimizes the influence of baseline confounding variables. The randomization scheme should be tamperproof. In small trials, stratified blocked randomization can reduce chance maldistributions of key predictors.
10. Blinding the intervention serves to control differential placebo effects, cointerventions, and biased ascertainment and adjudication of the outcome.
11. A pilot study can test the feasibility and estimate the time and costs of a trial but is too small to provide a precise estimate of the effect of an intervention.
12. It is essential to encourage participants to complete follow-up and adhere to treatment: incomplete follow-up and poor adherence can diminish or bias differences in the apparent efficacy and safety of an intervention.
13. A run-in period may exclude potential participants who do not adhere or are prone to immediate adverse effects of treatment.
14. Trials should be monitored with periodic unblinded analyses of the safety and efficacy of treatments by a DSMB. Trials may be stopped early if there are important differences in adverse effects or efficacy, or if continuing a trial is unlikely to demonstrate a difference.
15. Analysis of efficacy based on the original randomized assignment (intention-to-treat) preserves the value of randomization. Per-protocol analyses are a more conservative way to assess adverse effects.
16. Analyses of subgroups of participants can reveal differences in the effects of treatments on groups of patients. They can be misleading because these analyses have less statistical power to find differences and apparent differences may emerge by chance.

REFERENCES

1. The Women's Health Initiative Study Group. Design of the women's health initiative clinical trial and observational study. *Control Clin Trials.* 1998;19:61-109.
2. Califf R. Biomarker definitions and their applications. *Exp Biol Med.* 2018;243:213-221.
3. Black DM, Bauer DC, Vittinghoff, E, et al. Treatment-related changes in bone mineral density as a surrogate biomarker for fracture risk reduction: meta-regression analyses of individual patient data from multiple randomised controlled trials. *Lancet Diabetes Endocrinol.* 2020;8(8):672-682.
4. Nissen SE, Wolski K. Rosiglitazone revisited: an updated meta-analysis of risk for myocardial infarction and cardiovascular mortality. *Arch Intern Med.* 2010;170(14):1191-1201.
5. The Action to Control Cardiovascular Risk in Diabetes Study Group. Effects of intensive glucose lowering in type 2 diabetes. *N Engl J Med.* 2008;358:2545-2559.
6. Barter PJ, Caulfield M, Eriksson M et al. Effects of torcetrapib in patients at high risk for coronary events. *N Engl J Med.* 2007;357:2109-2122.
7. Self WH, Semler MW, Leither LM, et al. Effect of hydroxychloroquine on clinical status at 14 days in hospitalized patients with COVID-19: a randomized clinical trial. *JAMA.* 2020;324:2165-2176.
8. Ridker PM, Everett BM, Pradhan A, et al. Low-dose methotrexate for the prevention of atherosclerotic events. *N Engl J Med.* 2019;380(8):752-762.
9. Friedman LM, Furberg C, DeMets DL. *Fundamentals of Clinical Trials.* 4th ed. Springer; 2010.
10. Avins AL. Can unequal be more fair? Ethics, subject allocation, and randomised clinical trials. *J Med Ethics.* 1998;24:401-408.
11. Subak LL, Wing R, West DS, et al. Weight loss to treat urinary incontinence in overweight and obese women. *N Engl J Med.* 2009;360(5):481-490.
12. Prentice RL, Caan B, Chlebowski RT, et al. Low-fat dietary pattern and risk of invasive breast cancer: the women's health initiative randomized controlled dietary modification trial. *JAMA.* 2006;295:629-642.
13. CDP Research Group. The coronary drug project. Initial findings leading to modifications of its research protocol. *JAMA.* 1970;214:1303-1313.
14. Yu WY, Lu B, Tan D, et al. Effect of topical brimonidine on alcohol-induced flushing in Asian individuals: A randomized clinical trial. *JAMA Dermatol.* 2020;156(2):182-185.
15. Noseworthy JH, Ebers GC, Vandervoort MK, et al. The impact of blinding on the results of a randomized, placebo-controlled multiple sclerosis clinical trial. *Neurology.* 1994;44(1):16.
16. Al-Lamee R, Thompson D, Dehbi HM, et al. Percutaneous coronary intervention in stable angina (ORBITA): a double-blind, randomised controlled trial. *Lancet.* 2018;391(10115):31-40.
17. Cummings SR. Clinical trials without clinical sites. *JAMA Intern Med.* 2021;181:680-684.
18. Chesnut CH 3rd, Silverman S, Andriano K, et al. A randomized trial of nasal spray salmon calcitonin in postmenopausal women with established osteoporosis: the prevent recurrence of osteoporotic fractures study. PROOF Study Group. *Am J Med.* 2000;109(4):267-276.
19. Cummings SR, Chapurlat RD. What PROOF proves about calcitonin and clinical trials. *Am J Med.* 2000;109(4):330-331.
20. Huang AJ, Cummings SR, Schembri M, et al. Continuous transdermal nitroglycerin therapy for menopausal hot flashes: a single-arm, dose-escalation trial. *Menopause.* 2016;23(3):330-334.
21. Pfeffer M, Stevenson L. Beta-adrenergic blockers and survival in heart failure. *N Engl J Med.* 1996;334:1396-1397.
22. Armitage P, McPherson C, Rowe B. Repeated significance tests on accumulating data. *J R Stat Soc.* 1969;132A:235-244.
23. Parker MJ, Pryor G, Gurusamy K. Hemiarthroplasty versus internal fixation for displaced intracapsular hip fractures: a long-term follow-up of a randomised trial. *Injury.* 2010;41(4):370-373.
24. McClung MR, Boonen S, Torring O, et al. Effect of denosumab treatment on the risk of fractures in subgroup of women with postmenopausal osteoporosis. *J Bone Mineral Res.* 2012;27:211-218.
25. Wang R, Lagakos SW, Ware JH, et al. Statistics in medicine—reporting of subgroup analyses in clinical trials. *NEJM.* 2007;357:2189-2194.

APPENDIX 11A
Pilot Studies

Many studies, especially large cohort studies and clinical trials, benefit from the experience gained and data obtained from pilot studies performed before the main study begins or even before writing a proposal to fund a large study. A pilot study is often the best way to obtain trial information on the type, dose, and duration of the intervention; the feasibility of recruiting, randomizing, and maintaining participants in the trial; obstacles to making certain measurements; the likelihood of adherence; potential adverse events; and estimated costs of the study. Pilot studies vary from a brief test of the feasibility of making a measurement in a small number of volunteers to a longer study in hundreds of participants to prepare for a multicenter, multiyear investment.

An important goal of some pilot studies is to define the optimal intervention for a clinical trial while minimizing the chance of adverse events. For example, a pilot trial may compare several doses of a treatment for their effects on intermediate markers. When part of a sequence of trials to test a treatment for FDA approval, they are often called Phase II trials. A control group may not be needed if the purposes of the pilot study are limited to demonstrating the feasibility of the planned measurements, data collection instruments, and data management system; estimating the cost of the main trial; and obtaining data about change in a continuous outcome measurement.

Pilot studies are sometimes used to provide estimates needed for sample size calculations, such as the rate (or mean value) of the outcome in the placebo group and the intervention's anticipated effect size and statistical variability. In most situations, however, it's best to obtain these estimates from published studies of similar interventions in comparable participants. In the absence of such data, a pilot study may be helpful. In particular, the standard deviation of the change in a continuous measurement that will be the primary end point for a trial—which is often not available from previous studies—can be obtained by making repeat measurements over time in a small sample that resembles the expected participants in the main trial. However, a pilot study is *not* a reliable source of data about the expected effect size; after all, if it had the power to determine the effect size with any precision, it would have accomplished the aim of the main trial!

A good pilot study will require substantial time and resources but doing one will also improve the chances that the main trial will be funded and completed successfully. A pilot study for a large trial should have a short but complete protocol (approved by the IRB), data collection forms, and analysis plans; these will save time when starting the trial itself. Pilot study measurements may include the anticipated predictors and outcomes for the full-scale trial, as well as the number of participants available for recruitment, the proportions who respond to different recruitment techniques, the proportion eligible who would likely refuse randomization, the time and cost of recruitment and randomization, and estimates of adherence to the intervention and other aspects of the protocol, including study visits. It is usually helpful to debrief both participants and staff after the pilot study to obtain their views on how the trial methods could be improved.

APPENDIX 11B
Three Examples of Trials That Were Stopped Early

Below, we describe the evidence that led to the decisions to stop the trials and the effects of early termination.

- **Combination Antibiotic Therapy for Methicillin Resistant Staphylococcus Aureus Bacteremia: Early Termination for Harm** (1). This study compared two approaches to antibiotic treatment for hospitalized patients with methicillin-resistant *Staphylococcus aureus* (MRSA) bacteremia. The goal of this open-label randomized trial was to determine whether the addition of an anti-staphylococcal beta-lactam antibiotic to standard antibiotic therapy was more efficacious than standard antibiotic therapy alone. The investigators aimed to randomize 440 participants to detect a 12.5% absolute reduction in a composite outcome of mortality, persistent bacteremia after 5 days, microbiologic relapse, and microbiologic treatment failure. After the trial had enrolled and followed 343 participants, an interim analysis found no significant difference in this primary outcome, which was detected in 35% of participants assigned to combination therapy and 39% assigned to standard therapy (difference −4%, 95% confidence interval [CI]: –14% to 6%, $P = 0.42$). Analyses of five of the trial's seven prespecified secondary outcomes, including all-cause mortality, also showed no significant differences. However, one secondary outcome, acute kidney injury, was more common in the combination therapy group (23%) than in those receiving standard therapy (6%) (difference 17%; 95% CI: 9% to 25%), whereas persistent bacteremia at day 5, another secondary outcome, was less common in the combination group (11%) than in the standard therapy group (20%) (difference –9%, 95% CI: –17% to –1%). The difference in acute kidney injury was first noticed by the DSMB during a prior interim analysis of 220 participants; after further analysis of data from an additional 123 participants showed a higher rate of kidney injury and no decrease in 90-day mortality in the combination treatment group, the DSMB recommended stopping recruitment. The investigators explained that even though the reduction in persistent bacteremia could be interpreted as evidence of greater efficacy of combination treatment, they believed that it was offset by the potential harm associated with kidney injury. However, they acknowledged that the sample size may have been insufficient to detect other clinically important differences that favored combination antibiotic therapy.

- **Letrozole after Tamoxifen for Early Breast Cancer: Early Termination for Benefit** (2). At the time of this study, women with early-stage hormone-receptor-positive breast cancer were known to have better disease-free and overall survival if they took tamoxifen, an estrogen modulator, for 5 years. A double-blind, randomized, placebo-controlled trial was launched to determine whether an additional 5 years of another nonsteroidal aromatase inhibitor medication, letrozole, could improve disease-free survival among women who had completed 5 years of tamoxifen. The first interim analysis was conducted when 5157 participants had been enrolled, and the median follow-up time was only 2.4 years. At that time, recurrences of breast cancer or new primary cancers in the contralateral breast had occurred in 75 women in the letrozole group and 132 in the placebo group. The 4-year disease-free survival rates were 93% in the letrozole group and 87% in the placebo group ($P < 0.001$). On the basis of these interim results, the DSMB recommended that the findings be made public, the participants be notified of their treatment assignment, and those receiving placebo be given the opportunity to receive letrozole. This decision was consistent with the original statistical interim monitoring plan and early termination guidelines for the trial. However, some argued that ending the study after a median follow-up of only 2.4 years, when none of the participants had been followed for 5 years, decreased the usefulness of the results (3). Early termination of the trial also limited its ability to examine the potential long-term adverse effects of letrozole. At the time of early termination, there was a trend toward more self-reported diagnoses of osteoporosis in the letrozole group than the placebo group ($P = 0.07$), but early termination precluded obtaining more definitive evidence.

- **Pancreas Resection With and Without Routine Intraperitoneal Drainage: Early Termination of a Trial Subgroup for Harm** (4). This trial was designed to examine the common practice of placing drains in the abdominal cavity (ie, intraperitoneal drains) after surgical resection of the pancreas. Although many surgeons used drains to evacuate blood or pancreatic fluid after surgery, others were concerned that drains were associated with more serious postoperative complications such as pancreatic fistula (persistent drainage of fluid through a nonhealing drain wound tract). A randomized unblinded trial was launched to determine the effect of intraperitoneal drainage on the frequency and severity of postoperative complications in adults undergoing pancreatic resection, including those undergoing pancreaticoduodenectomy (PD; or resection of the head of the pancreas) or distal pancreatectomy (resection of the tail or body of the pancreas). The investigators planned to recruit 750 adults from 9 academic surgery centers in the United States to detect a 10% difference in grade 2 or higher complication rates (potentially life-threatening complications with the need of intervention or extended hospital stay) between the drain versus no drain groups. However, interim monitoring when the trial was at 18% of its target enrollment ($N = 282$, including 196 who had undergone PD) found 8 deaths (12%) in PD patients without drains and 2 deaths (3%) in PD patients with drains ($P = 0.10$). The DSMB recommended discontinuation of the trial in adults undergoing PD; the investigators continued to enroll participants undergoing distal pancreatectomy. When other clinical scientists expressed surprise at this decision because of the small number of deaths and requested more information about the interim monitoring plan, the investigators explained that while the trial had a preestablished interim statistical monitoring plan to guide early terminations for the primary outcome, there was no plan to monitor deaths (5). The investigators noted, however, that the DSMB members were aware of a newly published retrospective analysis of over a thousand patients undergoing pancreatic resection, which reported an excess mortality in patients undergoing PD without intraperitoneal drainage. Because of the trend toward increased death in participants undergoing PD without intraperitoneal drainage, the investigators added a new stopping plan specific to mortality into the trial. At the conclusion of follow-up, of 344 participants with distal pancreatectomy, no difference in the rate of mortality or grade 2 or higher complications were detected (6).

REFERENCES

1. Ton SY, Lye DC, Yahav D, et al. Effect of vancomycin or daptomycin with vs without an antistaphylococcal β-lactam on mortality, bacteremia, relapse, or treatment failure in patients with MRSA bacteremia: a randomized clinical trial. *JAMA.* 2020;323(6):527-537.
2. Goss PE, Ingle JN, Martino S, et al. A randomized trial of letrozole in postmenopausal women after five years of tamoxifen therapy for early-stage breast cancer. *N Engl J Med.* 2003;349(19):1793-1802.
3. Bryan J, Wormack N. Letrozole after tamoxifen for breast cancer—what is the price of success? *N Engl J Med.* 2003;349(19):1855-1857.
4. Van Buren G 2nd, Bloomston M, Hughes SJ, et al. A randomized prospective multicenter trial of pancreaticoduodenectomy with and without routine intraperitoneal drainage. *Ann Surg.* 2014;259(4):605-612.
5. Van Bruen G 2nd, Fisher WE. Pancreaticoduodenectomy without drains: interpretation of the evidence. *Ann Surg.* 2016;263(2):e20-e21.
6. Van Bruen G 2nd, Bloomston M Schmidt CR, et al. A prospective randomized multicenter trial of distal pancreatectomy with and without routine intraperitoneal drainage. *Ann Surg.* 2017;266(3):421-431.

APPENDIX 11C
Exercises for Chapter 11. Designing Randomized Blinded Trials

1. An herbal extract, huperzine, has been used in China as a remedy for dementia, and prelimi-nary studies in animals and humans have been promising. You would like to test whether this new treatment might decrease the progression of Alzheimer's disease. Studies have found that the plasma level of amyloid β protein 1-40 (Aβ40) is a biomarker for Alzheimer's disease: elevated lev-els are associated with a significantly increased risk of developing dementia and the levels of Aβ40 increase with the progression of dementia. In planning a trial to test the efficacy of huperzine for prevention of dementia in older patients with mild cognitive impairment, you consider two poten-tial outcome measurements: change in Aβ40 levels or incidence of a clinical diagnosis of dementia.
   a. List one advantage and one disadvantage of using change in Aβ40 levels as the primary outcome for your trial.
   b. List one advantage and one disadvantage of using the new diagnosis of dementia as the primary outcome for the trial.
2. The primary aim of your huperzine trial is to test whether this herbal extract decreases the incidence of a clinical diagnosis of dementia among older men and women with mild cogni-tive impairment. Describe the types of information that should be collected at baseline to achieve each of the following goals (list two potential variables for each goal):
   a. Maximize your study team's ability to follow up and retain participants;
   b. Enable clinicians and other researchers to assess whether your study sample is generalizable;
   c. Determine whether huperzine is efficacious in decreasing progression of Alzheimer's disease;
   d. Conduct future subgroup analyses to evaluate potential differences in treatment effects in certain groups; and
   e. Have data that your study can use to address other questions aside from the primary questions driving the trial.
3. People who carry an ApoE4 allele have an increased risk of dementia. You suspect that the effects of huperzine may differ among those with versus without the ApoE4 allele.
   a. How might you design your (1) screening and enrollment procedures and (2) random-ization strategy to address this question?
   b. What are the potential benefits and downsides of trying to address this question in an initial trial of huperzine?
4. A relatively large randomized, placebo-controlled trial of huperzine is being planned, with follow-up of participants over a 2-year period. Huperzine has the potential to cause gastroin-testinal symptoms, including diarrhea, nausea, and vomiting. Which of the following approaches to monitoring for potential gastrointestinal side effects of huperzine do you prefer, and why?
   a. Asking participants at the end of the trial if study treatment caused them to develop diar-rhea, nausea, or vomiting.
   b. Telling participants at the start of the trial that they should feel free to report any potential side effects of study treatment and waiting to see whether they report gastrointestinal symptoms.
   c. Asking participants at each follow-up visit if they have experienced gastrointestinal symptoms, using a checklist that includes diarrhea, nausea, and vomiting.
   d. Asking participants at each follow-up visit an open-ended question such as, "Have you experienced any new symptoms or health conditions since your last visit?"

5. Some participants stopped huperzine because they developed gastrointestinal symptoms. You are an interim monitor considering whether to recommend early termination of the trial due to the frequency of reports of stomach upset, nausea, or vomiting. What information about those with gastrointestinal symptoms might be useful to inform your decision (aside from how often this happened)? What potential alternatives to early termination might you consider?

6. During the trial of huperzine, 20% of the randomized participants do not return for the 1-year follow-up visit, and 40% stop study medication by 2 years. List one advantage and one disadvantage of analyzing the effect of treatment on gastrointestinal side effects by a strict intention-to-treat approach.

7. In an intention-to-treat analysis after 2 years, participants randomized to huperzine are less likely to be diagnosed with dementia than those randomized to placebo, but this difference is not statistically significant ($P = 0.08$). However, an additional analysis suggest that huperzine decreases the likelihood of dementia diagnosis by 25% more than placebo in participants younger than age 60 years ($P = 0.01$ in that subgroup). What are the potential problems with drawing the conclusion that huperzine is efficacious in preventing clinical dementia in individuals younger than age 60?

CHAPTER 12

Alternate Interventional Study Designs

Deborah G. Grady, Steven R. Cummings, and Alison J. Huang

In the last chapter, we discussed the classic individual-level, randomized, blinded, parallel group clinical trial. There are several other trial designs in which the investigator introduces an intervention, but some aspects of the classic randomized trial design are altered or missing. In this chapter, we describe alternative interventional study designs that are used commonly or have special advantages when the circumstances are right.

■ ALTERNATIVE RANDOMIZED DESIGNS

Factorial Design

A **factorial trial** aims to answer two (or more) distinct research questions in a single study (Figure 12.1). For example, the VITAL trial was designed to test the effects of vitamin D_3 and omega-3 fatty acid supplements on the risks of cardiovascular events and cancer. The participants were assigned randomly to one of four groups and four hypotheses were tested. At the end of the study, the rates of cardiovascular events and cancer in participants who had received vitamin D_3 were compared with the rates in participants receiving the equivalent placebo, disregarding that half of the participants in each of those groups received omega-3 fatty acids. Next, the rates of cardiovascular events and cancer in those who received omega-3 fatty acids were compared with those on the equivalent placebo, now disregarding that half also received vitamin D_3. The investigators studied two interventions (and two outcomes) for the price of one. Unfortunately, neither intervention was beneficial (1, 2).

A limitation of the factorial design, however, is the possibility of **effect modification**, for example, that the effect of vitamin D_3 on the risk of cardiovascular disease differed in those also treated with omega-3 fatty acids. If that were true, the effect of vitamin D_3 would have to be calculated separately for those who did—and did not—receive fatty acid supplements. This would reduce the power of these comparisons, because only half of the participants would be included in each analysis. Factorial designs can be used to study effect modification, but trials designed for this purpose are more complicated to implement and interpret, and larger sample sizes are required. Other limitations of the factorial design are that the same target population must be appropriate for both interventions, and that multiple treatments may interfere with recruitment and adherence.

Active Control Trials: Equivalence and Noninferiority

In an **active control trial**, the control group also receives an intervention that affects the condition of interest. This design, sometimes called a **comparative effectiveness trial** because two treatments are compared, may be optimal when there is a "standard of care" for a condition.

In some situations, the aim of an active control trial is to show that a new treatment is superior to an established treatment. In this case, the design and methods are similar to a placebo-controlled trial. Usually, however, investigators want to establish that a new therapy has

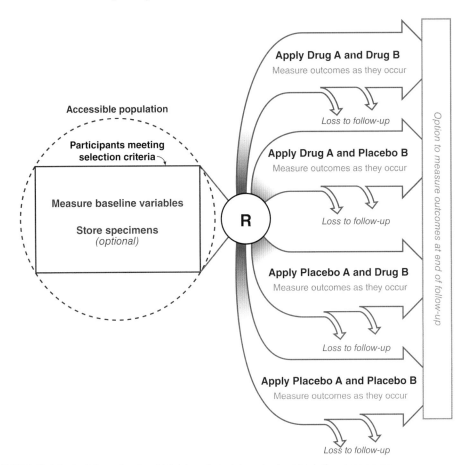

■ **FIGURE 12.1 Factorial randomized trial**. In a factorial randomized trial, the steps are to:
• Select a sample of participants from an accessible population suitable for receiving the interventions (drugs in this example).
• Measure baseline predictor variables and (if appropriate) the baseline level of the outcome variables.
• Consider the option of making additional measurements and storing specimens for later analysis.
• Randomly assign (represented by the letter R) two (or more) active drugs and their placebo controls to four (or more) groups.
• Follow the participants over time, minimize loss to follow-up, and assess adherence to the drug and placebo conditions.
• Measure the outcome variables.
• Analyze the results, first comparing the two drug A groups (combined) with the combined placebo A groups and then comparing the two drug B groups (combined) with the combined placebo B groups.

an advantage over an established therapy—because it is easier to use, less invasive, or safer—while having *similar* efficacy. (It is difficult to justify a trial to test a "me-too" treatment with none of these advantages.) In this case, an **equivalence** or **noninferiority** trial is more appropriate. For example, several studies had found that pelvic floor muscle training for individual women was efficacious for treating symptoms of urinary incontinence (3). A trial comparing individual to group training found that the group approach was not inferior to individual treatment (4), which could make training more widely available.

The statistical methods for equivalence or noninferiority trials are different than for trials designed to show that one treatment is better than another. In a trial designed to show that a treatment is superior, the standard analysis uses tests of statistical significance to reject the null hypothesis that there is no difference between groups. In a trial designed to show that a new treatment is equivalent to the standard treatment, on the other hand, the goal is to find that there is no difference. But proving that there is *no* difference between treatments (not even a tiny one) would require an infinite sample size. A practical solution is to design the sample size and analysis using a confidence interval for the effect of the new treatment compared with the standard treatment. The investigator specifies the difference in efficacy between the two treatments—called the **noninferiority margin** (delta or "Δ")—such that if the new treatment is less efficacious by delta or more, the investigator would conclude that the standard treatment was better (5, 6). On the other hand, **equivalence or noninferiority is established if the confidence interval for the difference in efficacy of the new compared to the established treatment does not include delta** (Figure 12.2). Usually, investigators are interested in showing that a new treatment is not inferior to the standard treatment and use a one-tailed confidence interval, which has the advantage of permitting a smaller sample size (Chapter 6).

Establishing the noninferiority margin is based on both statistical considerations and clinical judgments of the potential efficacy and advantages of the new treatment (7). One approach to setting delta is to perform a meta-analysis of previous trials of the established treatment compared to placebo and set delta at some proportion of the distance between the null and lower bound of the confidence interval for the treatment effect. Alternatively, since trials included in meta-analyses often vary in quality, it may be better to base delta on the results of the best quality randomized trial of the established therapy that has similar entry criteria, dosing of the established treatment, and outcome measures. It is important to set delta such that there is a high likelihood, taking all benefits and harms into account, that the new therapy is better than placebo (6, 8). Noninferiority trials are usually larger than placebo-controlled trials because the acceptable difference between a new and an established treatment is usually smaller than the expected difference between a new treatment and a placebo.

Noninferiority may not mean that the established and new treatments work—they could *both* be useless or even harmful. To ensure that a new treatment evaluated in a noninferiority trial is more efficacious than placebo, there should be strong prior evidence supporting the efficacy of the established treatment. This also means that the design of the noninferiority trial should be as similar as possible to trials that have established the efficacy of the standard treatment, including selection criteria, dose of and adherence to the established treatment, adherence to

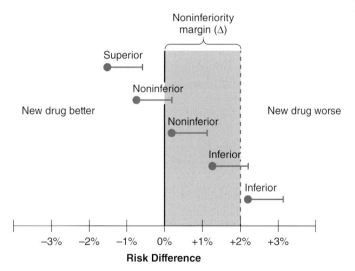

■ **FIGURE 12.2** Possible outcomes in a noninferiority trial comparing a new drug to warfarin as treatment to reduce stroke risk among patients with atrial fibrillation, with the noninferiority margin (delta) set at +2%. The one-sided 95% confidence intervals around the difference in stroke rate between warfarin and the new drug are shown illustrating the outcomes of superiority, inferiority, and noninferiority.

the standard treatment, length of follow-up, loss to follow-up, and so on (6, 8). Any problem that reduces the efficacy of the standard treatment (eg, enrolling participants unlikely to benefit, nonadherence, loss to follow-up) will make it more likely that the new therapy will not be inferior because the efficacy of the standard treatment has been reduced. A new, less efficacious treatment may appear to be noninferior when the findings just represent a poorly done study.

Adaptive Designs

Classic clinical trials are conducted according to a protocol that does not change during the study. However, for some types of treatments and conditions, **adaptive designs** that **allow changes to the trial protocol based on interim analyses of the results** may be preferable (9). For example, consider a trial of several doses of a new treatment for nonulcer dyspepsia. The initial design may plan to enroll 50 participants to a placebo group and 50 to each of three doses of the drug for 12 weeks of treatment over an enrollment period lasting 1 year. Review of the results after the first 10 participants in each group have completed 4 weeks of treatment might reveal that there is a trend toward relief of dyspepsia only in the highest dose group. It may be more efficient to stop assigning participants to the two lower doses and continue randomizing only to the highest dose and the placebo. Other facets of a trial that could be changed based on interim results include modifying the sample size or duration of the trial if interim results suggest that the effect size or rate of outcomes differ from the original assumptions.

Adaptive designs are feasible only for interventions that produce outcomes measured and analyzed early enough to make design changes possible. To prevent bias, rules for how such changes may be made should be established before the trial begins, and the interim analyses and consideration of any change in the design should be done by an independent data monitoring board. Statistical analyses must account for interim analyses that increase the probability of finding a favorable result that is due to chance.

Platform trials (and variants such as basket or umbrella trials) are adaptive trials that have a single master protocol that allows evaluation of multiple interventions, either simultaneously or sequentially (10). Platform trials generally evaluate intervention combinations, differences in intervention effects in subgroups, or multiple serial interventions. Adaptive platforms allow declaring one or more interventions (or doses) superior while continuing to evaluate other interventions, dropping interventions for lack of efficacy (or harm), and adding new interventions during the course of the trial while using the same master protocol and trial infrastructure. These trials may identify efficacious interventions more quickly and with fewer resources compared to traditional strategies investigating one intervention per trial. In addition, they do not require a new trial infrastructure for every intervention under investigation. For example, the Adaptive COVID-19 Treatment Trial (ACTT-1), sponsored by the National Institute of Allergy and Infectious Diseases, was a platform trial of serial treatments for severe acute respiratory syndrome coronavirus 2 (SARS-CoV2) or COVID-19. Remdesivir, the first drug studied, was associated with a shorter time to recovery compared to placebo. This platform trial was designed to drop the placebo arm when efficacious treatments were identified, but to continue to study beneficial treatments compared to other antivirals and modifiers of the immune response (11).

Bayesian trials differ from standard trials, which are sometimes called **frequentist trials**, by incorporating other evidence, such as previous studies of the same or similar interventions, in their design and analysis (Appendix 12A). For example, consider a frequentist trial that sets alpha at 0.05 to test whether the treatment reduces the risk of the outcome by at least 25%. If the trial found a 20% reduction in risk, with a P value of 0.09, that result would not be "statistically significant." In contrast, a Bayesian approach would apply the prior probability that the treatment was efficacious to the analysis (and design) of the trial. If previous studies had shown a 25% reduction in risk, for example, a **Bayesian analysis** of the same results might estimate that there is a 99% probability that the treatment reduces the risk of the outcome by at least 20%.

Bayesian trials often require enrollment of a flexible number of participants without a fixed sample size or budget. They do not have stopping rules based on *P* values adjusted for the number of looks. A Bayesian approach is sometimes used in adaptive trials that use results from prior studies to plan for the next trial.

Crossover Designs

In a **crossover study**, some participants are randomly assigned to start with the active intervention and then switch to the control intervention; the other participants begin with the control intervention and then switch to the active intervention (Figure 12.3). This approach permits **between-group** analyses (comparing the active treatment group with the control group), as well as **within-group** analyses (comparing each participant's results when he was treated with the intervention to when he was receiving the control). The advantages are substantial: because each participant serves as his own control, the paired analysis increases statistical power; crossover trials require fewer participants than parallel group trials. However, the disadvantages are also substantial: a doubling of the duration of the study, the added expense required to measure the outcome at the beginning and end of each crossover period, and the added complexity of analysis and interpretation created by potential **carryover effects**. A carryover effect is the residual influence of the intervention after it has been stopped—blood pressure not returning to baseline levels for months after a course of diuretic treatment, for example. To reduce carryover effect, the investigator can introduce an untreated "**washout period**" between treatments in the hope that the outcome variable will return to baseline before starting the next intervention, but it is difficult to know whether all carryover effects have been eliminated. In general, crossover studies are a good choice when the number of study participants is limited, and the outcome responds rapidly and reversibly to an intervention.

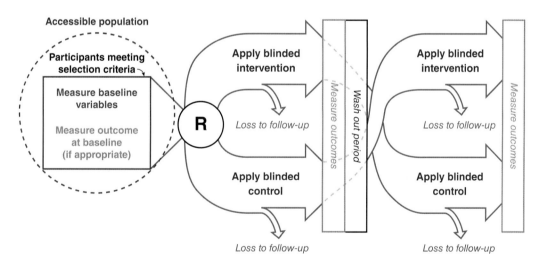

■ **FIGURE 12.3 Crossover trial**. In a crossover randomized trial, the steps are to:
- In a crossover randomized trial, the steps are to:
- Select a sample of participants from an accessible population suitable for receiving the intervention.
- Measure baseline predictor variables and (if appropriate) the baseline level of the outcome variables.
- Randomly assign (represented by the letter R) the blinded intervention and control condition.
- Follow the participants over time, minimizing loss to follow-up and assessing compliance with the intervention and control conditions.
- Measure the outcome variables.
- Discontinue the intervention and control condition and provide a washout period to reduce carryover effects, if appropriate.
- Apply intervention to former control group; apply control condition to former intervention group, then measure outcomes after following participants over time.

Wait-List Designs

A variation on the crossover design may be appropriate when the intervention to be studied cannot be blinded and the intervention, such as a new noninvasive procedure, is believed by participants to be more desirable than the control. In this situation, it may be very difficult to find eligible participants who are willing to be randomized to control. An excellent alternative may be randomization to receive the intervention at the start of the trial or to a wait-list control group that receives the intervention at the end of a defined period of time. Another situation in which a wait-list control may be appropriate is when a hospital, community, school, government, or similar entity has decided for political or fairness reasons that all members of a group should receive an intervention, despite limited evidence of efficacy. In this situation, randomization to a delayed intervention may be acceptable.

The **wait-list design** provides an opportunity for a randomized comparison between the immediate intervention and wait-list control groups. In addition, the two intervention periods (immediate intervention in one group and delayed intervention in the other) can be pooled to increase power for a within-group comparison before and after the intervention. For example, women with symptomatic uterine fibroids could be randomized to a new treatment such as uterine artery embolization versus a wait-list control group that was offered uterine artery embolization 6 months later. Subsequently, changes in fibroid symptom scores can be compared among those who were randomized initially to uterine artery embolization and those who were wait-listed initially, and within-group measurements of changes in symptom score can be pooled among all of the participants who received the intervention.

Wait-list designs require that the outcome occurs in a short enough period of time to keep the waiting period from becoming too long. In addition, providing the intervention to the control group at the end of the trial prolongs the length of follow-up and increases the cost of the trial.

N-of-1 Designs

N-of-1 designs (where N is an abbreviation for the sample size) resemble crossover trials that enroll only one person. Also called single patient trials, they generally aim to answer clinical questions about effectiveness or adverse effects in an individual patient. In the simplest N-of-1 trial, a patient is randomly assigned for a set period of time to a blinded treatment or to placebo (or a different active treatment), then crossed over to the alternative intervention for the same duration of time. Multiple crossovers can also be used; these provide stronger evidence on outcomes. For example, if a patient with frequent migraine headaches and his physician believe that treatment with gabapentin might reduce the frequency of headaches (but are not sure), they may agree to try an N-of-1 trial. The trial might include several periods in which the patient randomly receives gabapentin or placebo. The patient records the frequency of headaches at the beginning of the trial and periodically thereafter. Outcomes are typically chosen by the patient according to the most bothersome symptoms and scored using simple Likert scales. At the planned termination of the trial (typically after 2 to 5 crossover periods), the blind is broken and the data evaluated. Sometimes, simple inspection of the data is all that is needed to determine the best treatment, but statistics such as paired *t* tests or time series methods can also be used.

In comparison with trials that answer a clinical question for a group of participants, some of whom benefit while others do not, N-of-1 trials have the advantage that they may answer the question for a specific patient. However, N-of-1 trials are best suited to chronic or recurrent symptomatic conditions where the outcome occurs quickly in response to treatment and any effects resolve quickly after stopping treatment. As in crossover trials, a washout period can be included to try to minimize carryover effects of treatment, but the necessary duration of washout is often unclear. Patients must understand the requirements of the trial and be willing to undertake blinded treatment. If the treatment isn't blinded, the results may be no better than clinical judgment. N-of-1 trials are usually not feasible for an individual clinician to conduct without the assistance of a research pharmacy or "N-of-1 Service" (12).

Cluster Randomized Designs

Cluster randomized designs require that the investigator randomly assign naturally occurring groups or clusters of participants to the interventions, rather than individuals (Figure 12.4). A good example is a trial that enrolled players on 120 college baseball teams, randomly allocated half of the teams to an intervention to encourage cessation of spit-tobacco, and found that 35% of players at the intervention colleges quit compared to 16% at the control colleges (13).

Randomizing an intervention to groups of people may be more feasible and cost-effective than randomizing individuals one at a time, and it may better address research questions about the effects of public health programs in the population or quality improvement interventions within a health care delivery system. Some interventions, such as a low-fat diet, may be difficult to implement in only one member of a family. When participants in a natural group are randomized individually, those who receive the intervention are likely to discuss or share the intervention with family members, colleagues, team members, or acquaintances who have been assigned to the control group. Thus, the control group is likely to be exposed to the intervention, and this **contamination** can reduce the apparent efficacy of the intervention. Quality improvement interventions, such as electronic decision support or clinical process changes, may be especially difficult to randomize at the individual patient level, since a clinician, a clinic, or a clinical unit will likely have patients randomized to both the intervention and control groups, resulting in contamination of the intervention.

It is important to distinguish between a cluster randomized trial and a trial in which an intervention is delivered in groups. For example, in studies of yoga or tai chi, participants are commonly randomized individually, but the intervention may be delivered through group training

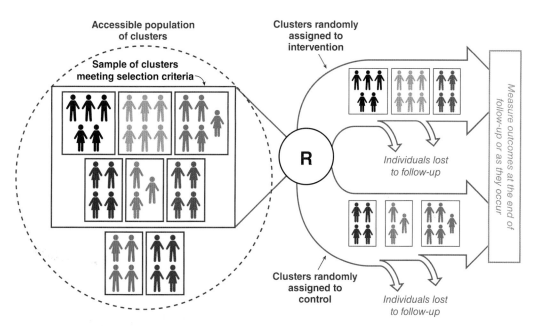

■ **FIGURE 12.4 Cluster-randomized trial.** In a cluster randomized trial, the steps are to:
- Select a sample of clusters from an accessible population suitable for receiving the intervention.
- Measure baseline predictor variables and (if appropriate) the baseline level of the outcome variables among members of the clusters.
- Randomly assign (represented by the letter R) the clusters to the blinded intervention or control condition.
- Follow the participants over time, minimizing loss to follow-up and assessing adherence to the intervention and control conditions.
- Measure the outcome variables.

sessions. This requires statistical adjustment to acknowledge potential clustering of intervention effects among participants within the same group of yoga or tai chi class, but this design is not a cluster randomized trial, because randomization is implemented at the individual level.

In the cluster randomized design, the units of randomization are groups, not individuals. The effective sample size is smaller than the number of individual participants, depends on the correlation of the effect of the intervention among participants in the clusters, and is somewhere between the number of clusters and the total number of participants (14). In general, power is higher if there are a large number of groups rather than a small number of groups with a larger sample per group (15).

Another potential problem in cluster randomized trials is imbalance in baseline characteristics between intervention arms. Randomization works best for balancing characteristics when there are many randomized units; cluster randomization decreases the number of randomized units. For example, a trial with thousands of persons clustered within four geographic areas, where one is very different than the other three, will result in imbalance between the randomized arms. Stratified or matched randomization (eg, on size, proportion of men, or prevalence of comorbidities) may help address the problem that clusters may have differences in important confounders, but it would not help in the example provided.

Other drawbacks to cluster randomization are that sample size estimation and data analysis are more complicated than for individual randomization (9).

Stepped Wedge Designs

A **stepped wedge trial** is a variation of the cluster randomized design in which a cluster, a group of clusters, or individual participants are randomized, not to intervention or control, but to the order in which they begin the intervention (16, 17). The trial begins with a baseline period of data collection during which no cluster receives the intervention. Subsequently, clusters randomly begin the intervention at set time intervals (called steps) throughout the trial. Once the intervention has started in a given cluster, it continues until the end of the trial. By the end of the trial, all clusters have received the intervention (Figure 12.5). Because all of the clusters experience both the control and intervention conditions, outcomes can be compared both between clusters and within clusters. Comparisons between clusters randomized to the intervention and control during the same period of time can control for temporal or cohort effects, and comparisons of changes in the outcome within the clusters can reduce potential confounding

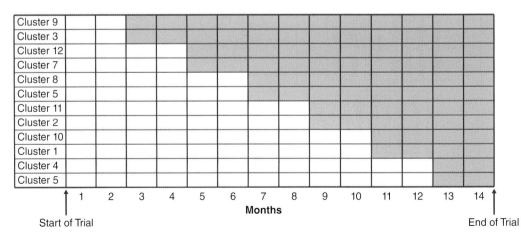

■ **FIGURE 12.5 Stepped wedge trial**. In a stepped wedge trial, all clusters (here 12) begin in the control condition (white). Some clusters (here 2) are randomly assigned to begin the intervention (blue) at fixed points in time (here every 2 months). Once a cluster has begun the intervention, it is continued until the end of the trial. The design is called "stepped wedge" because of the shape of the figure.

that might be introduced by differences between the clusters. Illustrations of these trial designs look like "stepped wedges" (Figure 12.5), which is where the design gets its name.

Stepped wedge designs are most often used for studies of clinical processes, public health interventions, or quality improvement. In addition to the benefits of clustered randomization described previously, the stepped wedge design may be more politically or culturally acceptable, feasible, and ethical. As in the wait-list design, stepped wedge designs may be most appropriate when a hospital, community, school, or government has decided that all members of a group should receive an intervention despite limited evidence of efficacy. In addition, limited resources or logistic complexity may make it impossible to roll out a large, complex intervention to an entire health system all at once. In this situation, a gradual rollout may be the most feasible approach. For example, in the Mesita Azul Intervention Study, researchers at UC Berkeley, in cooperation with a local nonprofit organization, did a stepped wedge trial to determine the efficacy of an ultraviolet disinfection water treatment system among 24 rural communities in Baja California Sur. The intervention, which was introduced in six clusters selected in random order, reduced the percentage of households that had *Escherichia coli* contamination of their drinking water, though it did not reduce the prevalence of diarrhea (18).

Like all cluster randomized trials, the sample size for a stepped wedge trial depends on correlations among members of the clusters and is somewhere between the number of clusters and the number of participants. Thus, stepped wedge trials may require a much larger sample size than individually randomized trials. Stepped wedge trials are typically large and complex, and require close collaboration with leaders of health systems or government. In a stepped wedge trial, data from the control condition are collected, on average, earlier than from the intervention condition. Thus, temporal changes in health care or data collection that have nothing to do with the intervention may confound the results. The analysis of a stepped wedge trial is complicated, as it must account both for the clustered design and for temporal trends in the outcome. Stepped wedge trials often use an intervention that is considered evidence-based and aimed to improve quality over usual care. In this situation, especially if the outcomes can be determined using data that are public or collected in the course of routine health care, individualized informed consent may be waived by the Institutional Review Board.

■ NONRANDOM INTERVENTIONAL DESIGNS

Trials that compare the effect of an intervention in groups that have not been assigned randomly—often called quasi-experimental or quasi-randomized designs—may be appropriate when randomized trials are not possible due to ethical, political, social, or logistical constraints. We introduced some of these designs in Chapter 10 when we called them "opportunistic" because they depend on an opportunity (perhaps created by a change in policy) to estimate the effect of change on an outcome. **Opportunistic designs** are observational—the investigator does not design or implement the change that he studies. In contrast, in this chapter, we address nonrandom interventional study designs in which an investigator designs and implements an intervention but does not apply the intervention randomly.

These types of trials are often employed to assess policy, health care practice changes, or implementation of evidence-based practices. However, nonrandomized trials are far less effective than randomized trials in controlling for confounding variables. For example, in a trial of the effects of coronary artery bypass surgery compared to percutaneous angioplasty, if clinicians are allowed to decide which patients undergo the procedures rather than using random allocation, patients chosen for surgery are likely to differ from those chosen for angioplasty. Analytic methods can adjust for measured baseline factors that are unequal in the two study groups, but this strategy does not deal with the problem of unmeasured confounding (see Chapter 10). When the findings of randomized and nonrandomized studies of the same research question are compared, the apparent benefits of intervention are often greater in the nonrandomized studies, even after adjusting statistically for differences in baseline variables (19).

Sometimes participants are allocated to study groups by a mechanism that mimics randomization. For example, every participant with an even hospital record number may be assigned to the treatment group. Such designs may offer logistic advantages, but pseudorandomization does not guarantee that the study groups are comparable at baseline, and the predictability of the study group assignment may permit the investigator or the study staff to manipulate the sequence or eligibility of new participants. For example, potential participants who are healthier than average may be enrolled preferentially if it is known that they will be in the active treatment group.

Nonrandomized designs are sometimes chosen in the mistaken belief that they are more ethical than randomization because they allow the participant or clinician to choose the intervention. We believe that studies are only ethical if they have a reasonable likelihood of producing the correct answer to the research question, and nonrandomized studies are less likely to lead to a correct result than randomized designs. Moreover, the ethical basis for any trial is the uncertainty as to whether the intervention will be beneficial or harmful. This uncertainty, termed **equipoise**, means that an evidence-based choice of interventions is not possible and justifies random assignment.

Nonrandomized Within-Group Designs

Before-After Trial Designs

Before-after (or pre-post) trial designs compare an outcome before and after an intervention is applied (Figure 12.6). The before-and-after study design amounts to a single-arm interventional trial with no control. Before-after designs are used widely, especially in studies of the effect of policy, process, and guideline changes, and in clinical quality improvement studies. The main advantages of before-after studies are that they may overcome ethical concerns related to randomized designs and are generally of low cost and simple to conduct (20).

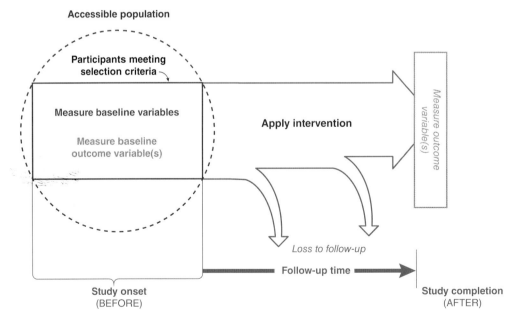

■ **FIGURE 12.6 Before-after trial**. In a before-after trial design, the steps are to:
• Select a sample of participants from an accessible population suitable for receiving the intervention.
• Measure the baseline predictor and outcome variables.
• Apply the intervention to the whole sample.
• Follow the sample over time, minimizing loss to follow-up and assessing adherence to the intervention.
• Measure the outcome after the intervention period.

If the same participants are measured before and after the intervention, each serves as his own control and individual characteristics like age, ethnicity, and genetic factors are not merely balanced (as they are in between-group randomized studies) but eliminated as confounding variables. For example, in a study of the effect of a training program, the ability of senior medical students to accurately interpret ECGs might be compared before and after the intervention. However, many before-after trials examine the outcome in different groups of people. If an intervention is introduced to reduce the incidence of hospital-acquired *Clostridium difficile* infections, the incidence before and after the intervention will likely have been measured among different patients. In this case, comparisons are susceptible to typical confounding variables, such as differences in age and severity of disease.

Causal inference in before-after study designs is also weakened substantially by the potential for temporal effects, **regression to the mean**, and **maturation effects**. Temporal or seasonal changes in disease incidence or clinical care might affect the outcome regardless of the intervention. There may be improvements in outcome over time in before-after studies due to changes in disease reporting, case definitions, and many other changes that are happening concurrent with the intervention. For example, in a study of the effect of introducing a new hand sanitizer to reduce the incidence of hospital-acquired infections, changes in staffing, staff education, increased use of personal protective equipment, or seasonal outbreaks might account for a change in rate of infections.

Changes before and after an intervention might also be due to regression to the mean—the tendency for a measurement to regress (move back) toward its mean value. Most measurements vary over time due to natural biologic variation and lack of precision of the measurement. If the cut point for inclusion in a study is set at the high (or low) end of this variation, subsequent measurements are likely to be closer to the overall mean. For example, if someone's systolic blood pressure varies randomly between 130 and 160 mm Hg, and enrollment in a trial requires that the blood pressure be >150 mm Hg, measurements made after enrollment are likely to be lower than that entry criterion simply due to regression to the mean, regardless of the effects of any intervention. The same problem occurs if an intervention is instituted due to a recent increase in the frequency of an outcome it is designed to prevent. For example, chance variability in rates of hospital-acquired infections may prompt infection control staff to institute an intervention when they observe a high rate of infections. The intervention may appear to be effective when in fact the reduction is due to regression to the mean.

People, staff, and clinicians tend to learn and improve over time (called the **maturation effect**) without any intervention. For example, in an uncontrolled before-after trial of an intervention to slow cognitive decline in patients with Alzheimer's disease, there may be a natural tendency for participants to improve their performance on cognitive function tests through increased familiarity with the tests. Finally, many before-after studies do not continue long enough to determine whether the effect of the intervention is sustainable.

Temporal changes, regression to the mean, and maturation effects can sometimes be minimized by **making several measurements of the outcome before the intervention** to ensure that it is stable. For example, in a before-after trial of a beta-blocker to reduce the frequency of migraine headache, the number of headaches per week might be averaged over several months in a group of patients before the intervention is applied. Another approach to strengthening causal inference is to add a prespecified **falsification test** to demonstrate that the intervention affects the outcome of interest, but not other outcomes that should not change due to the intervention. For example, in a before-after study of a new antiretroviral drug for preexposure prophylaxis to prevent HIV infection, investigators might also measure the incidence of other sexually transmitted diseases (STDs), which should not be affected by antiretrovirals. If there is a similar decrease in the incidence of HIV and other STDs after beginning treatment, it would suggest that the apparent benefit of the drug may have been due to a reduction in risky sexual behavior.

Interrupted Time Series Designs

Interrupted time series designs are similar to before-after designs, except that they require multiple measurements to estimate the preintervention trend (or slope) in the outcome, which is then "interrupted" by the intervention. Multiple postintervention measurements are then used to determine if there was a change in the level (a difference between the observed and predicted outcome level at the first postintervention time point) or trend of the outcome after the introduction of the intervention (Figure 12.7). The assumption is that the preintervention trend would have continued unchanged, except for the intervention (21).

Interrupted time series studies require clear differentiation of the pre- and postintervention periods. They work best with outcomes that change relatively quickly after the intervention. Conventionally, at least three measurements are needed before and after the intervention to calculate the trend in the outcome (more measurements provide more power). This may be hard to achieve in practice.

Like before-after studies, interrupted time series are often used to evaluate the impact of changes in policy, process, or practice when randomized trials are not possible. They have the advantage of accounting for trends in the outcome before the intervention. However, interrupted time series are prone to confounding by changes related to seasonality, data collection or classification methods, disease outbreaks, or other simultaneous changes in policy or practice. Some of these problems can be addressed by adding a control group that is similar to the intervention group, as discussed in the next section.

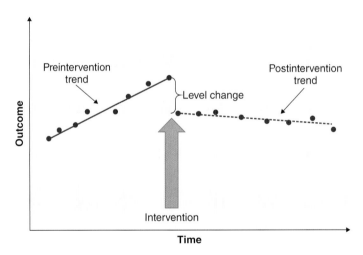

■ **FIGURE 12.7 Interrupted time series**. In an interrupted time series design the outcome is measured multiple times before the intervention to establish the preintervention trend or slope of the outcome (solid line). After the intervention is applied, the outcome is again measured multiple times to identify any abrupt change in the level of the outcome following the intervention (curly bracket) and to establish the postintervention trend of the outcome (dotted line). The intervention is said to "interrupt" the series of outcome measures.

Nonrandomized Within-Group Designs

Both before-after and interrupted time series studies may include a nonrandomized control group. A **controlled before-after study** (sometimes called a before-after study with nonequivalent control group) measures outcomes in two groups of participants concurrently before and after the intervention. Controls should be chosen from populations, regions, or clinics that are similar to the intervention group but did not receive the intervention. The main outcome is the difference in the change in outcomes between the intervention and control groups, often called a **"difference-in-differences"** analysis. If both groups experience the same seasonal, policy, and process changes, it is more plausible that any difference between groups in the outcome is due to the intervention. This design is often feasible if few measurements are required and available from the same sources (such as electronic health records) for both groups. Similarly, controlled interrupted time series designs add a nonrandomized control group, and the outcome is the difference between groups in the change in level or trend of the outcome.

Regression to the mean is still a major problem with controlled before-after studies, especially if the intervention group was selected due to an outbreak or high level of disease that did not occur in the control group. In both of these study designs, lack of randomization can result in differences between the intervention and control groups (such as seasonal, process, or data collection changes) that may confound the effect of the intervention.

■ SUMMARY

Variations on the classic individual-level, randomized, blinded, parallel group trial may be appropriate under the right circumstances:

1. A **factorial randomized trial** design aims to answer two (or more) separate research questions in a single trial by randomizing participants to multiple interventions, allowing the same trial to answer more than one research question. However, effect modification of one intervention by another can reduce the power of the trial, and the populations studied must be appropriate for each intervention.
2. **Noninferiority trials** are sometimes used to compare a new intervention to an established treatment to determine if the efficacy of the two treatments does not differ by more than a predetermined amount that is clinically important. Noninferiority trials may be appropriate when there is an established standard of care, but sample size is typically larger than for trials of a new intervention compared to placebo.
3. **Adaptive designs** that allow for changes to the trial protocol based on interim analyses of the results may be an efficient approach to studying certain interventions. Platform trials that have a single master adaptive trial protocol that allows evaluation of multiple interventions may identify efficacious interventions more quickly and with fewer resources compared to traditional trial designs.
4. In a **crossover design**, some participants are randomly assigned to start with the active intervention while others begin with the control intervention; each group then "crosses over" to the other intervention. Thus, each participant serves as his own control and the increased statistical power from paired analyses requires fewer participants than parallel group trials.
5. In a **wait-list trial**, participants are randomized to receive the intervention at the start of the trial or to a wait-list control group that receives the intervention after a defined period of time. This design has the advantage of making enrollment much more feasible if the intervention is highly desirable and of allowing a randomized comparison in situations where all eligible participants will eventually receive the intervention.
6. **N-of-1 designs** are crossover trials that enroll only one person. Such trials aim to answer clinical questions about effectiveness or adverse effects in an individual patient.
7. In a **cluster randomized trial**, groups, or clusters, of participants are randomly assigned to the interventions rather than individuals. Randomizing an intervention to groups of people may be more feasible and cost-effective than randomizing individuals one at a time.
8. In a **stepped wedge trial**, individuals, clusters, or groups of clusters are randomized to the order in which they begin the intervention. By the end of the trial, all participants will have received the intervention. Stepped wedge designs are most appropriate when political, cultural, or fairness concerns dictate that all members of a group should receive the intervention.
9. **Nonrandomized within-group designs**, which compare the effect of an intervention in groups that have not been randomized, may be appropriate when randomized trials are not possible due to ethical, political, social, or logistic constraints. These designs include:

a. **Before-after designs** in *individuals* measure the level or frequency of an outcome (such as body weight) before and after an intervention is applied to determine if the outcome changes after the intervention. Before-after designs in *populations* measure the frequency of an outcome in a population before and after an intervention.

b. **Interrupted time series designs** require multiple measurements before and after the intervention to estimate a change in the level of the outcome at the time of the introduction of the intervention or a change in the trend (slope) of the outcome after the intervention. In contrast to before-after studies, interrupted time series designs have the advantage of accounting for trends in the outcome before the intervention.

10. **Nonrandomized between-group designs.** Before-after and interrupted time series studies may include a nonrandomized control group. **Controlled before-after** studies measure outcomes in two groups of participants concurrently before and after an intervention. The main outcome is the **difference-in-differences**—the difference in the change over time in outcomes between the intervention and control groups. Including a control group may account for seasonal, policy and process changes and thus strengthen causal inference.

REFERENCES

1. Manson JE, Cook NR, Lee I-M, et al. Vitamin D supplements and prevention of cancer and cardiovascular disease. *N Engl J Med.* 2019;380:33-44.
2. Manson JE, Cook NR, Lee I-M, et al. Marine n–3 fatty acids and prevention of cardiovascular disease and cancer. *N Engl J Med.* 2019;380:23-32.
3. Dumoulin C, Cacciari LP, Hay-Smith EJC. Pelvic floor muscle training versus no treatment, or inactive control treatments, for urinary incontinence in women. *Cochrane Database Syst Rev.* 2018;10(10):CD005654.
4. Dumoulin C, Morin M, Danieli C, et al., for the Urinary Incontinence and Aging Study Group. Group-based vs individual pelvic floor muscle training to treat urinary incontinence in older women: a randomized clinical trial. *JAMA Intern Med.* 2020;180(10):1284-1293.
5. Piaggio G, Elbourne DR, Altman DG, et al. Reporting of non-inferiority and equivalence randomized trials. An extension of the CONSORT Statement. *JAMA.* 2006;295:1152-1160.
6. Piaggio G, Elbourne DR, Pocock SJ, et al. Reporting of non-inferiority and equivalence randomized trials. An extension of the CONSORT 2010 statement. *JAMA.* 2012;308:2594-2604.
7. D'Agostino RB Sr., Massaro JM, Sullivan LM, et al. Non-inferiority trials: design concepts and issues—the encounters of academic consultants in statistics. *Statist Med.* 2003;22:169-186.
8. Kaul S, Diamond GA. Good enough: a primer on the analysis and interpretation of non-inferiority trials. *Ann Intern Med.* 2006;145:62-69.
9. Chang M, Chow S, Pong A. Adaptive design in clinical research: issues, opportunities, and recommendations. *J Biopharm Stat.* 2006;16:299-309.
10. Berry SM, Connor JT, Lewis RJ. The Platform Trial: an efficient strategy for evaluating multiple treatments. *JAMA.* 2015;313:1619-1620.
11. Beigle JH, Tomashek KM, Dodd LE, et al., for the ACTT-1 Study Group Members. Remdesivir for the treatment of Covid-19—final report. *N Engl J Med.* 2020;383:1813-1826.
12. Guyatt G, Sackett D, Taylor DW, et al. Determining optimal therapy—randomized trials in individual patients. *N Engl J Med.* 1986;314:889-892.
13. Walsh M, Hilton J, Masouredis C, et al. Smokeless tobacco cessation intervention for college athletes: results after 1 year. *Am J Public Health.* 1999;89:228-234.
14. Donner A, Birkett N, Buck C, et al. Randomization by cluster: sample size requirements and analysis. *Am J Epidemiol.* 1981;114:906-914.
15. Cook AJ, Delong E, Murray DM, et al. Statistical lessons learned for designing cluster randomized pragmatic clinical trials from the NIH health care systems collaboratory biostatistics and design core. *Clin Trials.* 2016;13:504-512.
16. Hemming K, Haines TP, Chilton PJ, et al. The stepped wedge cluster randomised trial: rationale, design, analysis, and reporting. *BMJ.* 2015;350:h391.
17. Ellenberg SS. The stepped-wedge clinical trial. Evaluation by rolling deployment. *JAMA.* 2018;319:607-608.
18. Gruber JS, Reygadas F, Arnold BF, Ray I, Nelson K, Colford JM. A stepped wedge, cluster-randomized trial of a household UV-disinfection and safe storage drinking water intervention in rural Baja California Sur, Mexico. *Am J Trop Med Hyg.* 2013;89(2):238-245.
19. Chalmers T, Celano P, Sacks H, et al. Bias in treatment assignment in controlled clinical trials. *N Engl J Med.* 1983;309:1358-1361.
20. Sedgwick P. Before and after study designs. *BMJ.* 2014;349:g5074.
21. Bernal JL, Cummings S, Gasparrini A. Interrupted time series regression for the evaluation of public health interventions: a tutorial. *Int J Epidemiol.* 2017;46:348-355.

APPENDIX 12A
Bayesian Clinical Trials

Most clinical trials—such as a study of whether bisphosphonates reduce the risk of hip fracture in persons with Parkinson's disease—are designed to test whether a treatment has a specified effect, such as a 20% reduction in the risk of an outcome, at a given level of statistical significance (alpha). The study's sample size estimate as well as recruitment, follow-up plans, and budgets are made accordingly. When the study is completed, the investigators determine the *P* value for the test statistic comparing the risks of hip fracture in the intervention and control groups to see whether the results reached statistical significance. (If there are interim analyses, alpha can be divided by the number of such analyses or partitioned in another way.) This so-called **frequentist** approach to study design and data analysis is based on how frequently the study results (or ones even more extreme) would have been observed in the sample if the null hypothesis were true in the target population (see Chapter 5). It does not account for any prior information about the effects of bisphosphonates on hip fractures.

In contrast, a **Bayesian approach** (1-3) to the same research question would consider the many previous studies showing that bisphosphonates reduce hip fracture risk in people *without* Parkinson's disease (Table 12A.1). The approach begins by specifying a **prior probability** for each level of treatment efficacy in those *with* Parkinson's disease. As a simplified example, the prior probability might be 0.2 that bisphosphonates are not beneficial (or even harmful); 0.3 that the risk of hip fracture is reduced by up to 20%; and 0.5 that the risk of hip fracture is reduced by 20% or more. (The sum of these proportions must be 1.0.) As hip fractures occur during the study, the observed data would be combined with these prior probabilities to produce new likelihoods, called **posterior probabilities**. A Bayesian approach to clinical trials is analogous to what clinicians do when they combine the pretest probability of a disease with the results of a diagnostic test to determine the posttest probability of that disease (4).

The prior probability of a treatment's efficacy is not a single number—or even a few numbers as in the example earlier. Rather, it is expressed as a **prior distribution**, often a normal (bell-shaped) curve, that estimates the likelihood of efficacy as a continuous variable (Figure 12A.1). A prior distribution is narrow when a great deal is known about a treatment's effects and wide when that evidence is limited. Ideally, the prior distribution is based on the results of previous high-quality studies of similar research questions, but sometimes it must rely on expert opinions and subjective judgments.

How does one determine the prior distribution? Consider, for example, a new treatment that involves a minor modification to an existing drug that reduced the risk of the outcome of interest by about 15% in several well-done trials. In this situation, the new treatment is likely to have a similar effect, which may justify using an **optimistic prior distribution** located on the side of efficacy, say from a 7.5% to a 22.5% benefit. On the other hand, if prior studies of a similar drug were limited, for example, to its effects on biomarkers, a **skeptical prior distribution** centered around zero would be appropriate, with little possibility that the treatment will result in great benefit (or harm). Prior distributions are usually bell-shaped, but **uninformative priors** may be flat (ie, equally distributed at all reasonable levels of benefit and harm) to reflect the absence of information.

Often, the prior distribution obtained from previous study results is modified by mixing it with a skeptical or uninformative prior. The mixing proportion, which is based on expert judgment about the probability that the prior studies apply to the current clinical situation, generates a new prior distribution.

TABLE 12A.1 COMPARISON OF FREQUENTIST AND BAYESIAN APPROACHES TO CLINICAL TRIALS

CONCEPT	FREQUENTIST	BAYESIAN
Result of the trial	Treatment effect, expressed as a point estimate and confidence interval	Posterior distribution for the treatment effect, posterior mean or median treatment effect, credible interval
Consideration of prior evidence	Used subjectively, if at all, to interpret the *P* value	Analysis requires the prior probability distribution of efficacy. Absence of any evidence often implies a flat or skeptical prior (see text).
Statistical significance or sufficient evidence of efficacy	The *P* value for the null hypothesis is less than the prespecified threshold (often 0.05).	High posterior probability of efficacy; this may be more stringent when regulatory approval is sought for a new treatment.
Role of expert clinical opinion about efficacy	None	Sets the distribution of prior probabilities. Often involves specifying the degree to which previous study results are applicable to the current trial
Subjective decisions	Translating a *P* value into likelihood that there is a treatment effect. Specifications required for sample size estimates. Specifications for monitoring data. Choice of analytic model.	Choice of prior probability distribution. Choice of the analytic model.
Sample size	Specified in advance from effect size, alpha, and beta; effect size often a best guess.	May be left unspecified; participants accrued until a certain probability of efficacy (or harm or lack of efficacy) is achieved. Sometimes set by estimating the expected sample size needed for enough evidence.
Budget	Fixed sample size allows a fixed budget.	A fully sequential Bayesian design requires a flexible budget.
Monitoring and stopping rules	Data are analyzed at specified time points. Stopping rules based on *P* values are penalized for the number of interim analyses.	Results may be updated continuously without penalty; new posterior probabilities supersede previous ones.

When it is time to analyze the data, Bayesian trials do not test the statistical significance of a trial's result. Instead, that result is combined with the prior distribution to generate a **posterior distribution**, the range of the treatment's likely effect, often summarized as a **credible interval** or **highest posterior density interval**. For example, a 90% credible interval has a probability of 0.9 that the treatment effect lies within it, assuming the chosen prior distribution is valid. Alternatively, the results can be presented as the probability of a given treatment effect, for example, a probability of 0.94 that the treatment reduces the risk of the outcome by at least 30%, again assuming the selected prior distribution.

A Bayesian approach may lead to a different conclusion than a frequentist one. For example, Brophy (5) reanalyzed the results of a study that had randomly assigned patients with left main coronary artery disease to receive percutaneous coronary intervention (PCI) or coronary artery bypass graft (CABG) surgery. The study found that although the primary outcome (death, myocardial infarction, and stroke within 5 years) was substantially more common in patients receiving PCI than CABG, the 95% confidence interval for the increase in risk (−0.9% to 6.5%)

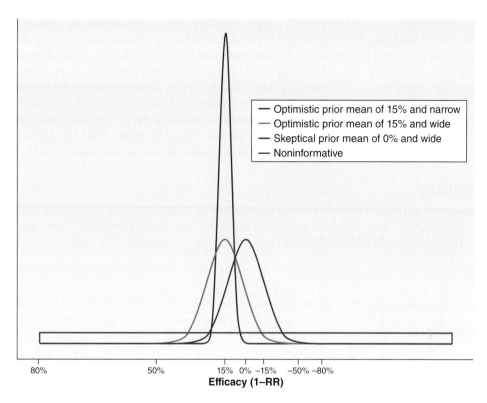

■ **FIGURE 12A.1** Examples of prior distributions. The *X*-axis represents the efficacy of a treatment; the *Y*-axis, the prior probability of a treatment's efficacy, defined as 1 − RR, where RR is the risk ratio comparing treatment with control. The red line shows a narrow prior distribution, centered on an efficacy of 15%; the green line shows a wider prior, centered on the same efficacy of 15%; the blue line shows a skeptical prior, centered on an efficacy of 0%; and the purple line shows a flat, uninformative prior, also centered on 0%. The area under each line equals 1.0.

included zero. Thus, using a frequentist approach, the study concluded that there was not a significant difference in outcomes between PCI and CABG, which conveys little take-home information. In contrast, a Bayesian approach that accounted for the results of previous trials with similar research questions estimated a likelihood of 0.96 that PCI *increased* the risk of the trial end points.

Designing a Bayesian trial differs in several ways from a classic randomized trial. Sample size for a Bayesian trial can sometimes be estimated based on the expected number of participants required to provide enough evidence to generate a "narrow enough" posterior distribution, but it need not be predetermined. Rather, in a sequential approach, as outcomes data are collected, the investigators update the probability that the treatment is efficacious or harmful; because Bayesian approaches do not rely upon *P* values and alpha, this can be done without the need to adjust for multiple looks (6). When that probability exceeds a preset threshold for efficacy, harm, or futility (meaning that the results are unlikely to answer the research question), enrollment may end. Of course, the investigators in a Bayesian trial must specify the prior distribution of treatment efficacy, how they will decide whether to modify it (eg, by mixing with a skeptical prior), as well as if and how they plan to update those decisions during the study.

Not having a fixed sample size (sometimes called a "fully sequential" design) requires a flexible approach to funding, since the sample size and follow-up time may not be known when the study begins. Instead of allocating a fixed budget, a study's funder must accept that it may continue longer, and thus cost more, than was hoped for—though it may also conclude earlier than expected.

In summary, Bayesian trials account for prior data about the efficacy of an intervention when they are designed and analyzed. A Bayesian approach may be appropriate when there is enough previous data to inform the prior distribution. Bayesian trials have the potential advantage of needing a smaller sample size if the observed results are consistent with prior expectations. In addition, presenting the study results as a range of probabilities for a treatment's efficacy may be more informative than a single P value or confidence interval. However, a Bayesian approach relies on subjective judgments about the prior distribution, including how well existing data apply to the target population and treatment. Bayesian trials also require flexibility in budgeting that may not be possible from conventional sources such as the National Institutes of Health (NIH).

REFERENCES

1. Harrell FE, Jr. Introduction to Bayes for Evaluating Treatments. http://hbiostat.org/doc/bayes/course.html
2. Diamond GA, Kaul S. Prior convictions: Bayesian approaches to the analysis and interpretation of clinical megatrials. *J Am Coll Cardiol.* 2004;43(11):1929-1939.
3. Berry DA. Bayesian clinical trials. *Nat Rev Drug Discov.* 2006;5:27-36.
4. Browner WS, Newman TB. Are all significant P values created equal? The analogy between diagnostic tests and clinical research. *JAMA.* 1987;257:2459-2463.
5. Brophy JM. Bayesian interpretation of the EXCEL trial and other randomized clinical trials of left main coronary artery revascularization. *JAMA Intern Med.* 2020;180:986-992.
6. Gelman A, Hill J, Yajima M. Why we (usually) don't have to worry about multiple comparisons. *J Res Educ Effective.* 2012;5:189-211.

APPENDIX 12B
Exercises for Chapter 12. Alternate Interventional Study Designs

1. Finasteride, a 5-alpha reductase inhibitor medication, is one of the only U.S. Food and Drug Administration (FDA)-approved medications for treating male-pattern hair loss. Used daily, the medication is modestly efficacious in promoting hair regrowth, although effects are lost after 6 months if it is discontinued. Another class of medications, statins, has been found to increase hair growth in rodents, through a different biologic pathway than finasteride. Imagine that a start-up company wants to collect evidence of the efficacy of a new topical statin medication (HairStat) for treatment of male pattern baldness. List at least one advantage and one disadvantage of the following approaches to conducting a trial for this purpose.
   a. Randomize men with male-pattern hair loss to use HairStat versus placebo, without offering finasteride to either group.
   b. Conduct a randomized trial of HairStat versus finasteride to compare the efficacy of these treatments.
   c. Randomize men to use HairStat versus placebo, but only recruit men who have previously failed to see a benefit from or tolerate finasteride.
   d. In a factorial trial design, randomly assign men to use (1) both finasteride and HairStat, (2) finasteride and a placebo-HairStat, (3) placebo-finasteride and HairStat, or (4) double placebo.
   e. Conduct a crossover trial in which men are randomized to start taking finasteride and then switched to HairStat after 3 months, or vice versa.

2. You work for a large multi-office company that is interested in decreasing obesity and promoting healthy dietary habits among its employees. A consultant recommends implementing a multicomponent dietary intervention consisting of distribution of nutrition brochures, workplace cafeteria nutrition promotions, educational posters in common areas, and dietary awareness workshops tailored to work-shift hours. You are interested in evaluating whether the intervention increases weight loss among employees who are overweight or obese. What are the potential advantages or disadvantages of the following approaches to implementing and evaluating this intervention?
   a. Randomize individual employees throughout the company to engage in the dietary support intervention versus no intervention and assess changes in their individual weight over 6 months.
   b. Implement the intervention simultaneously across all company offices for 6 months and examine change in employee weight pre- and postintervention.
   c. Conduct a stepped wedge trial in which the dietary intervention is sequentially introduced to all of the offices affiliated with the company in random order over a 6-month period.
   d. Conduct a cluster randomized trial in which different offices affiliated with the company are randomly assigned to implement the dietary support intervention versus no intervention.

CHAPTER 13

Designing Studies of Medical Tests

Thomas B. Newman, Michael A. Kohn, Warren S. Browner, and Mark J. Pletcher

Studies of medical tests, such as those performed to screen for a risk factor, diagnose a disease, or estimate a patient's prognosis, are an important aspect of clinical research. We include with tests risk scores made up of multiple primary measurements. The study designs discussed in this chapter can be used when studying whether, and in whom, a particular test should be performed.

Most designs for studies of medical tests resemble the observational designs in Chapters 8 and 9, with a few important differences. Most important, the goal of most observational studies is to identify statistically significant associations that represent causal effects. In contrast, demonstrating that a test result has a statistically significant association with a particular condition does not establish whether that test would be useful clinically, and for most studies of medical tests, causality is irrelevant. Thus, measures of association, statistical significance, and control of confounding are secondary considerations for these studies, which instead focus on *descriptive* parameters such as **sensitivity**, **specificity**, **receiver operating characteristic (ROC) curves**, and **likelihood ratios** (LRs), along with their associated confidence intervals (CI). Finally, studies of medical tests are almost always done on patients—the term we will use throughout this chapter.

■ DETERMINING WHETHER A TEST IS USEFUL

For a test to be useful it must pass muster on a series of increasingly difficult questions that address its **reproducibility, accuracy, feasibility,** and, most importantly, its **effects on clinical decisions and outcomes** (Table 13.1). Favorable answers to all these questions are necessary to be confident that a test is worth doing. After all, if a test gives very different results depending on who does it or where it is done, it is unlikely to be useful. If the test seldom supplies new information, it is unlikely to affect clinical decisions. Even if it affects decisions, if these decisions do not improve the clinical outcome of patients who were tested at reasonable risk and cost, the test still may not be useful.

If using a test improves the outcomes of tested patients, favorable answers to the other questions can be inferred. However, studies of whether doing a test improves patient outcomes are the most difficult to do. Instead, the potential effects of a new test on outcomes are usually inferred by comparing the accuracy, safety, or costs with those of existing tests. When developing a new diagnostic or prognostic test, it is helpful to consider what decisions it is intended to guide and what aspects of current practice are most in need of improvement. For example, are current tests unreliable, inaccurate, expensive, dangerous, or difficult to perform?

General Issues for Studies of Medical Tests

Before discussing issues specific to the different study designs described in Table 13.1, it is helpful to discuss several issues that apply generally to studying medical tests.

TABLE 13.1 QUESTIONS TO DETERMINE THE USEFULNESS OF A MEDICAL TEST, POSSIBLE DESIGNS TO ANSWER THEM, AND STATISTICS FOR REPORTING RESULTS

QUESTION	POSSIBLE DESIGNS	STATISTICS FOR RESULTS[a]
How reproducible is the test?	Studies of intra- and interobserver and intra- and interlaboratory variability	Proportion agreement, kappa, coefficient of variation, mean and distribution of differences, Bland-Altman plots (avoid correlation coefficient)
How accurate is the test at diagnosing disease?	Cross-sectional, case-control, or test-result-based sampling designs in which the test result is compared with a gold standard	Sensitivity, specificity, positive and negative predictive value, receiver operating characteristic (ROC) curves, and likelihood ratios
How accurate is the test or prediction model at predicting an outcome?	Cohort designs in which the test results are used to estimate the probability of developing an outcome	Risk ratios, hazard ratios, absolute risks, ROC curves, calibration plots, and net benefit calculations
How feasible and affordable is the test?	Prospective or retrospective studies comparing the test to the current standard of care	Mean costs, proportions experiencing adverse effects, proportions willing to undergo the test
How often do test results affect clinical decisions?	Diagnostic yield studies, studies of pre- and post-test clinical decision-making	Proportion abnormal, additional workup done in those testing positive, proportion of tests leading to changes in clinical decisions, cost per abnormal result or per decision change
Does doing the test improve clinical outcome or have adverse effects?	Randomized trials, cohort or case-control studies, or decision or cost-effectiveness analyses in which the predictor variable is receiving the test and the outcomes include morbidity, mortality, or costs related either to the disease or to its treatment	Risk ratios, odds ratios, hazard ratios, absolute risks, numbers needed to treat, rates and ratios of desirable and undesirable outcomes, such as cost or adverse effects per bad outcome prevented

[a]Most statistics in this table should be presented with confidence intervals.

Spectrum of Disease Severity and of Test Results

Because the goal of most studies of medical tests is to draw inferences about populations by making measurements on samples, the way the sample is selected has a major effect on the validity of the inferences. **Spectrum bias** occurs when the spectrum of disease (or nondisease) in the sample differs from that of the patients in the clinical population for which the test is intended. Early in the development of a test, it may be reasonable to investigate whether it can distinguish between patients with clear-cut, late-stage disease and healthy controls; if the answer is no, the investigator can go back to the lab to work on a modification or a different test. Later, however, when the research question addresses the clinical utility of the test, the spectra of both disease and nondisease should be representative of the patients in whom the test will be used. For example, a test that was developed by comparing patients with known pancreatic cancer to healthy controls could later be evaluated on a more difficult but clinically realistic sample, such as consecutive patients with unexplained abdominal pain or weight loss.

Spectrum bias can also occur from an inappropriate spectrum of test results. For example, consider a study of interobserver agreement among radiologists reading mammograms. If they are asked to classify the images as normal or abnormal, their agreement will be much higher if the investigator selects "positive" images that are clearly abnormal and "negative" images that are free of all suspicious abnormalities.

Importance of Blinding

Although many tests, such as those done by automated chemical analyzers, are objective, others, such as physical examinations and radiographs, involve subjective interpretation. Whenever possible, investigators should blind those interpreting subjective tests from other information about the patient being tested. In a study of the contribution of ultrasonography to the diagnosis of appendicitis, for example, those reading the sonograms should not know the results of the history and physical examination.[1] Similarly, although some **gold standards** (to which test results are compared) are objective (such as death), others are subjective, such as the pathologist's determination of who did and did not have appendicitis. When the gold standard is subjective, those applying it should not know the results of the test being evaluated. Blinding testers prevents biases, preconceptions, and information from other sources from affecting the test result; blinding those applying the gold standard prevents the test result from affecting the decision about who did and did not have the outcome.

Sources of Variability

For some research questions, differences among patients are the main source of variation in the results of a test. For example, the proportion of children with appendicitis who have high white blood cell (WBC) counts is not expected to vary much according to which laboratory does the blood count. On the other hand, many test results depend on the person doing the test or the setting in which the test is done. For example, the sensitivity, specificity, and inter-rater reliability of ultrasound for diagnosing appendicitis depend on the skill of the person doing the scan, the readers' skill and experience, and the quality of the equipment. When accuracy may vary from reader to reader or institution to institution, it is helpful to study different readers and institutions to assess the consistency of the results.

Imperfections in the Gold Standard

Some diseases have a gold standard that is generally accepted to indicate the presence or absence of the target disease, such as the pathologic examination of the appendix for appendicitis. Other diseases have gold standards that are defined arbitrarily, such as defining coronary artery disease as at least a 50% obstruction of one or more major coronary arteries as seen with coronary angiography. Still others, such as many rheumatologic diseases, require that a patient have a specified number of signs, symptoms, or laboratory abnormalities. Of course, if a sign, symptom, or laboratory test is part of the gold standard, it will be a good predictor of who has the disease. This is called **incorporation bias** because the test being studied (often called the **index test**) is incorporated into the gold standard. Incorporation bias can be avoided by using a gold standard that does not incorporate the index test; if this is not possible, then rather than investigating how well the index test predicts the gold standard, the investigator can determine how well the test results predict prognosis or response to treatment.

It is also important to consider whether the gold standard is truly gold. If the gold standard is imperfect, it can make a test either look worse than it really is (if in reality the index test outperforms the gold standard (1)) or look better than it really is (if the index test makes the same mistakes as the gold standard) (2).

---

[1]Alternatively, the accuracy of the history and physical examination alone could be compared with the accuracy of history and physical examination plus ultrasound.

Dangers of Overfitting

Tests are developed through research studies that are themselves imperfect. **Overfitting** occurs when the inevitable random variability and noise from sampling or measurement error is over-interpreted by test developers and incorporated into the test algorithm. Overfitting results in a test performing more poorly in reality than in the studies used to develop it and is an important reason to validate the performance of a test in a separate population.

For example, consider a study of 5 women with ovarian cancer and 95 without where a blood test was used to measure levels of 500 different metabolites present in serum. Many of the metabolites will be a bit higher in the women with ovarian cancer by chance alone; and it will almost certainly be possible to identify a very specific pattern of those 500 metabolites that would be present in all 5 women and not present in any of the controls. That pattern, however, would likely be useless as a screening test because it was the result of random variability. Although statistical procedures are useful for evaluating the role of chance, disciplined hypothesis testing often cannot keep up with the iterative process of test development nor overcome severe issues of multiple hypothesis testing.

Overfitting commonly occurs when multivariable models are used to combine multiple types of primary measurements into a test algorithm, as in the example mentioned previously. Overfitting can occur in simple tests as well, such as deciding on a particular cut point for a test (like a serum ferritin level) that has continuous results. When using such a test, it may be tempting for an investigator to look at all the results in those with the outcome (say, iron deficiency anemia) and those without the outcome (other types of anemia), and then select the best *apparent* cut point to define a positive test. However, this is a type of overfitting. Better approaches are to base the cut point on clinical or biologic knowledge from other studies or to divide continuous tests into intervals, then calculate likelihood ratios for each interval (see further). To minimize overfitting, cut points for defining intervals should be specified in advance or be reasonable round numbers. Model validation studies, designed to assess performance independent from model development, are discussed later in this chapter in the section focused on clinical prediction models.

■ STUDIES OF TEST REPRODUCIBILITY

Tests are **reproducible** if (absent a real change in the phenomena being measured) the test results do not vary according to when or where they were done or who did them. *Intraobserver* reproducibility describes the consistency of results when the same observer or laboratory performs the test on the same specimen at different times. For example, if a radiologist is shown the same chest radiograph on two occasions, what percent of the time will he agree with himself on the interpretation, assuming he is unaware of his prior interpretation? *Interobserver* reproducibility describes consistency between two or more observers: If another radiologist is shown the same image, how likely is he to agree with the first radiologist?

Often, the level of reproducibility (or lack thereof) is the main research question. In other cases, reproducibility is studied with the goal of quality improvement, either for clinical care or for a research study. When reproducibility is poor—because either intra- or interobserver variability is large—a measurement is unlikely to be useful, and it may need to be either improved or abandoned. Of course, all observers can agree with one another and still be wrong.

Designs

The basic design to assess test reproducibility involves comparing test results from more than one observer or that were performed on more than one occasion. For tests that involve several steps, differences in any one of which might affect reproducibility, the investigator will need to decide on the breadth of the study's focus. For example, measuring interobserver agreement of pathologists on a set of Pap smear slides in a single laboratory may overestimate the overall reproducibility of Pap smears because of failure to capture the variability in how the sample was obtained and how the slide was prepared.

The extent to which an investigator needs to isolate the steps that might lead to interobserver disagreement depends partly on the goals of his study. Most studies should estimate the reproducibility of the *entire* testing process because this is what determines whether the test is worth using. That said, an investigator who is developing or improving a test may want to focus on the specific steps that are problematic. In either situation, the investigator should lay out the exact process for obtaining the test result in the operations manual (Chapter 18) and then describe it in the methods section when reporting the study results.

Analysis

Categorical Variables

The simplest measure of interobserver agreement is the percent of observations on which the observers agree exactly. However, when the observations are not distributed evenly among the categories (eg, when the proportion that are "abnormal" on a dichotomous test is not close to 50%), the percent agreement can be hard to interpret, because it does not account for agreement that could result simply from both observers having some knowledge about the prevalence of abnormality. For example, if 95% of tests are normal, two observers who randomly choose which 5% of tests to call "abnormal" will agree that results are "normal" about 90% of the time. The percent agreement is also a suboptimal measure when a test has more than two possible results that are intrinsically ordered (eg, normal, borderline, abnormal), because it counts partial disagreement (eg, normal/borderline) the same as complete disagreement (normal/abnormal).

A better measure of interobserver agreement, called **kappa** (see Appendix 13A), measures the extent of agreement beyond what would be expected from the observers' estimates of the prevalence of abnormality[2] and can give credit for partial agreement. Kappa ranges from –1 (perfect disagreement) to 1 (perfect agreement). A kappa of 0 indicates no more agreement than would be expected from the observers' estimates of the prevalence of each level of abnormality. Kappa values above 0.8 are generally considered very good; levels of 0.6 to 0.8 are good.

Continuous Variables

When a study measures the agreement between two machines or methods (eg, paired temperatures on a series of patients obtained from two different thermometers), a simple way to describe the data is to compute the difference between the two measurements (made at close to the same time in the same person) and simply describe those differences (eg, by calculating the mean difference and its standard deviation). Those differences can also be plotted as a function of the mean of the two measurements, a so-called Bland-Altman plot that provides information about how reproducibility (or lack thereof) may be different in different ranges of the measurement (3). Alternatively, investigators can report how often the difference between the two measurements exceeds a clinically relevant threshold. For example, if a clinically important difference in body temperature is 0.3 °C, a study comparing temperatures from no-contact infrared thermometers and electronic axillary thermometers could estimate both the mean and standard deviation of the difference between the two techniques and report how often the two measurements differed by >0.3 °C.[3]

---

[2]Kappa is often described as the extent of agreement beyond that expected by chance, but the estimate of the agreement expected by chance is calculated from the prevalence of abnormality assigned by each observer, as if it were fixed and known to them, which it generally is not.

[3]Although commonly used, the correlation coefficient is best avoided in studies of the reliability of laboratory tests because it is highly influenced by outlying values and does not allow readers to determine how frequently differences between the two measurements are clinically important. Confidence intervals for the mean difference should also be avoided because their dependence on sample size makes them potentially misleading. A narrow confidence interval

Often variability in a measurement increases as the value of the measurement increases. For example, blood pressure may vary by ± 4 mm Hg when it is about 120/80 and ± 6 mm Hg when it is 180/120. This relationship can be seen clearly in a Bland-Altman plot. When this is the case, results can be summarized using the **coefficient of variation (CV)**, the standard deviation of all the results obtained from a single specimen divided by the mean value (Chapter 4). This measure of reproducibility is often used to examine the interassay, interobserver, or interinstrument variability of tests across a large group of different technicians, laboratories, or machines. Often, the CVs of two or more different assays or instruments are compared; the one with the smallest CV is the most precise (though it may not be the most accurate).

■ STUDIES OF THE ACCURACY OF TESTS

Studies in this section address the question, "How often does the test give the right answer?" This assumes, of course, that a gold standard is available to reveal what the right answer is.

Designs

Designs for studies of test accuracy depend on whether the test is *diagnostic* (intended to diagnose disease already present, ie, prevalent disease) or *prognostic* (intended to predict an outcome that has not yet occurred, ie, incident outcomes).[4] A **diagnostic test study** has a cross-sectional time frame and measures how well the test identifies a target condition as determined by an independent gold standard. A prognostic test study has a longitudinal time frame and measures both how well the test separates those who develop the outcome from those who don't (**discrimination**) and how accurately it predicts risk in groups of patients (**calibration**).

Sampling

Most studies of diagnostic test accuracy have designs analogous to case-control or cross-sectional studies. In the case-control design of a diagnostic test study, those with and without the disease are sampled separately, and the test results in the two groups are compared.

As previously noted, case-control sampling may be appropriate early in the development of a diagnostic test, when the research question is whether the test warrants further study, especially if the disease is rare. Later, when the research question relates to the clinical utility of the test, the spectra of disease and nondisease should resemble those of the people to whom the test will be applied clinically, that is, people in whom the diagnosis is not yet known. This is more difficult to achieve with case-control sampling because the cases will already have been diagnosed, and it may be hard to find controls in whom the diagnosis was considered but then ruled out. Studies of tests that use case-control sampling are also subject to bias in the measurement or reporting of the test result, because those performing and/or interpreting the test may already know the diagnosis (a reason for blinding).

As described in Chapter 3, consecutive sampling is a good approach for developing a representative sample. A consecutive sample of patients being evaluated for a particular diagnosis will generally provide representative spectra of both diseased and nondiseased participants. For example, Tokuda et al. (5) found that the degree of chills (eg, feeling cold vs. whole-body shaking under a thick blanket) was a strong predictor of bacteremia in febrile adults in an emergency department (ED). Because the patients were enrolled before it was known whether they were bacteremic, they should be reasonably representative of similar patients who present to EDs with fever.

---

for the mean difference between the two measurements does not imply that they generally closely agree—only that the mean difference between them is being measured precisely. See Bland and Altman (3) or Newman and Kohn (4) for additional discussion of these points.

[4]Another distinction often made between types of tests is between diagnostic and screening tests; the latter are used in people who have no known signs or symptoms of the condition being tested for. To simplify this discussion, our use of "diagnostic tests" will generally include screening tests.

As discussed later (see Section "Differential Verification Bias"), applying an invasive gold standard to people whose index test is negative may not be ethical or feasible. Even when the gold standard is not invasive, however, it may be inefficient to apply it to everyone in the study if negative test results are common. In that situation, analogous to the double-cohort design presented in Chapter 8, those with positive and negative test results can be sampled separately, so-called **test-result-based sampling**. For example, the investigators could apply the gold standard to all patients who test positive, but to only a random sample of those who test negative. Simple algebra can then be used to estimate the test's sensitivity, specificity, and likelihood ratios.

A relatively efficient sampling scheme that we call **tandem testing** is sometimes used to compare two (presumably imperfect) tests with one another. Both tests are done on a representative sample of patients and the gold standard is selectively applied to those with positive results on either or both tests. The gold standard should also be applied to a random sample of patients with concordant negative results, to make sure that they really don't have the disease. This design, which allows the investigator to determine which test is more accurate without the expense of doing the gold standard test in all those with negative results, has been used in studies comparing different cervical cytology methods (6).

Studies of prognostic test accuracy require cohort designs. In a prospective design, the test is done at baseline, and the cohort is then followed to see who develops the outcome of interest. A retrospective cohort or nested case-control design can be used when a new test becomes available, such as serum neurofilament light chain (sNfL) levels as an early sign of multiple sclerosis (7), if a previously defined cohort with banked blood samples is available. Then the sNfL level can be measured in the stored blood to see whether it predicts onset of multiple sclerosis. The **nested case-control design** (Chapter 9) is particularly attractive if the outcome of interest is rare and the test is expensive.

Predictor Variable: The Test Result

Although it is simplest to think of the results of a diagnostic test as being either positive or negative, many tests have categorical, ordinal, or continuous results. In order to take advantage of all available information in the test, investigators should generally report the results of ordinal or continuous tests rather than dichotomizing as "normal or abnormal." Most tests are more indicative of disease if they are very abnormal than if they are slightly abnormal and have a borderline range in which they do not provide much information.

Outcome Variable: The Disease (or Its Outcome)

The outcome variable in a diagnostic test study is the presence or absence of the disease, which is best determined with a gold standard. Wherever possible, the assessment of outcome should not be influenced by the results of the diagnostic test being studied. This is best accomplished by blinding those applying the gold standard so that they do not know the results of the test under study.

Sometimes, particularly with screening tests, uniform application of the gold standard is not ethical or feasible. For example, Smith-Bindman et al. (8) studied the accuracy of mammography. Women with positive mammograms were referred for further tests, eventually with pathologic evaluation of a biopsy specimen as the gold standard to distinguish mammograms that were **true-positives** from those that were **false-positives**. However, it is not reasonable to do breast biopsies in women whose mammograms are negative. Therefore, to determine whether these women had **false-negative** or **true-negative** mammograms, the authors linked the mammography results with local tumor registries to determine whether breast cancer was diagnosed in the year following mammography. This solution assumed that all breast cancers that exist at the time of mammography would be diagnosed within 1 year, and that all cancers diagnosed within 1 year were present at the time of the mammogram. Measuring the gold standard differently depending on the result of the test creates a potential for bias, discussed in more detail at the end of the chapter, but sometimes it is the only feasible option.

The outcome variable in a **prognostic test study** involves what happens to patients with a disease, such as how long they live, what complications they develop, or what additional treatments they require. Again, blinding is important, especially if clinicians caring for the patients may make decisions based upon the prognostic factors being studied.

One problem is that a poor prognosis can become a self-fulfilling prophesy, making a prognostic test appear to be a stronger predictor of outcome than it would otherwise be. For example, Rocker et al. (9) found that attending physicians' estimates of prognosis, but not those of bedside nurses, were associated with intensive care unit mortality. This could be because the attending physicians were more skilled at estimating severity of illness, but it could also be because their prognostic estimates had a greater effect than those of the nurses on decisions to withdraw life support. To distinguish between these possibilities, it would be helpful to obtain estimates of prognosis from attending physicians other than those involved in making or framing decisions about withdrawal of support.

On the other hand, prognostic tests or scores will be less predictive of outcome if their worrisome results lead to treatment decisions that then improve the prognosis. For example, the ability of a positive test for HIV to predict 10-year mortality is much reduced if patients have access to highly effective antiretroviral treatment.

Analysis

Sensitivity, Specificity, Positive and Negative Predictive Values, and Accuracy

The comparison of a dichotomous test with a dichotomous gold standard can be summarized in a 2×2 table (Table 13.2). The **sensitivity** of a test is defined as the proportion of patients *with* the disease in whom the test gives the right answer (ie, is positive); **specificity** is the proportion of patients *without* the disease in whom the test gives the right answer (ie, is negative). If the study sample is representative of the population for which the test is intended, two additional parameters can be calculated. The **positive predictive value** is the proportion of those with positive tests who have the disease, and the **negative predictive value** is the proportion of those with negative tests who don't have the disease.

Another measure that is sometimes used for diagnostic tests is **accuracy**: the overall proportion of the patients in whom the test gave the right answer. As such, accuracy is the average of sensitivity and specificity, weighted by the proportion in the sample with the disease. For this reason, accuracy is not a very helpful statistic: a worthless test can be >99% accurate for a disease with <1% prevalence simply by always having a negative result.

TABLE 13.2 SUMMARIZING RESULTS OF A STUDY OF A DICHOTOMOUS TEST IN A 2 × 2 TABLE

		GOLD STANDARD			
		DISEASE	NO DISEASE	TOTAL	
TEST	**POSITIVE**	a True-positive	b False-positive	a + b	Positive predictive value* = a/(a + b)
	NEGATIVE	c False-negative	d True-negative	c + d	Negative predictive value* = d/(c + d)
	TOTAL	a + c	b + d	a + b + c + d	
		Sensitivity = a/(a + c)	Specificity = d/(b + d)		Accuracy = $\dfrac{a + d}{a + b + c + d}$

*Positive and negative predictive values can be calculated from a 2 × 2 table like this *only* when the prevalence of disease is (a + c)/(a + b + c + d). This will not be the case if those with and without disease are sampled separately (eg, 100 of each in a study with case-control sampling).

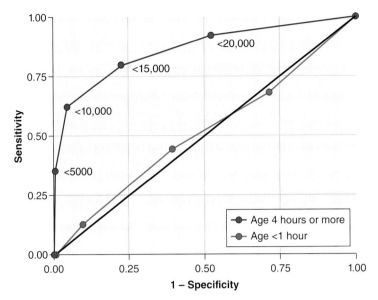

■ **FIGURE 13.1** Receiver operating characteristic curves for the white blood cell count (per μL) as a predictor of infection in newborns (10). Each point represents a different cutoff for calling the test abnormal. At ≥4 hours of age, the test is pretty good, but at <1 hour of age, it is worthless.

Receiver Operating Characteristic Curves

Many diagnostic tests yield ordinal or continuous results. With such tests, several values of sensitivity and specificity are possible, depending on the cut point chosen to define a positive test. This trade-off between sensitivity and specificity can be displayed using a graphic technique originally developed in electronics: **receiver operating characteristic (ROC) curves**. The investigator selects several cut points and determines the sensitivity and specificity at each. He then graphs the sensitivity (or true-positive rate) on the Y-axis as a function of $1 -$ specificity (the false-positive rate) on the X-axis. For example, the upper line in Figure 13.1 shows the cut points (per μL) for considering the WBC count positive as a test for infection in newborns aged ≥4 hours, alongside the corresponding points on the ROC curve. (Lower values of the WBC are more indicative of infection at this age.)

A perfectly accurate test is one that reaches the upper left corner of the graph (100% true-positives and no false-positives). A worthless test follows the diagonal from the lower left to the upper right corners: at any cut point the true-positive rate is the same as the false-positive rate. Figure 13.1 also shows that unlike the situation when performed at ≥4 hours, when performed at <1 hour of age, the WBC count is worthless for predicting infection.

The area under the ROC curve (abbreviated AUROC and also called the C statistic) provides a summary estimate of test **discrimination**—how well the test can discriminate (tell the difference) between people who do and do not have the disease—and can be used to compare two or more tests.[5] The area ranges from 0.5 for a useless test to 1.0 for a perfect test. (If the area is <0.5, it means you need to switch your definition of what direction of results [higher or lower] is more indicative of disease.) The AUROC for the WBC count at age ≥4 hours was 0.86, whereas at age <1 hour, it was 0.51.

---

[5]The AUROC is a good measure of the discrimination of a test only when the slope is monotonically decreasing, that is, the higher (or lower, for tests more abnormal when low) the test result, the more likely the disease. When test results in a middle range are normal and both low and high results can suggest a disease, the AUROC curve is not a good measure of discrimination. For ROC curves with monotonically decreasing slopes, the AUROC can also be used to compare diagnostic tests; the greater the AUROC, the better the test discriminates between those with and without the disease.

Likelihood Ratios

Although the accuracy of a diagnostic test with continuous or ordinal results can be summarized using sensitivity and specificity at a single chosen cut point, there is a better way. **Likelihood ratios** allow the investigator to take advantage of all information in a test. For each test result, the LR is the ratio of the likelihood of that result in someone with the disease to the likelihood of that result in someone without the disease.

$$\text{Likelihood ratio (LR)} = \frac{P(\text{Result}|\text{Disease})}{P(\text{Result}|\text{No Disease})}$$

The *P* is read as "probability of" and the "|" is read as "given." Thus, P(Result|Disease) is the probability of the result given disease, and P(Result|No Disease) is the probability of that result given no disease. The LR is a ratio of these two probabilities.[6] One way to remember it is with the acronym WOWO, which stands for With Over WithOut, as in the probability of a particular result in those *with* disease *over* the probability of that result in those *without* the disease.

If the result is more likely among people with the disease than among people without it, the LR will be greater than one; the higher the LR, the better that test result is for **ruling in** a disease. On the other hand, if the result is less likely among people with disease than among people without it, the LR will be less than one; the lower the LR (the closer it is to 0), the better the test result is for **ruling out** the disease. An LR of 1 means that the test result provides no information at all about the likelihood of disease; LRs close to 1 (say from 0.5 to 2.0) provide little helpful information.

An example of likelihood ratios is shown in Table 13.3, which presents data used to create the upper ROC curve in Figure 13.1. At ≥4 hours of age, a WBC count <5000 cells/µL was much more common among infants with serious infections than among other infants. The calculation of LRs simply quantifies this: about 36% of the infants ≥4 hours old with infections had WBC counts <5000 cells/µL, compared with only 0.44% of those without infections.

TABLE 13.3 CALCULATION OF LIKELIHOOD RATIOS FROM A STUDY OF WHITE BLOOD CELL COUNTS TO PREDICT SERIOUS INFECTIONS IN NEWBORNS (10)

WBC INTERVAL (PER µL)	N WITH INFECTION IN INTERVAL	% OF THOSE WITH INFECTION WITH RESULT IN INTERVAL	N WITH NO INFECTION IN INTERVAL	% OF THOSE WITH NO INFECTION WITH RESULT IN INTERVAL	INTERVAL LR
0 to <5000	32	36	104	0.44	82
5000 to <10,000	24	27	980	4.1	6.5
10,000 to <15,000	16	18	4305	18	1.0
15,000 to <20,000	11	12	7060	30	0.4
≥20,000	7	8	11,376	48	0.2
Total	90	100	23,825	100	

LR, likelihood ratio; WBC, white blood cell count.

---

[6]For dichotomous tests, the likelihood ratio for a *positive* test is $\dfrac{\text{Sensitivity}}{1-\text{Specificity}}$ and the likelihood ratio for a *negative* test is $\dfrac{1-\text{Sensitivity}}{\text{Specificity}}$.

Therefore, the LR for that test result is 36%/0.44% = ~82.[7] (This first LR corresponds to the first line segment on the upper ROC curve of Figure 13.1, which goes from the origin to the <5000 point, where sensitivity was 36% and 1 − specificity was 0.44%. In fact, the slopes of the line segments on the ROC curve correspond to the LRs for intervals defined by the surrounding cut points!)

When tests are used clinically, the LR for the test result can be combined with previous information (the pretest or **prior probability**) using Bayes' theorem to estimate the probability that the patient has the disease taking the test result into account (the post-test or **posterior probability**). The formula for doing this is:

$$\text{Pretest odds} \times \text{LR} = \text{Post-test odds}$$

where odds are related to probability by odds $= \dfrac{P}{1-P}$ and $P = \dfrac{\text{Odds}}{1+\text{Odds}}$. For example, in a newborn whose pretest probability of serious infection was 1% (pretest odds 1%/99% =0.0101), if the WBC were <5000 cells/μL, the post-test odds of infection would be $0.0101 \times 82 = 0.83$ and the post-test probability of infection ($= \dfrac{\text{Odds}}{1+\text{Odds}}$) would be 0.83/1.83 = 0.45 = 45%.

See the text by Newman and Kohn (11) or its website (www.ebd-2.net) for more on calculating and using LRs.

Absolute Risks, Risk Ratios, Risk Differences, and Hazard Ratios

The analysis of studies of prognostic tests is similar to that of other cohort studies. If everyone in a prognostic test study is followed for a set period (say 1 year) with few losses to follow-up, then the results can be analyzed as a simple cohort study with absolute risks, risk ratios, and risk differences. Especially when follow-up is complete and of short duration, results of studies of prognostic tests are sometimes summarized like those of diagnostic tests, using sensitivity, specificity, predictive value, LRs, and ROC curves. On the other hand, when the study participants are followed for varying lengths of time, a survival-analysis technique that accounts for the length of follow-up time and estimates hazard ratios is preferable.

Calibration

For prognostic tests, which aim to inform decisions by estimating the probability that an outcome will occur within a defined period, the test must have more than good discrimination (ie, have different results for people who do and do not subsequently develop the outcome, as measured by the AUROC). It must also have good calibration: the predicted probability of an outcome should be close to the true probability. Quantifying calibration requires that the study sample be divided into groups (say, deciles) with similar predicted probabilities of the event. Predicted probabilities in each decile are then compared with the proportion of individuals in that decile who experienced the event. Results are typically summarized in a **calibration plot**, in which observed probabilities are plotted as a function of predicted probabilities; if deciles are used, such a plot will have 10 points. Perfect calibration would lead to plots along the diagonal (with slope = 1). See Newman and Kohn for a review of additional measures of calibration, including the mean bias, the mean absolute error, the Brier Score, and net benefit calculations (12).

---

[7]To get the exact LR you could calculate 32/90/(104/23,825) = 81.453. We rounded up because we thought more people trying to understand the calculation would just divide the percentages: 36%/0.44% = 81.8.

■ STUDIES TO CREATE CLINICAL PREDICTION MODELS

Developing Prediction Models

Studies to create **clinical prediction models** have the goal of improving clinical decisions by using mathematical methods to develop a new (composite) test that combines multiple types of primary measurements into a test algorithm. The proliferation of clinical prediction models (many overly optimistic) has led to guidelines for reporting their results (13) and assessing them for risk of bias (14); and the U.S. Food and Drug Administration (FDA) has started regulating them under a "Software as a Medical Device" paradigm (15). Investigators considering such studies should consult these guidelines, in addition to the brief discussion below.

Patients for these studies should be similar to those in whom the model will be applied. A clinical prediction model, and any "rules" that result from the model, is likely to be most helpful when intended to guide a specific decision, such as whether to start treatment with statins (for which the American College of Cardiology/American Heart Association risk prediction tool (16) is often used). Therefore, models should be studied in patients similar to those in whom a specific clinical decision needs to be made, including those in whom that decision is currently difficult or uncertain (17). Models developed using data from multiple centers are more likely to be generalizable.

Mathematical methods for creating prediction rules generally involve a multivariable technique for selecting candidate predictor variables and combining their values to generate a prediction. The candidate variables should include known and plausible predictor variables that can be easily, reliably, and inexpensively measured. A multivariable model, such as logistic regression or the Cox (proportional hazards) model, can quantify the independent contribution of candidate predictor variables for predicting the outcome. Those most consistently available and strongly associated with outcome can be included in the model. For example, Puopolo et al. (18) used a logistic regression model to create a prediction score for early-onset neonatal sepsis using data available from the mother's electronic medical record at the time of birth. This prior probability of infection can then be combined with objective newborn clinical findings for a revised estimate of the probability of infection that can guide treatment decisions (19, 20).

Recursive partitioning, or classification and regression tree (CART) analysis, is an alternative technique that can generate rules of high sensitivity without requiring an underlying model. The technique creates a tree that asks a series of yes/no questions, taking the user down different branches depending on the answers. At the end of each branch will be an estimated probability of the outcome. The tree can be designed to have high sensitivity by instructing the software to make the penalty for false-negatives higher than that for false-positives. For example, a study of infants <60 days old from the Pediatric Emergency Care Applied Research Network (PECARN) (21) used a penalty ratio of 100:1 for false-negatives compared with false-positives to create a prediction rule to identify those at very low risk of serious bacterial infection (Figure 13.2).

Both multivariable models and recursive partitioning have the advantage of transparency. The user can look at the model or tree and see what variables contributed to a particular person's probability estimate. There are several machine learning techniques for prediction that do not share this feature, including random forests and neural networks (22). These "black box" methods are evaluated based on discrimination and calibration, just as more transparent methods are. However, their opacity may make it harder to detect biases such as those caused by structural racism in the data-generating process (23). Users of these methods must decide whether any improvement in predictive performance attained through the use of these methods offsets the inability to understand how they arrive at their predictions and the potential biases to which they are susceptible.

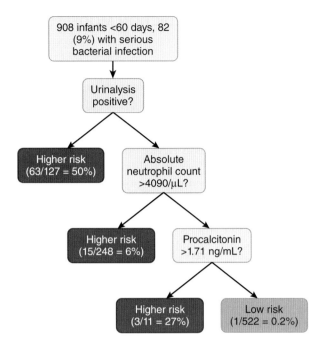

■ **FIGURE 13.2** Example of a classification and regression tree to identify febrile infants <60 days old at low risk of serious bacterial infections. Light blue boxes with questions divide infants into those at higher risk of bacterial infection (red boxes) and those at low risk (green box); the numbers show the proportions with "serious bacterial infections" in the red and green "terminal branches" of the tree. Data from Kuppermann N, Dayan PS, Levine DA, et al. A clinical prediction rule to identify febrile infants 60 days and younger at low risk for serious bacterial infections. *JAMA Pediatr.* 2019;173(4):342-351.

Model Validation

Regardless of the method chosen to develop the prediction model, it must be validated in a group of patients different from those in whom it was derived. This avoids the overly optimistic estimates of model performance resulting from **overfitting**, which, as previously discussed, involves overinterpretation of random variability in a sample (24). The classification tree from the PECARN study in Figure 13.2 illustrates this: the specific cut points selected for absolute neutrophil count (4090/μL) and procalcitonin (1.71 ng/mL) were presumably identified by the recursive partitioning software because rounder numbers for the cut points did not perform quite as well.

Split sample validation, the simplest method, allows estimation of the degree of overfitting by randomly dividing the cohort into **derivation** (typically 50% to 67% of the sample) and **validation data sets**, and testing the rule derived from the derivation cohort on the validation cohort. In the PECARN study, the clinical prediction rule was validated in a separate 50% sample. Impressively, performance in the validation set was only a little worse than in the derivation set: sensitivity declined from 98.8% to 97.7% and specificity from 63.1% to 60.0%.

Split sample validation sacrifices some sample size to preserve a separate validation set. In contrast, **K-fold cross validation** efficiently uses all observations in the sample both for model derivation and for validation. The study sample is divided into k groups and a *process* (eg, stepwise logistic regression) is used to select variables and derive the best model on $k - 1$ of these groups and test it on the remaining group. This is repeated k times. For example, one might randomly divide the sample of 1000 patients into 5 groups of 200. For each of the 5 groups, you would derive the model using the *other* 4 groups and generate predicted values for the left out group (for a total of 5 rounds of derivation and testing). The final model is obtained using the process on the full data set, but the AUROC and other estimates of model performance are based on the predicted and observed values in the k different left out groups, which together make up the full sample. These estimates of model performance should be more realistic than the overly optimistic estimates that would be produced from the entire sample.

Both split sample and K-fold cross validation should be considered **internal validation** because they validate estimates of model performance using the same overall study sample (25). To address external validity, it is also important to determine how well the rule performs at different times, in different settings, or in different populations ("prospective or external validation"). Many clinical prediction models fail at this stage.

■ STUDIES OF THE EFFECT OF TEST RESULTS ON CLINICAL DECISIONS

A test may be accurate, but if the disease is very rare, the test may be so seldom positive that it is hardly ever worth doing. Other tests may not affect clinical decisions because they do not provide new information beyond what was already known (eg, from the medical history and physical examination). The study designs in this section address the **yield** of diagnostic tests and their **effects on clinical decisions**.

Diagnostic Yield Studies

Diagnostic yield studies address such questions as:

- When a test is ordered for a particular indication, how often is it abnormal?
- Can abnormal results be predicted from other information available at the time of testing?
- Do abnormal test results lead clinicians to make different decisions about further evaluation or treatment?

Diagnostic yield studies estimate the proportion of positive tests among patients with an indication for the test. Showing that a test is often positive is not enough to indicate the test should be done. In fact, it might suggest the opposite! For example, Tarnoki et al. (26) performed whole-body magnetic resonance imaging (MRI) scans on 22 healthy adult volunteers (18 men, age 47 ± 9 years, "mainly managers, lawyers, accountants, chief executive officers, [and] company directors"). They reported, "Incidental findings would have needed diagnostic workup at a urologist (17 lesions), rheumatologist (15 lesions), internist (13 lesions), otorhinolaryngologist (6 lesions), pulmonologist (6 lesions), surgeon (5 lesions), gynecologist (4 lesions), and dermatologist (1 lesion)." This is quite a yield: a total of 67 lesions requiring further evaluation, an average of >3 per (presumably well-insured) patient.

On the other hand, a diagnostic yield study showing a test is almost always negative may be sufficient to question its use for that indication. For example, Siegel et al. (27) studied the yield of stool cultures in hospitalized patients with diarrhea. Although not all patients with diarrhea receive stool cultures, it seems reasonable to assume that those who do are, if anything, more likely to have a positive culture than those who do not. Overall, only 40 (2%) of 1964 stool cultures were positive and none of those were obtained in the 997 patients who were tested after being in the hospital for >3 days. The authors concluded that stool cultures are of little value among patients with diarrhea who have been in the hospital for >3 days, because a negative stool culture is unlikely to affect their management. More recently, the low yield of identified stool pathogens in patients hospitalized for ≥3 days was confirmed using a molecular diagnostic test for 22 gastrointestinal pathogens (28).

Before/After Studies of Clinical Decision-Making

These designs directly address the effect of a test result on clinical decisions. The design generally involves a comparison between what clinicians do (or say they would do) before and after obtaining the results of a diagnostic test. For example, Lam et al. (29) prospectively studied the effect of point-of-care ultrasound (POCUS) on treatment decisions in 209 pediatric emergency department patients with skin and soft-tissue infections. They found that POCUS changed the initial treatment plan in almost one-quarter of the patients.

Of course (as discussed later), altering a clinical decision does not guarantee that a patient will benefit, and some altered decisions could be harmful. Studies that demonstrate effects on decisions are most useful when the natural history of the disease and the efficacy of treatment are clear or when outcome data are available. In the study just described, the investigators compared outcomes of the children who received POCUS with those of 90 children with similar lesions and comorbidities who did not receive POCUS. They found no differences in treatment failures within 7 days or in any other outcome (29).

■ STUDIES OF FEASIBILITY, COSTS, AND RISKS OF TESTS

Another important area for clinical research relates to the practicalities of diagnostic testing. For example, if you mail patients a fecal occult blood test kit, what proportion will return it with a valid stool sample? What additional tests are done to follow-up abnormal low-dose computed tomography (CT) scans for lung cancer screening, and how often do they lead to complications? How do false-positive fetal ultrasound scans affect the fetus's mother? What proportion of colonoscopies are complicated by colonic perforation?

Designs

Studies of the feasibility, costs, and (short-term) risks of tests are generally *descriptive*: the goal is to estimate how often something happens and how bad it is, not so much whether the test caused it. The sampling scheme is important because tests often vary among the people or institutions doing them and among the patients receiving them.

A straightforward choice is to study everyone who receives the test, as in a study of home fecal occult blood test kits. Alternatively, for some questions, the study may only include those with positive or falsely positive results. For example, Viaux-Savelon et al. (30) studied 19 mothers of infants who had false-positive "soft markers" on fetal ultrasound scans—findings like echogenic bowel or nuchal translucency that may increase the risk for severe abnormalities, but usually turn out to be false alarms. They found much higher risks of clinically significant anxiety and depression among women with the false-positive scans compared with a matched control group, even 2 months after the birth of a healthy baby.

Adverse effects can occur not just from false-positive results but also from the testing itself. For example, Thulin et al. (31) studied the risks of perforation from 593,308 colonoscopies performed in Sweden. The found that the risk of perforation varied about 14-fold across counties, from ~2 to ~28 per 10,000 colonoscopies.

Adverse effects are sometimes delayed (eg, cancer from radiologic tests), in which case the link between testing and the outcome may not be obvious and considerations discussed in the following section (Studies of the Effect of Testing on Outcomes) apply.

Analysis

Results of these studies can usually be summarized with simple descriptive statistics like means and standard deviations, medians, ranges, and frequency distributions. Dichotomous variables, such as the occurrence of adverse effects, can be summarized with proportions and their 95% CIs. For example, in the aforementioned Swedish colonoscopy study, the lowest perforation risk was 3/15,908 (2 per 10,000; 95% CI: 0.4 to 6 per 10,000) and the highest was 37/13,732 (28 per 10,000; 95% CI: 19 to 38 per 10,000).[8]

---

[8]The authors did not calculate these CIs, but they provided numerators and denominators, so we were easily able to do so. There's a calculator for CIs for proportions at sample-size.net.

■ STUDIES OF THE EFFECT OF TESTING ON OUTCOMES

The best way to determine the value of a medical test is to see whether patients who are tested have a better clinical outcome (eg, live longer or with better quality of life) than those who are not. Randomized trials are the ideal design for making this determination, but trials of diagnostic tests are often difficult to do. The value of tests is therefore usually estimated from observational studies. It is sometimes useful to conduct a formal decision analysis (or cost-effectiveness analysis if cost is an issue), which allows investigators to combine information from different sources (eg, different kinds of observational studies) to project the net impact on outcomes and weigh potential trade-offs. In any case, the key difference between the designs described in this section and the designs discussed elsewhere in this book is that the predictor variable for this section is *performing* the test, rather than a treatment, risk factor, or the result of a test.

Choice of Outcome

Testing itself is unlikely to have any direct benefit on the patient's health. It is only when a test result leads to effective preventive or therapeutic interventions that the patient may benefit (32). Therefore, one important caveat about outcome studies of testing is that the predictor variable actually being studied is not just a test (eg, a fecal occult blood test), but also all of the medical care that follows (eg, colonoscopy, surgery).

The outcome variables for these studies should include a measure of morbidity or mortality, not just a diagnosis or stage of disease. For example, showing that men who are screened for prostate cancer have a greater proportion of cancers diagnosed at an early stage does not establish the value of screening: many of those so-called cancers would not have caused any problem if they had not been detected, a problem called **overdiagnosis** (33, 34).

The outcomes measured should also include plausible adverse effects of testing and treatment, such as psychological as well as medical effects of testing. For example, a study of the value of prostate-specific antigen screening for prostate cancer should include treatment-related impotence or incontinence in addition to cancer-related morbidity and mortality. When many more people are tested than are expected to benefit (as is usually the case), even minor adverse outcomes among those without the disease may be important, because they occur frequently. Although negative test results may be reassuring and comforting to some patients (35), in others the psychological effects of labeling or false-positive results, loss of insurance, and troublesome (but nonfatal) side effects of preventive medications or surgery may outweigh infrequent benefits (33).

Observational Studies

Observational studies are generally quicker, easier, and less costly than clinical trials. However, they have important disadvantages, especially because patients who are tested tend to differ from those who were not tested in important ways that may be related to the risk of a disease or its prognosis. For example, those getting the test could be at relatively *low* risk of an adverse health outcome, because people who volunteer for medical tests and treatments tend to be healthier than average. On the other hand, those tested may be at relatively *high* risk, because patients are more likely to be tested when there are indications that lead them or their clinicians to be concerned about a disease, an example of **confounding by indication** for the test (Chapter 10).

An additional problem with observational studies of testing is the changes in care that follow positive results may be poorly standardized and documented. If a test does not improve outcomes in a particular setting, it could be because follow-up of abnormal results was poor, because patients were not compliant with the planned intervention, or because the intervention used in the study was applied by people not very good at it.

As discussed in Chapter 10, it is helpful to consider a target clinical trial when designing and evaluating an observational study of testing. In such a trial, outcomes are measured from the time of testing (or not testing, in the comparison group) and all patients are followed, not just those diagnosed with disease.

Clinical Trials

The most rigorous design for assessing the benefit of a diagnostic test is a clinical trial, in which patients are randomly assigned to receive or not to receive the test, the result of which is used to guide subsequent management. A variety of outcomes can be measured and compared in the two groups. Randomized trials minimize or eliminate confounding and selection bias and standardizing the testing and intervention process enables others to reproduce the results.

Unfortunately, randomized trials of diagnostic tests are often not practical, especially for tests already in use. They are generally more feasible and important for tests that might be used in large numbers of apparently healthy people, such as new screening tests.

Randomized trials may bring up ethical issues about withholding potentially valuable tests. Rather than randomly assigning patients to undergo a test or not, one approach to minimizing this ethical concern is to randomly assign some patients to receive an intervention that increases the use of the test, such as frequent postcard reminders and assistance in scheduling. The primary analysis must still follow the "intention-to-treat" rule—that is, the entire group that was randomized to receive the intervention to encourage testing must be compared with the entire control group. However, this rule will tend to create a conservative bias; the observed efficacy of the test-facilitating intervention will underestimate the actual efficacy of the test, because some of those in the control group will get the test and some in the intervention group will not.[9]

Analysis

Analyses of studies of the effect of testing on outcome are those appropriate to the specific design used—odds ratios for case-control studies, and risk ratios or hazard ratios and risk differences for cohort studies or clinical trials. A convenient way to express the results of cohort studies or randomized trials is to project the results of the testing procedure to a large group of people and list the number of initial tests, follow-up tests, people treated, side effects of treatment, costs, and deaths in tested and untested groups (in a cohort study) or treatment arms (in a randomized trial), say per 1000 patients.

Decision Analysis

An alternative approach to estimating the effect of using a test on outcomes is decision analysis, whereby an investigator can model the downstream impact of a test (36). Decision analysis models typically combine results from multiple sources of information, along with assumptions that may be more or less evidence-based, to simulate the results of a randomized trial. Cost-benefit models and cost-effectiveness models incorporate cost information and produce estimates of value (eg, cost per unit improvement in health). For example, when investigators compared the potential benefits of measuring coronary calcium to improve targeting of statin therapy against direct harms of testing, indirect harm from unnecessary follow-up testing, and costs, they found coronary calcium screening would be cost effective only if statin therapy were expensive or significantly reduced quality of life (37).

---

[9]This problem can be addressed in secondary analyses that include testing rates in both groups and assume all the difference in outcomes between the two groups is due to different rates of testing. The actual benefits of testing as a result of the intervention can then be estimated algebraically using instrumental variable methods, where the instrument is random allocation to the intervention designed to encourage testing.

■ PITFALLS IN THE DESIGN OR ANALYSIS OF DIAGNOSTIC TEST STUDIES

As with other types of clinical research, compromises in the design of studies of diagnostic tests may threaten the validity of the results, and errors in analysis may hinder their interpretation. Some of the most common and serious of these, along with steps to avoid them, are outlined in this section.

Inadequate Sample Size

When the disease or outcome is rare, a very large number of people may be needed to study a test. Many laboratory tests, for example, are not expensive, and a yield of 1% or less might justify doing them, especially if they can diagnose a serious treatable illness. For example, Sheline and Kehr (38) reviewed routine admission laboratory tests, including the Venereal Disease Research Laboratory (VDRL) test for syphilis, among 252 psychiatric patients and found that the laboratory tests identified one patient with previously unsuspected syphilis. If this patient's psychiatric symptoms were indeed due to syphilis, it would be hard to argue that it was not worth the $3186 spent on VDRLs to make this diagnosis. But if the true rate of unsuspected syphilis were close to the 0.4% seen in this study, a study of this sample size could easily have found no cases.

Inappropriate Exclusion

When calculating proportions, it is inappropriate to exclude patients from the numerator without excluding similar patients from the denominator. For example, in a study of routine laboratory tests in emergency department patients with new seizures (39), 11 (8%) of 136 patients had a correctable laboratory abnormality (eg, hypoglycemia) as a cause for their seizure. In 9 of the 11 patients, however, the abnormality was suspected based on the history or physical examination. The authors therefore reported that only 2 (1.5%) of the 136 patients had unsuspected abnormalities. But if all patients with suspected abnormalities are excluded from the numerator, then similar patients should have been excluded from the denominator as well.

Dropping Borderline or Uninterpretable Results

Sometimes a test may fail to give any answer at all, such as if the assay failed, the test specimen deteriorated, or the test result fell into a gray zone of being neither positive nor negative. These problems should not be ignored, but how to handle them depends on the specific research question and study design. In studies dealing with the expense or inconvenience of tests, failed attempts to do the test are clearly important results. Patients with "nondiagnostic" imaging studies or a borderline result on a test need to be counted as having had that specific result on the test, changing a dichotomous test (positive, negative) to an ordinal one—positive, indeterminate, and negative. ROC curves can then be drawn and LRs can be calculated for "indeterminate" as well as positive and negative results.

Partial Verification Bias: Selective Application of a Single Gold Standard

A common sampling strategy for studies of medical tests is to study *only* patients who are tested for a disease who *also* receive the gold standard for diagnosis. However, this causes a problem if the test being studied is used to decide who gets the gold standard. For example, consider a study of the accuracy of a urinalysis (UA) as a test for urinary tract infection, defined by a positive urine culture, among children with painful urination. If those with a positive UA were more likely to get a urine culture, patients with a negative UA will be underrepresented in the study. This will lead to fewer false-negatives (thus increasing sensitivity) as well as fewer true-negatives (thus decreasing specificity). **Partial verification bias** can be avoided by using strict criteria for application of the gold standard that do not include the test or finding being studied. If this is not practical, it is possible to estimate and correct for partial verification bias using test-result-based sampling, applying the gold standard to all who test positive and to a random sample of those who test negative.

Differential Verification Bias: Different Gold Standards for Those Testing Positive and Negative

It is not difficult to do urine cultures on everyone who has a UA, but if the gold standard is something more costly or invasive than a urine culture, it may not be feasible or ethical to do it on people whose index test is negative. We previously mentioned this issue in the section on outcome variables for studies of diagnostic test accuracy, when we noted that although a biopsy for breast cancer is appropriate in those with positive mammograms, it would be inappropriate to apply that gold standard to people with negative mammograms. Instead, diagnosis of breast cancer in the following year was used as the gold standard for those with negative mammograms (8).

However, this can cause **differential verification bias**, also called double gold standard bias (2, 40). This bias can occur any time the gold standard among those with positive results differs from the gold standard for those with negative test results (assuming that the two gold standards do not always give the same answer). For example, let us suppose Overdiagnosed Olga has a breast lesion that would be diagnosed as breast cancer if she had a biopsy but would never cause a problem if she did not. If Olga's mammogram is positive, she will get a biopsy, it will be positive, and it will appear that the mammogram got the right answer. If Olga's mammogram is negative, she won't be diagnosed with breast cancer in the next year, her follow-up will be negative, and, once again, it will appear that the mammogram got the right answer. For spontaneously resolving or extremely indolent lesions, if the mammogram guides the gold standard selection, it can never be wrong!

Differential verification bias can be avoided by applying the same gold standard to everyone or by using test-result-based sampling and applying the gold standard to a random sample of those who test negative. When neither of these designs is feasible, investigators should make every effort to estimate the likelihood and significance of overdiagnosis and spontaneously resolving disease. For example, overdiagnosis is suggested by temporal trends showing an increase in diagnoses but no change in mortality from a disease (41) or autopsy studies reporting a high prevalence of previously undiagnosed and asymptomatic pathology (42).

■ SUMMARY

1. The usefulness of medical tests can be assessed using designs that address a series of increasingly stringent questions (Table 13.1).
2. A diagnostic test should be studied in patients who have a spectrum of disease and non-disease appropriate for the research question, reflecting the anticipated use of the test in clinical practice.
3. If possible, the investigator should blind those interpreting the test results and determining the gold standard from other information about the patients being tested.
4. Measuring the reproducibility of a test, including the intra- and interobserver variability, is often a good first step in evaluating a test.
5. Studies of the accuracy of tests require a gold standard for determining if a patient has, or does not have, the disease or outcome being studied.
6. The results of studies of the accuracy of diagnostic tests can be summarized using sensitivity, specificity, predictive value, ROC curves, and LRs and their CIs.
7. Results of studies of prognostic tests can be summarized with risk ratios, hazard ratios, and risk differences and their CIs, as well as ROC curves and calibration plots.
8. Studies to develop new clinical prediction models are subject to problems of overfitting and lack of generalizability, requiring that new rules be validated in separate samples.

9. The most rigorous design for studying the utility of a diagnostic test is a clinical trial, with participants randomized to receive the test or not, and with mortality, morbidity, cost, and quality of life among the outcomes.

10. If trials are not ethical or feasible, observational studies and decision- and cost-effectiveness analyses of benefits, harms, and costs, with appropriate attention to possible biases, can be helpful.

REFERENCES

1. Limmathurotsakul D, Turner EL, Wuthiekanun V, et al. Fool's gold: why imperfect reference tests are undermining the evaluation of novel diagnostics: a reevaluation of 5 diagnostic tests for leptospirosis. *Clin Infect Dis.* 2012;55(3):322-331.

2. Newman T, Kohn M. *Evidence-Based Diagnosis: An Introduction to Clinical Epidemiology.* 2nd ed. Cambridge University Press; 2020:89-91.

3. Bland JM, Altman DG. Statistical methods for assessing agreement between two methods of clinical measurement. *Lancet.* 1986;1(8476):307-310.

4. Newman T, Kohn M. *Evidence-Based Diagnosis: An Introduction to Clinical Epidemiology.* 2nd ed. Cambridge University Press; 2020:110-137.

5. Tokuda Y, Miyasato H, Stein GH, Kishaba T. The degree of chills for risk of bacteremia in acute febrile illness. *Am J Med.* 2005;118(12):1417.

6. Sawaya GF, Washington AE. Cervical cancer screening: which techniques should be used and why? *Clin Obstet Gynecol.* 1999;42(4):922-938.

7. Bjornevik K, Munger KL, Cortese M, et al. Serum neurofilament light chain levels in patients with presymptomatic multiple sclerosis. *JAMA Neurol.* 2020;77(1):58-64.

8. Smith-Bindman R, Chu P, Miglioretti DL, et al. Physician predictors of mammographic accuracy. *J Natl Cancer Inst.* 2005;97(5):358-367.

9. Rocker G, Cook D, Sjokvist P, et al. Clinician predictions of intensive care unit mortality. *Crit Care Med.* 2004;32(5):1149-1154.

10. Newman TB, Puopolo KM, Wi S, Draper D, Escobar GJ. Interpreting complete blood counts soon after birth in newborns at risk for sepsis. *Pediatrics.* 2010;126(5):903-909.

11. Newman T, Kohn M. *Evidence-Based Diagnosis: An Introduction to Clinical Epidemiology.* 2nd ed. Cambridge University Press; 2020:16-22.

12. Newman T, Kohn M. *Evidence-Based Diagnosis: An Introduction to Clinical Epidemiology.* 2nd ed. Cambridge University Press; 2020:144-167.

13. Moons KG, Altman DG, Reitsma JB, et al. Transparent reporting of a multivariable prediction model for Individual Prognosis or Diagnosis (TRIPOD): explanation and elaboration. *Ann Intern Med.* 2015;162(1):W1-W73.

14. Moons KGM, Wolff RF, Riley RD, et al. PROBAST: a tool to assess risk of bias and applicability of prediction model studies: explanation and elaboration. *Ann Intern Med.* 2019;170(1):W1-W33.

15. Food and Drug Administration. *Software as a Medical Device* (SaMD). https://www.fda.gov/medical-devices/digital-health-center-excellence/software-medical-device-samd

16. Goff DC Jr, Lloyd-Jones DM, Bennett G, et al. 2013 ACC/AHA guideline on the assessment of cardiovascular risk: a report of the American College of Cardiology/American Heart Association Task Force on Practice Guidelines. *Circulation.* 2014;129(25 Suppl 2):S49-S73.

17. Grady D, Berkowitz SA. Why is a good clinical prediction rule so hard to find? *Arch Intern Med.* 2011;171(19):1701-1702.

18. Puopolo KM, Draper D, Wi S, et al. Estimating the probability of neonatal early-onset infection on the basis of maternal risk factors. *Pediatrics.* 2011;128(5):e1155-e1163.

19. Escobar GJ, Puopolo KM, Wi S, et al. Stratification of risk of early-onset sepsis in newborns ≥34 weeks' gestation. *Pediatrics.* 2014;133(1):30-36.

20. Kuzniewicz MW, Walsh EM, Li S, Fischer A, Escobar GJ. Development and implementation of an early-onset sepsis calculator to guide antibiotic management in late preterm and term neonates. *Jt Comm J Qual Patient Saf.* 2016;42(5):232-239.

21. Kuppermann N, Dayan PS, Levine DA, et al. A clinical prediction rule to identify febrile infants 60 days and younger at low risk for serious bacterial infections. *JAMA Pediatr.* 2019;173(4):342-351.

22. Newman T, Kohn M. *Evidence-Based Diagnosis: An Introduction to Clinical Epidemiology.* 2nd ed. Cambridge University Press; 2020:175-200.

23. Robinson WR, Renson A, Naimi AI. Teaching yourself about structural racism will improve your machine learning. *Biostatistics.* 2020;21(2):339-344.

24. Steyerberg EW, Bleeker SE, Moll HA, Grobbee DE, Moons KG. Internal and external validation of predictive models: a simulation study of bias and precision in small samples. *J Clin Epidemiol*. 2003;56(5):441-447.

25. Steyerberg EW, Harrell FE Jr. Prediction models need appropriate internal, internal-external, and external validation. *J Clin Epidemiol*. 2016;69:245-247.

26. Tarnoki DL, Tarnoki AD, Richter A, Karlinger K, Berczi V, Pickuth D. Clinical value of whole-body magnetic resonance imaging in health screening of general adult population. *Radiol Oncol*. 2015;49(1):10-16.

27. Siegel DL, Edelstein PH, Nachamkin I. Inappropriate testing for diarrheal diseases in the hospital. *JAMA*. 1990;263(7):979-982.

28. Hitchcock MM, Gomez CA, Banaei N. Low yield of FilmArray GI panel in hospitalized patients with diarrhea: an opportunity for diagnostic stewardship intervention. *J Clin Microbiol*. 2018;56(3).

29. Lam SHF, Sivitz A, Alade K, et al. Comparison of ultrasound guidance vs. clinical assessment alone for management of pediatric skin and soft tissue infections. *J Emerg Med*. 2018;55(5):693-701.

30. Viaux-Savelon S, Dommergues M, Rosenblum O, et al. Prenatal ultrasound screening: false positive soft markers may alter maternal representations and mother-infant interaction. *PLoS One*. 2012;7(1):e30935.

31. Thulin T, Hammar U, Ekbom A, Hultcrantz R, Forsberg AM. Perforations and bleeding in a population-based cohort of all registered colonoscopies in Sweden from 2001 to 2013. *United European Gastroenterol J*. 2019;7(1):130-137.

32. Zapka J, Taplin SH, Price RA, Cranos C, Yabroff R. Factors in quality care—the case of follow-up to abnormal cancer screening tests—problems in the steps and interfaces of care. *J Natl Cancer Inst Monogr*. 2010;2010(40):58-71.

33. Welch HG, Schwartz LM, Woloshin S. *Overdiagnosed: Making People Sick in Pursuit of Health*. Beacon Press; 2011.

34. Esserman LJ, Thompson IM, Reid B, et al. Addressing overdiagnosis and overtreatment in cancer: a prescription for change. *Lancet Oncol*. 2014;15(6):e234-e242.

35. Detsky AS. A piece of my mind. Underestimating the value of reassurance. *JAMA*. 2012;307(10):1035-1036.

36. Pletcher MJ, Pignone M. Evaluating the clinical utility of a biomarker: a review of methods for estimating health impact. *Circulation*. 2011;123(10):1116-1124.

37. Pletcher MJ, Pignone M, Earnshaw S, et al. Using the coronary artery calcium score to guide statin therapy: a cost-effectiveness analysis. *Circ Cardiovasc Qual Outcomes*. 2014;7(2):276-284.

38. Sheline Y, Kehr C. Cost and utility of routine admission laboratory testing for psychiatric inpatients. *Gen Hosp Psychiatry*. 1990;12(5):329-334.

39. Turnbull TL, Vanden Hoek TL, Howes DS, Eisner RF. Utility of laboratory studies in the emergency department patient with a new-onset seizure. *Ann Emerg Med*. 1990;19(4):373-377.

40. Kohn MA, Carpenter CR, Newman TB. Understanding the direction of bias in studies of diagnostic test accuracy. *Acad Emerg Med*. 2013;20:1194-1206.

41. Welch HG, Kramer BS, Black WC. Epidemiologic signatures in cancer. *N Engl J Med*. 2019;381(14):1378-1386.

42. Bell KJ, Del Mar C, Wright G, Dickinson J, Glasziou P. Prevalence of incidental prostate cancer: a systematic review of autopsy studies. *Int J Cancer*. 2015;137(7):1749-1757.

APPENDIX 13A
Calculation of Kappa to Measure Interobserver Agreement

Consider two observers listening for an S4 gallop on cardiac examination. They either hear it or not (Table 13A.1). The simplest measure of interobserver agreement is the proportion of observations on which the two observers agree. This proportion can be obtained by summing the numbers along the diagonal from the upper left to the lower right and dividing it by the total number of observations. In this example, out of 100 patients there were 10 patients in whom both observers heard a gallop, and 75 in whom neither did, for (10 + 75)/100 = 85% agreement.

TABLE 13A.1 INTEROBSERVER AGREEMENT ON PRESENCE OF AN S4 GALLOP

| | OBSERVER #1 | | |
OBSERVER #2	GALLOP	NO GALLOP	TOTAL, OBSERVER 2
Gallop	10	5	15
No gallop	10	75	85
Total, observer 1	20	80	100

Especially when the observations are not evenly distributed among the categories (eg, when the proportion "abnormal" on a dichotomous test is substantially different from 50%), or when there are more than two categories, another measure of interobserver agreement, called *kappa* (κ), is sometimes used. Kappa measures the extent of agreement beyond what would be expected from the observed **marginal values** (ie, the row and column totals). Kappa ranges from –1 (perfect disagreement) to 1 (perfect agreement). A kappa of 0 indicates that the amount of agreement was exactly that expected from the row and column totals. Kappa is estimated as:

$$\kappa = \frac{\text{Observed agreement (\%)} - \text{Expected agreement (\%)}}{100\% - \text{Expected agreement (\%)}}$$

The "expected" proportion in each cell is simply the proportion in that cell's row (ie, the row total divided by the sample size) times the proportion in that cell's column (ie, the column total divided by the sample size). The (total) expected agreement is obtained by adding the expected proportions in the cells along the diagonal of the table, in which the observers agreed.

For example, in Table 13A.1 the observers appear to have done quite well: They have agreed (10+75)/100 = 85% of the time. But how well did they do as compared with the agreement expected from their marginal totals? By chance alone (given the observed marginal values) they will agree about 71% of the time: (20% × 15%) + (80% × 85%) = 71%. Because the observed agreement was 85%, kappa is (85% – 71%)/(100% – 71%) = 0.48—respectable, but less impressive than 85% agreement.

When there are more than two categories of test results, it is important to distinguish between ordinal variables, which are intrinsically ordered, and nominal variables, which are not. For ordinal variables, kappa as calculated above fails to capture all the information in the data, because it does not give partial credit for coming close. To give credit for partial agreement, a *weighted* kappa should be used. (See Newman and Kohn (1) for a more detailed discussion.)

REFERENCE

1. Newman T, Kohn M. *Evidence-Based Diagnosis: An Introduction to Clinical Epidemiology*. 2nd ed. Cambridge University Press; 2020:110-137.

APPENDIX 13B
Exercises for Chapter 13. Designing Studies of Medical Tests

1. You are interested in studying the usefulness of the erythrocyte sedimentation rate (ESR) as a test for pelvic inflammatory disease (PID) in women with abdominal pain.
   a. To do this, you will need to assemble groups of women who do and do not have PID. What would be the best way to sample these women?
   b. How might the results be biased if you used final diagnosis of PID as the gold standard and those assigning that diagnosis were aware of the ESR?
   c. You find that the sensitivity of an ESR of at least 20 mm/hour is 90%, but the specificity is only 50%. On the other hand, the sensitivity of an ESR of at least 50 mm/hour is only 75%, but the specificity is 85%. Which cut point should you use to define an abnormal ESR?

2. You are interested in studying the diagnostic yield of CT head scans in children presenting to the ED with head injuries. You use a database in the radiology department to find reports of all CT scans done on patients <18 years old and ordered from the ED for head trauma. You then review the ED records of all those who had an abnormal CT scan to determine whether the abnormality could have been predicted from the physical examination.
   a. Out of 200 scans, 20 show one or more abnormalities. However, you determine that in 10 of the 20, there had been either a focal neurologic examination or altered mental status. Because only 10 patients had abnormal scans that could not have been predicted from the physical examination, you conclude that the yield of "unexpected" abnormal CT scans is only 10 in 200 (5%) in this setting. What is wrong with that conclusion?
   b. What is wrong with using "one or more abnormalities" on CT scan as the outcome variable for this diagnostic yield study?
   c. What would be some advantages of studying the effects of the CT scan on clinical decisions, rather than just studying its diagnostic yield?

3. You now wish to study the sensitivity and specificity of focal neurologic findings to predict intracranial injuries. (Because of the small sample size of such injuries, you increase the sample size by extending the study to several other EDs.) One problem you have when studying focal neurologic findings is that children who have them are much more likely to get a CT scan than children who do not. Explain how and why this will affect the sensitivity and specificity of such findings if:
   a. Only children who had a CT scan are included in the study.
   b. Eligible children with head injuries who did not have a CT scan are included and assumed not to have had an intracranial injury if they recovered without neurosurgical intervention.

CHAPTER 14

Qualitative Approaches in Clinical Research

Daniel Dohan

Interviews, **focus groups**, and other qualitative approaches can provide information about areas of clinical practice and research for which reliable tests, surveys, or other numeric measures are impossible, impractical, or not yet developed. They also furnish a holistic view of the complex reality of the clinical world in its social and contextual richness—a specific kind of **interpretation** that is not possible with numeric data. Qualitative approaches have been used to study conditions or situations that are socially sensitive or stigmatized, to include vulnerable populations or groups that have been underrepresented in research, and to translate research-derived evidence into the messy reality of everyday practice (1-3).

Although qualitative research uses commonsense procedures, such as asking **open-ended questions** and observing clinical interactions, it remains controversial in health research (4, 5). This chapter addresses the assumptions that underlie qualitative research, how it differs from quantitative research, and provides examples of how qualitative studies are useful. It also discusses practical issues in designing, executing, and disseminating qualitative research.

■ WHAT IS QUALITATIVE RESEARCH?

Qualitative research provides insights into experiences, meanings, and culture without using numeric measures, predesigned tests, or closed-ended surveys. Rather, the investigator engages with research participants to collect data and then interprets their narrative responses. The following three examples illustrate how investigators participate in and shape qualitative studies.

Example 14.1 Trials Knowledge: Exploring What Cancer Patients Know About Clinical Trials

Ethnography is a qualitative social science method for documenting the social interactions and behaviors of a group, team, organization, or community. It involves gathering qualitative data to provide a detailed, holistic analysis of a culture (6). For example, an ethnographic study explored how oncologists enroll patients in early-phase clinical research by conducting in-depth interviews with 78 patients who had advanced cancer (7). The study team began by observing appointments in oncology clinics and speaking with clinicians who recruited patients. The team learned that informal aspects of trials recruitment started long before a clinician asked a patient to sign a consent form. Oncologists reported that they thought about who would be a "good study patient" before even discussing research participation (8). This brought up several questions, such as whether patients were aware this was happening and what they knew about clinical trials before being asked to participate.

An interview protocol was constructed to probe this topic. To avoid biasing patients' responses, interviewers did not discuss the topic of trial participation unless the patient raised it. Most patients did so during their first interview. Many described participating in studies at earlier stages of their disease. Some expressed enthusiasm about these past experiences and looked forward to joining a future study. Others had more mixed feelings or worried that they might not be eligible to join a study. The team also discovered that there was often a mismatch between how much patients thought they knew about trials and the accuracy of their knowledge. Comfort with—or even mastery of—the technical language of oncology did not equate to substantive understanding of clinical trials.

These findings serve as a reminder of the difference between what patients say and what they understand. Patients may make efforts to appear knowledgeable, perhaps to present themselves as "good study patients" who would be offered a clinical trial. But taking them at face value may do patients and the clinical trials process a disservice.

Example 14.2 Deimplementing the Medical Home: Describing Why a New Care Delivery Model Was Undone

Key informant interviews are a qualitative tool for learning about the views and perspectives of experts. Such interviews are typically open-ended, following a semi-structured format: The interviewer formulates his own questions about prespecified topics and decides when to address them; interviewees respond in their own words. As in all qualitative research, when interesting but unanticipated issues come up, the interviewer is free to develop new questions to explore them. This approach is particularly valuable to learn what experts think of a topic in which they have deep knowledge, as well as for exploring how leaders arrive at consequential decisions.

Key informant interviews with 38 leaders, managers, clinicians, and staff helped explain why a large medical group abandoned a new policy initiative, the Patient Centered Medical Home (9). For policymakers, their decision had raised a troubling question: Why did the Medical Home initiative not achieve its goal of encouraging, incentivizing, and supporting patient-centered care?

It became clear that within the organization, stakeholders never connected patient-centered care to the Medical Home policy. Clinicians, leaders, and staff believed that their practice remained committed to implementing patient-centered care even as their Medical Home designation was allowed to lapse. Inside the organization, one set of managers was responsible for ensuring patient-centered care, while another group oversaw efforts to earn formal Medical Home recognition. Senior clinicians and leaders argued that patient-centered care remained an organizational priority, but managers who had led the effort to earn accreditation did not connect their work to this core value. Rather, they thought that the organization had sought Medical Home accreditation because a large employer group offered an incentive to do so. When it came time to renew accreditation, the incentive had expired, so practice managers prioritized other work and the designation lapsed. Policymakers had reason to be concerned: The Medical Home policy never achieved legitimacy within the organization. But failure to renew accreditation did not indicate the organization had drifted from prioritizing patient-centered primary care.

Example 14.3 EngageUC: Comparing Perspectives on Biobanking Research Among Diverse Communities

Qualitative researchers gather a focus group of 4 to 10 people to take the temperature of a community on a topic. The group answers a set of questions posed by a moderator. (There are often two moderators—one to keep the conversation moving and another to attend to the nonverbal aspects of the group's interactions and make sure that all voices are heard.) When the University of California (UC) wanted to expand its research biobanks and make them more inclusive of California's diverse populations, they pulled together focus groups with community members in both the Northern and Southern parts of the state to gauge their views and elicit their recommendations (10).

The goal of the project was to identify ways for UC to be more responsive to the needs of the state's populations. All told, 51 community members—selected intentionally from dozens of communities with distinct racial/ethnic histories and traditions to represent a cross-section of California's diversity—participated in the focus groups, which were conducted in English and Spanish. Content experts educated the participants about the technicalities of biobank operations and experienced facilitators guided community members in their discussions.

Though it might seem more efficient to interview a group of people all at once rather than conduct individual interviews, the focus groups brought their own complexities, including extensive travel for the research team and managing logistics of transportation, meals, and compensation for participants. The team also had to wrangle the technical issues of recording, transcribing, translating, and analyzing the vast trove of qualitative data that emerged. On the concluding day, participants were asked to propose and vote on recommendations for UC biobank leaders. Twenty-three consensus recommendations were identified; 24 others were endorsed without achieving consensus.

For the study team and UC biobanking leaders, the focus groups provided insights into how Californians view the university and state's biobanking research efforts. This diverse group of laypeople found important areas of consensus: broader education about biobanking, strong support for sharing information and data freely, a desire for more researcher oversight and accountability, and a preference for a consent process that went beyond legal requirements to engage with patients who contributed samples to the biobank.

These examples highlight some of the core features of qualitative approaches in clinical research. In each, study participants were chosen using **purposeful selection**, rather than randomly. The study team worked closely with participants to collect data; they even tailored their questions for each patient in the oncology study. The Medical Home study, which had focused first on implementation, turned into a study of deimplementation as data collection procedures were altered to pursue emerging insights. EngageUC sought to tap into participants' everyday perspectives to understand how biobanking was viewed in different California communities.

The central characteristics of qualitative research raise tricky questions: What constitutes an unbiased research study when the investigator has such an intimate role in the research? Can an investigator who asks open-ended questions be unbiased in the same way as a closed-ended survey? How does interpreting a narrative response compare to interpreting a clinical test?

To address these questions, qualitative researchers begin with an explicit consideration of what types of questions can be addressed (11). Some qualitative researchers pursue an objective, unbiased approach—as in most medical research—embracing a **positivist research paradigm**. Positivists believe the universe is governed by objective laws that science can identify. Positivist research projects attempt to use precise, unbiased measurements to address hypothesis-driven questions. Answering these questions allows scientists to identify universal laws. Given its emphases on precise measurement and hypothesis testing, few qualitative researchers embrace positivism.

Some qualitative researchers believe the universe is governed by objective laws, but do not believe science can identify those laws with certainty. **Post-positivists** argue that science, like any human activity, is carried out within a particular social context. Thus, positivists' claims to unbiased measurement must be greeted skeptically. Post-positivists believe research can help understand our world more accurately, but that hypothesis-driven designs are not the only helpful tools in that pursuit. Post-positivist projects strive to be unbiased and to answer research questions with objectivity, while recognizing that the context of a study is always central for understanding its findings.

Other research paradigms in qualitative research emphasize the importance of context even more strongly, to the point of questioning the notion that research should focus on discovering a set of universal laws. **Constructivism** believes individuals and groups socially construct different versions of objective reality, and critical theory research focuses on how the nature of objective reality reflects power relationships in society (12).

In each of these paradigms, qualitative research can use the logic of **deduction** (the study's hypotheses specify the measurements) as well as **induction** (hypotheses are formed from observations). Qualitative research often uses data that emerge during a study to derive new ideas and hypotheses; even study questions, protocols, and sites can change. Rather than trying to define variables in terms of numbers, qualitative research aims to provide rich description, often based on narrative reports. Samples for qualitative research are usually small, based on how many participants are thought to be necessary to understand the concepts, issues, and processes being studied. Qualitative investigators achieve rigor and reproducibility by selecting purposeful samples and interacting with participants to collect data. Important differences between quantitative and qualitative research are displayed in Table 14.1.

TABLE 14.1 COMPARISON OF QUANTITATIVE AND QUALITATIVE STUDIES

	QUANTITATIVE STUDIES	QUALITATIVE STUDIES
Research focus	(See Chapter 2) The research question is established a priori.	Research question may change or even be discovered during the study
Study participants	(See Chapter 3) • Specification—selection (inclusion and exclusion) criteria that specify who is eligible to participate • Sampling—representative of target population	• Flexible inclusion and exclusion criteria designed to be inclusive; may change during the study • Purposeful, snowball, may be nonrepresentative
Designs	(See Chapters 8-12) Cross-sectional study Cohort study Case-control study Randomized trial	Observational Exploratory Descriptive Comparative
Sample size estimate	(See Chapters 5-6) Based on estimated effect size and its variation, alpha and beta	Enough to understand concepts, issues, and processes fully

TABLE 14.1 COMPARISON OF QUANTITATIVE AND QUALITATIVE STUDIES (*continued*)

	QUANTITATIVE STUDIES	QUALITATIVE STUDIES
Measurements and data	(See Chapter 4)	Flexible, interactive with field notes, audio or video taping
	Set procedures with standardized data collection forms	Ethnographic observation
	Structured questionnaires	In-depth interviews
	Physical exams	Focus groups
	Laboratory/imaging tests	Analysis of written/electronic documents
	Outcome ascertainment	
	Predictor and outcome variables, with covariates	Memos on data collection context and processes
Data management	(See Chapter 19)	Standard data format
	Standard database software	Coding scheme
	Coding	Code data
	Data cleaning	
Analyses	Preplanned hypothesis testing using statistical inference	Iterative review of coded output and memos to identify findings and counterexamples

Qualitative studies advance clinical research by providing insights into the experiences of individuals, the dynamics of organizations, and the nature of the structural determinants of health.

- At the individual level, qualitative data are essential for understanding how patients, caregivers, and clinicians experience illness and care. These understandings can be the crucial ingredient for developing ideas about how to develop or interpret quantitative measures of health, illness, and care among diverse or vulnerable populations.
- At the organizational level, qualitative approaches provide insights into the complex dynamics of health care delivery organizations, which help clinical researchers implement strategies to improve the delivery of care.
- In community-engaged research, qualitative approaches capture perspectives of those affected by health care and clinical research. Using qualitative approaches, clinical researchers can gain an appreciation for how the health of community members reflects culture and institutions. Such insights may improve the validity of researchers' conceptual models and the plausibility of their hypotheses. They can also generate ideas about the causes and consequences of a disease, and suggest strategies and approaches for tailoring health improvement interventions (see Chapter 15).

Three Approaches in Qualitative Research Studies

It is helpful to distinguish between three types of qualitative research goals, each of which necessitates a somewhat different approach to study design and methods (13). In the context of qualitative research, these terms have a specialized meaning compared with how they are used in quantitative research.

- **Exploratory studies**: All qualitative research projects include some degree of inquiry, but an exploratory study involves a topic without any prior research. Exploratory studies focus on describing a new landscape. Investigators know where to start—perhaps with a puzzling clinical finding or the unexpected failure of a promising intervention—but they cannot anticipate what they might find. Unsure where their explorations will take them, research protocols are at best tentative; they will be revised, refocused, and expanded during the study. It is not possible to develop a sampling frame for an unknown topic, so investigators rely on **snowball data collection**, meaning they ask study participants to suggest others (14). Similarly, there is no basis for proposing a study analysis plan, so **grounded theory**, a set of inductive data analysis procedures, is often used to uncover new theories and understandings (15, 16).

• **Descriptive studies**: These studies take another step. There is enough knowledge to focus on a particular area of inquiry, but not yet enough to propose a comprehensive study protocol. This is a common approach when an investigator wishes to adapt a research instrument or protocol to a new target population. He may know how the instrument behaves in one group of respondents and needs to explore whether those same experiences and understandings apply in a socially or culturally distinct group.

• **Comparative studies**: These are closest, in their logic of inquiry, to quantitative studies. Well-designed comparative studies aim to articulate how study sites or participants are similar, as well as to identify important differences. They thus include an element of deductive logic that allows investigators to describe the study sites, data collection procedures, and analytical approaches before starting the study. The quantitative parallels end there, however. Comparative qualitative studies do not propose or test hypotheses: Non-numeric data do not permit tests of statistical significance. Moreover, investigators remain open to discovering new inductive findings that can change study questions, protocols, or field sites—flexibility that is rarely possible in a quantitative study.

Comparing Exploratory, Descriptive, and Comparative Approaches

Exploratory, descriptive, and comparative studies can be used to address questions in clinical research, implementation science, and community-engaged research (Table 14.2).

TABLE 14.2 EXAMPLES OF RESEARCH QUESTIONS IN CLINICAL RESEARCH, IMPLEMENTATION SCIENCE, AND COMMUNITY-ENGAGED RESEARCH, BY STUDY DESIGN

STUDY DESIGN	CLINICAL RESEARCH	IMPLEMENTATION SCIENCE	COMMUNITY-ENGAGED RESEARCH
Exploratory	How do patients make sense of a health condition or health care experience? *(see Trials Knowledge in Example 14.1)*	How does a clinic engage with an intervention as they put it into practice?	Which aspects of a health condition do members of a community consider most important, and why is that the case?
Descriptive	What do researchers need to know about how participants complete an instrument to enhance its validity and reliability?	What accounts for an organization's decision to deimplement a program that it had embraced with enthusiasm? *(see Medical Home in Example 14.2)*	How are health concerns of one community understood and responded to in other communities?
Comparative	How do patient and organizational cultures combine to shape decision-making among nursing home residents?	How do organizational dynamics support (or undermine) implementation success in a group of similar clinics?	What are areas of consensus for how to improve the practice of health science among diverse communities? *(see EngageUC in Example 14.3)*

Exploratory studies have a common look and feel. They often use a constructivist research paradigm. Questions are broad and open-ended, reflecting the descriptive and discovery aims of this design; they do not suggest that the investigator expects to find any particular associations, causal or not, among study concepts.

Descriptive qualitative studies often examine existing findings in a new target population or examine how a study instrument developed with one population will be received by a different one. A descriptive study may explore how a community makes sense of health concerns that surfaced elsewhere. In implementation science, a descriptive study might examine patient-provider communication in clinics that have different clinical outcomes, such as in diabetes control.

Comparative designs anticipate which groups are worth comparing and how those groups might differ. These designs are often theory-driven with purposeful sampling, such as when a qualitative study compares selected members of the intervention and control groups in a randomized trial. Their findings contribute to explaining what accounts for patterns of behavior, beliefs, and outcomes across groups.

Comparing Qualitative Approaches with Quantitative Techniques

All qualitative studies focus on explaining health and health care, such as how a patient decides on a particular treatment, how a clinic grapples with evidence-based practice changes, or why a community suffers disproportionately from a particular disease. Qualitative researchers study these questions observationally, as they exist in daily life, to complement findings made using quantitative methods. They often provide individual-level data that can help make sense of group-level findings. Qualitative data often form a valuable adjunct in quantitative studies, whether in the form of a mixed-methods study (which includes both qualitative and quantitative methods) or as an independent exploratory arm of a larger effort. Relatively small troves of qualitative data can provide insights that improve the validity of the quantitative study or allow the parent study to avoid unanticipated pitfalls.

■ WHEN TO USE QUALITATIVE METHODS

Qualitative data can contribute to developing measurements, capturing complex concepts, and exploring new ideas.

Developing New Measurements or Improving Existing Ones

Qualitative approaches can be helpful in the development of **closed-ended questions**. At an early stage of research, qualitative data from semi-structured interviews can identify what matters to potential participants about a topic. Interviews and focus groups can help gauge the appropriateness of items for different respondents, reveal ways in which items might be misunderstood, and guide investigators toward refining final items. They can also inform the interpretation of quantitative results. For example, ethnographic data that analyze everyday culture can provide insights into why an intervention produced the results it did. Because developing and refining measures involve building on existing knowledge, descriptive designs—in which investigators seek to deepen their understanding of a phenomenon—are often an appropriate research vehicle.

Capturing Complex Concepts That Are Difficult to Measure Quantitatively

Quantitative measures are ill-suited to measure some concepts of interest to clinical researchers. These types of difficult-to-measure concepts fall into three domains:

- At an **individual level**, clinical researchers may be interested in the meaning of a behavior for a research participant. For example, studies of patient decision-making may benefit from qualitative data that go beyond the decision itself by exploring how a patient decided.
- Capturing the nuances of **dyadic interaction**, such as between patients and providers or between patients and family caregivers, is difficult to accomplish with quantitative measures.

Qualitative data, particularly when collected from the perspectives of both people in a relationship and can thus be **triangulated**, often constitute a good source of information about the dynamics of the dyad.

* **Complex systems**, such as clinics, communities, or health care delivery organizations, generate and sustain their own culture. **Ethnography** and other qualitative measures are considered the gold standard for this type of work due to their ability to capture the richness and subtleties of culture.

Exploring New Ideas

Qualitative approaches can identify novel aspects of clinical medicine, as exemplified by groundbreaking studies including *Boys in White* (how medical school socializes students into the physician role) (17), *Awareness of Dying* (how patients, caregivers, and clinicians navigate the experience of death in the hospital) (18), and *Forgive and Remember* (how surgeons manage error) (19). Indeed, clinicians can use qualitative research tools—observation and note taking or asking open-ended questions and probing the meaning of the responses—in the course of patient care and in their roles as educators and health system leaders. Such activities can provide new insights into the experiences of patients, students, and colleagues that enrich their ability to conduct studies with an enhanced degree of rigor, replicability, and impact.

■ MATCHING DESIGN TO QUESTION

Most of the conventions used in quantitative research—such as the value of randomization and blinding, the need to measure and adjust for confounders, and the importance of estimating the sample size—do not have ready parallels in qualitative research. In the absence of such guideposts, researchers must use reflection and anticipation—about the study questions, about what is known about study sites and participants, about the intended audience for the results, and about how the study might unfold—to guide study design.

An exploratory study investigates the new and unknown, so its design needs to focus on why and how the novelty matters. From the earliest moments of research design, investigators who embark on an exploratory study must consider the audience for their results. Consider a hypothetical study that explores unmet health care needs among a vulnerable population. One audience may be those who are already familiar with the problem and understand its importance. For this audience, an exploratory study should collect data to identify new issues, using inductive logic to manage and analyze the data. The study might include in-depth interviews with a small group of key informants, expanding to include others based on what is discovered in the first set of interviews. The researcher might emphasize collective review of data through team meetings and the development of analytical **memos**—short essays that identify emerging topics of interest and guide ongoing data collection.

The same research question may merit a different exploratory design when it aims to provide preliminary data for a subsequent study to change clinical practice, which would need to convince an audience of practitioners, who may view small qualitative studies with skepticism. A design for this audience would likely have to include a larger number of participants, even if that meant getting less data from each respondent. Open-ended survey questions or structured open-ended interview protocols, as well as a rigorous approach to data management and analysis, may work better than an in-depth ethnography of a single clinic.

An exploratory study aimed at providing new insights into a previously unstudied topic must focus on gaining access to sites and participants. The investigator will likely need to leverage existing relationships to pursue the study, and the design should show how the researcher will engage participants as the study proceeds. Exploratory designs focus on the process of research, which extends to describing how a decision will be made to stop data collection. Oftentimes, an exploratory study is constrained by logistics or funding; in this situation, the investigator must acknowledge these constraints and show how the time available is sufficient to accomplish the study goals. In other circumstances, the study will continue until the investigator reaches **thematic (or data) saturation**—roughly, the point at which collecting more data yields few new insights.

Comparative designs must collect enough data to support cross-site or cross-participant analysis while remaining mindful of how access to enough participants will be achieved. To thread this needle, investigators need a purposeful sampling strategy, starting with a conceptual model that illustrates how each site (or group) addresses the project's analytical needs. Based on the needs described in this model, investigators can reflect on how results from each site may guide project findings and adjust data collection and analysis under different scenarios.

For example, comparative investigators may want to gather qualitative data to understand how care processes (say, control of diabetes and hypertension) in high-quality clinics differ from those in low-quality ones, with the ultimate aim of importing lessons from the high-quality group. Armed with quantitative measures of quality, an investigator may pick one clinic from each group and start collecting data. But what if the measures of quality turn out to be poor indicators of more holistic aspects of clinic operations? Perhaps the high-quality clinics serve more advantaged patients or were savvier in how they recorded quality-related data—not necessarily in how well they provided care. These findings suggest the investigators started the study with a faulty conceptual model. Data from previous exploratory or descriptive qualitative studies should have sensitized them to the ways in which social advantage confounds quality measurement and alerted them to consider that clinics might "game" quality measurement systems. This understanding should also guide them toward better ways to select clinics that have authentic differences in care processes—perhaps by selecting clinics embedded in different types of health care systems or with different leadership structures. Incorporating these insights would improve their conceptual model and lead to study findings that more effectively achieved their aim of identifying processes to translate from high-quality settings.

■ COLLECTING DATA

Once settled on a qualitative study design, investigators face decisions about the logistics and mechanics of data collection.

Determining the Sample Size

"What is an appropriate sample size?" is the most common question asked about qualitative research. The goal is not to have adequate power to detect a specified effect size, but to understand selected concepts, issues, and processes. There is a sense among many qualitative social scientists that including 30 to 40 people is a sensible start for a modest qualitative study carried out by a single investigator. Ultimately, the right sample size depends on the research question, the intended audience for the results, and logistics of the study; a well-designed qualitative sample balances all three.

- **Question:** Exploratory questions typically use small samples; a rule of thumb from grounded theory analysis is that 20 to 25 interviews are needed. Descriptive and comparative studies recruit from multiple sites or populations and thus tend to include larger samples. Iterative data collection and analysis allow investigators to tailor their recruitment to tackle emerging questions. As descriptive and comparative investigators gain deeper insights into the study questions, conducting 15 interviews at the first site, 10 at the second, and 5 at the third may be enough. Circling back for a set of confirmatory interviews may require 10 more, which brings the total back to the "Goldilocks" estimate of 30 to 40 individuals.
- **Audience:** An important aim of qualitative research is to convince policymakers, clinicians, researchers, and journal editors that the findings are valid. Because those audiences are used to larger studies, small selected samples may cause concern. Although increasing sample

size—or having a similar number of participants in each group—may not be necessary to achieve a study's qualitative aims, doing so can be a practical way to anticipate those concerns and bolster a study's chance of publication.

• Logistics: Qualitative research is labor-intensive. It takes time to gain and maintain access to field sites and participants. Many times, qualitative studies are undertaken by a solo investigator, but even in team projects, the principal investigator shoulders the responsibility to build and maintain relationships with sites. Investigator time is often a rate-limiting factor in carrying out a qualitative study, which mitigates against increasing sample size beyond what is necessary scientifically.

Interviews or Focus Groups?

Another frequent question is whether to use interviews or focus groups. Focus groups may seem attractive as a more efficient way to gather data, because the process involves interviewing six to eight people at a time. But interviews and focus groups collect different kinds of qualitative data, and the choice between them should be based on the research question, rather than perceptions of efficiency and scale. An interview reveals individual perspectives, beliefs, and experiences, whereas a focus group reveals the reactions and responses of the group to one another and the facilitator.

Investigators who want to understand the perspectives of individuals from different communities or groups are often best served by conducting a series of individual interviews. Focus groups have their own internal dynamics, for example, participants who talk frequently may shape the collective views. A skilled facilitator can overcome these tendencies to some extent, but focus groups are the right tool to reveal group interactions, not to explore individual perspectives. For example, the biobanking study described in Example 14.3 aimed to elicit community recommendations about biobanking; thus, focus groups were the right way to hear how individuals from different communities discussed biobanking among themselves and arrived at particular recommendations.

Managing Field Sites and Study Participants

Qualitative interviews require substantial time commitments from participants and investigators. Often, the work of collecting data falls on the principal investigator, who may be the only member of the research team. Moreover, in-depth interview studies don't lend themselves to divisions of labor parallel to those used for collecting biologic specimens or administering closed-ended questionnaires. Each interview unfolds somewhat differently, and interviewers need to be competent and agile at handling a semi-structured protocol. Even when a study is large enough to merit a multiperson team, training and supervising field workers involves lots of hands-on engagement from the study lead.

Protecting Confidentiality

Qualitative data create unique challenges related to data anonymization and protection of confidentiality. Some participants may be identified readily from how they described their position or the stories they told. Qualitative investigators may ask sensitive questions, such as whether a group of patients experienced unequal treatment or why a quality improvement initiative failed. It may also be necessary to develop protocols that enable the team to cross-check insights from one interview with others without breaching confidence.

Qualitative researchers must protect participants' confidentiality. Most investigators are aware of the importance of not taking advantage of participants with limited power, but effective qualitative research may also pose hidden risks for people who have power and privileged social status. In studies with clinicians or health organization leaders, skilled investigators create relationships of trust with privileged informants, who may share confidences about stigmatized behaviors or attitudes that they otherwise would keep confidential. Should these data become public, the negative impact on an informant's reputation could be profound.

Interview Guides

Developing an interview guide is a chance to improve a project's execution and to envision and navigate potential pitfalls. Commonly, investigators develop an initial interview guide that they revise throughout the project. The guide ensures that interviewers will explore the main research questions while leaving open the possibility that unexpected topics will arise.

Many qualitative studies benefit from a **stem and probe approach** to designing interview (and focus group) questions. A stem introduces a core study question, which is followed by probes—questions, prompts, or statements to ensure a thorough and thoughtful response. In the study of what cancer patients knew about clinical trials (Example 14.1), for example, a productive stem was, "Tell me what happened at your last visit with your oncologist." This was followed by probes to find out what the patient heard the oncologist say about their diagnosis, prognosis, and treatment choices, whether they felt they had had a chance to raise topics of concern, and if the oncologist had heard and responded to their questions.

- **Exploratory study guides** typically have a small number of topic areas (10 or fewer) that investigators want to learn more about. Stems need not be formal questions, as an exploratory study interview unfolds ideally as a conversation between interviewer and respondent. The interviewer uses the guide as a reminder to cover all relevant topics, but it is common for an exploratory interview to follow its own logic rather than a preset structure.
- **Descriptive interviews** have more structure. The guide may list stem questions that touch on issues investigators have prioritized, with probes that lead respondents to expand on topics of interest.
- **Comparative studies** often include a structured guide that focuses on questions about how respondents' experiences resemble or differ from those at other sites. The guide may include instructions for how interviewers should ask each question, which help focus data analysis.

Before entering the field, an interview guide illustrates study procedures to potential funders and collaborators. As the project enters the field, the investigators use the guide in pilot interviews and to train interviewers. The guide will change and improve during these processes: Its length will be adjusted, unclear questions will be revised, and the order of the questions may change. Once in the field, the guide may be revised further in response to emerging findings, and some questions or topics will be set aside as redundant or uninteresting. The final version will be used to describe the study during manuscript development and revision.

Data Collection

Quantitative data collection strategies strive for samples that are representative of the target population and use set procedures to eliminate bias during data collection (Table 14.3). In contrast, **qualitative investigators achieve rigor and reproducibility by selecting purposeful samples and participating actively in the collection of data.** Representativeness and bias are familiar principles in clinical research; purposefulness and participation less so. In purposeful sampling, investigators consider how the sites and participants they engage will provide information to address the study question. Flexible data collection strategies allow investigators to uncover unexpected findings that challenge their theories.

In the EngageUC study (Example 14.3), for example, investigators sought to include Spanish-speaking respondents—who had not been included fully in prior discussions of genomic research—in focus groups. Logistically, this meant planning for simultaneous interpretation throughout the study. It also led to discussions within the research team about whether breakout groups should be bilingual (with interpretation) or monolingual (without).

TABLE 14.3 RIGOROUS AND REPRODUCIBLE DATA COLLECTION IN QUANTITATIVE AND QUALITATIVE RESEARCH

RESEARCH ACTIVITY	QUANTITATIVE RESEARCH	QUALITATIVE RESEARCH
Select research participants	*Representativeness*: Random samples of representative groups	*Purposefulness*: Sites and participants selected according to theoretical need
Obtain data	*Limit bias*: Fixed data collection procedures not influenced by investigators	*Facilitate participation*: Flexible data collection strategies that involve interactions between investigators and participants

Ultimately, the participants themselves helped decide the issue when they expressed their desire for free-flowing discussion afforded by monolingual breakouts.

■ DATA MANAGEMENT, ANALYSIS, AND REPORTING

Managing and analyzing qualitative data retain a feeling of mystery for new and experienced investigators alike. Investigators accustomed to cleaning and analyzing numeric data using statistical software may find themselves adrift as transcripts arrive for analysis. Experienced investigators report that immersing themselves in qualitative data and developing interpretative analyses involves intellectual processes that are difficult to characterize.

Software for qualitative data analysis (QDA) helps manage textual data, but it does not actually analyze data. Rather, it is a tool to help an analyst organize the data (even a modestly sized qualitative project can produce hundreds of pages of data) and monitor ongoing results.

Goals of Qualitative Analysis

Both quantitative and qualitative research use data analysis to accomplish two crucial scientific tasks: to avoid erroneous findings and to communicate findings in ways readers find credible (Table 14.4). Qualitative investigators use an iterative process of data review and inquiry to refine results and reduce interpretive errors. This process begins with data collection and continues throughout a project. A key step is to develop data **codes**. Codes capture the analytical and conceptual issues a project will examine during the course of analysis. Each project has a unique set of codes, and the number of codes and how they are defined reflect the size and goals of the project as well as the research paradigm of the investigator and the extent to which the project follows a deductive versus inductive logic. As a rule, smaller projects—including projects that have less empirical data or are less ambitious conceptually—tend to have fewer codes, as do deductive projects in the post-positivist tradition. A complete code includes a specific definition, inclusion and exclusion criteria that demarcate how the code resembles and is

TABLE 14.4 RIGOROUS AND REPRODUCIBLE DATA ANALYSIS IN QUANTITATIVE AND QUALITATIVE RESEARCH

RESEARCH ACTIVITY	QUANTITATIVE RESEARCH	QUALITATIVE RESEARCH
Avoid chance findings	*Statistics*: Hypothesis testing using statistical inference	*Process*: Iterative review of data (often including coding and memos) to refine results
Convince others of findings	*Transparency*: Present data in standard, well-known formats	*Context*: Provide results with enough narrative context for interpretation

distinguished from conceptually related codes; examples of data to which the code should be applied (and data to which it should not be applied if necessary or helpful); and a data **memo** that describes the origins of the code and the history of its development and use during the iterative process of data collection and analysis.

Investigators organize codes into a **codebook**. Similar to a codebook of variables for a quantitative dataset, the qualitative codebook is a repository for code definitions, exemplars, and other information. Codebooks also illustrate relationships among project codes. They typically have a hierarchical structure in which more specific codes are grouped within larger analytical categories. Oftentimes, codebooks are shown with a tree structure. Codebooks provide one mechanism for operationalizing a project's conceptual model. The central elements of the conceptual model should be reflected in the codebook structure, which will evolve as new codes are discovered and defined and as the study team gains insights into new conceptual relationships in the study site. As a study reaches the point of thematic or data saturation, the codebook is finalized. At that point, there should be no need to add new codes, and the relationships among study concepts should allow the team to publish a final codebook that can be used to definitively code all study data. This is a major turning point in any qualitative study.

With codes and codebook in hand, the study team can focus on coding the data. Some codes will identify key study themes while others may be used to sort or organize the data, for example, some projects may apply a specific code to document where an observed interaction took place. Such organizational codes are particularly useful as the team begins to explore the patterns that emerge from the coded data. The team documents these patterns in *analytical memos*. (Earlier in the analysis process, *data memos* document the evolution of codes.) During this phase of analysis, analytical memos document the evolution of study findings. Analytical memos capture the emerging insights and ideas of study analysts. Some of these emerging ideas may lead nowhere. Additional data may reveal that the data that generated the insight were a one-time occurrence or that they are contradicted by other data. When other team members discuss the memo, they may recognize that the insight should be integrated into other findings, or they may conclude that it represents the singular interpretation of one analyst but not an interpretation the study team can endorse.

Some analytical memos will capture core ideas that evolve into study findings. For example, in the Trials Knowledge project (Example 14.1), an analytical memo from one interview noted the irony that a patient who was familiar with many of the obscure technical aspects of a clinical trial study drug nevertheless seemed confused about the basic goal of clinical research in general and of early-phase clinical research studies in particular. Other analysts agreed with this interpretation, which led to an examination of coded data to explore whether other patients displayed similar patterns of knowledge about clinical trials. Eventually, this insight emerged as one of the study's central findings about what patients with advanced cancer understand about clinical trials processes.

The textual and narrative data produced by qualitative research do not fit well with standardized reporting formats that provide transparency and foster reproducibility. Rather, qualitative analysts provide contextual details that illustrate their interpretations and findings so they can convince others of the validity of their results.

Using Qualitative Data Analysis (QDA) Software

Computer-assisted QDA has become common, but it has not changed the fundamental process of managing qualitative data. Prior to QDA, qualitative analysts organized and made sense of data by reading, tagging, and sorting results, as well as by writing memos to document these intellectual processes and refine their research findings. These steps are still essential to help researchers avoid arbitrary findings and convince others of what they have discovered. They are carried out by writing annotations in the margins of interview transcript printouts using colored pens, by making copies of transcripts and sorting them into different piles, or even by using general purpose office software such as Microsoft Word and Excel.

QDA software is primarily a database for *storing* qualitative data that incorporates annotation, sorting, and filtering capacities. Most QDA software is based on grounded theory tradition and has been designed to facilitate exploratory coding and analyzing data for thematic content. In exploratory projects with these goals, QDA software can be an effective tool for:

- **Maintaining data integrity** through version control when several team members are involved in data coding;
- **Facilitating the calculation of quantitative scores** for **intercoder reliability** to document the validity of coding;
- **Creating and maintaining the thematic codes** that an exploratory study may produce, especially when many codes emerge during data management and analysis; and
- **Generating reports** on individual codes as well as on groups of codes that are documented in the codebook; this includes exporting raw data with particular codes or from particular sections of the codebook.

The Process of Managing and Analyzing Qualitative Data

The data management protocol explains how interviews, focus groups, and other field data will be converted into a consistent format for analysis. These processes begin with descriptions of how the researchers will gain access to field sites and respondents, obtain and document informed consent, and collect narrative data using digital recorders (preferably two, to avoid loss of information if one device fails) or by taking notes. Processing this raw data into a standard format involves transcribing interviews, describing how the identity of speakers will be ascertained in focus groups, and clarifying how field notes will be transcribed from notebooks (or recorders) into word-processed documents.

Setting up the QDA database also requires investigators to decide how to organize and name data files. An initial codebook includes the deductive questions that motivated a descriptive or comparative study and may also signal the themes that investigators anticipated uncovering in an exploratory study. In every project, however, codebooks evolve over time. Finalizing a coding scheme is often a bottleneck. Investigators may convene multiple times during active fieldwork to review data and discuss coding approaches. These are opportunities to refine analytic concepts and incorporate unexpected findings. Reading, discussion, and rereading are essential; paper-based hand coding and a whiteboard to track concepts, codes, and ideas can be helpful.

With the data management protocol and codebook in hand, investigators launch into the heart of data analysis, either in QDA software or by hand. A key decision is whether investigators will emphasize inductive or deductive analysis. Inductive analysis is more common in exploratory studies, such as those that use grounded theory analysis: Data are coded inductively to discover themes, and these themes are then pulled together to propose new theories.

Comparative or descriptive studies incorporate deductive analysis, at least to some degree. This begins with a set of concepts or themes, similar to the variables in a quantitative analysis, to be examined. For example, researchers might use **framework analysis**, in which each row represents a study concept and each case study contributes a column to the grid, to compare case studies to each other. Qualitative data, such as an interview quote or other data that illustrate a particular concept, are entered into the cells (20).

Investigators should pay attention to whether their study is better suited for induction or deduction and select an analytical strategy to match. A pitfall to avoid in qualitative analysis is to use an inductive approach, such as grounded theory, to analyze data from studies with a deductive character, for example, a study where analysts could articulate their expected findings. In this situation, an inductive analysis may (falsely) suggest that emerging insights have confirmed researchers' expectations. A more defensible analytical approach in this situation is to recognize that the interview guide (or other aspects of study design or procedures) may coax respondents toward confirmatory findings. A deductive analytical approach that places more emphasis on discovering and examining contradictory data is more likely to generate compelling research findings. Consulting with mentors and trained qualitative researchers can help recognize when a study may be vulnerable to this type of error and how to avoid it.

Writing and Sharing Results

Data management protocols and the memos that document the team's intellectual processes can serve as a rough draft of the methods section for a manuscript, while the data management and analysis processes form the core of the results section.

- In an **exploratory study**, the results include inductively discovered themes. Studies identify more findings than can be reported, so investigators need to prioritize those that are most relevant for the intended audience. There is nothing improper about selecting exemplars that will be most compelling, but researchers must also provide contradictory results, if any, to ensure accurate interpretation.
- In a **descriptive design**, results should include findings that fit the themes the investigators thought they would identify, as well as any unexpected results. Inductive findings may also discuss ways in which the study evolved in response to the analysis of emerging data.
- Results from **comparative studies** focus mostly on the similarities and differences among the study sites that the investigators had inquired about, particularly those that illustrate the main themes of the study. Unexpected findings should also be included.

Qualitative investigators often share findings with study stakeholders, including participants, and those who helped the study in other ways. Participants often want to hear how their stories and insights were understood by investigators and how their experiences compared with those of other participants. When sharing findings with these audiences, participants' identities must be shielded: Anodyne findings for researchers may be controversial among stakeholders, and viewpoints that participants share in one-on-one interviews or focus groups may spark concern when disclosed publicly.

For the foreseeable future, qualitative studies will continue to represent a small segment of published clinical research. Most journals limit a manuscript's maximum word count, which makes it difficult to convey the narrative richness and contextual particularity that makes qualitative results convincing. In addition, journal editors and reviewers may not have exposure and expertise with qualitative studies. Navigating these hurdles can benefit from creativity in how a manuscript is prepared. For example, some journals do not count text within tables and boxes against their word limit, so authors should consider placing quotes and other supporting evidence therein. Investigators should select table headings thoughtfully. Quotes that illustrate a related cluster of themes work well for an exploratory study; descriptive and comparative studies may sort evidence according to site or based on whether the finding was anticipated or not. When deciding which journal to target for a submission, it may be wise to reach out to the editor with a pre-submission inquiry. Editors may also appreciate suggestions of qualified reviewers.

Finally, a word of caution about submitting a qualitative manuscript to a high-impact journal. It is common for clinical researchers to start at the top, and if unsuccessful, try a lower-rated journal. For qualitative studies, however, revising a manuscript for a new journal with a different audience may involve substantial rewriting, especially if that journal has a different maximum word count. Eliminating pages from an already-pithy manuscript may be painful and time-consuming. Targeting the initial submission to a more receptive journal is usually a better approach.

■ SUMMARY

1. Qualitative approaches allow investigators to examine complex, context-dependent, or sensitive topics holistically.
2. Qualitative research is used to explore a new phenomenon, to describe the application of existing concepts or instruments in new settings or populations, and to compare complex social processes and organizations.
3. Qualitative research requires self-reflection, starting with selection of an appropriate exploratory, descriptive, or comparative research design.
4. When collecting qualitative data, researchers select research sites and participants with attention to the research question and use flexible strategies to engage participants to ensure collection of rich data.
5. Qualitative studies use an iterative process of data collection, review, and analysis and report findings with contextual detail.

REFERENCES

1. Hoff TJ, Witt LC. Exploring the use of qualitative methods in published health services and management research. *Med Care Res Rev.* 2000;57(2):139-160.
2. Mays N, Pope C. Rigour and qualitative research. *BMJ.* 1995;311(6997):109-112.
3. Weiner BJ, Amick HR, Lund JL, Lee SYD, Hoff TJ. Review: use of qualitative methods in published health services and management research: a 10-year review. *Med Care Res Rev.* 2011;68(1):3-33.
4. Devers KJ. How will we know "good" qualitative research when we see it? Beginning the dialogue in health services research. *Health Serv Res.* 1999;34(5):1153-1188.
5. Greenhalgh T, Annandale E, Ashcroft R, et al. An open letter to the BMJ editors on qualitative research. *BMJ.* 2016;352:i563.
6. Reeves S, Kuper A, Hodges BD. Qualitative research methodologies: ethnography. *BMJ.* 2008;337:a1020.
7. Garrett SB, Koenig CJ, Trupin L, et al. What advanced cancer patients with limited treatment options know about clinical research: a qualitative study. *Support Care Cancer.* 2017;25(10):3235-3242.
8. Joseph G, Dohan D. Diversity of participants in clinical trials in an academic medical center: the role of the "good study patient?" *Cancer.* 2009;115(3):608-615.
9. Dohan D, McCuistion MH, Frosch DL, Hung DY, Tai-Seale M. Recognition as a patient-centered medical home: fundamental or incidental? *Ann Fam Med.* 2013;11(Suppl_1):S14-S18.
10. Dry SM., Garrett SB, Koenig BA, et al. Community recommendations on Biobank Governance: results from a deliberative community engagement in California. *PLOS One.* 2017;12(2):e0172582.
11. Teherani A, Martimianakis T, Stenfors-Hayes T, Wadhwa A, Varpio L. Choosing a qualitative research approach. *J Grad Med Educ.* 2015;7(4):669-670.
12. Brown MEL, Dueñas AN. A medical science educator's guide to selecting a research paradigm: building a basis for better research. *Med Sci Educ.* 2020;30(1):545-553.
13. Rendle KA, Abramson CM, Garrett SB, Halley MC, Dohan D. Beyond exploratory: a tailored framework for designing and assessing qualitative health research. *BMJ Open.* 2019;9(8):e030123.
14. Goodman LA. Snowball sampling. *Ann Math Stat.* 1961;32:148-170.
15. Charmaz K. *Constructing Grounded Theory.* Sage Publications; 2014.
16. Glaser BG, Strauss AL. *The Discovery of Grounded Theory: Strategies for Qualitative Research.* Aldine Publishing Company; 1967.
17. Becker HS, Geer B, Hughes EC, Strauss AL. *Boys in White; Student Culture in Medical School.* University of Chicago Press; 1961.
18. Glaser BG, Strauss AL. *Awareness of Dying.* Aldine Pub. Co.; 1965.
19. Bosk C. *Forgive and Remember: Managing Medical Failure.* University of Chicago Press; 1979.
20. Gale NK, Heath G, Cameron E, Rashid S, Redwood S. Using the framework method for the analysis of qualitative data in multi-disciplinary health research. *BMC Med Res Methodol.* 2013;13(1):117.

APPENDIX 14A
Exercises for Chapter 14. Qualitative Approaches in Clinical Research

1. In the context of historical and contemporary discrimination, it has been well documented that Black Americans have limited trust in medicine and medical research. An investigator is planning a qualitative study to learn more about how the nature and experience of mistrust may vary among different Black populations. The study will include recent immigrants from Ghana, second- and third-generation Afro-Caribbeans from the Dominican Republic, and African Americans who have lived in the United States for multiple generations. Suggest and justify an appropriate qualitative research design (exploratory, descriptive, comparative).

2. Example 14.3 describes the EngageUC study that used focus groups to elicit recommendations about how the University of California could better engage diverse California communities in biobanking research. Select the best justification for using focus groups for this study:
   a. Given the size in California, focus groups allowed investigators to include a large number of participants in the study in an efficient fashion.
   b. Focus groups allowed EngageUC investigators to examine and understand how members of diverse communities made sense of biobanking among themselves.
   c. Using focus groups allowed research participants to speak more freely because they felt more safe doing so within a group context.

3. Most qualitative studies involve both inductive and deductive analysis. Consider the studies in Examples 14.1 (Trials Knowledge) and 14.2 (Deimplementing the Medical Home). What type of analysis was most appropriate in the Trials Knowledge study? Which type was more appropriate for the Deimplementing study? Of the two studies, which included a combination of the two types of analysis? Explain your answer.

Approaches and Implementation

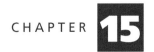

Community-Engaged Research

Alka M. Kanaya

Most clinical research is conceived of and takes place in academic medical centers or other research institutes. Such sites offer many advantages for conducting research, including having experienced investigators and support staff. In addition, an established culture, reputation, and infrastructure for research facilitates the work of everyone from novice investigator to tenured professor. However, these enabling factors may come at the cost of poor generalizability and inadequate dissemination of academic research into communities; they may also have the unintended consequence of exacerbating health disparities. To overcome these limitations, there has been substantial growth in federal funding for community engagement in research through the National Institutes of Health's Clinical Translational Science Awards (CTSAs) and the Patient-Centered Outcomes Research Institute (PCORI). This chapter describes research that involves stakeholders from diverse backgrounds, who collaborate to design, conduct, interpret, disseminate, and implement research results done with communities.

We define **community-engaged research** as research designed to meet the needs of the communities where it is conducted. Community can be defined in many ways, from individuals who live in a geographic area, those with a certain disease, people of a certain gender or ethnic identity, nonprofit organizations or advocacy groups, health care providers within a health system, policymakers, or a combination of these groups. A community-based approach to research involves **collaboration between relevant community stakeholders and investigators from a research center**. Such collaborations are critical for solving local health problems and promoting health equity, and they can be extraordinary opportunities for mutual learning and capacity building. However, they can be challenging because of the time and energy needed to create trusting relationships, manage timelines and expectations, and address existing imbalances in power.

■ WHY DO COMMUNITY-ENGAGED RESEARCH?

Collaborative research is often the only way to answer research questions that involve special settings, specific populations, or new or re-emerging diseases. Research in academic medical centers tends to focus on priorities that may be quite different from local community needs. Participation in research has benefits for a community and for academic researchers that go beyond the value of the information collected in a particular study. Lasting relationships, a sense of pride, and the development of economic and logistical capacity may result from community research done with care and concern for promoting health equity.

Local Questions and Local Knowledge

Conducting community-engaged research ensures that questions of local importance and relevance are prioritized, like the examples in Table 15.1. National- or state-level data from central sources may not reflect local disease burdens or the distribution of risk factors in the community. Interventions, especially those designed to change behavior, may not have the same effect in different settings. For example, public health campaigns for smoking cessation may be ineffective in reaching important demographic groups with high smoking rates,

TABLE 15.1 EXAMPLES OF RESEARCH QUESTIONS REQUIRING COMMUNITY-ENGAGED RESEARCH

What are the vaping rates among adolescents in low-income neighborhoods in Chicago?

Can culturally targeted outreach improve colorectal cancer screening among Asian American populations?

What is the impact of a worksite-based sexually transmitted infection prevention campaign for migrant farm workers in Texas?

Can a community health worker intervention improve type 2 diabetes management in the Puerto Rican community?

such as the Vietnamese American populations. Therefore, studies have used community-engaged methods to understand which messages will be most effective for smoking cessation (1) and then test these culturally focused interventions within the communities where they are most likely to have impact (2).

Local knowledge can identify novel problems and more democratic solutions (3). The understandings and practices related to health, health care, and illness can differ significantly across different communities (4). For example, structural barriers that result in social, political, and economic causes of health disparities may prevent optimal blood pressure control in Black men in traditional health care settings. An example of an academic and community partnership was conducted in a trusted setting, namely Black-run barbershops in Los Angeles County. The study used barbers—community members who had long-term relationships with their clientele—as the main delivery agents of the study intervention (5). In a cluster-randomized trial (the barbershop was the unit of randomization), patrons with uncontrolled hypertension either met with a pharmacist in the barbershop who prescribed medications and monitored their blood pressure and electrolytes (intervention) or were encouraged by the barber about lifestyle modification and making doctor appointments (active control group). After 6 months, the intervention group had an impressive 22 mm Hg greater mean reduction in systolic blood pressure and better measures of self-rated health and patient engagement than the control group.

Greater Generalizability

Research within communities is useful for producing results that may be more **generalizable** to groups that are not well-represented among patients at academic medical centers. For example, patients with back pain who are seen at referral hospitals are very different from those seen by primary care providers. Studies of the natural history of back pain or response to treatment at a tertiary care center therefore may be of limited use for clinical practice in the community.

Partly in response to this problem, several **practice-based research networks** have been organized in which physicians from community settings work together to study research questions of mutual interest (6). An example is the response to treatment of patients with carpal tunnel syndrome. Previous studies had recommended early surgical intervention based on studies of patients treated at a major referral center. But most patients treated in primary care practices improved with conservative therapy; few required referral to specialists or sophisticated diagnostic tests (7).

Building Local Capacity and Program Sustainability

Conducting research in community settings in collaboration with community stakeholders ensures that questions of local importance will be prioritized. The value of community participation in research goes beyond the specific information collected in each study. It also raises local scholarly standards and encourages creativity and independent thinking. Each project builds skills and confidence that allow local researchers to see themselves as partners and leaders in the scientific process, not just as consumers of knowledge produced elsewhere. This in turn encourages more research. Furthermore, participating in research can bring intellectual and financial resources to a community and help to encourage local empowerment and self-sufficiency.

Community-engaged research can also implement and test programs that can be sustained beyond the duration of a study. Having community partners provide foundational input for what, when, how, and by whom an intervention is conducted gives the community more ownership of the program. This approach can lead to much greater buy-in and longer term sustainability of the program.

Promoting Health Equity

Another important reason to conduct community-engaged research is to **reduce health disparities in affected communities** (8). Several aspects of working collaboratively with communities, from identifying the questions that matter most to them, determining local solutions, and building capacity for effective and sustainable programs, can help to promote health equity. When solutions are found for the most pressing problems within a community, there will be more trust and buy-in, leading to better outcomes and fewer health disparities. The most just approaches involve collaborative efforts among community, academic, and other stakeholders who gather and use research and data to build on strengths and priorities of the community to improve health and social equity (9).

Research in community settings can lead to better health policy. An example was the collective impact effort of the Tenderloin Healthy Corner Store Coalition in San Francisco. Building upon community-engaged research findings, stakeholders from community organizations, local businesses, academic partners, the health department, and advocacy groups focused their efforts to reduce tobacco and alcohol advertising and sales, and improving access to healthy, affordable, and sustainable food in one of the poorest neighborhoods in the city (10).

■ APPROACHES TO COMMUNITY-ENGAGED RESEARCH

Potential approaches include *any* research method or study design, from qualitative interviews, focus groups, and ethnographic observations, to quantitative data collected from epidemiologic surveys or large datasets, to clinical trials. Although the traditional observational and experimental study designs described in prior chapters can be used with stakeholder input throughout the research process, often there is also a need to develop study questions based on assessment of community needs and open-ended feedback to help interpret study results. Most community-engaged research studies employ mixed methods, with some stages of research requiring qualitative study designs (Chapter 14) and others requiring quantitative designs.

In theory, the process of starting such a project is the same as for any other study. In practice, the greatest challenge for young academic investigators is finding colleagues or mentors with community relationships with whom to interact and learn. Such help may not be available locally or through the academic center. This often leads to an important early decision for would-be community investigators: to work alone or in collaboration with more established investigators, who may not have direct ties with local community organizations.

Getting Started

Getting started in community-engaged research without the help of a more experienced colleague is like teaching oneself how to swim: It is not impossible, but it is difficult and sometimes fraught with unforeseen dangers. Following a few steps may make the process easier.

- **Network.** As discussed in Chapter 2, networking is important for any investigator. A good way to begin research in a community is often in collaboration with more experienced researchers with established relationships built upon trust in the target communities. New investigators should contact researchers who are addressing similar research questions or working with a specific community of interest. Attending a scientific conference in one's field of interest is a good way to make contacts and identify colleagues with similar interests locally. Many academic centers have community engagement offices as part of their clinical research infrastructure, with staff who can help junior investigators make connections with local and regional community partners. Searching for groups or programs that have worked on the topic area can open avenues to other community resources.

- **Start simple.** It is seldom a good idea to begin research in a community with a randomized controlled trial. Small descriptive studies producing useful local data may make more sense and will build a foundation for future collaborations with community partners. More ambitious projects can be saved for later. For example, a descriptive study of heart disease knowledge among immigrant South Asians in Chicago (11) served as the first step toward a larger behavioral intervention for cardiovascular disease prevention in this community (12).

- **Think about local advantages.** What questions can investigators answer in their local setting better than anywhere else? It is often best for a young investigator to focus on health problems or populations that are common in the local community, obtaining their input to identify the most relevant and important questions.

A Continuum of Collaborative Research

The intensity of community engagement (Figure 15.1) should be considered (13).

Studies with a *modest level* of community engagement originate in academic centers and involve community partners in the recruitment of participants for the study. This occurs, for example, when researchers work with community partners and staff to develop culturally tailored and in-language recruitment materials. In this level of community engagement, the academic investigators are usually responsible for designing the study and then obtaining the necessary funding and clearances to carry it out. Ways to involve partners include **community engagement studios** that provide feedback early in the research planning phase (Table 15.2). Community partners receive funding and resources to help with **community outreach** and recruitment, and develop experience working on research studies.

Studies with *substantial* community engagement involve stakeholders in the design and implementation of the research protocol. In this scenario, the community partner is often a subcontractor on the grant, working collaboratively with the academic research team to deliver the study program, like an educational or counseling intervention in the community setting. **Community advisory boards** are often used throughout the research process to provide input on elements of the study such as the protocol and recruitment materials. They also participate in dissemination of the results and planning for the next steps for partnership (Table 15.2). Advantages of this level of engagement include the intrinsic scientific merit of conducting a study in the community, coauthorship of resulting publications, the satisfaction of building

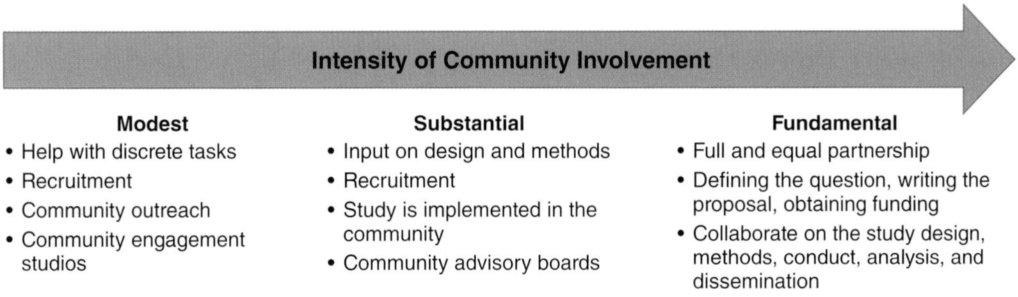

Intensity of Community Involvement

Modest	Substantial	Fundamental
• Help with discrete tasks	• Input on design and methods	• Full and equal partnership
• Recruitment	• Recruitment	• Defining the question, writing the proposal, obtaining funding
• Community outreach	• Study is implemented in the community	• Collaborate on the study design, methods, conduct, analysis, and dissemination
• Community engagement studios	• Community advisory boards	

■ **FIGURE 15.1** Community-engaged research continuum.

TABLE 15.2 COMMUNITY-ENGAGED RESEARCH APPROACHES

Community Outreach	Members of the research team (both community and academic) can give talks to increase awareness of key issues facing the community. This approach can engage community members, help in recruitment and retention for studies, and generate new ideas for future research.
Community Engagement Studios	This is a structured process that may be a service provided by institutions to facilitate project-specific input from relevant community and patient stakeholders to enhance research design, implementation, and dissemination (14). Investigators give a brief presentation and present a few questions to the studio panel, which is composed of community members. The panel members provide feedback, allowing colearning, and process evaluation.
Community Advisory Boards (CABs)	CABs serve as liaisons between the community and researchers. Most CABs include representatives from different community constituents (clients and staff of a community organization, members of religious groups, schools, media). CABs are convened early in the study; members review and provide input into elements of the study and meet throughout its life.

a collaborative community-academic partnership, and helping a community develop its own research capacity.

An example of a moderate intensity of community engagement was the Live Well Be Well study (15) that included an academic and community organization partnership with shared governance and divided responsibilities. The community partners were the staff at the California Department of Public Health (DPH) in the city of Berkeley who provided input into the methods of a diabetes prevention trial, conducted the telephone-based intervention, and assisted with the dissemination of the study findings. Academic partners were investigators at the University of California, San Francisco, who assisted with community outreach and recruitment, and conducted the program evaluation and data analysis. In this randomized controlled trial, the telephone-based lifestyle intervention resulted in significant reductions of weight and triglyceride levels and improved diet among community participants with prediabetes (16). Because of the DPH involvement from the inception of the program with the trial, this program was built to be sustainable and complementary to other programs that the health department offers routinely, and it continues to be offered years after trial completion.

Fundamental community engagement occurs when academic researchers work collaboratively with stakeholders to build the infrastructure to support research and identify opportunities for mutual benefit. In the most rigorous model, the community participates in all aspects of the research, from conception to the dissemination of findings. **Community-based participatory research (CBPR)** is based on community priorities with decision-making authority shared between community and academic researchers (9). The ultimate goal and reward is improved community-based outcomes and health equity. Some examples of long-term CBPR-oriented research are Asian American Network for Cancer Awareness, Research and Training San Francisco, a collaboration to promote cancer awareness and prevention (17), and Project GRACE in rural African American communities in North Carolina, whose projects were first focused on HIV awareness and prevention and have since evolved to cardiovascular disease prevention (18, 19).

Many studies funded through the federal PCORI have explicit requirements to include patients, family, community members, and health care stakeholders in all aspects of study development, governance, implementation, and dissemination (20). As an example, patient and health care stakeholders (nonclinical population health management staff doing routine patient outreach for primary care clinics) helped to choose and refine the weight loss intervention for a three-arm cluster-randomized trial among overweight patients with hypertension or type 2 diabetes. The trial compared usual care with either an online weight management program alone or a combined intervention with an online program and population health management staff. They found that the combined intervention led to greater weight loss than the online program or usual care (21). An advantage of this trial was that the researchers worked with existing population health teams that were already integrated in routine care in the clinics, using staff input to create a program that could be embedded in their workflow. This trial showed that systems-level changes in primary care clinics are feasible and effective, and can be scaled and sustained to improve patient health.

■ CHALLENGES OF COMMUNITY-ENGAGED RESEARCH

Without a thorough understanding of a community's cultural perspectives, many studies fail, despite careful planning and advanced technologies. Researchers must appreciate the local understandings and practices of disease and develop culturally sound approaches to their collaborative research. Lack of frequent communication and delayed response to queries are signs that a collaboration may be in trouble.

Building Trust

Trust between academic and community partners in is foundational and should be bidirectional. The community stakeholders and researchers must trust each other, and both partners need to believe that their collaboration will bring mutual benefit. Relationships with partners should be built before a research agenda is established. Threats that undermine trust can occur at individual, interpersonal, societal, and structural levels. Many communities have been neglected, condescended to, or exploited in the past by academic researchers, creating a legacy of distrust (22). Academic investigators have to put conscious efforts into repairing and strengthening these relationships with acknowledgment of past wrongs, honest dialogue, humility, and respect for all voices and experiences (23).

Academic investigators often have a position of power and privilege: They come from a well-resourced institution and have experience and training in clinical research and other tangible support. Acknowledging this privilege and sharing assets such as knowledge, skills, opportunities, and funding with community partners is essential to building trust in long-term relationships.

It takes time and effort needed to build trust with partners. Working with colleagues who have already established a trusting relationship with a community partner can be helpful. However, the junior investigator should also develop independent lines of clear and consistent communication and show commitment to community partners. One method to ensure good communication with community partners is to schedule regular meetings—preferably with food and refreshments, as well as time for socializing—for both parties to provide updates and give input into challenges and next steps.

Managing Timelines and Expectations

Planning meetings with community partners and stakeholders may be difficult to arrange; often meetings on weekends and in the evenings are necessary. Once a project is started, the community partner needs to find time and space in which to accommodate the research work in the organization's overall portfolio of activities. These issues need to be determined and agreed upon early in the planning period or they can derail any internal or funder-driven timelines. In general, it is good to expect delays in **study start-up** and with recruitment and to get early and ongoing input from the community stakeholders on what they think will be the most feasible timeline given their prior experience.

There are hierarchical structures of power in academia and in most community settings. However, some communities may have no formal organization or structure, making it difficult to find partners. In this case, the investigator should seek advocacy groups or other social services that interact with the community. However, working with representatives who do not represent the interests of the most vulnerable individuals in a community can exacerbate inequalities rather than increasing community capacity.

Other areas to clarify in the planning process of any new partnership are the roles and expectations of each of the parties. In most academic-based clinical studies, each subcontracting site has a scope of work, with tasks and deliverables. A clear communication of expectations with community partners is important especially if there is not a formal subcontract. In that circumstance, the investigator should consider developing a **Memorandum of Understanding (MOU)** that documents the scope of work, including the deliverables and general timeline, and is created and signed by both parties.

Academia rewards scientific productivity as measured by research grants and the number and quality of publications and presentations. In contrast, the rewards for nonacademic stakeholders are different, such as creation of sustainable programs that improve health, create jobs, and reduce disparities. Investigators who align their priorities and long-term goals with their community partners obtain the most reward and personal growth, especially if academic medical centers align their internal culture to be more flexible and inclusive of community input (24). All stakeholders stand to gain through increased collaboration and expanded research opportunities.

■ SUMMARY

1. Community-engaged research can help to identify cultural and other local factors that determine which interventions are most needed—and will be effective—in specific communities.
2. Participation in clinical research can benefit community partners by generating more applicable findings, creating local capacity and sustainable programs, and promoting health equity.
3. Although the design and ethical issues are similar to those related in any clinical research, practical issues such as building community partnerships and finding mentorship can be more difficult in a community setting. Tips for success include networking, starting small, and identifying local advantages.
4. Collaboration between academic centers and community researchers spans a continuum of intensity from modest (community investigators assist with discrete tasks that originate from the academic partner), to substantial (community investigators collaborate on outreach and conduct of the study), to fundamental (community and academic investigators collaborate equally in all aspects of the research).
5. Specific approaches include community outreach, community engagement studios, and community advisory boards.
6. Challenges include the time required to build trusting relationships and adequate management of timelines and expectations.

REFERENCES

1. Kenny JD, Tsoh JY, Nguyen BH, Le K, Burke NJ. Keeping each other accountable: social strategies for smoking cessation and healthy living in Vietnamese American men. *Fam Community Health*. 2021;44(3):215-224.
2. Tong EK, Saw A, Fung LC, Li CS, Liu Y, Tsoh JY. Impact of a smoke-free-living educational intervention for smokers and household nonsmokers: a randomized trial of Chinese American pairs. *Cancer*. 2018;124(Suppl 7):1590-1598.
3. Corburn J. Bringing local knowledge into environmental decision making: improving urban planning for communities at risk. *J Plan Educ Res*. 2003;22(4):420-433.
4. Griffith BN, Lovett GD, Pyle DN, et al. Self-rated health in rural Appalachia: health perceptions are incongruent with health status and health behaviors. *BMC Public Health*. 2011;11:229.
5. Victor RG, Lynch K, Li N, et al. A cluster-randomized trial of blood-pressure reduction in black barbershops. *N Engl J Med*. 2018;378:1291-1301.
6. Nutting PA, Beasley JW, Werner JJ. Practice-based research networks answer primary care questions. *JAMA*. 1999;281:686-688.
7. Miller RS, Ivenson DC, Fried RA, et al. Carpal tunnel syndrome in primary care: a report from ASPN. *J Fam Pract*. 1994;38:337-344.

8. Cooper L. Rethink how we plan research to shrink COVID health disparities. *Nature*. 2021;590:9.
9. Wallerstein N, Duran B, Oetzel J, Minkler M, eds. *Community-Based Participatory Research for Health: Advancing Social and Health Equity*. 3rd ed. Jossey-Bass; 2018.
10. Flood J, Minkler M, Hennessey Lavery S, et al. The Collective Impact Model and its potential for health promotion: overview and case study of a healthy retail initiative in San Francisco. *Health Educ Behavior*. 2015;42(5):654-668.
11. Kandula NR, Tirodkar MA, Lauderdale DS, et al. Knowledge gaps and misconceptions about coronary heart disease among U.S. South Asians. *Am J Prev Med*. 2010;38(4):439-442.
12. Kandula NR, Patel Y, Dave S, et al. The South Asian Heart Lifestyle Intervention (SAHELI) study to improve cardiovascular risk factors in a community setting: design and methods. *Contemp Clin Trials*. 2013;36(2):479-487.
13. Pasick R, Oliva G, Goldstein E, Nguyen T. Community-engaged research with community-based organizations: a resource manual for UCSF researchers. In: Fleisher P, ed. *UCSF Clinical and Translational Science Institute (CTSI) Resource Manuals and Guides to Community-Engaged Research*. Clinical Translational Science Institute Community Engagement Program, University of California San Francisco; 2010. http://ctsi.ucsf.edu
14. Joosten YA, Israel TL, Williams NA, et al. Community Engagement Studios: a structured approach to obtaining meaningful input from stakeholders to inform research. *Acad Med*. 2015;90(12):1646-1650.
15. Delgadillo AT, Grossman M, Santoyo-Olsson J, et al. Description of an academic-community partnership lifestyle program for lower-income, minority adults at risk for diabetes. *Diabetes Educ*. 2010;36(4):640-650.
16. Kanaya AM, Santoyo-Olsson J, Gregorich S, et al. A telephone-based lifestyle intervention trial to lower risk factors in ethnic minority and lower socioeconomic status adults at risk of diabetes: the live well be well study. A randomized controlled trial. *Amer J Public Health*. 2012;102(8):1551-1558.
17. McPhee SJ, Nguyen TT, Mock J, et al. Highlights/best practices of San Francisco's Asian American Network of Cancer Awareness, Research, and Training (AANCART). *Cancer*. 2005;104(12):2920-2925.
18. Corbie-Smith G, Adimore AA, Youmans S, et al. Project GRACE: a staged approach to development of a community-academic partnership to address HIV in rural African American communities. *Health Promot Pract*. 2011;12(2):293-302.
19. Corbie-Smith G, Wiley-Cene C, Bess K, et al. Heart Matters: a study protocol for a community-based randomized trial aimed at reducing cardiovascular risk in a rural, African American community. *BMC Public Health*. 2018;938.
20. Hickam D, Totten A, Berg A, et al. *The PCORI Methodology Report*. Patient-Centered Outcomes Research Institute; 2013.
21. Baer HJ, Rozenflum R, De La Cruz BA, et al. Effect of an online weight management program integrated with population health management on weight change. A randomized clinical trial. *JAMA*. 2020;324(17):1737-1746.
22. Pacheco CM, Daley SM, Brown T, et al. Moving forward: breaking the cycle of mistrust between American Indians and researchers. *Am J Public Health*. 2013;103:2152-2159.
23. Moreno-John G, Gachie A, Fleming CM, et al. Ethnic minority older adults participating in clinical research: developing trust. *J Aging Health*. 2004;16(5 Suppl):93S-123S.
24. Michener L, Cook J, Ahmed SM, et al. Aligning the goals of community-engaged research: why and how academic health centers can successfully engage with communities to improve health. *Acad Med*. 2012;87(3):285-291.

APPENDIX 15A
Exercise for Chapter 15. Community-Engaged Research

1. A new investigator wants to find ways to improve breast cancer screening among immigrant Asian women. She is early in her planning process for this study and is considering ways to include community partners for this study.
   a. Describe different approaches that the investigator can use for modest or substantial community involvement in this project.
   b. What are the advantages and the challenges of using the modest versus substantial intensities for community engagement?

CHAPTER 16

Research Using Existing Data or Specimens

Mark J. Pletcher, Deborah G. Grady, and Steven R. Cummings

Many research questions can be answered quickly and efficiently using precollected research data or specimens. An investigator may access such data to do a **secondary data analysis** or combine existing data with new measurements in an **ancillary study**. An existing data source that is continuing to follow participants can be used to collect outcome data for a new prospective cohort study or randomized trial.

Data are also collected for reasons other than research. Health care delivery, for example, generates massive amounts of health-related data; and all our interactions with the internet or internet-connected devices like smartphones are tracked and recorded.

While studies using existing data have major advantages, such as speed and economy, they also have disadvantages. The accessible population, sample, and measurements are all predetermined. The sample may be narrower than desired (eg, only women ages 50 to 64 years old), the measurement approach may not be what the investigator would prefer (a history of hypertension in place of actual blood pressure), and the quality of the data may be poor (with many missing or incorrect values). Important confounders and outcomes may not have been measured adequately. **All these factors contribute to the main disadvantage of using existing data: the lack of control over what is available.** Nonetheless, making creative use of existing data and specimens is a fast and effective way for new investigators with limited resources to address important research questions, and it is the primary method for some types of research, such as studying health care delivery and "real-world" use of medical products (1).

In this chapter, we first discuss studies that involve the analysis of existing data, including their advantages and pitfalls (Table 16.1). We then review creative ways to use and enhance existing data, including meta-analysis, ancillary studies, combining different sources of data, and using an existing data collection mechanism for prospective studies including randomized trials.

■ EXISTING DATA SOURCES

Studies that rely on existing data depend heavily on where, when, how, and in whom those data were assembled. Such data sources have distinct advantages and disadvantages.

Data Collected for Research Purposes

Collecting data for research requires substantial resources and time. Use of existing research data helps investigators and funders maximize the value of their investments and honors the donation of time and energy from research participants.

National Surveys

All investigators should be aware of national surveys and other data collected by the government and made available for research. These surveys are either conducted in all available persons

TABLE 16.1 USES, ADVANTAGES, AND PITFALLS OF DIFFERENT TYPES OF EXISTING DATA

TYPE OF EXISTING DATA	USES/ADVANTAGES	PITFALLS
Research Data		
National surveys	• National scope • Sampling methods often allow generalization to U.S. population. • Well-documented and easily accessible	• Multilevel cluster sampling requires special analytic methods. • Limited set of measurements and participants • Another researcher may be doing a similar analysis and publish it sooner.
Registries	• Curated data elements from a focused target population (eg, patients with a particular disease)	• Inclusion of persons in a registry and data collection typically depends on nonrandom engagement from participants, health systems, or other institutions.
Other research studies	• Research-grade measurements are available, well-documented, and ready for statistical analysis.	• Volunteer participants in research studies differ from the general population. • Measurements made in the context of a research study may not reflect usual participant experience or physiology. • The investigator has no control over the study sample or measurements.
Health Care Delivery Data		

EHR data	• Extensive information is available on medical encounters, procedures, diagnoses, medications, laboratory measurements and outcomes.
	• Good for health care utilization, health services, disparities in health care delivery
		• Deriving useful data elements from complex EHR data is challenging.
		• Patients are included in EHR databases for specific reasons (they are sick, desire specific services, receive care) and must have access to the health system.
		• Interventions are not random, measurements are not systematic, but are performed because of the patient's personal/health characteristics, so:
		  • Evaluation of intervention effectiveness is subject to confounding by indication.
		  • Missing measurements are frequent and difficult to impute.
		  • Incomplete exposure and (especially) outcome ascertainment often occurs because patients receive care at multiple health care delivery systems
		• Data are sensitive, protected by HIPAA, and challenging to access.
		• Different EHR systems produce data that are structured in different ways and difficult to combine.

TABLE 16.1 USES, ADVANTAGES, AND PITFALLS OF DIFFERENT TYPES OF EXISTING DATA (*continued*)

TYPE OF EXISTING DATA	USES/ADVANTAGES	PITFALLS
Health care claims, billing, and other administrative data	• Extensive information is available on medical diagnoses and procedures (including laboratory measurements ordered) and limited information about medical encounters. • Good for health care utilization, health services, disparities in health care delivery • Relatively complete outcome ascertainment	• No clinical measurements are available (eg, lab values or blood pressure measurements). • Samples are typically limited (eg, >65 years old for Medicare data, few poor patients in private health plan data sets). • Data are sensitive, protected by HIPAA, and often expensive to obtain.
	***Internet and Device Data***	
Smartphone data	• Smartphone sensors collect data on location via global positioning system, movement via triaxial accelerometers, image data via cameras, and social interactions via call and text, and Bluetooth data from other devices. • Smartphone apps interact with users to gather additional subjective information (eg, diet records), deliver interventions, and synthesize data.	• Smartphone technology varies (iPhone vs. Android vs. text-only without internet access) and is associated with user characteristics. • Measurement presence, accuracy, and frequency depends on technology. • Users often engage with apps only transiently.
Consumer electronics data	• Consumer electronic devices connected to the internet can collect data actively (blood pressure or weight measurements) or passively (step counts, sleep). • Rapidly advancing technology	• Technology and measurements are highly variable and strongly associated with user characteristics. • Measurements are derived from proprietary algorithms and often not validated. • Users often engage with devices only transiently, do not recharge batteries, or otherwise disengage.
Social media	• Combination of structured (friend and group relationships) and unstructured (text content) data rich in information about user interests, habits, sentiments, mood, and social connections	• Measurement utility dependent on degree of user engagement. • May be sensitive and difficult to access.

EHR, electronic health record; HIPAA, Health Insurance Portability and Accountability Act.

(eg, a census or registry) or use sampling schemes designed to yield results that are nationally representative. As such, they have high potential value for research. Notable examples are below.

• **The National Health and Nutrition Examination Survey (NHANES)** employs population-based cluster random selection to identify a representative sample of the U.S. population and collects data from self-report (eg, demographic, socioeconomic, dietary, and health-related behaviors), physical examinations, laboratory tests, and other measurements. NHANES data can provide population-based estimates of disease prevalence, risk factors, and other variables. Data and documentation from NHANES are maintained by the National Center for Health Statistics (NCHS, cdc.gov/nchs), which also conducts other population-based surveys such as the National Health Interview Survey (NHIS).

- **The National Ambulatory Medical Care Survey (NAMCS)** is a nationally representative study of outpatient visits to office-based practices in the United States. NAMCS abstracts and codes information from medical records, including reasons for the visit, vital signs, presence and severity of pain, medications prescribed, and diagnoses. NAMCS and the National Hospital Ambulatory Medical Care Survey (NHAMCS, which includes nearly identical surveys of outpatient visits to hospital emergency departments and clinics) are coordinated and maintained by the NCHS.
- **The Medical Expenditure Panel Survey (MEPS)** is designed to measure utilization of health care services, their costs, how they are paid for, and availability and costs of health insurance in the United States. The survey is maintained by the Agency for Healthcare Research and Quality, which also supports the Healthcare Cost and Utilization Project (hcup-us.ahrq.gov) to provide access to health care databases such as the National Inpatient Sample (NIS) and the National Ambulatory Surgery Sample (NASS), as well as some state-level data.
- **The U.S. Census Bureau (census.gov)** attempts to collect survey data every 10 years from every person residing in the United States and makes much of it available along with more detailed survey information collected on a rolling sample of the U.S. population via the American Community Survey (2).
- **NCHS also maintains vital statistics for the U.S. population,** including records of all births and deaths. The National Death Index (NDI) is a centralized database of death certificate data, including date and cause of death. Deaths occurring during follow-up in a research study can be ascertained by submitting social security numbers, names, and/or dates of birth to the NDI when a participant has been lost to follow-up.
- **The Centers for Disease Control and Prevention's Wide-ranging ONline Data for Epidemiologic Research (CDC WONDER)** is a web-based system for accessing vital statistics and other public health data, including cancer and reportable infectious diseases (wonder.cdc.gov).

National survey data can be used for many purposes. For example, investigators used NHANES to describe normal values of bone mineral density of the hip in the United States and helped define "osteoporosis" as 2.5 standard deviations below the young adult average (3); used NHAMCS to demonstrate disparities in opioid prescribing for pain in U.S. emergency departments (4); and used the NDI to complete follow-up for vital status in a randomized trial of a wearable defibrillator for prevention of sudden cardiac death (5).

New investigators are encouraged to consider whether an analysis of national survey data in their area of interest might be worthwhile. One challenge of using national survey data is using the correct statistical methods to account for any cluster sampling methods, but this is overcome easily with statistical support. It is also possible to get "scooped" by another investigator because the data are so accessible.

Registries

Registries identify persons belonging to a specific population (eg, women with newly diagnosed breast cancer) and collect information designed to facilitate future research analyses (6). Registry data can be analyzed to answer a specific research question, linked with other data sources, or used for participant recruitment. Unlike national survey data, registries do not use random sampling methodology, but instead are constructed through participation of willing health systems or other institutions, or through direct engagement of the target population.

Cancer registries have collected population-based data on cancer incidence, treatment, and outcomes since 1973 via the Surveillance, Epidemiology, and End Results (*SEER*) program. SEER registries cover many states and regions and three Native American populations (seer.cancer.gov/registries); the National Program of Cancer Registries helps collect data for other parts of the United States (cdc.gov/cancer/npcr). Investigators used the SEER registry to show that the incidence of estrogen receptor–positive breast cancer declined in postmenopausal women between 2001 and 2003, a trend that paralleled the reduction in the use of hormone replacement therapy, suggesting a causal association (7). The Greater Bay Area and Los Angeles SEER registries were used to recruit and interview a sample of women with breast cancer who had completed primary treatment within 5 years. The investigators found that low-acculturated Chinese women had worse physical functioning but better emotional functioning and lower anxiety than White women (8).

Cardiovascular disease registries are also well-developed in the United States. The American College of Cardiology supports the National Cardiovascular Data Registry (cvquality.acc .org/NCDR-Home) program, which maintains registries for patients with various conditions (such as chest pain or myocardial infarction and atrial fibrillation) or who have received certain treatments (such as percutaneous coronary interventions [PCIs], implanted cardioverter-defibrillators, and outpatient prevention). These data have been used by investigators to show that although appropriate treatment of patients with atrial fibrillation with oral anticoagulant therapy has been increasing, only half of high-risk patients receive a prescription (9).

The National Institutes of Health (NIH) maintains a list of registries with links to web materials and study contact information (10), but these represent only a subset of what enterprising investigators may find in their fields. The Patient-Centered Outcomes Research Institute funded a large set of "patient-powered" registries that include patient-reported information and outcomes with engagement through online portals (11). For example, the **Health eHeart Study** (health-eheartstudy.org) is a large online registry of persons interested in heart health and technology, many donating data from their smartphones and wearable devices; and the Pride Study (pridestudy.org) is a registry of self-identified LGBTQ+ persons interested in contributing their data for research and participating in ancillary studies. Health eHeart Study data collected from use of a smartphone app designed to measure pulse via placing a finger on the camera lens were used to develop a "digital biomarker" associated with self-reported diabetes status that was then validated in several external populations (12).

The **United Kingdom Biobank** enrolled 500,000 volunteers with linked data from questionnaires and electronic health records (EHRs) and has developed an extensive set of measurements including whole genome sequencing; metabolomics; and brain, heart, and body magnetic resonance imaging (ukbiobank.ac.uk). Using these data, investigators estimated that overall physical activity levels are about 20% heritable in a genome-wide association study of device-measured physical activity (13). The NIH's **All of Us Research Program** supports a registry (allofus.nih.gov) that will collect data from self-report, EHRs, devices, and biospecimens including genetic materials from a large cohort of participants.

Registries depending on active participant engagement typically recruit samples that are more White and more highly educated than the underlying population (14), and resulting analyses must be interpreted accordingly.

Other Research Studies

Most research studies store data for future use. The NIH and other major funders require data management and sharing plans for funded projects, and journals often require authors to provide access to data for secondary analyses. For some NIH-funded studies, a key project goal is to support secondary data analyses. For example, the Coronary Artery Disease In Young Adults (CARDIA) study (cardia.dopm.uab.edu), a multicenter cohort study funded by NIH to investigate the development and determinants of coronary artery disease, has well-documented procedures for requesting data and proposing ancillary studies, a publications committee to approve requests and resulting manuscripts, and analysts that verify study results before publication. The rich, unique, and repeated measurements collected by CARDIA over decades have been used for over 700 publications including many unrelated to coronary artery disease, such as a study that used pulmonary function test measurements and survey data to demonstrate that smoking marijuana at usual levels does not impact pulmonary function, in contrast to smoking tobacco (15). The NIH-funded Osteoarthritis Initiative hosts an extensive online resource for learning about and accessing research data including images of osteoarthritic knees (nda. nih.gov/oai). The Alzheimer's Disease Neuroimaging Initiative, which has data from patients with Alzheimer's disease as well as others with mild or no cognitive impairment, includes radiologic images, genetics, cognitive tests, and cerebrospinal fluid and blood biomarkers (adni.loni. usc.edu). The NIH also hosts extensive indexed repositories for genomic and phenotypic data (dbGaP at ncbi.nlm.nih.gov/gap) and for data from research studies funded by the National Heart, Lung, and Blood Institute (BioLINCC at biolincc.nhlbi.nih.gov/home).

In addition, smaller research studies also usually collect more data than they can analyze; though they tend to have less formal mechanisms for requesting access to data, many investigators are open to reasonable requests for collaboration.

Getting Started with Research Data

After choosing a research topic and becoming familiar with the literature in that area, new investigators should look into whether their research question can be addressed through secondary analysis of existing data, including data collected for unrelated reasons. Experienced research mentors can be invaluable in identifying—and gaining access to—an appropriate data set, whether at their own institution or elsewhere.

For example, the Osteoporotic Fractures in Men Study enrolled community-dwelling older men to study risk factors for osteoporotic fractures. A new investigator, with the help of mentors, accessed these data and demonstrated that frailty was more common in men with lower urinary tract symptoms (16). The Heart and Estrogen/Progestin Replacement Study (HERS), a clinical trial of hormone replacement to prevent additional coronary events in women with coronary heart disease (17), required participants to have a normal Pap test to enter the trial and annually thereafter. A new investigator used HERS data to document that although 110 Pap tests were abnormal among the 2763 women screened, only one woman had abnormal follow-up histology (ie, all but one of the abnormal Pap tests were falsely positive) (18). This study influenced the subsequent U.S. Preventive Services Task Force recommendation that Pap tests should not be performed in low-risk women over age 65 years with previous normal tests.

Sometimes an internet search is all that is required to find an accessible source of existing data. NHANES and BioLINCC, for example, have websites that provide open access to study data. Other studies like CARDIA or the Framingham Heart Study (framinghamheartstudy. org), which launched the field of cardiovascular epidemiology, have procedures for requesting data that welcome new investigators. When the data are not available online, phone calls or e-mail messages to the authors of previous studies or to government officials may be helpful. It is a good practice to use official titles and your institutional domain name on correspondence or e-mail and to copy your mentor as someone who will be recognized in the field. New investigators should determine if their mentors are acquainted with the investigators who developed the database, as an introduction may be more effective than a cold contact. That said, most investigators are surprisingly cooperative when contacted by a younger colleague with an interesting research question and will either provide the requested data themselves or suggest other places to try.

It is helpful to find an investigator on the original study team who is willing to become a collaborator. This investigator can facilitate access to the data and ensure understanding of the study methods and how the variables were measured. It is wise to define collaborative relationships early on, including who will be first and last author of planned publications. Developing collaborative relationships with investigators at other institutions is gratifying and valuable for both parties and helps new investigators develop opportunities and independence from mentors at their home institution.

Health Care Delivery Data

An abundance of data is stored in EHRs, generated from billing and claims sent to health care payers, and exchanged within the complex network of hospitals, clinics, pharmacies, laboratories, and other entities that comprise the U.S. health care delivery system. Health care delivery data, and other "real-world data" collected outside the context of a research study (1), have three major advantages: they are not limited to self-selected altruistic participants willing to donate their time and energy to science, the measurements collected are less subject to distortion from participants knowing they are being observed for a research study, and the number of observations tends to be large. On the other hand, health care delivery data are hard to access, challenging to analyze, incomplete, and reflect the complexity and fragmentation of medical care in the United States. Below are some examples of how they can be used.

- EHR data can be used to study how clinicians work, how they use EHR systems, and their impact on clinical care and clinician well-being. For example, investigators analyzed EHR audit logs and found that time spent working in the EHR after hours on clinical days was associated with burnout measured by a clinician survey (19).
- Health care delivery data can be used to study time trends, disparities, and other patterns in how health services are delivered to a population. For example, investigators analyzed opioid prescribing orders in EHR data from a large network of community health centers and found higher rates of prescribing in non-Hispanic White patients than other racial/ethnic groups and a substantial decrease in opioid prescriptions per capita from 2009 to 2018 (20).
- Health care delivery data can be used to evaluate quality of care. For example, investigators used Medicare claims data to show that individual surgeons with a high volume of surgery had substantially lower operative mortality than low-volume surgeons for many high-risk procedures ranging from aortic valve replacement to pancreatic cancer resection (21).
- Though it is fraught with potential for bias and misinterpretation (22), health care delivery data are also sometimes used to make inferences about the effectiveness and safety of medical products or other interventions. For example, investigators used EHR data from the Veterans Affairs Health System to study elderly veterans who were new users of statins, compared them to nonusers with propensity score weighting, and found that statin initiation was associated with reduced mortality (23). However, the likelihood that the association represents a causal effect seems low, in part because the effect size was more than five times larger for noncardiovascular than for cardiovascular mortality (24). Other investigators used a combined sample of claims and EHR data to compare monotherapy with different types of antihypertensive medications and found lower rates of myocardial infarction, heart failure, and stroke in new users of thiazide or thiazide-like diuretics when compared with new users of angiotensin-converting enzyme inhibitors (25).

Making inferences about effectiveness of medical interventions using observational data is susceptible to confounding. In the real world (ie, not in a randomized controlled trial), patients exposed to a medical product or other medical intervention differ from patients who are not exposed: they have access to care, a perceived medical indication for the intervention, and must start and then adhere to the intervention over time. These factors themselves (rather than the intervention) may be strongly associated with outcomes, resulting in confounding by indication and healthy user effects (26). Various methods, including multivariable adjustment, propensity scores-weighted or matched samples, and "trial emulation" methods may make users more comparable to nonusers in an analysis (see Chapter 10). Residual confounding, however, is *always* a challenge and may be insurmountable (22).

Analyzing trends over time within and between groups can also be used to evaluate interventions. Health care delivery organizations often modify procedures, for quality improvement or other organizational imperatives. Investigators can analyze outcomes before and after such modifications occur to make inferences about their effects. As described in Chapter 12, these designs may be useful when modifications occur abruptly in time and variably across clinical units or institutions, but confounding can occur due to co-occurring time trends.

Use of existing data from health care delivery for research is also fraught with problems from selection bias, missing data, and loss to follow-up. Health care data should be used cautiously to make inferences about a population because persons who seek and obtain health care are different from those who do not. Health care–related measurements, like laboratory tests, are performed for clinical reasons, so the presence and timing of a measurement are often more informative than the result of the measurement itself (27). Also, because patients may obtain health care from multiple institutions, outcome ascertainment during follow-up is often incomplete when EHR data from a single institution are used for research. Health care claims data available from Medicare or private insurers may be more complete in this regard, but the fragmentation of the U.S. health care system makes complete outcome ascertainment a challenge. EHRs work well for short cohort studies of hospitalized inpatients where follow-up is complete upon discharge. Health systems integrated with a health plan, like Kaiser Permanente, can also provide reliable follow-up data for cohort studies of outpatients.

Deriving usable variables from health care delivery data is challenging. EHR data are structured primarily to collect data to support billing and secondarily to support convenient data entry and retrieval by clinicians in a myriad of different clinical contexts. As such, similar data elements like clinical diagnoses or medication codes are often found in many different data tables. For example, medication codes can be found in tables storing historical medications, current medication lists, prescription orders, administration events, and dispensing events. Coding systems may be designed to provide specificity (eg, about a specific brand, dose, and formulation of a medication) or hierarchical consistency (eg, ICD10 = S93.4 is used for an encounter for an ankle sprain; S93.421A is for an initial encounter for sprain of the deltoid ligament of the right ankle); however, they are used inconsistently by clinicians and are challenging to group into meaningful concepts. For example, defining a simple indicator variable for presence of type 2 diabetes using EHR data can require complex logic involving diabetes-related diagnosis codes, medications used only or mostly by diabetic patients, and lab tests that might indicate the presence of untreated and undiagnosed diabetes.

EHR systems and data structures are customized for each institution where they are installed to support local clinical workflows and preferences. This is true even if they use the same EHR system vendor (eg, Epic). The result is that extraction and analysis code written for one institution may not work for any other. Research networks have developed to support common data models with harmonized table and variable names and definitions to facilitate use of EHR data and claims data for research across institutions. For example, the University of California's six medical centers support transforming their EHR data into the OMOP (Observational Medical Outcomes Partnership) Common Data Model (promoted by the Observational Health Data Sciences and Informatics program [ohdsi.org]) and pooling those data in a single data warehouse (data.ucop.edu). The Veterans Affairs Health System and other institutions also use OMOP. The Patient-Centered Outcomes Research Institute supports PCORnet, the National Patient-Centered Clinical Research Network (pcornet.org), which includes the PCORnet Common Data Model and a network of contractual relationships to facilitate multicenter studies. Common data models make multicenter research with EHR data possible, but they are expensive to develop and maintain and lack much of the detail and specificity that is present in the native data tables.

Getting Started with Health Care Delivery Data

Access to health care delivery data is controlled to protect privacy and confidentiality and due to its perceived institutional value. According to the Health Insurance Portability and Accountability Act (HIPAA), a patient's health care data can be accessed for research when that patient signs a consent and **HIPAA authorization**, or with a waiver of consent and authorization that can be granted in a limited set of circumstances by an institutional review board. HIPAA requires that data derived from EHRs be accessed through honest brokers that provide only the **minimum necessary** data for a project. Many institutions also create **deidentified** versions of their health care delivery data sets that are stripped of the 18 elements of **protected health information**; **limited data sets** that are deidentified except for dates and zip codes can be accessed with a **data use agreement**. Understanding the basics of HIPAA helps investigators interested in analyzing health care delivery data navigate the processes required for accessing these data.

Large health care claims data sets have been assembled by payers, including Medicare and private insurers. Medicare and Medicaid claims data sets can be purchased through government agencies (data.medicare.gov). For-profit companies like Optum and Truven Health Analytics bundle and sell access to large sets of claims data from private insurance companies.

Analyzing these large data sets can be a technical challenge. Database programs often require use of structured query language to extract data into a manageable form for statistical analysis (Chapter 19). Informatics training is useful for understanding and navigating coding systems used in health care data. Getting help from specialized analysts with experience is recommended.

Internet and Device Data

Data derived from interactions with the internet and internet-connected devices are collected and used by companies to target advertising, increase consumer engagement, and otherwise support business goals. Some companies make their data available to their consumers or to other entities including researchers. Below are examples of how internet and device data can be used for research.

- Use of the internet—conducting searches for information, reading news, shopping and interacting via social media—generates data that may be useful for research. For example, an investigator used free text data from Twitter to create and validate an algorithm that detected negative racial sentiments in tweets and used the algorithm to demonstrate a large increase in negative tweets referencing Asian Americans following emergence of the COVID-19 pandemic [28].
- Smartphones employ a variety of sensors including audio, video (from the camera), location (from global positional systems), movement (from triaxial accelerometers), and Bluetooth receivers to gather data. Some smartphone applications ("apps") use proprietary algorithms to convert raw signal from these sensors into health information. For example, accelerometer data can be used to track step counts and time spent exercising, and video from the camera can be used to detect the pulse in a user's fingertip. Investigators collaborated with a technology company with a free and popular smartphone app to show widespread global reductions in physical activity during the COVID-19 pandemic [29].
- Other electronic devices collect data either actively (eg, a Bluetooth-connected scale in your bathroom to measure body weight) or passively (an activity tracker on your wrist). These devices send data to centralized servers, usually via an internet-connected smartphone. For example, a wristwatch device connected to a smartphone can detect irregular pulse. Investigators collaborated with the company making the device, provided an ECG patch for up to 7 days to persons with an apparently irregular pulse, and diagnosed atrial fibrillation in 34% [30].

Internet and device data from a single source tend to be limited to a small set of measurements, but they are often repeated over time, sometimes with very high frequency. Users of internet-connected consumer devices tend to be different from the general population, so results from research studies using convenience samples of device users may not generalize. Although most adults in the United States now own a mobile phone, their phone type, internet access, and data plans vary by socioeconomic status. Also, usage of many internet services, smartphone apps, and wearable devices that require active engagement (eg, charging the device and putting it on) tends to wane quickly over time. Investigators interested in systematic collection of internet or device data for a research study may need to supply devices to study participants and incentivize their ongoing use.

Getting Started with Internet and Device Data

Getting access to internet and device data can be a challenge. Some companies are willing to collaborate and provide access to their data directly; a few, like Twitter, make their data publicly available.

A special mechanism for obtaining internet and device data involves active authorization by users. Technology companies often make data available to other applications their customers use, for example, by enabling their cloud-based servers to communicate with other servers via an **application programming interface (API)**. Researchers can access these data with permission from participants, though doing so requires specialized programming and infrastructure. The **Eureka Research Platform** (info.eurekaplatform.org), an NIH-funded platform available for use by funded investigators, specializes in mobile health (mHealth) data collection via API-based interaction with commercial platforms along with electronic consent (eConsent), online surveys, and smartphone app-based data collection directly from engaged research participants.

■ CREATIVE USES OF EXISTING DATA

Existing data alone may suffice for answering a research question. Sometimes, however, doing so requires more creative use, augmentation with other data sources, or special methods.

Meta-Analysis

When more than one study has data on a similar research question (such as whether statins are effective in the elderly), existing data may be combined in a **meta-analysis** to develop a single summary estimate. Often, this process begins with a **systematic review** of the published literature, accomplished by taking a comprehensive and specified approach to identify all studies of a given research question, with clear criteria that define which studies to include, and standardized methods to extract data from those studies.

When participant-level data from the reviewed studies are available, a single large data set may be created and analyzed de novo in a "pooled" meta-analysis. For example, by combining data from randomized trials of statin therapy, the Cholesterol Treatment Trialists' Collaboration showed evidence of statin efficacy even in participants older than 75 years, who had comprised a very small proportion of study participants in the trials (31).

More often, only the results of the reviewed studies (without participant-level data) are available from published articles. By combining results from different studies, summary estimates may be obtained that are more precise than any study could produce alone. Special analysis techniques must be used to combine estimates from different studies in order to account for the precision of each estimate. Studies that are larger result in more precise estimates (with narrower confidence intervals), and the estimates from these studies carry more weight in meta-analysis. For example, investigators used meta-analysis of subgroup findings from 40 randomized trials (each of which included only a limited number of older adults) to demonstrate that exercise programs lasting at least 1 year resulted in lower risks of falls and injurious falls in persons 60 years of age and older (32).

The inevitable differences among studies must be considered in a meta-analysis. Meta-analysis techniques produce estimates of **heterogeneity** (how different results are across studies). When substantial heterogeneity is present—meaning that different studies may not reflect estimates of the same underlying phenomenon—it may not be reasonable to report a single summary estimate that averages results across studies. Analyzing subsets of studies that have more similar characteristics can be useful, as can **meta-regression**, which accounts for study characteristics simultaneously. For example, the meta-analysis described earlier conducted a series of meta-regressions suggesting an optimal exercise frequency of two to three times per week (32). Meta-regression, however, requires either individual-level data or data from many studies.

A more pernicious problem is **publication bias**, which occurs when studies that are published (or otherwise available for inclusion in a meta-analysis) do not represent all completed studies, typically because positive studies are more likely to be published than negative ones. Investigators undertaking a meta-analysis should: (1) do a systematic review of the published literature to identify all relevant published studies; (2) look for evidence of unpublished studies (eg, by asking investigators in the field and reviewing abstracts, meeting presentations, and doctoral theses) and obtain the results whenever possible; and (3) use special meta-analytic techniques to analyze study results for evidence of publication bias (eg, when there appears to be an unexpected dearth of small studies with less favorable results) (33).

New investigators may gain much from undertaking a systematic review and meta-analysis, including a deep understanding of published literature in their field of interest and a publication of their own that can help establish them as an expert. However, even though systematic reviews may not require much funding, they require substantial time and effort. Investigators undertaking a systematic review should consider resources published by the Cochrane network, including the *Cochrane Handbook for Systematic Reviews* (http://handbook.cochrane.org), and seek out help or additional training in meta-analysis techniques.

Ancillary Studies

In an ancillary study, the investigator designs and adds measurements to an existing research study to answer a new research question. Ancillary studies have many of the advantages of secondary data analysis with fewer constraints. They can be added to any type of study, but are particularly well suited for prospective cohort studies and randomized trials. For example, in the HERS trial of the effect of postmenopausal hormone therapy (17), an investigator added measurements of the frequency and severity of urinary incontinence, thereby creating a large trial of the effect of hormone therapy on urinary incontinence, with little additional time or expense (34).

Ancillary studies are usually most informative when measurements are added before enrollment begins, and it may be difficult for an outsider to identify a potential "host" study that is still in the planning phase. Even when a variable was not measured at baseline, however, adding a single measurement during or at the end of a trial can produce useful information. By measuring cognitive function at the end of the HERS trial, for example, investigators were able to compare the cognitive function of elderly women treated with hormone therapy for 4 years to those treated with placebo (35).

Investigators responsible for a study must balance participant burden with the scientific gains from data collection. Adding ancillary measurements may upset that balance and even lead to participant dissatisfaction and dropout. New investigators should be sensitive to this issue and design ancillary studies that participants will find engaging and that will not be detrimental to the main study.

Ancillary studies can also use the banks of biospecimens, images, and other materials that are collected by most large clinical trials and cohort studies. Making new measurements in these stored specimens can be a cost-effective approach to answering a novel research question that does not add any burden to participants. Often it is possible (and efficient) to make these measurements on a subset of specimens using a nested case-control or case-cohort design (Chapter 9). In HERS, for example, a nested case-control study carried out genetic analyses on stored specimens and showed that the excess number of thromboembolic events in the hormone-treated group was not due to an interaction with factor V Leiden (36).

Most large, multicenter studies require a written application for an ancillary study that is reviewed by a committee that can approve, reject, or revise the study plan; some require collaboration with a study investigator. Many ancillary measurements require additional funding, and the ancillary study investigator must find a way to pay these costs. (Of course, the marginal cost of an ancillary study is far less than the cost of conducting the same study independently.)

Ancillary studies are well suited for some types of NIH funding that provide modest support for measurements and analyses but substantial support for career development (Chapter 20). Some large studies have their own mechanisms for funding ancillary studies, especially if the research question is important and considered relevant by the funding agency.

Combining Data from Multiple Sources

Two or more existing data sets may be linked to create a new one. For example, investigators who were interested in how military service affects health used data from the 1970 to 1972 draft lottery (the first data set), which determined the order, based on their birthdates, in which 20-year-old American men were drafted for military service during the Vietnam War. Data about mortality were ascertained from death certificate registries from California and Pennsylvania (the second source of data). The predictor variable (date of birth) was a randomly assigned proxy for military service. The study found that men who had been randomly assigned to be eligible for the draft had significantly greater mortality from suicide and motor vehicle accidents in the ensuing 10 years (37). The study was done inexpensively, yet it was a more unbiased approach to examining the effect of military service on specific causes of subsequent death than other studies with much larger budgets.

Location-based data can be combined profitably with data from other sources. For example, investigators obtained information on deaths from asthma by location in Philadelphia (the first data source) as well as information about crowding, poverty, and other demographic information about census tracts in Philadelphia from the 1990 U.S. Census (the second data source) and found a strong association between living in a census tract with high levels of poverty and mortality from asthma (38). Other investigators combined step count data collected from Fitbit devices in the Health eHeart Study (the first data source), linked it with air quality sensor data over time (the second data source), and demonstrated an 18% reduction in daily step counts associated with poor versus reasonable air quality during the 2017 to 2018 wildfire seasons in California (39).

Linking data sources by institution is sometimes possible. For example, investigators obtained discharge data from emergency departments from the California Office of Statewide Health Planning and Development (OSHPD, the first data set), linked those data by institution over time to ambulance diversion data collected from California local emergency medical services agencies (the second data set), and showed no increase in readmissions on days when emergency departments are overcrowded (40).

When data sources are combined and analyzed only at an aggregate level (not using individual-level data), inferences about causal relationships at an individual level are relatively weak and subject to what is known as the **ecologic fallacy**. For example, investigators demonstrated that breast cancer incidence rates, which varied more than fivefold across 21 countries, increased with per capita intake of dietary fat (41). However, analyses of high-quality dietary and outcome data on individual participants in the Nurses' Health Study did not support this increase (relative risk of breast cancer per 5% increase in total fat intake = 0.96; 95% confidence interval: 0.93 to 0.99) (42). The apparently incorrect result from the ecologic analysis was blamed on severe confounding by country-level differences in breast cancer risk factors such as later onset of menses and use of hormone replacement therapy that were also correlated with per capita fat intake (42).

Randomized Trials Using Existing Data Collection Mechanisms

Sometimes an existing data collection mechanism can be used for prospective data collection in a cohort study or randomized trial.

A **randomized registry trial**, for example, adds a randomized intervention to the ongoing data collection within a registry (43). For example, the Swedish Coronary Angiography and Angioplasty Registry collects data prospectively for patients undergoing percutaneous coronary intervention (PCI). Investigators randomly assigned some patients in the registry to undergo thrombus aspiration at the time of PCI and used the registry to compare clinical outcomes including recurrent myocardial infarction and stroke. They found no difference in outcomes when the thrombus aspiration patients were compared with those randomized to PCI only (44).

EHR-embedded randomized trials use EHR data collection systems to compare outcomes among subsets of patients, encounters, clinicians, or clinical units that are randomly assigned to receive different interventions. For example, investigators conducted a cluster-randomized trial in five intensive care units to compare use of saline versus balanced crystalloids and found a slightly lower risk of major adverse kidney events in patients who received balanced crystalloids (45).

In a **randomized quality improvement trial**, investigators implement a quality improvement intervention only partially—with some patients or providers randomly receiving the intervention and others not, often using a stepped wedge design (Chapter 12)—to determine whether it is effective and has no unintended consequences. This helps determine whether the intervention should be implemented fully (ie, for all patients/providers). For example, investigators randomly assigned a lower default quantity for opioid prescriptions (but still allowed clinicians to decide on the prescribed dose) and showed that doing so reduced the average quantity of opioids dispensed (46).

Randomized quality improvement trials are particularly useful for studying interventions that use an EHR system to prompt providers to follow guidelines, provide clinical decision support, or otherwise take actions likely to improve care. These trials **may be embedded entirely in the EHR system**, with patient selection, randomization, intervention delivery, and follow-up conducted automatically, but several ethical implications and methodologic challenges must be considered (47). EHR-embedded randomized trials and randomized quality improvement trials are part of the National Academy of Medicine's vision for a "learning health system" (48).

■ SUMMARY

1. **Prior research studies** are a rich and varied source of data. New investigators, working with mentors, should always determine whether data from a prior research study might be used to answer their research questions. Using data collected by mentors is a good way to start a research career.

2. **Health care delivery data** from EHR systems, health care claims, or other administrative sources can be used to study health care utilization, health services, and quality improvement. They are challenging to analyze and interpret due to potential selection bias and confounding.

3. **Internet and device data** collected by companies for business purposes can sometimes be accessed and used for research.

4. Conducting a **systematic review and meta-analysis**, combining results from several studies of the same basic research question, can be a good way for a new investigator to become an expert in a field of research. Meta-analyses should include assessment of heterogeneity and publication bias.

5. **Ancillary studies** allow investigators to leverage an existing study by adding one or more measurements. They are often inexpensive and efficient.

6. **Combining data from multiple sources** often allows an investigator to answer novel research questions. Aggregate-level associations can be subject to the *ecologic fallacy* and should be interpreted with caution.

7. **Randomized trials using existing sources of data collection**, when possible, can efficiently generate strong clinical evidence.

REFERENCES

1. US Food and Drug Administration. Real-World Evidence. Accessed April 4, 2021. https://www.fda.gov/science-research/science-and-research-special-topics/real-world-evidence

2. US Census Bureau. American Community Survey (ACS). Accessed April 30, 2021. https://www.census.gov/programs-surveys/acs.

3. Looker AC, Johnston CC, Jr., Wahner HW, et al. Prevalence of low femoral bone density in older U.S. women from NHANES III. *J Bone Miner Res*. 1995;10(5):796-802.

4. Pletcher MJ, Kertesz SG, Kohn MA, Gonzales R. Trends in opioid prescribing by race/ethnicity for patients seeking care in US emergency departments. *JAMA*. 2008;299(1):70-78.

5. Olgin JE, Pletcher MJ, Vittinghoff E, et al. Wearable cardioverter-defibrillator after myocardial infarction. *N Engl J Med*. 2018;379(13):1205-1215.

6. Workman TA. Engaging Patients in Information Sharing and Data Collection: The Role of Patient-Powered Registries and Research Networks. Agency for Healthcare Research and Quality; 2013.

7. Kerlikowske K, Miglioretti DL, Buist DS, et al. Declines in invasive breast cancer and use of postmenopausal hormone therapy in a screening mammography population. *J Natl Cancer Inst*. 2007;99(17):1335-1339.

8. Wang JH, Gomez SL, Brown RL, et al. Factors associated with Chinese American and White cancer survivors' physical and psychological functioning. *Health Psychol*. 2019;38(5):455-465.

9. Hsu JC, Maddox TM, Kennedy KF, et al. Oral anticoagulant therapy prescription in patients with atrial fibrillation across the spectrum of stroke risk: insights from the NCDR PINNACLE registry. *JAMA Cardiol*. 2016;1(1):55-62.

10. National Institutes of Health. List of Registries. Accessed April 30, 2021. https://www.nih.gov/health-information/nih-clinical-research-trials-you/list-registries.

11. PCORnet PPRN Consortium, Daugherty SE, Wahba S, Fleurence R. Patient-powered research networks: building capacity for conducting patient-centered clinical outcomes research. *J Am Med Inform Assoc*. 2014;21(4):583-586.

12. Avram R, Olgin JE, Kuhar P, et al. A digital biomarker of diabetes from smartphone-based vascular signals. *Nat Med*. 2020;26(10):1576-1582.

13. Doherty A, Smith-Byrne K, Ferreira T, et al. GWAS identifies 14 loci for device-measured physical activity and sleep duration. *Nat Commun*. 2018;9(1):5257.

14. Guo X, Vittinghoff E, Olgin JE, Marcus GM, Pletcher MJ. Volunteer participation in the health eheart study: a comparison with the US population. *Sci Rep*. 2017;7(1):1956.

15. Pletcher MJ, Vittinghoff E, Kalhan R, et al. Association between marijuana exposure and pulmonary function over 20 years. *JAMA*. 2012;307(2):173-181.

16. Bauer SR, Scherzer R, Suskind AM, et al. Co-occurrence of lower urinary tract symptoms and frailty among community-dwelling older men. *J Am Geriatr Soc*. 2020;68(12):2805-2813.

17. Hulley S, Grady D, Bush T, et al. Randomized trial of estrogen plus progestin for secondary prevention of coronary heart disease in postmenopausal women. Heart and Estrogen/progestin Replacement Study (HERS) Research Group. *JAMA*. 1998;280(7):605-613.

18. Sawaya GF, Grady D, Kerlikowske K, et al. The positive predictive value of cervical smears in previously screened postmenopausal women: the Heart and Estrogen/progestin Replacement Study (HERS). *Ann Intern Med*. 2000;133(12):942-950.

19. Adler-Milstein J, Zhao W, Willard-Grace R, Knox M, Grumbach K. Electronic health records and burnout: time spent on the electronic health record after hours and message volume associated with exhaustion but not with cynicism among primary care clinicians. *J Am Med Inform Assoc*. 2020;27(4):531-538.

20. Muench J, Fankhauser K, Voss RW, et al. Assessment of opioid prescribing patterns in a large network of US community health centers, 2009 to 2018. *JAMA Netw Open*. 2020;3(9):e2013431.

21. Birkmeyer JD, Stukel TA, Siewers AE, Goodney PP, Wennberg DE, Lucas FL. Surgeon volume and operative mortality in the United States. *N Engl J Med*. 2003;349(22):2117-2127.

22. Collins R, Bowman L, Landray M, Peto R. The magic of randomization versus the myth of real-world evidence. *N Engl J Med*. 2020;382(7):674-678.

23. Orkaby AR, Driver JA, Ho YL, et al. Association of statin use with all-cause and cardiovascular mortality in US veterans 75 years and older. *JAMA*. 2020;324(1):68-78.

24. Digitale JC, Newman TB. New statin use and mortality in older veterans. *JAMA*. 2020;324(18):1907-1908.

25. Suchard MA, Schuemie MJ, Krumholz HM, et al. Comprehensive comparative effectiveness and safety of first-line antihypertensive drug classes: a systematic, multinational, large-scale analysis. *Lancet*. 2019;394(10211):1816-1826.

26. Shrank WH, Patrick AR, Brookhart MA. Healthy user and related biases in observational studies of preventive interventions: a primer for physicians. *J Gen Intern Med*. 2011;26(5):546-550.

27. Agniel D, Kohane IS, Weber GM. Biases in electronic health record data due to processes within the healthcare system: retrospective observational study. *BMJ*. 2018;361:k1479.

28. Nguyen TT, Criss S, Dwivedi P, et al. Exploring U.S. shifts in anti-Asian sentiment with the emergence of COVID-19. *Int J Environ Res Public Health*. 2020;17(19).

29. Tison GH, Avram R, Kuhar P, et al. Worldwide effect of COVID-19 on physical activity: a descriptive study. *Ann Intern Med*. 2020;173(9):767-770.

30. Perez MV, Mahaffey KW, Hedlin H, et al. Large-scale assessment of a smartwatch to identify atrial fibrillation. *N Engl J Med*. 2019;381(20):1909-1917.

31. Cholesterol Treatment Trialists Collaboration. Efficacy and safety of statin therapy in older people: a meta-analysis of individual participant data from 28 randomised controlled trials. *Lancet*. 2019;393(10170):407-415.

32. de Souto Barreto P, Rolland Y, Vellas B, Maltais M. Association of long-term exercise training with risk of falls, fractures, hospitalizations, and mortality in older adults: a systematic review and meta-analysis. *JAMA Intern Med.* 2019;179(3):394-405.

33. Lin L, Chu H. Quantifying publication bias in meta-analysis. *Biometrics.* 2018;74(3):785-794.

34. Grady D, Brown JS, Vittinghoff E, et al. Postmenopausal hormones and incontinence: the Heart and Estrogen/Progestin Replacement Study. *Obstet Gynecol.* 2001;97(1):116-120.

35. Grady D, Yaffe K, Kristof M, Lin F, Richards C, Barrett-Connor E. Effect of postmenopausal hormone therapy on cognitive function: the Heart and Estrogen/progestin Replacement Study. *Am J Med.* 2002;113(7):543-548.

36. Herrington DM, Vittinghoff E, Howard TD, et al. Factor V Leiden, hormone replacement therapy, and risk of venous thromboembolic events in women with coronary disease. *Arterioscler Thromb Vasc Biol.* 2002;22(6):1012-1017.

37. Hearst N, Newman TB, Hulley SB. Delayed effects of the military draft on mortality. A randomized natural experiment. *N Engl J Med.* 1986;314(10):620-624.

38. Lang DM, Polansky M. Patterns of asthma mortality in Philadelphia from 1969 to 1991. *N Engl J Med.* 1994;331(23):1542-1546.

39. Rosenthal DG, Vittinghoff E, Tison GH, et al. Assessment of accelerometer-based physical activity during the 2017–2018 California wildfire seasons. *JAMA Netw Open.* 2020;3(9):e2018116.

40. Hsia RY, Asch SM, Weiss RE, et al. Is emergency department crowding associated with increased "bounceback" admissions? *Med Care.* 2013;51(11):1008-1014.

41. Prentice RL, Kakar F, Hursting S, Sheppard L, Klein R, Kushi LH. Aspects of the rationale for the Women's Health Trial. *J Natl Cancer Inst.* 1988;80(11):802-814.

42. Holmes MD, Hunter DJ, Colditz GA, et al. Association of dietary intake of fat and fatty acids with risk of breast cancer. *JAMA.* 1999;281(10):914-920.

43. Lauer MS, D'Agostino RB, Sr. The randomized registry trial—the next disruptive technology in clinical research? *N Engl J Med.* 2013;369(17):1579-1581.

44. Frobert O, Lagerqvist B, Olivecrona GK, et al. Thrombus aspiration during ST-segment elevation myocardial infarction. *N Engl J Med.* 2013;369(17):1587-1597.

45. Semler MW, Self WH, Wanderer JP, et al. Balanced crystalloids versus saline in critically ill adults. *N Engl J Med.* 2018;378(9):829-839.

46. Montoy JCC, Coralic Z, Herring AA, Clattenburg EJ, Raven MC. Association of default electronic medical record settings with health care professional patterns of opioid prescribing in emergency departments: a randomized quality improvement study. *JAMA Intern Med.* 2020;180(4):487-493.

47. Pletcher MJ, Flaherman V, Najafi N, et al. Randomized controlled trials of electronic health record interventions: design, conduct, and reporting considerations. *Ann Intern Med.* 2020;172(11 Suppl):S85-S91.

48. Friedman CP, Wong AK, Blumenthal D. Achieving a nationwide learning health system. *Sci Transl Med.* 2010;2(57):57cm29.

APPENDIX 16A
Exercises for Chapter 16. Research Using Existing Data or Specimens

1. The research question is: "Do Latinos in the United States have higher rates of gallbladder disease than other ethnicities and races?" What existing databases might enable you to determine race/ethnicity-, age-, and sex-specific rates of gallbladder disease at low cost in time and money?

2. A research fellow became interested in the question of whether mild or moderate renal dysfunction increases risk for coronary heart disease events and death. Because of the expense and difficulty of conducting a study to generate primary data, he searched for an existing database that contained the variables he needed to answer his research question. He found that the Cardiovascular Health Study (CHS), a large, NIH-funded multicenter cohort study of predictors of cardiovascular disease in older men and women, provided all of the variables required for his planned analysis. His mentor was able to introduce him to one of the key investigators in CHS who helped him prepare and submit a proposal for analyses that was approved by the CHS Steering Committee.

   a. What are the advantages of this approach to study this question?

   b. What are the disadvantages?

3. An investigator is interested in whether the effects of treatment with postmenopausal estrogen or selective estrogen receptor modulators (SERMs) vary depending on endogenous estrogen levels. How might this investigator answer this question using an ancillary study?

4. A group of investigators interested in use of sodium glucose cotransporter 2 (SGLT2) inhibitors during the COVID-19 pandemic has access to EHR data from a large academic health system that cares for many thousands of diabetic patients.

   a. A mechanistic hypothesis arose during the pandemic that SGLT2 inhibitors might make diabetic patients infected with COVID-19 more susceptible to severe disease. Describe how the investigators might use EHR data to address this mechanistic question, how confounding by indication might pose a threat to their ability to make causal inferences, and what analytic approach might be used to mitigate this threat.

   b. Because the mechanistic hypothesis was reported in the popular press, the investigators believe that SGLT2 inhibitor usage patterns may have changed. Describe how they might use EHR data to investigate this health care utilization hypothesis.

CHAPTER 17

Designing, Selecting, and Administering Self-Reported Measures

Alison J. Huang, Steven R. Cummings, and Michael A. Kohn

Much of the information used in clinical research is gathered using **self-reported measures** in which participants describe their own behaviors, attitudes, medical history, symptoms, functioning, or quality of life. For many studies, the validity of the findings depends on how well this information is ascertained.

Self-reported data can be collected in many ways, including paper-based or online questionnaires, diaries or logs completed on paper or using electronic devices, and structured interviews conducted in person or over the telephone. Regardless of how they are administered, good self-reported measures share the same design principles: **clear instructions or well-phrased questions that elicit informative responses**. Good self-reported measures are also **tailored to their target population**, including respondents' expected literacy levels and cultural assumptions.

In this chapter, we describe common types of self-reported measures, review the core elements of self-reported questions and response options, examine aspects of self-reported measures that may affect the quality of the data they yield, and outline procedures for selecting, adapting, and administering the right measures for a study.

■ COMMON TYPES OF SELF-REPORTED MEASURES

Self-reported data can be collected in multiple ways and for different purposes, such as:

- Structured interviews in which a study coordinator asks screening questions to assess whether a potential participant is eligible for a study
- E-mailed surveys, created using software like Qualtrics, SurveyMonkey, and REDCap, that allow participants to answer questions about their health history
- Paper-based questionnaires completed by participants at home or during study visits to describe their health-related quality of life
- Diaries that record the type and frequency of episodic symptoms for future data abstraction
- Electronic logs in which participants use a mobile phone or other portable electronic device to indicate when they perform a health-related behavior

■ BASIC ELEMENTS OF SELF-REPORTED QUESTIONS AND RESPONSES

Open- and Closed-Ended Questions

Structured self-reported measures use one of two basic formats. **Open-ended questions** invite free-form answers, allowing participants to respond in their own words, with fewer limits than is possible with a discrete list of answers. For example:

What habits do you believe increase a person's chance of having a stroke?

However, **open-ended questions may yield variable and unpredictable responses**, which means that they do not provide reliable information about the frequency of any one specific response. For example, the question above does not prompt respondents to identify smoking as a risk factor for stroke, even if they might have done so had it been suggested as an explicit response option. Open-ended questions also tend to require qualitative methods or special systems, such as coding dictionaries, to code and analyze the diverse responses they generate (Chapter 14).

Closed-ended questions include a list of possible answers for participants to choose, ensuring that each possibility is considered. This format may also help to clarify the meaning of an unclear question, and the selected answer(s) can be tabulated quickly. On the other hand, **closed-ended questions offer only answers that the researcher has anticipated and listed.** As a result, they lead participants in prespecified directions and do not allow them to express their own, potentially more accurate or informative answers.

Closed-Ended Question Response Options

When a single response to a closed-ended question is desired, the respondent should be instructed to "Choose one option only." For an online survey, the question should be programmed to accept only one response. The set of response options should also be **mutually exclusive** (ie, there should not be any meaningful overlap between response categories) to prevent confusion about which response to select.

Alternately, a closed-ended question (eg, "Which of the following do you believe increases the risk of stroke?") may invite more than one answer by instructing the respondent to choose "All that apply." However, this approach does not force the respondent to consider each possible response, so that an unselected response may represent either a "no" answer or an overlooked possibility. Instead, separate "yes" and "no" boxes for each response are preferable (Chapter 19).

When possible, response options for closed-ended questions should also be **collectively exhaustive** (ie, include all possible response options). If other potential responses are anticipated, questions may include an option such as "Other (please specify)" to elicit additional open-ended responses.

Ordered Response Options for Closed-Ended Questions

Many closed-ended questions are designed to capture the amount, frequency, or intensity of self-reported phenomena. These questions can yield ordered categorical data or can elicit responses that lie along a continuous scale.

For questions that involve ordered categorical response scales, respondents select a response from a ranked list. For example:

How severe was your pain in the past 7 days?
○ 1 = no pain
○ 2 = very mild
○ 3 = mild
○ 4 = moderate
○ 5 = severe
○ 6 = very severe

With a **Likert scale**, response options are arranged in bilaterally symmetric distances about a middle or "neutral" value option to accommodate participants with neutral or undecided feelings as well as those with more extreme feelings:

> **How satisfied are you with control of your pain in the past 7 days?**
> ○ 1 = very satisfied
> ○ 2 = satisfied
> ○ 3 = neither satisfied nor dissatisfied
> ○ 4 = dissatisfied
> ○ 5 = very dissatisfied

Another approach elicits responses along a continuous numerical scale, such as asking respondents to rate their pain severity from 0 (least) to 10 (most). Words or phrases may be added to anchor both the extreme ends and internals along the scale:

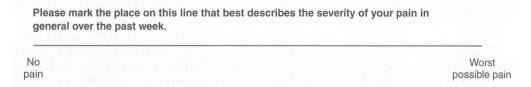

How severe was your pain in the past 7 days?

0	1	2	3	4	5	6	7	8	9	10
No pain		Mild pain		Moderate pain		Intense pain		Severe pain		Worst possible pain

A visual analog scale (VAS) asks for responses along a continuum, using lines or other figures. The participant is asked to mark a line at a spot along the continuum from one extreme to the other that best represents his answer. Once again, words that anchor each end describe the most extreme values for the item of interest, but intermediary descriptive terms are not usually included. VASs may be more sensitive to small changes than ratings based on categorical lists.

Please mark the place on this line that best describes the severity of your pain in general over the past week.

No pain   Worst possible pain

Branching Questions

Sometimes researchers wish to follow up certain answers to an initial question with more detailed questions. This can be accomplished by branching questions, in which the answer to an initial question (often referred to as a "screener") determines whether additional questions need to be answered. Branching questions can save time and allow respondents to avoid irrelevant or redundant questions.

On a paper-based instrument, a branching question must direct the respondent to the next appropriate question using an arrow that points from the initial response to the follow-up question and including directions such as "*Go to question 11*":

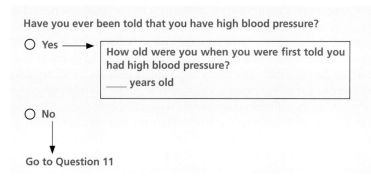

Have you ever been told that you have high blood pressure?

○ Yes → | How old were you when you were first told you had high blood pressure?
          | ____ years old

○ No
  ↓
Go to Question 11

One advantage of online instruments is that they can be programmed to incorporate automatic skip logic. For example, branching logic can be used so that participants who report never being told that they have high blood pressure are not asked *when* they were first told they had it. However, any skip logic programmed into branching questions must be validated during the study's pretesting phase, because complex skip logic can result in dead ends and "orphan" questions that are never reached.

Optimal Wording of Questions

Good self-reported questions are simple and free of ambiguity; they also encourage accurate and honest responses without embarrassing or offending the respondent.

- **Clarity.** Questions should be clear and specific, using concrete rather than abstract terms whenever possible. For example, asking, "How much exercise do you usually get?" may yield unreliable information if respondents have different ideas about what constitutes exercise. Better alternatives would be to ask a series of questions like "During a typical week, how many hours do you spend in vigorous walking?" to address all relevant forms of exercise, or to provide a clear and inclusive definition of exercise with examples (eg, "Exercise includes any physical activity done to improve your health and fitness, such as walking, swimming, yoga, playing a sport, or lifting weights.").
- **Simplicity.** To prevent confusion, questions should use common words and grammar, avoiding technical terms. A rule of thumb for measures designed for U.S. adults is to avoid using language above an eighth-grade reading level; for studies focusing on older or more vulnerable populations, questions should avoid language above a sixth-grade reading level. When developing questions, investigators may take advantage of tools for monitoring reading grade level in word-processing software programs, such as the "readability statistics" option in the proofing settings of Microsoft Word.
- **Neutrality.** Question stems should avoid "loaded" words and stereotypes that suggest a desirable answer. For example, asking "During the last month, how often did you drink too much alcohol?" may discourage respondents from admitting that they drink a lot of alcohol. "During the last month, how often did you drink five or more drinks in one day?" is a less judgmental and more definitive question.

Sometimes it is useful for a question to start with a preamble that permits the respondent to admit to behaviors and attitudes that may be considered undesirable. For example, when asking about a participant's adherence to prescribed medications, an interviewer may use an introduction: "People sometimes forget to take medications their doctor prescribes. Does that ever happen to you?" To elicit honest responses, questions should make participants feel that it is acceptable to choose any of the responses without leading them to choose any one response.

Common Pitfalls in Question Design

- **Double-barreled questions.** Questions should contain only one concept, issue, or behavior. Consider this question designed to assess satisfaction with the care received from health care providers during a recent hospital stay: "How satisfied were you with the care you received from the doctors and nurses?" A participant who was satisfied with the care he received from nurses but not from doctors might have difficulty providing a single response. Two separate questions, one for doctors and one for nurses, would yield more accurate information.
- **Hidden assumptions.** Questions can be difficult to answer if they make assumptions that may not apply to all participants. For example, consider a depression item that asks how often, in the past week, "I felt down or depressed even with help from my family." This assumes that respondents have families and ask for emotional support. Those who don't have a family (or seek help from their family) may not know how to answer the question.

- **Incongruous question and answer options.** Answer options should match the question stem. For example, for the question "Have you had pain in the last week?", response options of "never," "seldom," "often," "very often" may produce confusing responses. Instead, the question stem could be rephrased as "How often have you had pain in the last week?"
- **Medical or scientific jargon.** Questions should reflect the expected **health literacy** (and overall literacy) level of respondents. Many health-related terms that are familiar to investigators are confusing to participants who lack biomedical training. For example, it may be clearer to ask about "high blood pressure" instead of "hypertension," or about "rapid heart rate" instead of "tachycardia."

Question Time Frames

When assessing characteristics that may vary over time, questions should guide participants in considering an appropriate unit of time in their response. Sometimes researchers pose a question assuming that a behavior or characteristic—such as the number of tablets of a medication taken each day—is the same day after day: "How many tablets do you take a day?" However, if use of a medication varies over time, the question may yield more reliable information if a time frame is specified: "In the past 2 weeks, how many tablets of the medication did you usually take each day?"

Questions are most likely to elicit useful information if they specify the shortest recent segment of time during the period of interest that a respondent can recall accurately. The optimal length of time depends on the variable. For example, although questions about sleep habits during the past week may represent patterns of sleep during an entire year, the frequency of unprotected sex often varies from week to week, requiring questions that cover longer intervals. If participants are asked to consider too long a time period (such as to report sexual activity during the previous entire year), their recollection may not be accurate.

Questions about average behavior can be asked in two ways: asking about "usual" or "typical" behavior or counting actual behaviors during a period of time. For example, an investigator may determine average intake of beer by asking participants to estimate their usual intake:

> **About how many beers do you have during a typical week (one beer is equal to one 12-oz can or bottle, or one large glass)?**
>
> [___] beers per week

Although this question format is simple and brief, it assumes that participants can average their behavior into a single estimate. Because drinking patterns often change markedly over even brief intervals, the participant may have a difficult time deciding what is a typical week. Faced with questions that ask about typical behavior, people often report the things they do most commonly and ignore the extremes. Thus asking about drinking on typical days would underestimate alcohol consumption if a participant drinks large amounts on weekends.

Finally, if a series of questions are asked (say, about how often a participant consumes alcohol, marijuana, and other substances), the same approach and time period should be used for each question.

Multi-item Scales to Measure Abstract Variables

Some self-reported measures assess an abstract concept, such as quality of life, that can be difficult to capture in a single question; instead, scores from a series of questions are summarized as a multi-item scale (1, 2). By combining questions to create a multi-item instrument, the researcher enriches the assessment of the concept being measured. In addition, multi-item scales often have a greater range of possible score values (eg, a multi-item quality-of-life scale might generate scores from 1 to 100, whereas a single question might produce only a few responses, from "poor" to "excellent"). This may increase the sensitivity of the resulting measure to detect differences.

For example, consider a questionnaire designed to measure the strength of a person's opinion that a diet high in fruits and vegetables improves health:

For each item, circle the one number that best represents your opinion:

		STRONGLY AGREE	AGREE	NEUTRAL	DISAGREE	STRONGLY DISAGREE
a.	Eating more fruits and vegetables reduces the risk of heart disease.	1	2	3	4	5
b.	Vegetarians are generally healthier than people who include meat in their diet.	1	2	3	4	5
c.	Increasing the intake of fruits and vegetables slows the rate of aging.	1	2	3	4	5

A researcher can compute an overall score by averaging the scores for all nonmissing items, assuming that all items have the same weight and measure the same general characteristic. For example, a respondent who answers that he strongly agrees that eating more fruits and vegetables reduces the risk of heart disease (one point) and that vegetarians are generally healthier than people who include meat in their diet (one point), but disagrees that increasing the intake of fruits and vegetables slows aging (four points) would have a total score of 6.

Multi-item measures are also associated with less random error (ie, greater **reliability**), because random error in any one item is offset by the other items. On the other hand, multi-item scales with more complex scoring algorithms can produce results (eg, a quality-of-life score of 46.2) that are difficult to understand intuitively.

The **internal consistency** of a multi-item scale can be evaluated statistically using metrics, such as Cronbach's alpha (3), that assess the degree to which different items in the scale yield similar responses. Cronbach's alpha, which ranges from 0 to 1.0, is calculated from the correlations between scores on individual items, with higher values indicating greater consistency. No two items would be expected to produce identical responses from all participants; however, low values for internal consistency (such as Cronbach's alpha <0.70) indicate that some of the items measure different characteristics, suggesting that combining them into a single scale may be inappropriate.

Formatting of Multi-item Instruments

The format of an instrument should make it easy for respondents to complete all questions in the correct sequence. If the format is too complex, participants or interviewers may skip questions, provide the wrong information, or fail to complete the instrument.

To ensure accurate and standardized responses, all instruments should include initial instructions specifying how they should be completed. Clear instructions are important not only for self-administered measures but also for measures in which research staff pose the questions and record responses. Sometimes it is helpful to provide an example of how to complete a question, using one that is answered easily:

INSTRUCTIONS ON HOW TO FILL OUT A QUESTIONNAIRE THAT ASSESSES DIETARY INTAKE

These questions are about your usual eating habits during the past 12 months.
Please mark your usual serving size and write down how often you eat each food in the boxes next to the type of food.
For example, if you drink a medium (6 oz) glass of apple juice about three times a week, you would answer:

Apple Juice	○ Small (3 oz)	[3] time(s) per	○ Day
	⊙ Medium (6 oz)		⊙ Week
	○ Large (9 oz)		○ Month
			○ Year

Questions that address similar topic areas or use the same question format should be grouped together. Each set of questions addressing a new topic—or using a different format—should be introduced by brief instructions, a short descriptive statement, or a heading.

The order of questions may also account for whether some questions are more difficult or sensitive to answer. Respondents may be more likely to provide complete and honest responses if instruments present emotionally neutral questions first (like date of birth and size of household) and more sensitive questions later (eg, about income or sexual behavior).

Diaries and Logs

Diaries or logs may offer a more accurate approach to keep track of events, behaviors, or symptoms that happen only episodically (such as falls) or that vary from day to day (such as menstrual bleeding). This may be valuable if the timing or duration of an experience matters or if the occurrence is forgotten easily. Participants can record diary data on paper or enter data electronically into online forms or apps for mobile electronic devices. Data from diaries can then be abstracted to allow researchers to calculate the average frequency of the event or behavior over a relevant time interval, such as daily or weekly.

However, this approach is more time-consuming for participants than just asking retrospective questions. Participants may find it burdensome to keep detailed diaries for extended periods, resulting in "diary fatigue" that can cause higher rates of missing or inaccurate data. As a result, **diaries and logs should be reserved for behaviors or events—like a key predictor or outcome—that are essential to a study**, and participants should be asked to collect diary data for the shortest amount of time that is informative.

Because participants are usually asked to record information in diaries while carrying out their usual activities, they may not have the benefit of real-time guidance from study personnel in making diary entries. As a result, clear instructions and examples are especially important to minimize incomplete or uninterpretable responses.

For example, for clinical trials evaluating treatments for urinary incontinence, voiding diaries are often used to assess the frequency, timing, severity, and type of participants' urinary symptoms (4). Because of the complex information assessed, however, participants may require not only detailed instructions but also examples of completed diary entries to fill out diaries accurately:

SAMPLE VOIDING DIARY ENTRY

1. Time	2. Did you have an urge to urinate?				3. Did you urinate in the toilet?		4. Did you leak urine?		If yes	4a. Reason for leakage (DK = Don't Know)		
	No	Mild	Mod.	Severe								
<u>10:30</u>	☐	☐	☒	☐	☐	☒	☐	☒	→	☒	☐	☐
☒ AM	1	2	3	4	No	Yes	No	Yes		Urge	Stress	DK
☐ PM												

For paper-based diaries or logs, research staff may need to abstract data for subsequent quantitative analysis. This creates the need for a separate diary abstraction form or questionnaire for research staff in addition to the diary completed by the participant:

SAMPLE VOIDING DIARY ABSTRACTION FORM

	URINATIONS IN TOILET	URINE LEAKAGES	REASON(S) FOR LEAKAGE(S)		
			URGE	STRESS	OTHER
DAYTIME Total:	☐☐	☐☐	☐☐	☐☐	☐☐
NIGHTTIME Total:	☐☐	☐☐	☐☐	☐☐	☐☐

An advantage of electronic or online diaries or logs is that they can eliminate this step by generating summed or averaged data from participants' diary entries.

■ DESIGNING NEW MEASURES VERSUS USING EXISTING MEASURES

Designing New Measures

If no standardized questionnaire, diary, or interview approach is available to measure an important characteristic, a researcher may have no choice but to develop a new self-reported instrument. The task of developing a new measure can range from the creation of a single new question about a minor variable in a small study to designing and testing a new multi-item scale for measuring the primary outcome for a multicenter investigation.

At the simplest end of this spectrum, an investigator may use good judgment and basic principles of writing to develop an item that can be **pretested** to make sure it is clear and produces appropriate answers. At the other extreme, it can take years of effort to develop, refine, and validate a new instrument to measure an important study concept (5).

The latter process often begins by clarifying the construct being measured and then generating potential items for the instrument from qualitative interviews or **focus groups** (small groups of people with relevant experience or characteristics who are invited to spend 1 or 2 hours discussing specific topics pertaining to the study with a group facilitator). Based on the insights from this formative qualitative research, an initial pool of items may be developed and then refined iteratively from pretesting in additional participants.

The researcher may go on to draft a multi-item instrument that encompasses the most promising items, followed by critical review by peers, mentors, and experts. The researcher must then proceed with the iterative process of additional pretesting, revising, shortening, and evaluating properties of the instrument described in the next section (and illustrated by Example 17.1).

The process of developing and validating a new instrument is time-consuming, so it should be used only when existing measures are not adequate for an essential variable, such as a study's main predictor or outcome.

Using Existing Measures

Whenever possible, researchers should use or adapt an existing measure, thus benefiting from prior work and making it easier for findings to be compared across studies. Researchers seeking to measure a characteristic for a new study are often surprised at the number and variety of self-reported instruments, many of which are available for free in the public domain. Some have been developed by consensus organizations to advance research and care in their fields (Table 17.1).

Not all self-reported measures are in the public domain. When in doubt, researchers should contact the authors or publishers to request permission to use or adapt them in new target populations, because copyright protections apply regardless of whether notices are published with measures. Even when instruments are made available for use without charge, researchers should acknowledge or cite the origin of measures in any reports arising from their research.

Using existing instruments without modification is ideal if their properties have been evaluated. However, if some of the items are inappropriate (as may occur when a questionnaire developed for one cultural group is applied to a different setting), it may be necessary to delete, change, or add a few items.

If an established instrument is too long, researchers may consider contacting its developers to see if there are shorter versions that retain the strengths of the original. Deleting items from an established scale risks changing the meaning of its scores, endangering comparisons of the findings with results from studies that used the intact scale, and diminishing its reproducibility and sensitivity to detect changes. However, some instruments include multiple discrete sections or "subscales" that can be scored separately, allowing investigators to drop nonessential subscales but leave others intact.

EXAMPLE 17.1 Development of a New Multi-item Instrument

The Day-to-Day Impact of Vaginal Aging (DIVA) questionnaire exemplifies the iterative process of developing, testing, and evaluating the properties of a multi-item instrument. At the time, an expert panel convened by the National Institutes of Health (NIH) had expressed concern about the lack of robust measures for assessing postmenopausal vaginal symptoms across diverse populations of women (6). The DIVA questionnaire was designed to serve as a self-reported measure of the impact of common postmenopausal vaginal symptoms on multiple dimensions of functioning and well-being important to community-dwelling women and was developed and tested over multiple years. The investigators began by conducting focus groups of symptomatic postmenopausal women from three racial/ethnic groups to discuss the impact of their symptoms on their activities, feelings, and relationships (7). They developed a pool of 100 potential questionnaire items that were refined or eliminated based on input from clinical experts and additional symptomatic women. This resulted in a 25-item questionnaire that was administered to hundreds of women in a multiethnic cohort study in northern California. Respondent data were used to consolidate the list to 23 items, which were organized into four domain scales—activities of daily living, emotional well-being, sexual functioning, and self-concept and body image—based on evaluation of item and scale variability, internal consistency, reliability, and construct validity (8). Subsequent incorporation of the questionnaire into the NIH-funded Menopause Strategies: Finding Lasting Answers for Symptoms and Health (MsFLASH) Vaginal Health multicenter trial network allowed for further evaluation of construct validity in additional women in other geographic U.S. regions (9), as well as evaluation of sensitivity to change and potential minimal clinically important differences in domain scale scores after treatment (10). Continued administration of the questionnaire to other participant samples in the United States and other countries has enabled further evaluation of its psychometric properties over time, including the development of shorter or more specific versions designed for special populations such as women with cancer (11).

TABLE 17.1 SAMPLE DATABASES OF PUBLICLY AVAILABLE SELF-REPORTED MEASURES

DATABASE AND URL	DESCRIPTION
PhenX toolkit https://www.phenxtoolkit.org/	Provides established and broadly validated measures relevant to biomedical research, with special collections in substance abuse and addiction, mental health, blood sciences, and social determinants of health
National Institutes of Health toolbox http://www.healthmeasures.net/exploremeasurement-systems/nih-toolbox	Includes measures assessing cognitive, sensory, motor, and emotional function across the lifespan, developed and validated in nationally representative samples
PROMIS (Patient-Reported Outcomes Measurement Information System) http://www.healthmeasures.net/exploremeasurement-systems/promis	Provides self-report measures of physical, mental, and social health for use with the general population and those with chronic conditions
Science of Behavior Change Measures Repository https://scienceofbehaviorchange.org/measures	Contains measures of mechanisms of behavior change used by Science of Behavior Change Network investigators; includes evidence of psychometric adequacy in specific populations

(continued)

TABLE 17.1 SAMPLE DATABASES OF PUBLICLY AVAILABLE SELF-REPORTED MEASURES (*continued*)

DATABASE AND URL	DESCRIPTION
National Institutes of Health Common Data Element (CDE) Resource Portal https://www.nlm.nih.gov/cde	Includes lists of CDEs, surveys, questionnaires, instruments, instrument items, and other methods of data collection
Neuro-QoL Neurologic Quality of Life Measures http://www.healthmeasures.net/exploremeasurement-systems/neuro-qol	Provides self-report measures assessing quality of life across physical, mental, and social health among adults and children with neurologic disorders
REDCap HealthMeasures https://www.healthmeasures.net/implement-healthmeasures/administration-platforms/redcap	Includes self- and proxy-report measures, including those from PROMIS and Neuro-QoL, for administration through the REDCap online surveys and database application
Rand Health https://www.rand.org/health-care/surveys_tools.html	Includes surveys designed for assessing patients' health, screening for mental health conditions, and measuring quality of care and quality of life

Adapted with permission from Anita Stewart, PhD.

◼ RECOMMENDED STEPS FOR SELECTING AND ADAPTING MEASURES

The following step-by-step approach can be used to select, review, and adapt self-reported measures for inclusion in a new study. This process can be applied to each variable or construct to be measured, whether it is a predictor, outcome, or potential confounder. The goal is to assess the strengths and weaknesses of existing instruments for collecting key data to answer the research question in the target population.

Step 1: Define Variables or Constructs

Create a list of the important variables or constructs you want to measure. Consider writing a short definition of each variable and assess whether any more complex variables may have more than one underlying dimension or "subconstruct" that should be measured separately.

Step 2: Compile Existing Measures

Assemble files of available questions or instruments for measuring each variable or construct. Start by collecting instruments from other studies that examined the same phenomena of interest and searching common repositories (see Table 17.1). Compile any original and subsequent publications that provide information about each measure's development. When there are several alternatives, create a folder of candidate questions and instruments for each variable.

Step 3: Review Underlying Concepts

For each measure, review the way the concept being measured is defined, including more specific concepts examined in any domains or subscales. Consider how similar these definitions are to what you intend to measure in your study, based on a review of the measure's instructions, item stems, and response scales.

Step 4: Examine Scale Construction and Score Interpretability

Review the range of scores each measure is designed to produce and the direction of scoring (eg, the meaning of a high vs. a low score). Consider whether the numeric value of the measure's score is intuitively meaningful. Examine any special methods that were used to develop the scale for the measure (eg, factor analysis). Check whether a user manual or guide is available to indicate how to generate scores from the measure.

Step 5: Review Previous Administration Methods and Target Populations

Assess whether the measure was developed or tested in a group that is similar to your target population; if not, determine where the differences matter. Examine past methods of administration for this measure (self- or interviewer-administered, in person or by telephone, etc.) and consider whether changes may be necessary in your study. If translations are needed, check whether a version is available in the languages of interest.

Step 6: Review Psychometric Characteristics

For instruments designed to assess complex constructs, review information about the way it performed in respondents similar to the target population. That information, also known as a measure's **psychometric characteristics** (Table 17.2), can indicate whether it is likely to yield

TABLE 17.2 COMMON PSYCHOMETRIC PROPERTIES OF SELF-REPORTED MEASURES

Variability	Initial assessment of the variability of scores can confirm whether a self-reported measure produces an adequate distribution of responses. If responses have a highly skewed distribution that may result in "ceiling" or "floor" effects, it may be difficult to detect differences among subgroups or change in response to interventions.
Test-Retest Reliability	A self-reported measure should produce the same or similar responses if repeated over an interval that is short enough that no underlying change in the characteristic of interest should occur, but long enough that respondents would not be expected to recall their initial response. Higher correlation between the initial and repeat assessments indicates greater test-retest reliability, suggesting that responses to the measure are reproducible if administered under the same conditions.
Validity	Evidence of validity of a measure often starts with face validity, the subjective but important judgment that items assess the characteristics of interest. For example, a new instrument designed to measure vision-related functioning should include questions that have face validity to people with common visual disorders ("Are you able to read a newspaper without glasses or contact lenses?"). Further efforts may include other assessments of content validity and construct validity, through assessment of whether answers to this questionnaire are correlated with other measures of overlapping constructs. For example, researchers may demonstrate that scores from a new measure correlate with scores from existing measures of similar constructs (convergent validity) and that they do not correlate with scores from other measures of dissimilar constructs (divergent validity).
Sensitivity to Change	If the goal of a study is to measure change, then the responsiveness of a measure can be evaluated by applying it to participants before and after receiving interventions considered effective. For example, scores from a questionnaire assessing vision-related functioning (such as the ability to drive after dark) can be examined in adults before and after cataract surgery. Those with improvement in visual acuity after cataract surgery (say, from 20/60 to 20/30) would also be expected to show improvement in their questionnaire scores (and those who do not experience improvement in visual acuity would *not* be expected to show such improvement).
Minimal Clinically Important Difference	For measures that yield numerical scores and are designed to serve as outcome measures, it can be useful to determine the minimal clinically important difference in the score that corresponds to an improvement (or deterioration) in the outcome that is meaningful. For example, for a questionnaire designed to assess vision-related functioning, the minimal clinically important change could represent the magnitude of change in score that corresponds to another accepted metric of treatment success (such as participants' overall satisfaction with the change in their vision after cataract surgery or their stated willingness to repeat the surgery).

dependable, useful, and relevant information. Questionnaires and other self-reported measures can be assessed for **variability** (whether they produce an appropriate range of responses), **reliability** (whether they reproduce consistent responses under the same conditions), **validity** (whether they represent the underlying phenomena they are intended to measure), and **sensitivity to change** (Chapter 4).

Step 7: Revise and Shorten the Set of Instruments

Resist the temptation to include additional measures "just in case" they might produce interesting data. Long interviews, questionnaires, and examinations may tire respondents and thereby decrease the accuracy and reproducibility of their responses. Questions that are not essential to answering the main research question increase the amount of effort involved in obtaining, entering, cleaning, and analyzing data. A good maxim for deciding which items to include is: When in doubt, leave it out.

Step 8: Pretest Instruments

When possible, pretest instruments by administering them in a small sample of people who resemble your target population. Pretesting can provide valuable information about the time required to administer self-reported measures, especially if measures are new or will be used in a new population. Following pretesting, consider modifying items that produce missing or confusing responses and improving the instructions and formatting of instruments. For key measures, large-scale pretesting may be necessary to confirm that each question or scale produces an adequate range of responses, as well as to assess other psychometric characteristics.

■ EVALUATING MEASURES FOR DIVERSE POPULATIONS

Many self-reported measures are developed and tested in mainstream, well-educated groups of respondents. As a result, little information is available on the appropriateness, reliability, validity, or responsiveness of these measures in other populations.

Biased responses to self-reported measures can arise from cultural differences in the perceived meaning of concepts, the way participants cognitively process questions, or their familiarity with common data collection methods (12). For example, in a study of depression among ethnically diverse adults, responses to questions can be influenced by differences in cultural norms about expressing negative feelings, participants' comfort level with being interviewed by strangers about their emotional well-being, and nuances in the meaning of the word "depression" in languages other than English.

When adapting a measure for use in a new population, researchers may need to assess its **conceptual adequacy** in the population—that is, whether the underlying concept is still relevant, meaningful, or acceptable in that group. It may also be necessary to confirm the **conceptual equivalence** of the measure across groups—that is, whether the concept being measured is fundamentally the same in one cultural group as another (13). Specific items may need to be retested if they rely on cultural assumptions that may not apply to members of the target group.

The **psychometric adequacy** of the measure may also need to be reevaluated to confirm that it still yields reliable and valid data in a new cultural group. Although this may require more time and effort, it can help ensure that measures are appropriate for use across all groups under study. If researchers wish to use a measure to draw comparisons between cultural groups, then they should feel confident that the measure has **psychometric equivalence** across groups. Otherwise, any differences in scores derived from the measure may simply reflect differences in the measures' performance characteristics between these groups.

■ ADMINISTERING MEASURES

Administration Platforms

Self-reported measures can be distributed using a wide array of platforms. Respondents may complete questionnaires on paper or using a computer tablet or workstation during study visits. They may click on a questionnaire link provided on the study website or sent to them via e-mail. They may complete and mail back paper diaries or forms using prestamped envelopes.

E-mailed and online questionnaires have several advantages over those administered on paper. First, answers can be integrated directly into an electronic study database, eliminating the expense and potential errors associated with transferring data from paper forms (14). Answers can be checked automatically for missing and out-of-range values, the errors pointed out to the respondent in real time, and the responses accepted only after the errors are corrected. Electronic survey software can be programmed to send reminders to participants who do not complete measures within a specified time, as well as to notify staff when answers are incomplete.

However, e-mailed or online measures are not accessible to individuals who lack access to the internet or electronic devices, which may decrease enrollment or follow-up in populations with less widespread use of digital communication technology, such as older adults and economically vulnerable participants. Researchers may need to give or lend participants portable electronic devices for the duration of a study, or invite participants to come to a study site to complete measures.

A self-reported measure that is designed for one administration platform, such as paper, may need to be reformatted if it is to be administered for another, such as online. On paper, measures should involve well-spaced questions and response options that appear in a large and easy-to-read font, such as black type on white forms. For online measures, investigators must consider the type of device that will be used, ensuring that the items are formatted for the size of the respondent's screen: Participants may miss important response options if they are cut off from view or require excessive scrolling.

Self- Versus Interviewer Administration

Self-administered (or participant-administered) measures provide an efficient and uniform way to administer simple questions, such as those about basic demographic information. They tend to require less research staff time, particularly if data are captured electronically and do not need to be entered into a database later. They may also elicit more honest responses to potentially sensitive questions, such as those about symptoms or behaviors associated with social stigma.

In contrast, interviewer-administered measures are better for collecting answers to complicated questions that require explanation or more detailed instructions. Interviewers may also be needed when participants have variable ability to read and understand questions or when researchers want to confirm in real time that participants' responses are complete. However, interviewer-based administration of measures is more costly and time-consuming. Moreover, the responses may be influenced by the relationship between the interviewer and respondent, and they are inevitably administered at least a little differently each time, because of minor variations in the way the interviewer presents the questions or response options.

Both self- and interviewer-administered approaches are susceptible to errors caused by imperfect respondent memory. They are both also affected by a respondent's tendency to give socially acceptable answers, although this may be more pronounced for interviewer-administered measures where respondents respond directly to researchers.

An alternative to interviewer administration of measures is to allow participants to complete measures on their own, but ask them to do this during study visits in which research personnel are present. Administering measures during a study visit allows researchers to explain the instructions before participants start answering questions. Questionnaires can also be sent in advance of a visit, with the answers checked for completeness before participants leave.

Interviewing Approaches

For interviewer-administered measures, the skill of the interviewer can have a substantial impact on the quality of the responses. Standardizing the interview approach from one interview to the next is the key to maximizing reproducibility, with uniform wording of questions and uniform nonverbal signals during the interview. **Interviewers must strive to avoid introducing their own biases into the responses by changing the words or the tone of their voice.** For the interviewer to comfortably read the questions verbatim, the interview should be written in language that resembles common speech. Questions that sound unnatural or stilted when said aloud will encourage interviewers to improvise their own, more natural but less standardized ways of asking them.

Sometimes it is necessary for interviewers to follow up on respondents' answers to encourage them to give more appropriate answers or to clarify the meaning of responses. This process of "probing" can also be standardized by writing standard phrases in the margins or beneath the text of each question. To a question about how many cups of coffee respondents drink on a typical day, some respondents might respond, "I'm not sure; it's different from day to day." The instrument could include the follow-up probe: "Do the best you can; tell me about how many you drink on a typical day."

Interviews can be conducted in person, by videoconference, or over the telephone. However, in-person interviews may be appropriate if the study requires direct observation of participants to collect other data, as well as for participants who do not or cannot use phones.

■ ALTERNATIVE MEASUREMENT STRATEGIES

Physiologic instruments and biologic assays may provide alternatives to self-reported instruments for measuring some common conditions and exposures. For example, direct measurement of physical activity with small, wearable accelerometers yields a more objective and precise estimate of the total amount and patterns of physical activity and energy expenditure than questionnaires (15). Actigraphy and other sensors worn at night measure duration and disruption of sleep more accurately than self-reported sleep diaries (16). Researchers should be alert for new technologies that measure characteristics that could only be assessed previously by self-report.

However, self-reported measures frequently provide unique or complementary information that cannot be replaced by physiologic or laboratory data. For example, a researcher conducting a study about insomnia may find it valuable to describe participants' perceptions of their sleep quality or the impact of their daytime sleepiness even if actigraphy offers an objective measure of sleep duration or disruption. More importantly, some health conditions, such as generalized anxiety disorder or irritable bowel syndrome, are defined primarily by patients' perception of their symptoms. In that case, self-reported instruments provide the best, if not the only, measure of participants' experiences.

■ SUMMARY

1. The **validity of a study's results** often depends on the quality and appropriateness of self-reported data collected by questionnaire, diary, or interview.
2. Questions used in self-reported measures should be **clear, simple, neutral, and appropriate** for the target population. They should be examined from the viewpoint of participants, looking for ambiguous terms and pitfalls such as double-barreled questions, hidden assumptions, response options that do not match the question, and medical jargon.
3. To measure abstract variables such as attitudes or health status, **questions can be combined into multi-item scales**, assuming that the questions measure a single characteristic and responses are internally consistent.

4. An investigator should **search for existing instruments** that are likely to produce valid and reliable results among their target participants.

5. **Developing a new measure starts by clarifying the concepts, reviewing existing measures, and generating potential items** for pretesting and subsequent refinement. The most promising items should undergo critical peer review, followed by more pretesting, revision, and evaluation.

6. **Instruments used in a study should be pretested;** the time required to administer them should be assessed before the study begins.

7. Measures designed for one target population may not be appropriate for respondents from a different cultural background.

8. Compared with interviewer-administered questionnaires, **self-administered** ones are **more economical and easier to standardize;** the added privacy can enhance validity. Interviewer administration can promote more complete responses and clarify respondents' understanding of measures.

9. Electronic or online administration of instruments can enhance the efficiency of a study and the accuracy of the data collected, but requires that respondents have access to digital communication.

10. **Questions used in self-reported measures should be easy to read, and interviewer-administered questions should be comfortable to read out loud.** Measures should be formatted for the expected platform of administration.

REFERENCES

1. McDowell I. *Measuring Health: A Guide to Rating Scales and Questionnaires.* 3rd ed. Oxford University Press; 2006.
2. Streiner DL, Norman GR. *Health Measurement Scales: A Practical Guide to Their Development and Use.* 4th ed. Oxford University Press; 2009.
3. Bland JM, Altman DG. Cronbach's alpha. *Br Med J.* 1997;314:572.
4. Food and Drug Administration. Guidance for Industry and Food and Drug Administration Staff: Clinical Investigations of Devices Indicated for the Treatment of Urinary Incontinence. March 2011. FDA-2008-D-0457.
5. Food and Drug Administration. Guidance for Industry: Patient-Reported Outcome Measures: Use in Medical Product Development to Support Labeling Claims; 2009.
6. Santoro N, Sherman S. *New Interventions for Menopausal Symptoms Meeting Summary.* National Institutes of Health; 2007.
7. Huang AJ, Luft J, Grady D, et al. The day-to-day impact of urogenital aging: perspectives from racially/ethnically diverse women. *J Gen Intern Med.* 2010; 25(1):45-51.
8. Huang AJ, Gregorich SE, Kuppermann M, et al. Day-to-day impact of vaginal aging questionnaire: a multidimensional measure of the impact of vaginal symptoms on functioning and well-being in postmenopausal women. *Menopause.* 2015; 22(2):144-154.
9. Hunter MM, Guthrie KA, Larson JC, et al. Convergent-divergent validity and correlates of the day-to-day impact of vaginal aging domain scales in the MsFLASH vaginal health trial. *J Sex Med.* 2020;17(1):117-125.
10. Gibson CJ, Huang AJ, Larson JC, et al. Patient-centered change in the day-to-day impact of postmenopausal vaginal symptoms: results from a multicenter randomized trial. *Am J Obst Gynecol* 2020;223(1):99.e1-99.e9.
11. Toivonen K, Santos-Iglesias P, Walker LM. Impact of vulvovaginal symptoms in women diagnosed with cancer: a psychometric evaluation of the day-to-day impact of vaginal aging questionnaire. *J Women Health (Larchmt).* 2021;30(8):1192-1203.
12. Sanchez A, Hidalgo B, Rosario AM, Artiles L, Stewart AL, and Nápoles A. Applying self-report measures in minority health and health disparities research. In: Dankwa-Mullan I, Pérez-Stable EJ, Gardner KL, Zhang X, and Rosario AM, Eds. *The Science of Health Disparities Research.* 1st ed. John Wiley & Sons, Inc. 2021;153-169.
13. Stewart AL, Thrasher AD, Goldberg J, and Shea JA. A framework for understanding modifications to measures for diverse populations. *J Aging Health.* 2012;24(6):992-1017.
14. Dillman DA, Smyth JD, Christian LM. *Internet, Mail, and Mixed-Mode Surveys: The Tailored Design Method.* 3rd ed. Wiley, 2008.
15. Mackey DC, Manini TM, Schoeller DA, et al. Validation of an armband to measure daily energy expenditure in older adults. *J Gerontol Ser A Biol Sci Med Sci.* 2011;66:1108-1113.
16. Girshik J, Fritschi L, Heyworth J, Waters F. Validation of self-reported sleep against actigraphy. *J Epidemiol.* 2012;22:462-468.

APPENDIX 17A
Exercises for Chapter 17. Designing, Selecting, and Administering Self-Reported Measures

1. As part of a study of alcohol and muscle strength, an investigator plans to use the following item in a self-reported measure to determine current alcohol use:
   "How many drinks of beer, wine, or liquor do you consume each day?" Check one circle.
   ○ 0
   ○ 1 to 2
   ○ 3 to 4
   ○ 5 to 6
   Briefly describe at least two problems with this item.
2. Write several questions for a self-reported measure that will better assess current alcohol use.
3. In an observational study of young adults, you want to collect information about behaviors that may put the participants at risk of sexually transmitted infections. Comment on the advantages and disadvantages of assessing the frequency of unprotected sexual intercourse using a self-administered questionnaire, versus an interviewer-administered questionnaire, versus a diary in which participants record the dates and context of sexual activity.
4. You are planning a study of a community-based exercise program for low-income older adults with chronic back pain and would like to evaluate the impact of this program on their pain-related functioning and quality of life. Searching the literature, you find that another researcher has recently developed a 10-item structured self-reported measure, the "Impact of Chronic Back Pain" (ICBP) questionnaire, that is designed to generate a total score from 0 (minimal impact) to 40 (most severe impact). You review the publication about this measure to assess whether it may be appropriate for use in your research. What potential issues are suggested by following information published about this measure?
   4a. This ICBP measure was developed by an orthopedic surgeon who evaluated its properties among patients seen in a private practice.
   4b. In a sample of patients who were seeking consultation about surgical treatment for their back pain, the mean (±standard deviation) ICBP score was 10 ± 6, with a range from 4 to 24.
   4c. The Cronbach's alpha for internal consistency of this questionnaire is 0.59.
   4d. In a sample of respondents who also completed a different, well-established, more generic measure about the severity and impact of pain, the Brief Pain Inventory (BPI), no correlation between ICBP and BPI scores was found.

CHAPTER 18

Study Implementation and Quality Control

Deborah G. Grady and Alison J. Huang

Most of this book deals with matters of study design. In this chapter, we focus on issues related to study implementation and **quality control**. All clinical research studies pose challenges for implementation, but those that involve direct recruitment of participants for data collection are the most complicated to implement. For these, even the best of plans assembled thoughtfully in an armchair may work out differently in practice. Skilled research staff may be unavailable, study space less than optimal, participants less willing to enroll, follow-up more difficult than anticipated, interventions poorly tolerated, and measurements challenging to obtain. The conclusions of a well-designed study can be marred by ignorance, carelessness, lack of training and **standardization**, and other errors in finalizing and implementing the protocol.

Successful study implementation begins with **assembling the resources needed for the study**, including space, equipment, staff, and financial management. The next task is to **finalize the protocol by pretesting recruitment mechanisms, measurement procedures, and intervention plans**, if applicable, to avoid the need for protocol revisions after data collection has begun. Detailed instructions for study procedures should be spelled out in an **operations manual**, which may require updating after the start of the study. The study is then carried out with a **systematic approach to quality control** of data collection and data management.

Most of the strategies in this chapter are aimed at single-center studies carried out by a small research team. But many of the strategies also pertain to major studies with large research teams distributed across multiple sites and led by several investigators.

■ GETTING STARTED

Study Start-Up

At the beginning of the study, the **principal investigator** (PI) and staff must be trained on the protocol, finalize the budget, develop and sign any necessary contracts, define staff positions, hire and train staff, identify and equip space, obtain institutional review board (IRB) approval, purchase materials, write the operations manual, develop and test the data collection forms and database, and plan participant recruitment strategies and materials. This period of study activity before the first participant is enrolled is referred to as **study start-up** and requires intensive effort. Adequate time and planning for study start-up are important to the conduct of a high-quality study—often requiring several months of effort.

The Research Team

Although research teams range in size from just the investigator and a part-time research assistant to hundreds of full-time staff, they must carry out similar activities, even if one person fills several roles. The PI must ensure that each of the functions described in Table 18.1 is accomplished. Some team members, such as the financial and human resources managers, are usually

TABLE 18.1 FUNCTIONAL ROLES FOR MEMBERS OF A RESEARCH TEAM

ROLE	FUNCTION	COMMENT
Principal investigator (PI)	Ultimately responsible for the design, funding, staffing, conduct, quality of the study, safety of the study participants, and for reporting findings	
Project director/clinic coordinator	Provides day-to-day management of all study activities	Should be experienced, responsible, meticulous, and with good interpersonal and organizational skills
Recruitment coordinator	Ensures that the desired number of eligible participants are enrolled	Should be experienced with a range of recruitment techniques
Clinical research coordinator/clinic staff	Carries out study visit procedures and makes measurements	May require special licenses or certification for physical examination or other specialized procedures
Clinical research associate	Monitors study site activities (especially in multicenter studies)	Conducts site visits and reviews study documents to ensure proper progress, regulatory compliance, and record keeping of study sites
Regulatory affairs manager/Quality control coordinator	Processes/submits necessary documents to institutional review boards (IRBs) and government agencies, ensuring compliance and timelines; ensures that all staff follow standard operating procedures (SOPs) and oversees quality control	Performs IRB and regulatory submission/maintains approvals; observes study procedures to ensure adherence to SOPs, may supervise audit by external groups such as U.S. Food and Drug Administration
Data manager	Designs, tests, and implements the data entry, editing, and management system	Maintains and manages ongoing data cleaning, data reporting, and query/data editing systems
Programmer/analyst	Produces study reports that describe recruitment, adherence, and data quality; conducts data analyses	Works under the supervision of the PI and statistician
Statistician	Collaborates on study design, estimates sample size and power, designs analysis plan and data and safety monitoring guidelines, interprets findings	Involved in overall study design, conduct, interim monitoring, data analyses, and presentation of results
Administrative assistant	Provides administrative support, sets up meetings, etc.	
Financial manager	Prepares budget and manages expenditures	Provides projections to help manage budget
Human resources manager	Assists in preparing job descriptions, hiring, evaluations	Helps manage personnel issues and problems

employed by the investigator's institution to provide support for all investigators and staff in a particular unit.

After deciding on the number of team members and the distribution of duties, the next step is to work with a departmental administrator to prepare and post job descriptions, and then evaluate responses and interview candidates. Hiring research staff can be challenging, because formal training may not be available for all research functions, and job requirements may vary from one study to the next. The crucial position of project director—who provides day-to-day management of study activities—may be filled by a person with a background in nursing, pharmacy, public health, laboratory services, or pharmaceutical research; the duties of this position can vary widely. Another important position is the clinical research coordinator (CRC), who carries out day-to-day study procedures and makes measurements. The CRC usually has the most contact with study participants and is thus the "face" of the study. To ensure optimal recruitment and retention, the CRC must be able to build a good rapport with study participants and be responsive to participants' needs. Many institutions offer training programs and certification for research staff, including CRCs.

Although most institutions have formal methods for posting job openings, other avenues, like online job listings and social media/LinkedIn outreach, can be useful. The safest approach is to find staff of known competence, such as someone working for a colleague whose project has ended. Some institutions support a pool of experienced research coordinators and other staff who can be hired part-time.

Leadership and Team-Building

The quality of a study begins with the **integrity and leadership of the PI**, who must ensure that all staff are trained properly and are certified to carry out their duties. The PI should convey the message that protection of human participants, maintenance of privacy, completeness and accuracy of data, and fair presentation of research findings are paramount. Though PIs cannot watch every measurement made by colleagues and staff, they can create a sense of being aware of all study activities and believing strongly in the protection of participants and the quality of the data; most staff will respond in kind. A good leader is adept at delegating authority appropriately while setting up a system of supervision that ensures oversight of the study.

From the outset of planning the study, the investigator should lead **regular staff meetings** with all members of the research team. An agenda should be distributed in advance, with progress reports from those who have been given responsibility for specific areas of the study. These meetings provide an opportunity to discover and solve problems, as well as to involve everyone in the process of developing the project and conducting the research. Staff meetings can be enhanced by scientific discussions and updates related to preliminary findings of the project. Regular staff meetings are a great source of establishing camaraderie, good morale, and interest in the goals of the study, while also providing on-the-job education and training.

Investigators may need to supplement group team meetings with periodic one-on-one meetings to allow staff members to bring up concerns and elicit suggestions for improving study processes that they are not comfortable raising in group settings. Feedback to staff members on job performance should be delivered *individually*, rather than in group meetings. Meeting individually with research team members can take time and energy—but it is important because the investigator serves as the team leader as well as the employer.

Many research institutions provide a wide range of **resources for conducting clinical research**, such as database management services, professional recruiter services, core laboratories where specialized measurements can be performed, analysts with expertise regarding U.S. Food and Drug Administration (FDA) or other regulatory issues, and libraries of study forms and documents. How to access this infrastructure may not be apparent in a large sprawling institution, so investigators should become familiar with their local resources before trying to reinvent the wheel.

Space and Equipment

Some clinical research studies involve participant visits in an area that is dedicated solely to research or in facilities that are also used for clinical care. Others rely on remote platforms for data collection, such as web-based interactive systems, mailed interventions, telephone- or videoconference-based visits, home-based study measurements, and online or mobile device–based data entry. Even when many study activities rely on remote platforms, staff will require dedicated space in which to conduct their behind-the-scenes work and store, organize, and process study materials.

If **physical space** for study visits or procedures is needed, it should be accessible, attractive, affordable, and sufficient. Failing to secure space early in the planning process can result in difficulty enrolling participants, poor adherence to study visits, incomplete data, and unhappy staff. Clinical research space must be easy for participants to find and have adequate parking or proximity to public transportation. The space should be spacious enough to accommodate staff, measurement equipment, and storage of study drug and study-related files. If the research requires physical examination, provision for privacy and handwashing must be available. If the participants must go to other places for tests (such as the hospital laboratory or radiology department), these should also be accessible.

Many clinical studies also require **dedicated equipment**, such as computers, laboratory equipment, and devices used for physical exam measurements. Start-up activities for a new research study may involve purchase of equipment and creation of a schedule for its maintenance, calibration, and quality checks. For expensive items, researchers should allocate time to obtain cost quotes from different vendors and special approval, if needed, from their institutions.

Investigators may find it more convenient to use **centralized clinical research facilities**, if available, rather than setting up and equipping their own research space. However, most clinical research centers require reimbursement for their services, as well as an application and review process.

Study Budget

Adequate funding for conducting the study is crucial. The PI will have prepared a budget at the time of submitting a proposal for funding, well in advance of starting the study (Chapter 20). Most research institutions employ staff with financial expertise to assist in the development of budgets (the **pre-award manager**). It is worthwhile to get to know these staff well, to discuss regulations related to various sources of funding in advance and to **respect their stress levels around deadlines** by meeting timetable goals. The PI should make financial plans that take into account the rules for spending research funds, which vary depending on the funding organization.

Sometimes investigators do not receive the full amount of requested funds or the estimated costs of some research activities change after an award is made. In general, the total amount of awarded funds usually cannot be increased if the work turns out to be more costly than predicted, and shifting money across categories of expense (eg, personnel, equipment, supplies, travel) or making substantial reductions in the percent effort of key personnel requires approval by the sponsor. Institutions typically employ financial personnel whose main responsibility is to ensure that funds available to an investigator through grants and contracts are spent appropriately. This **post-award manager** should prepare regular financial reports and projections that allow the investigator to make the best use of the available funds during the life of the study, ensuring that the budget will not be overdrawn at its end. A modest surplus at the end of the study can be a good thing, as sponsors often approve "**no-cost extensions**" that allow the use of the surplus funds to complete or extend the work described in the scope of the award.

The budget for a study supported by a pharmaceutical or other private or industry funder is often part of a contract that incorporates the protocol and a clear delineation of the tasks to be carried out by the investigator and the sponsor. Contracts are legal documents that obligate the investigator and institution to conduct activities, often describing the timing and amount of payment in return for specified "deliverables," such as meeting recruitment milestones and submitting progress reports. Legal assistance is often needed to help develop such contracts and ensure that they protect the investigator's intellectual property rights, access to data, and publication rights. However, lawyers are generally unfamiliar with the tasks required to complete a specific study, and input from the investigator is crucial, especially with regard to the scope of work and deliverables.

Data Collection Platforms

A critical step in study planning is determining the most appropriate methods or platforms for collecting study data and administering any study interventions. For this, researchers must balance the needs of scientific rigor and precision, participant convenience and access, and cost or burden to study staff. Many research measurements that once required in-person participant assessments can now be captured using remote platforms, including web-based questionnaire platforms, wearable electronic monitors or devices, or telehealth- or videoconference-based examinations.

However, researchers may need to invest substantial time and effort into developing and testing **remote data collection procedures**. This includes time to prepare detailed instructions to guide participants in accessing remote platforms or using and returning loaned devices, as well as staff procedures for ensuring the security and quality of remotely collected data. Researchers may also need to create informed consent procedures that meet regulatory standards for electronic documentation, such as FDA's 21 CFR Part 11 regulations.

Sometimes, early in-person contact with participants may help establish rapport, particularly in studies that require extended effort over time, even if it is not necessary for data collection. After meeting study staff in an initial in-person visit, participants may develop a stronger personal connection to study staff or a greater investment in the study; as a result, they may be more likely to complete subsequent follow-up activities even if they involve no in-person contact with the study team.

Institutional Review Board Approval

For most studies, PIs must obtain approval from their IRBs for the study protocol, consent form, and recruitment materials before recruitment can begin (Chapter 7). Any questionnaires, data forms, study websites, or other materials intended for participants (ie, "participant facing" materials) usually need to be reviewed by the IRB before they are used. Investigators should be familiar with the requirements of their local IRB and the time required to obtain approval. This can be substantial, particularly if IRB members have questions or believe that materials should be modified before being deployed. To prevent delays, study team members should **contact IRB staff early** to discuss any procedural issues and design decisions that affect study participants.

Coverage Analysis

Many studies include imaging, blood tests, and other procedures that may be paid for by a participant's health insurance unless they were obtained primarily for research purposes. Most institutions require an independent review of clinical research studies (called coverage analysis) to **determine if procedures and services should be billed to insurance** or to the study sponsor. For example, in studies of new drugs for treating cancer, the coverage analysis would determine if imaging studies required to measure the main outcome of change in tumor size can be billed to the patient's insurance.

Operations Manual and Forms Development

The study protocol can be expanded to create an **operations manual**, which includes the protocol, information on study organization and policies, and a more detailed description of the study methods (Appendix 18A). It specifies how to recruit and enroll study participants and describes all activities that occur at each visit. For example, in a randomized trial, this might include how randomization and blinding will be achieved, how each variable will be measured, quality control procedures, data management practices, the statistical analysis plan, and the plan for data and safety monitoring (Chapter 11). It should also include a list or chart of all of the questionnaires and measurements that will be administered in the study, with instructions on contacting the study participants, carrying out any study interviews, completing and coding study forms, entering and editing data, and collecting and processing any specimens.

An operations manual is **especially important for collaborative research projects** carried out at several sites or when the study will take place over an extended period of time. It provides a consistent guide to procedures regardless of where they are conducted or whether there is turnover in the research team.

Even when a single investigator does all the work of the study, **written operational definitions help reduce random variation and changes in measurement technique** over time. They also ensure that the investigator has thought through the operational details of a study. Often, investigators become aware of unrecognized logistical challenges or the need to modify procedures during the process of writing the operations manual.

Design of the data collection forms affects the quality of the data and the success of the study (Chapter 19). Before the first participant is recruited, **all forms should be pretested**. Any data entry that involves subjective judgment requires an explicit operational definition that should be summarized on the form itself and set out in more detail in the operations manual. Pretesting forms will ensure that their meaning is clear and that they are easy to use. Labeling each page with its completion or study visit date, as well as the ID numbers of the participant and staff member filling out the form, safeguards the integrity of the data. Web-based digital forms, handheld tablets, and other mobile devices for collecting data must be pretested during study start-up and directions for their use included in the operations manual.

Database Design

Before the first participant is recruited, the database that will be used to enter, edit, store, monitor, and analyze the data should be developed and tested (Chapter 19). Development and testing of the data entry and management system can require weeks to months, even after staff with the appropriate skills have been hired and trained. Many institutions provide services to help investigators develop an appropriate database. For very large studies, investigators may benefit from professional database design and management services, but their costs must be anticipated in the study budget. Early-stage investigators may want to get advice on these options from trusted in-house technical experts and senior advisors.

Investigators eager to begin a study sometimes record data on paper forms or in a spreadsheet rather than in an actual database program. This approach, although easier initially, may cost much more in time and effort when it is time to clean and analyze the data. The advantage of **setting up a database early** is that it prompts the investigator to consider what values are acceptable for each variable and disallow or generate alerts for out-of-range, illogical, or missing values. High-quality data entry and management systems improve quality control during data collection and entry, as well as reduce the time needed for data cleaning. But the greatest value of using a data management system is to avoid discovering late in a study that there are a large number of missing, out-of-range, or illogical values that cannot be corrected.

Recruitment and Retention

Timely recruitment is the most difficult aspect of many studies. Adequate time, staff, resources, funding, and expertise are essential and should be planned well in advance of study start-up. Many investigators underestimate (and rarely do investigators overestimate) the time, cost, and effort required to reach a study's recruitment goal. Approaches to recruiting the goal number of study participants are described in Chapter 3.

Once study recruitment has begun, investigators should **monitor the success of different recruitment approaches**, including the number of eligible participants yielded by each approach relative to its cost. Over the course of a study, investigators may discontinue some recruitment approaches or reallocate funds to new ones. Sometimes it is useful to question those who decline to enroll; this may yield information to guide future study recruitment strategies.

For studies involving prospective follow-up, careful plans for promoting and monitoring retention are also important. This begins with a protocol to **minimize participant dropout** by planning frequent follow-up contact with participants to maintain their interest in the study without overburdening them. If participants are provided incentives for agreeing to enroll in the study, they should also receive additional incentives for follow-up. As a study continues, if retention is lower than expected, investigators may need to increase the frequency or method of participant contact or the incentive schedule, or eliminate burdensome follow-up procedures.

Other strategies for **promoting retention** include:

- Providing vouchers for parking or transportation to offset the burden of site-specific follow-up visits or procedures
- Sending participants periodic information about the results of their study measurements (eg, results of their bone density tests or summary results from their questionnaires) to retain their interest
- Sending birthday or holiday cards from the study, or newsletters about interim accomplishments from the research
- Providing food and beverages for long or tiring visits and procedures
- Creating more flexible options for study visit times, such as evenings or weekends

■ FINALIZING THE PROTOCOL

Pretests, Dress Rehearsals, and Pilot Studies

Pretests, dress rehearsals, and pilot studies are designed to evaluate the feasibility, efficiency, and cost of study methods; the reproducibility and accuracy of measurements; and likely participant recruitment rates. The nature and scale of pretests and pilot studies depend on the study design and the needs of the study. For most studies, pretesting study procedures may suffice, but for large, expensive studies, a full-scale pilot study may be appropriate. It may be desirable to spend up to 10% of the eventual cost of the study on a pilot to make sure that recruitment strategies will work, sample size estimates are realistic, study measurements are appropriate, and participant burden is minimized.

Pretests are evaluations of specific questionnaires, measures, or procedures that can be carried out by study staff to assess their functionality, appropriateness, and feasibility. For example, the data entry and database management system can be pretested by having study staff complete forms with missing, out-of-range, or illogical data; entering these data; and testing to ensure that the data editing system identifies the errors.

Before a study begins, it is a good idea to test plans for clinic visits and other study procedures in a **full-scale dress rehearsal**. Having the PI or staff members go through a **complete mock study visit** can help iron out problems with the final set of instruments and procedures. What appears to be a smooth, problem-free protocol on paper usually reveals logistic and substantive problems in practice, and the dress rehearsal will generate improvements in the approach.

Pilot studies, which are preliminary efforts to obtain information to guide the design and conduct of a full-scale study, are often crucial to the success of a full-scale study (see Chapter 11 for a description of pilot studies for clinical trials). They are used to learn about the feasibility of tasks such as recruiting participants, randomizing them to interventions (if appropriate), making study measurements, collecting data, and maintaining participants in the study, as well as estimating the costs of all of these activities.

Minor Protocol Revisions Once Data Collection Has Begun

No matter how carefully a study is designed and its procedures pretested, problems often appear once the study is underway. The general rule is to make as few changes as possible after participant recruitment has begun. Sometimes, however, protocol modifications can strengthen the study. The decision as to whether a minor change will improve the integrity of the study is often a trade-off between the benefit that may arise from the improved methodology and the disadvantages of altering the uniformity of the study methods, as well as the time and money necessary to implement the change, and the possibility of greater confusion for the team.

Decisions that involve making an operational definition more specific are relatively easy. For example, in a study that excludes persons with alcohol abuse, can a person who has been abstinent for several years be included? This decision should be made in consultation with coinvestigators and then communicated through memos and documented in the operations manual to ensure that it is applied uniformly by all staff for the remainder of the study.

Often minor adjustments of this sort do not require IRB approval, particularly if they do not involve any increase in the risk to participants or changes to the protocol that has been approved by the IRB, but the PI should **ask an IRB staff member if there is any uncertainty**. Any change to the protocol, informed consent form, operations manual, or other study documents should be identified by **giving the revised document a new version number and date**. Researchers should also ensure that systems are in place to prevent research personnel from using out-of-date versions of documents.

Substantive Protocol Revisions Once Data Collection Has Begun

Major changes in the study protocol, such as revising the study's eligibility criteria or changing the intervention or outcome, are a serious issue. Although there may be good reasons for making these changes, they must be undertaken with a view **to analyzing and reporting the data collected before and after the change separately** if this will lead to a more appropriate interpretation of the findings.

The judgments involved are illustrated by two examples from the Raloxifene Use for The Heart (RUTH) trial, a multicenter clinical trial of the effect of treatment with raloxifene on coronary events in 10,101 women at high risk for coronary heart disease. The initial definition of the primary outcome was the occurrence of nonfatal myocardial infarction (MI) or coronary death. Early in the trial, the rate of this outcome was lower than expected, probably because new procedures such as thrombolysis and percutaneous angioplasty lowered the risk for MI. After careful consideration, the RUTH Executive Committee decided to change the primary outcome to include acute coronary syndromes other than MIs. This change was made early in the trial, allowing for a consistent approach to the primary outcome for the remainder of the study. Also, appropriate information had been collected on potential cardiac events to determine if these met the new criteria for acute coronary syndrome, allowing the study database to be searched for acute coronary syndrome events that had occurred before the change was made (1).

Also early in the RUTH trial, results from the Multiple Outcomes of Raloxifene Evaluation (MORE) trial showed that the risk of breast cancer was reduced markedly by treatment with raloxifene (2). These results were not conclusive, because the number of breast cancers was small, and there were concerns about generalizability because all women enrolled in MORE had osteoporosis. To determine if raloxifene would also reduce the risk of breast cancer among older women without osteoporosis, the RUTH Executive Committee decided to add breast cancer as a second primary outcome (1).

Each of these changes required a protocol amendment, approval of the IRB at each clinical site, approval of the FDA, and revision of many forms and study documents. These substantive revisions enhanced the study without compromising its overall integrity. Substantive revisions should only be undertaken after weighing the pros and cons with members of the research team and appropriate advisors such as the Data and Safety Monitoring Board (DSMB) or funding agency. The investigators must then deal with the potential impact of the changes when analyzing the data and drawing the study conclusions.

Closeout

At some point in all longitudinal studies, follow-up of participants stops. The period during which participants complete their last visit in the study—often called "**closeout**"—presents several issues that deserve careful planning (3). At a minimum, at the closeout visit staff should thank participants for their time and effort and inform them that their participation was critical to the success of the study. In addition, closeout may include the following activities:

- Notification of participants (and often their clinicians) of the results of clinically relevant laboratory tests or other measurements that were performed during the study, either in person at the last visit (with a copy in writing) or later by mail
- In a blinded clinical trial, notification of participants of their intervention status, either at the last visit or at the time all participants have completed the trial and the main data analyses are complete or published
- Archival of study hard copy and electronic data according to regulatory requirements or description in the protocol
- Closeout of the IRB record once analyses of study data are complete
- Provision for maintenance of archived specimens that may be used to address future or ancillary research questions
- Mailing of a copy of the main published manuscript from the study to participants and a press release or other description of the findings written in lay language, with a phone number for participants who have questions

■ QUALITY CONTROL DURING THE STUDY

Good Clinical Practice

A crucial aspect of clinical research is the approach to ensuring that all aspects of the study are of the highest quality. Guidelines for high-quality research, called **Good Clinical Practice** (GCP), were developed for clinical trials that test drugs requiring approval by the FDA or other regulatory agencies. They are defined as "an international ethical and scientific quality standard for designing, conducting, recording, and reporting trials that involve the participation of human subjects." Compliance with this standard provides public assurance that the rights, safety, and well-being of trial participants are protected (4).

These principles are applied increasingly to all types of clinical trials sponsored by federal and other public agencies and to research designs other than trials (Table 18.2). GCP requirements are described in detail in the FDA Code of Federal Regulations Title 21 (4, 5). The International Conference on Harmonization (6) provides quality control guidelines used by regulatory agencies in Europe, the United States, and Japan.

GCP is best implemented by having clear, detailed, written guidelines for all aspects of study conduct, also known as **standard operating procedures** (SOPs). The study protocol, operations manual, statistical analysis plan, and data and safety monitoring plan can be considered SOPs, but often do not cover areas such as how staff are trained and certified, how the database is developed and tested, or how study files are maintained, kept confidential, and backed up. Many institutions have staff who specialize in processes for meeting GCP guidelines and can

---

TABLE 18.2 ASPECTS OF THE CONDUCT OF CLINICAL RESEARCH THAT ARE COVERED BY GOOD CLINICAL PRACTICE

- The design is supported by preclinical, animal, and other data as appropriate.
- The study is conducted according to ethical research principles.
- A written protocol is carefully followed.
- Investigators and those providing clinical care are trained and qualified.
- All clinical and laboratory procedures meet quality standards.
- Data are reliable and accurate.
- Complete and accurate records are maintained.
- Statistical methods are prespecified and carefully followed.
- The results are clearly and fairly reported.

provide templates and models for SOPs. In this chapter, we focus on quality control of study procedures and data management; the related topic of ethical conduct of research is addressed in Chapter 7.

Quality Control for Clinical Procedures

One member of the research team should be designated as the **regulatory affairs manager** or **quality coordinator** who is responsible for implementing appropriate quality control techniques for all aspects of the study, including supervising staff training and certification; maintaining study staff certification, staff ID, and delegation logs; preparing regulatory submissions; and monitoring the use of quality control procedures during the study. The goal is to detect possible problems before they occur and prevent them. The quality control coordinator may also be responsible for preparing for and acting as the contact person for audits by the IRB, FDA, or study sponsor. Quality control begins during the planning phase and continues throughout the study (Table 18.3).

TABLE 18.3 QUALITY CONTROL OF CLINICAL PROCEDURES[a]

Steps that precede the study	Develop an operations manual.
	Define recruitment strategies.
	Create operational definitions of measurements.
	Create standardized instruments and forms.
	Create quality control systems.
	Create systems for blinding participants and investigators.
	Appoint quality control coordinator.
	Train the research team and document this.
	Certify the research team and document this.
Steps during the study	Provide steady and caring leadership.
	Hold regular staff meetings.
	Create special procedures for drug interventions.
	Recertify the research team.
	Undertake periodic performance review.
	Compare measurements across technicians and over time.

[a]Clinical procedures include blood pressure measurement, structured interview, chart review, etc.

- **The operations manual.** The operations manual is essential for quality control (Appendix 18A). To illustrate, consider measuring height in a study where it will be used as a predictor of osteoporosis. The operations manual should give specific instructions for the type of measurement device to be used (eg, brand and model of stadiometer), as well as instructions on preparing the participant for the measurement (remove shoes and socks), positioning the patient on the device, and making and recording the measurement.
- **Calibration, training, and certification.** Measurement devices (scales, stadiometers, imaging equipment, laboratory equipment, etc.) should be calibrated before beginning the study and periodically during the study. All staff involved in the study should receive appropriate training and be certified as to competence in using equipment before the study begins. The certification procedure should be supplemented during the study by scheduled recertifications, and a log of training, certification, and recertification should be maintained at the study site.
- **Performance reviews and observations.** Supervisors should review the way clinical procedures are carried out by sitting in on representative clinic visits or telephone calls. After obtaining the study participant's permission, the supervisor can be present for at least one

complete example of every kind of interview and technical procedure each member of his research team performs.

- **Standardized checklists** (provided in advance and based on the protocol and operations manual) can help guide these observations. Afterward, communication between the supervisor and the research team member can be facilitated by reviewing the checklist and resolving any quality control issues that were noted in a positive and nonpejorative fashion. The timing and results of performance reviews should be recorded in training logs.

- **Involving peers from the research team** as reviewers is useful for building morale and teamwork, as well as for ensuring the consistent application of standardized approaches among members of the team who do the same thing. One advantage of using peers as observers in this system is that all members of the research team acquire a sense of ownership of the quality control process. Another advantage is that the observer often learns as much from observing someone else's performance as the person at the receiving end of the review procedure.

- **Periodic data reports.** Tabulating data on the technical quality of the clinical procedures and measurements at regular intervals can give clues to the presence of missing, inaccurate, or variable measurements. Differences among the members of a blood pressure screening team in the mean levels observed over the past 2 months, for example, can lead to the discovery of differences in their measurement techniques. Similarly, a gradual change over a period of months in the standard deviation of sets of readings can indicate a change in the technique for making the measurement. Periodic reports should also address the success of recruitment, the timeliness of data entry, the proportion of missing and out-of-range variables, the time to address data queries, and the success of follow-up and adherence to the intervention.

- **Special procedures for drug interventions.** Clinical trials that use drugs require special attention to the quality control of labeling, drug delivery, and storage; dispensing the medication; and collecting and disposing of unused medication. Providing the correct drug and dosage is ensured by planning the drug distribution approach with the manufacturer or research pharmacy, by overseeing its implementation, and by testing the composition of the blinded study medications to make sure they contain the correct constituents. Drug studies also require clear procedures and logs for tracking receipt of study medication, storage, distribution, and return by participants.

Quality Control for Laboratory Procedures

The quality of laboratory procedures can be controlled using many of the approaches described in Table 18.3 for clinical procedures. However, specimen collection poses unique issues for quality control, as specimens can be mishandled or mislabeled. The technical nature of laboratory testing can also create a need for several special strategies to promote quality:

- **Attention to labeling.** When a specimen obtained from a participant is labeled mistakenly with another individual's study ID, it may be impossible to correct or even discover the error later. Prevention is key: study staff should avoid mislabeling and transposition errors by checking the participant's name and ID number as each specimen is obtained. Preprinted labels with bar/QR codes for specimen tubes and records can speed the process of labeling and avoid mistakes that can occur when numbers are handwritten.

- **Blinding.** The task of blinding an observer is easy when it comes to measurements on specimens as opposed to participants, and it is always a good idea to label specimens so that the technician has no knowledge of the study group or the values of other key variables. Even for apparently objective procedures, like an automated blood glucose determination, this precaution reduces opportunities for bias. However, blinding laboratory staff means that there must be clear procedures for reporting abnormal results to a member of the staff who is qualified to review the results and decide if the participant should be notified or other action should be taken. In clinical trials, there must also be strategies in place for (sometimes emergent) unblinding if laboratory measures indicate abnormalities that might be associated with study interventions and require immediate action.

- **Blinded duplicates, standard pools, and consensus measures.** When specimens or images are sent to a central laboratory for chemical analysis or interpretation, it may be desirable to send blinded duplicates—a second specimen from a random subset of participants that is assigned a separate and fictitious ID number—through the same system. This strategy gives a measure of the precision of the technique. Another approach is to prepare a pool of specimens at the outset, freeze them, and send aliquots labeled with fictitious ID numbers for periodic testing. Measurements carried out on the specimen pool at the outset, using the best available technique, establish its values; the pool is then used as a gold standard during the study, providing estimates of accuracy and precision. A third approach, for measurements that have inherent variability such as a Pap test or mammography readings, is to involve two independent, blinded readers. If both agree within predefined limits, the result is established. Discordant results may be resolved by discussion and consensus, or the opinion of a third reader.
- **Commercial laboratory contracts.** Some studies use commercial laboratories to measure values in blood, sera, or tissue samples. The lab must be licensed and certified, and a copy of these certifications should be on file in the study office. Commercial labs should provide data on the reproducibility of their measurements, such as coefficients of variation. They should also guarantee timely service and provide standardized procedures for handling coded specimens, notifying investigators of abnormal results, and transferring data to the main database.

Quality Control for Data Management

Investigators should create and pretest the data management system before the study begins (Chapter 19). This includes designing the forms for recording measurements; choosing computer hardware and software for data entry, editing, and management; designing the data editing parameters for missing, out-of-range, and illogical entries; and planning dummy tabulations to ensure that the appropriate variables are collected (Table 18.4).

TABLE 18.4 QUALITY CONTROL OF DATA MANAGEMENT: STEPS THAT PRECEDE THE STUDY

Be parsimonious: collect only needed variables.

Select appropriate computer hardware and software for database management.

Program the database to flag missing, out-of-range, and illogical values.

Test the database using missing, out-of-range, and illogical values.

Plan analyses and test with dummy tabulations.

Design paper or electronic forms that are:

   Self-explanatory

   Coherent (eg, multiple-choice options are exhaustive and mutually exclusive)

   Formatted clearly for data entry with arrows directing skip patterns

   Printed in lower case using capitals, underlining, and bold font for emphasis

   Pleasing to look at and easy to read

   Pretested and validated (see Chapter 15)

   Labeled on every page with date, study ID number, and/or bar code

- **Missing data.** Missing data can be disastrous if a large proportion of the measurements are affected, and even a few missing values can sometimes bias the conclusions. A study of the long-term sequelae of a procedure that has a delayed mortality of 5%, for example, could seriously underestimate this complication if 10% of the participants were lost to follow-up and death were a common reason for that loss. Erroneous conclusions because of missing data can sometimes be corrected after the fact—in this case by an intense effort to track down the missing participants—but often the measurement cannot be replaced. Although there are statistical techniques for **imputing missing values** based on other information from baseline or other follow-up visits or from mean values among other participants, they do not guarantee conclusions free of nonresponse bias if there are substantial missing observations. The only good solution is to design and carry out the study in ways that minimize missing data, for example, by having a member of the research team check forms for completeness before the participant completes the study visit, designing electronic data entry interfaces that do not allow skipped entries, and designing the database so that missing data are immediately flagged for attention by study staff (Table 18.5). Missing clinical measurements should be addressed while the participant is still in the clinic, when it is easy to correct errors that are discovered.

• **Inaccurate and imprecise data.** This is an insidious problem that often remains undiscovered, particularly when more than one person is involved in making the measurements. In the worst case, a measurement may be biased seriously by the consistent use of an inappropriate technique. The investigator will assume that the variables mean what they were intended to and, ignorant of the problem, may draw erroneous conclusions from the study.

  Staff training and certification, periodic performance reviews, and regular evaluation of differences in mean or range of data generated by different staff members can help identify or prevent these problems. Another approach is interactive editing, using data entry and management systems programmed to flag or reject forms with missing, inconsistent, and out-of-range values. A standardized procedure should be in place for changing original data on any data form. Generally, this should be done as soon after data collection as possible and with a process that includes an "audit trail," such as marking through the original entry (not erasing it) and then signing and dating the change. Similar processes should be included in electronic data entry and editing systems. The audit trail justifies changes in data and can help prevent data falsification.

  Periodic tabulation and inspection of frequency distributions of important study variables allow the investigator to assess the completeness and quality of the data at a time when correction of past errors may still be possible (eg, by contacting the participant by e-mail or phone, or requesting that the participant return to the study offices) and when further errors in the remainder of the study can be prevented.

• **Fraudulent data.** Clinical investigators who lead research teams should keep in mind the possibility of an unscrupulous colleague or employee who fabricates study data. Approaches to guarding against such a disastrous event include taking great care in choosing colleagues and staff, developing strong relationships with team members to promote ethical behavior by all, staying alert to the possibility of fraud when data are examined, and making unscheduled checks of the primary source of the data to be sure that they are real.

TABLE 18.5 QUALITY CONTROL OF DATA MANAGEMENT: STEPS DURING THE STUDY

Flag or check for omissions and major errors while participant is still in the clinic.

No errors or transpositions in ID number or date on each page

All the correct forms for the specified visit have been filled out.

No missing entries or faulty skip patterns

Entries are legible.

Values of key variables are within permissible range.

Values of key variables are consistent with each other (eg, age and birth date).

Carry out periodic frequency distributions and variance measures to discover aberrant values.

Create other periodic tabulations to discover errors.

Collaborative Multicenter Studies

Many research questions require larger numbers of participants than are available at a single center; these are often addressed in collaborative studies carried out by research teams in several locations. Sometimes study activities are all based in the same city or state, and a single investigator can oversee all the research teams. Often, however, collaborative studies are carried out at locations thousands of miles apart, and each site has its own funding, administration, and regulatory structures.

Multicenter studies require special steps to ensure that all centers are using the same study procedures and producing comparable data that can be combined in the analysis of the results. A **coordinating center** establishes the study communication network; coordinates the development of the operations manual, forms, and other standardized quality control aspects of the trial; trains staff at each center who will make the measurements or administer interventions; and oversees data management, analysis, and publication. Collaborative studies generally use **distributed electronic data entry systems** connected through the internet.

Such studies may also require a governance system with a **steering committee** made up of the PIs and representatives of the funding institution and with various subcommittees. One subcommittee needs to be responsible for quality control issues, including developing the standardization procedures and the systems for training, certification, and performance review of study staff. These can be complicated and expensive, requiring centralized training for relevant staff from each center, site visits for performance review, and data audits by coordinating center staff and peers. Other potential subcommittees include groups that oversee participant recruitment and clinical activities, that review and approve publications and presentations, and that consider proposed ancillary studies.

In a multicenter study, changes in operational definitions and other study methods often result from questions raised by a clinical center that are answered by the relevant study staff or committee. These changes should be posted on the study website or on a shared document in a running list, to make sure that everyone involved in the study is aware of the changes. If a substantial number of changes accumulate, revised pages in the operations manual and other study documents should be prepared and dated. Small single-site studies can follow a simpler procedure, making notes about changes that are dated and retained in the operations manual.

Multicenter studies may also involve clinical research associates, also known as clinical monitors, who are tasked with monitoring compliance with the study protocol and regulatory requirements. Clinical monitors may work directly for the sponsor of a clinical study or as an independent or contracting consultant. Although they are not usually involved in collecting the study data, they may conduct site visits, review study records, and communicate with the project managers or CRCs responsible for the day-to-day work of the study.

A Final Thought

A common error in research is the **tendency to collect too much data**. Investigators may be tempted to include every baseline variable that might conceivably be of interest and then to include additional follow-up visits to collect even more data. Aside from the direct time and costs required to measure less important items, this risks tiring out and annoying participants, who may drop out of the study, leading to deteriorating data quality for more important measurements. In addition, the greater size and complexity of the study database make quality control and data analysis more difficult.

It is wise to **question the need for every variable** that will be collected and to eliminate many that are optional. Including a few intentional redundancies can improve the validity of important variables, but parsimony should be the rule.

■ SUMMARY

1. Successful study implementation begins with assembling resources including staff, space, and funding for the study and its start-up, all of which require strong leadership by the PI.

2. Study start-up requires managing the budget, obtaining IRB approval, and finalizing the protocol and operations manual through a process of pretesting the appropriateness and feasibility of plans for recruitment, interventions, predictor and outcome variable measurements, forms, and the database; the goal is to minimize the need for subsequent protocol revisions once data collection has begun.

3. Minor protocol revisions after the study has begun, such as adding an item to a questionnaire or modifying an operational definition, are accomplished easily, though IRB approval may sometimes be required and data analysis may be affected.

4. Major protocol revisions after the study has begun, such as a change in the nature of the intervention, inclusion criteria, or primary outcome, have major implications and should be carefully considered. Major changes require the approval of key bodies such as the DSMB, IRB, and funding institution.

5. Closeout procedures should be designed to properly inform participants of study findings and to manage transition of and implications for their care.

6. Quality control during the study should be ensured with a systematic approach under the supervision of a quality control coordinator, following the principles of GCP, and including:

   - SOPs with an operations manual; staff training, certification, and performance review; periodic reports (on recruitment, visit adherence, and measurements); and regular team meetings.

   - Quality control for laboratory procedures—blinding and labeling specimens taken from study participants, and using standard pools, blinded duplicates, and consensus measures.

   - Quality control of data management—designing forms and electronic systems to enable oversight of the completeness, accuracy, and integrity of collecting, entering, editing, and analyzing the data.

   - Collaborative multicenter studies create subcommittees and other distributed systems for managing the study and quality control.

REFERENCES

1. Mosca L, Barrett-Connor E, Wenger NK, et al. Design and methods of the Raloxifene Use for The Heart (RUTH) Study. *Am J Cardiol.* 2001;88:392-395.

2. MORE Investigators. The effect of raloxifene on risk of breast cancer in postmenopausal women: results from the MORE randomized trial. Multiple Outcomes of Raloxifene Evaluation. *JAMA.* 1999;281:2189-2197.

3. Shepherd R, Macer JL, Grady D. Planning for closeout—from day one. *Contemp Clin Trials.* 2008;29:136-139.

4. U.S. Food and Drug Administration. CFR - Code of Federal Regulations Title 21. https://www.accessdata.fda.gov/scripts/cdrh/cfdocs/cfcfr/cfrsearch.cfm

5. U.S. Food and Drug Administration. Good Clinical Practise. https://www.fda.gov/about-fda/center-drug-evaluation-and-research-cder/good-clinical-practice.

6. European Medicines Agency. Good clinical practice. https://www.ema.europa.eu/en/human-regulatory/research-development/compliance/good-clinical-practice

APPENDIX 18A
Example of an Operations Manual Table of Contents for a Randomized Trial[a]

Chapter 1. Study protocol
Chapter 2. Organization and policies
    2.1   Participating units (clinical centers, laboratories, coordinating center, etc.) and the investigators and staff administration and governance (committees, funding agency, data and safety monitoring, etc.)
    2.2   Policy guidelines (publications and presentations, ancillary studies, conflict of interest, etc.)
Chapter 3. Recruitment
    3.1   Eligibility and exclusion criteria
    3.2   Sampling design
    3.3   Recruitment approaches (publicity, referral contacts, screening, etc.)
    3.4   Informed consent
Chapter 4. Clinic visits
    4.1   Content of the baseline visit
    4.2   Content and timing of follow-up visits
    4.3   Follow-up procedures for nonresponders
Chapter 5. Randomization and blinding procedures
Chapter 6. Predictor variables
    6.1   Measurement procedures
    6.2   Intervention, including drug labeling, delivery, and handling procedures
    6.3   Assessment of adherence
Chapter 7. Outcome variables
    7.1   Assessment and adjudication of primary outcomes
    7.2   Assessment and management of other outcomes and adverse events
Chapter 8. Quality control
    8.1   Overview and responsibilities
    8.2   Training in procedures
    8.3   Certification of staff
    8.4   Equipment maintenance
    8.5   Peer review and site visits
    8.6   Periodic reports
Chapter 9. Data management
    9.1   Data collection and recording
    9.2   Data entry
    9.3   Editing, storage, and backup
    9.4   Confidentiality
Chapter 10. Data analysis plans
Chapter 11. Data and safety monitoring guidelines
Appendices
    A.1   Letters to participants, primary providers, etc.
    A.2   Questionnaires, forms
    A.3   Details on procedures, criteria, etc.
    A.4   Recruitment materials (advertisements, fliers, letters, etc.)

[a]This is a model for a large multicenter trial. The operations manual for a small study may be less elaborate.

APPENDIX 18B
Exercises for Chapter 18. Study Implementation and Quality Control

1. An investigator carried out a study of the research question: "What are the predictors of death following hospitalization for myocardial infarction?" Research assistants abstracted detailed data from participants' medical charts and recorded the data on paper forms, as well as conducted extensive interviews with 120 hospitalized patients followed over the course of 1 year. About 15% of the patients died during the follow-up period. When data collection was complete, one of the research assistants entered the data into a computer using a spreadsheet. When the investigator began to run analyses of the data, he discovered that 10% to 20% of some predictor variables were missing, and others did not seem to make sense. Only 57% of the sample had been seen at the 1-year follow-up, which was now more than a year overdue for some participants. You are called in to consult on the project.

   a. What can the investigator do now to improve the quality of his data?
   b. Briefly describe at least three ways that he could reduce missing values and errors in his next study.

2. You are preparing an application for funds to carry out a single-center randomized trial of a new medication to improve sleep quality in older adults with insomnia. You already have research assistants in your study team who have worked with you in previous studies about other topics and interventions, but not about insomnia. One of the required components of the application is a project or study timeline indicating how long it will take for the study team to complete important study tasks. Your draft timeline includes the following activities in the first project year. What other activities might be important to account for in study planning?

Month 1	Month 2	Month 3	Month 4	Month 5	Month 6
Finalize Study Protocol and Consent					
Confirm IRB and DSM Approval		IRB Modification for Final Approval			
		Finalize ClinicalTrials.gov Registration			

CHAPTER 19

Data Management

Michael A. Kohn and Thomas B. Newman

Undertaking a clinical research project requires choosing a study design, defining the target population, and specifying the predictor and outcome variables. Ultimately, most information about the participants and variables will reside in a database that will be used to store, update, and monitor the data, as well as format it for statistical analysis. The study database may also store administrative data, such as call logs, visit schedules, and reimbursement records.

In many clinical trials, especially those preparatory to application for regulatory approval of a drug or device, the specialists who create data entry forms, manage and monitor the data collection process, and format and extract the data for analysis are referred to as **clinical data managers** (1). Pharmaceutical companies devote substantial resources and personnel to clinical data management. Although the scale is smaller, beginning investigators also need to attend to data management issues. After all, the conclusions of a study depend on the accuracy, completeness, and security of the study data.

A simple study database consisting of a single data table can be maintained using a spreadsheet or **statistical program**. More complex databases use **database management software** to define the **data tables**, develop the **data entry system**, and monitor the data.

■ DATA TABLES

All computer databases consist of data tables with rows that correspond to individual **records** (which may represent participants, events, or transactions) and columns that correspond to **fields** (attributes of those records). For example, the simplest study database consists of a single table in which each row represents a study participant, and each column contains a participant-specific attribute, such as name, date of birth, sex, or outcome status. In general, the first column in a data table is a unique **participant identification number** (such as "ParticipantID"). Assigning each participant a unique identifier, such as sequential integers (eg, 1, 2, 3, …), with no intrinsic meaning makes it easier to maintain participant confidentiality.

Figure 19.1 shows a simplified data table for a hypothetical cohort study (inspired by a real study (2)) of the association between elevated neonatal bilirubin levels and IQ score at 5 years of age. Each row in the table corresponds to a study participant and each column corresponds to an attribute of that participant. The binary predictor is whether the participant had hyperbilirubinemia ("Hyperbili_ind"), and the continuous outcome is "IQ," which is the participant's IQ on exam at age 5. If the study data are limited to a single two-dimensional table, like the one in Figure 19.1, it is easily accommodated in a spreadsheet or statistical package, and often referred to as a flat file.

If a study tracks multiple lab results, medications, or other repeated measurements for each participant, a single data table will not be adequate. Rather, data management software will need to be used to store those repeated measurements in separate tables distinct from the table of study participants (3, 4). Each row in one of these separate tables corresponds to an individual measurement including what was measured, its date and time, and the result. One field in the row includes the participant identification number to link the measurement back to the participant table. In this **relational database**, because one participant can have many

ParticipantID	FName	DOB	Sex	Hyperbili_ind	ExDate	ExWght	ExHght	IQ
2101	Robert	1/6/2010	M	1	1/29/2015	23.9	118	104
2322	Helen	1/6/2010	F	0	1/29/2015	18.3	109	94
2376	Amy	1/13/2010	F	1	3/22/2015	18.5	117	85
2390	Alejandro	1/14/2010	M	0				
2497	Isiah	1/18/2010	M	0	2/18/2015	20.5	121	74
2569	Joshua	1/23/2010	M	1	2/13/2015	24.8	113	115
2819	Ryan	1/26/2010	M	0				
3019	Morgan	1/29/2010	F	0	2/9/2015	19.1	105	105
3031	Cody	2/15/2010	M	0	4/16/2015	15.2	107	132
3290	Amy	2/16/2010	F	1	4/12/2015	18.0	102	125
3374	Zachary	2/21/2010	M	1				
3625	David	2/22/2010	M	1	2/10/2015	19.2	114	134
3901	Jackson	2/28/2010	M	0				

■ **FIGURE 19.1** Simplified data table in "datasheet view" for a cohort study of the association between neonatal hyperbilirubinemia and IQ score at age 5. The binary predictor is "Hyperbili_ind," defined as whether the total bilirubin rose to 25 mg/dL or more in the first 10 days after birth, and the continuous outcome is "IQ," the participant's IQ score at age 5. Participants 2390, 2819, 3374, and 3901 were not examined at age 5.

measurements, the relationship between the participant table and the measurement table is termed **one-to-many**. The first column in each of the measurement tables should be a unique record identifier, called the table's **primary key**. In Figure 19.2, the primary key is ExamID.

Although the participants in the infant jaundice study had only one IQ test, most had other examinations during which, for example, height and weight were assessed and used to calculate body mass index (BMI) and growth curve percentiles. (See "Extracting Data [Queries]" later in this chapter.) This type of data is best accommodated in a separate Exam table in which each row corresponds to a discrete examination and the columns represent examination date, examination results, and the participant identification number (Figure 19.2). Because a participant can have several examinations, the relationship between participant and exam tables is one-to-many. The field that links the exam-specific data to the participant-specific data is called a **foreign key**; in the Exam table of Figure 19.2, ParticipantID serves as the foreign key that enables each measurement to be linked to a specific participant.

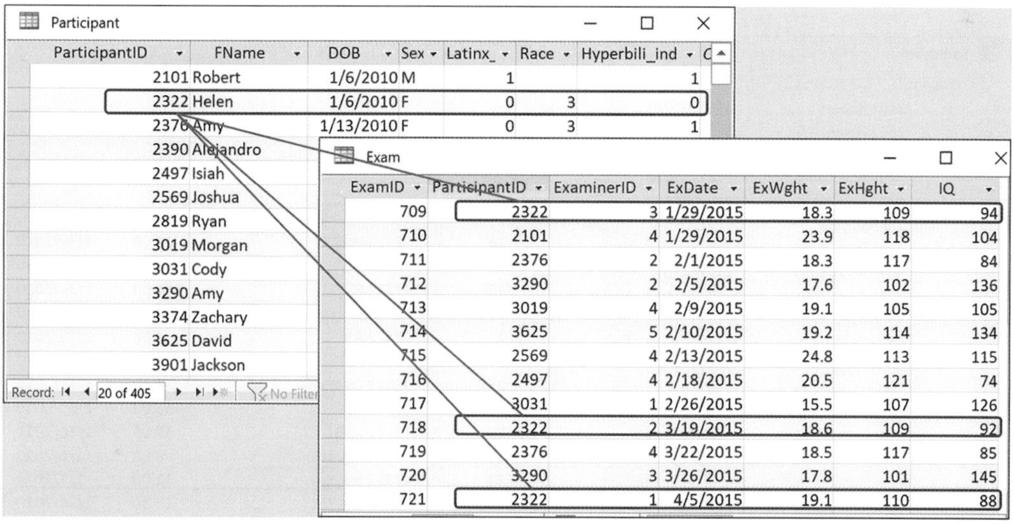

Participant

ParticipantID	FName	DOB	Sex	Latinx_	Race	Hyperbili_ind
2101	Robert	1/6/2010	M	1		1
2322	Helen	1/6/2010	F	0	3	0
2376	Amy	1/13/2010	F	0	3	1
2390	Alejandro					
2497	Isiah					
2569	Joshua					
2819	Ryan					
3019	Morgan					
3031	Cody					
3290	Amy					
3374	Zachary					
3625	David					
3901	Jackson					

Record: 20 of 405 No Filter

Exam

ExamID	ParticipantID	ExaminerID	ExDate	ExWght	ExHght	IQ
709	2322	3	1/29/2015	18.3	109	94
710	2101	4	1/29/2015	23.9	118	104
711	2376	2	2/1/2015	18.3	117	84
712	3290	2	2/5/2015	17.6	102	136
713	3019	4	2/9/2015	19.1	105	105
714	3625	5	2/10/2015	19.2	114	134
715	2569	4	2/13/2015	24.8	113	115
716	2497	4	2/18/2015	20.5	121	74
717	3031	1	2/26/2015	15.5	107	126
718	2322	2	3/19/2015	18.6	109	92
719	2376	4	3/22/2015	18.5	117	85
720	3290	3	3/26/2015	17.8	101	145
721	2322	1	4/5/2015	19.1	110	88

■ **FIGURE 19.2** A two-table infant jaundice study database with a table of study participants (in which each row corresponds to a single study participant) and a table of examinations (in which each row corresponds to a particular examination). For example, Participant 2322 is identified as Helen, date of birth 1/6/2010, in the first table, and has three exams in the anonymous second table. Note that ExWght and ExHght are entered in the exam table, not the participant table.

In a two-table database structure with a participant and an exam table, locating all exams performed within a time period requires searching just a single exam date column. Changes to a participant-specific field, like date of birth, are made in one place, and consistency is preserved. Fields holding personal identifiers, such as name and date of birth, appear only in the participant table; the exam table links back to this information via the ParticipantID. The database can still accommodate participants (such as Alejandro, Ryan, Zachary, and Jackson) who have no exams.

Detailed tracking of lab results would require a separate table. For example, if the investigators needed the entire trajectory of bilirubin levels after birth, then the database should include a separate lab result table with one record per lab result and fields for date/time of lab test, lab test type (total bilirubin), test result (bilirubin level), and ParticipantID, the foreign key for linking back to the participant-specific information, as in Figure 19.3.

A study's administrative data, such as call logs, visit schedules, and reimbursement records, also require separate tables. In the infant jaundice study, just a few calls were made to the parents of some study participants, but 50 or more calls were made to those who were harder to reach. It would be difficult to track these calls in a data table with one row per study participant, because such a table would need to have enough columns to accommodate the participant with the highest number of calls, and those columns would be empty for most participants. It is much easier to have a separate table with one row per call; ParticipantID links the data to the study participant about whom the call was made.

The process of putting fields for which each participant has only a single value in one table (such as birth date, birth weight, and sex assigned at birth) and fields that take on multiple and variable numbers of values per participant in another table (such as phone calls or bilirubin levels) is part of database **normalization**. A key feature of normalization is that the only participant-specific field in new tables should be the ParticipantID to link back to the participant record. All other participant-specific fields (such as date of birth and sex) are stored in a table with only one record per participant. Normalization eliminates redundant storage and the opportunity for inconsistencies. Relational database software can be set to maintain **referential integrity** that will not allow creation of an exam, lab result, or call record for someone who is not already listed in the participant table. Similarly, it prevents deletion of a participant unless all that participant's exams, lab results, and calls have also been deleted.

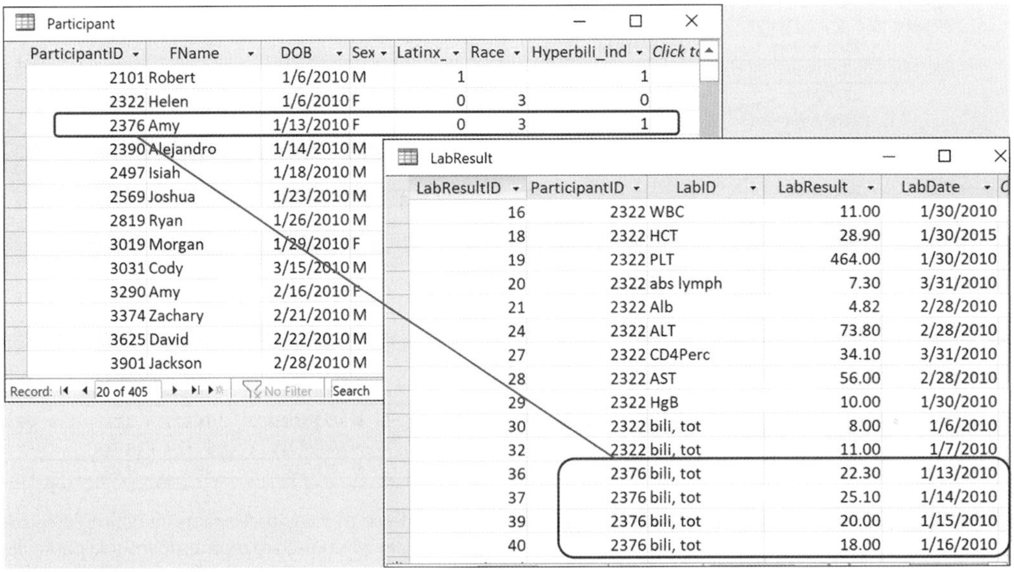

■ FIGURE 19.3 The linkage between the table of participants and the table of lab results. The lab results capture the trajectory of Amy's total bilirubin levels during the first 4 days after birth.

Data Dictionaries, Data Types, and Domains

Each column or field in a database must have a name, data type, and definition. For example, in the participant table of Figure 19.2, "FName" is a **text field** that contains the participant's first name, "DOB" is a **date field** that contains the participant's birth date, and "Hyperbili_ind" is a **yes/ no field** that indicates whether the bilirubin exceeded 25 mg/dL. In the exam table, "ExWght" is a (continuous) **number field** for weight in kilograms and "IQ" is a (discrete) **integer** IQ score. The data types and definitions should be made explicit for every field in a **data dictionary**. The data dictionary is referred to as **metadata**, because it contains information about the database itself.

Figure 19.4 shows the participant and exam tables in table design (or "data dictionary") view. The data dictionary is itself a table, with rows for each field and columns for the field name, data type, and field description, as well as a range of allowed values. For example, in the infant jaundice database, the allowed values for the "Sex" field were "M" and "F"; other values cannot be entered in this field.[1] Similarly, the "IQ" field allowed only integers between 40 and 200. Data managers often refer to validation rules as "edit checks" (1), because they afford some protection against data entry errors. Some data types come with automatic validation rules; for example, database software will always reject a date of April 31.

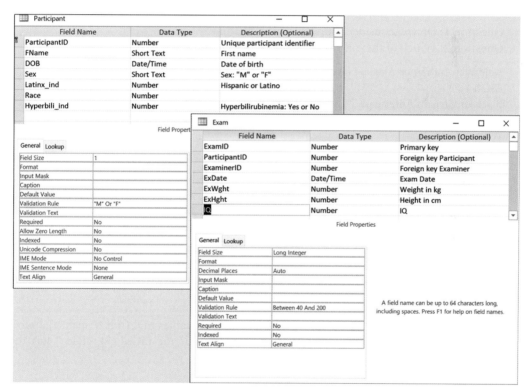

■ **FIGURE 19.4** Table of study participants ("Participant") and the table of measurements ("Exam") in "data dictionary view." Each variable has a name, a data type, a description, and a domain or set of allowed values.

Variable Names and Coding Conventions

Variable names should be short enough to type quickly, but long enough to be self-explanatory. Avoid using spaces and special characters; separate the words in a variable name either by using (aptly named) "InterCaps" or "camelCase," or with an underscore character. Binary indicator variables should be named for the *yes* or *present* condition (eg, "EverSmoker_ind") and valued

---

[1] A more inclusive way to code sex is suggested later.

as 1 for *yes* or *present* and 0 for *no* or *absent*. With this coding, the average value of the variable is simply the proportion with the attribute. Appending "_ind" to binary indicator variables allows them to be identified readily. Most software packages allow users to designate a longer, more descriptive, and easier-to-read **variable label** to use on data entry forms and reports instead of the compact variable name.

In coding response options, one convention is to use the digit 9 (or 99) for "Unknown," "Does Not Apply," "Not Answered," etc., and 8 (or 88) for "Other (Specify)." Coding sex, ethnicity, and race often uses the approach of the National Center for Health Statistics (5), which has been incorporated into several electronic health records.

For sex, use the following standard codes:

0 Female
1 Male
4 Transgender Female to Male
5 Transgender Male to Female
8 Nonbinary
9 Unknown

For ethnicity and race, the standardized approach is to ask two questions:

Question 1: Do you consider yourself Hispanic/Latino?
Question 2: Which of the following five racial designations best describes you?

American Indian or Alaska Native
Asian
Black or African American
Native Hawaiian or Other Pacific Islander
White

This approach allows multiple responses to Question 2 (Figure 19.5); it is also possible to add options for "Other (includes more than one race)" and "Unknown/Not Reported" and then allow only one response.

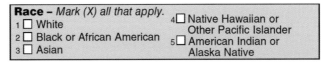

■ **FIGURE 19.5** Coding of Race on the National Hospital Ambulatory Medical Care Survey (6) of the National Center for Health Statistics.

The ethnicity field name, "EthnLatino_ind," has allowed values of 0 (not Hispanic/Latino), 1 (Hispanic/Latino), and 9 (Unknown/Decline to state). For the race field, "Race" has the following codes:

1. White
2. Black or African American
3. Asian
4. Native Hawaiian or Other Pacific Islander
5. American Indian or Alaska Native
6. Other (includes more than one race)
7. Unknown/Not Reported

Common Data Elements

Several funding and regulatory organizations, including the National Institute of Neurologic Disorders and Stroke (NINDS) (7), the National Cancer Institute (8), the U.S. Food and Drug

Administration (FDA) (9), the European Medicines Agency, and nongovernmental, nonprofit associations such as the Clinical Data Interchange Standards Consortium (CDISC) (10), have launched initiatives to develop common data elements for study databases.

Standardizing record structures, field names/definitions, data types/formats, and data collection forms will eliminate the problem of "reinventing the wheel" for every new study and enable sharing and combining data across studies. This entails establishing a data dictionary and a set of data collection instruments with accompanying instructions that all investigators in a particular area of research are encouraged to use.

■ DATA ENTRY

Whether the study database consists of one or many tables, or whether it uses spreadsheet, statistical, or database management software, a way to populate the data tables (enter the data) is needed. In the past, the most common method for populating a study database was to collect data on a paper form, called a case report form (CRF) in clinical trials. Study personnel then transcribed the information into computer tables, preferably using on-screen forms that made data entry easier and included automatic data validation checks.

Electronic Data Capture

Handwriting data onto a paper form is increasingly rare. In general, research studies should collect data primarily using online forms, in clinical trials called electronic case report forms (eCRFs). Online forms may be viewed, and data entered on portable, wireless devices such as a tablet (iPad), smartphone, or notebook computer. Data entry via online forms has many advantages:

- The data are keyed directly into the data tables without a second transcription step, removing that source of error.
- The computer form can include validation checks and provide immediate feedback when an entered value is out of range.
- The computer form can also incorporate skip logic. For example, a question about packs per day appears only if the participant answered "yes" to a question about cigarette smoking.

When using online forms for electronic data capture, it sometimes makes sense to print a paper record of the data immediately after collection that can be verified by the study participant. It may be used as the original or source document if a paper version is required for auditing purposes.

Online data collection forms provide two main formats for displaying *mutually exclusive* (no overlap) and *collectively exhaustive* (all-encompassing) response options: **drop-down list** or **option group** (Figure 19.6A and B). These formats will be familiar to any research participant or data entry person who has worked with an online form.

A question with a set of mutually exclusive responses corresponds to a single field in the data table. In contrast, the responses to an "All that apply" question are not mutually exclusive; rather, they correspond to as many yes/no fields as there are possible responses. By convention, response options for "All that apply" questions use **square check boxes** rather than the **round radio buttons** used for mutually exclusive responses. "All that apply" questions should be avoided; requiring a yes or no response to each item is preferable. Otherwise an unmarked response could either mean "does not apply" or "not answered."

Importing Measurements and Laboratory Results

Much study information, such as baseline demographic information, lab results, and measurements made by dual-energy x-ray absorptiometry (DEXA) scanners and Holter monitors, is often already in digital format in a hospital's electronic health record. Whenever possible, these data

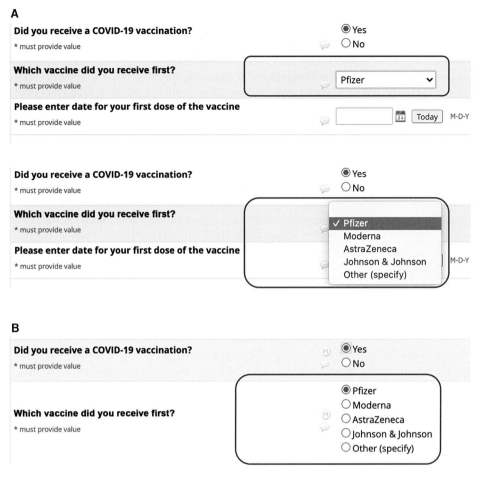

■ **FIGURE 19.6** Formats for entering from a mutually exclusive, collectively exhaustive list of responses. The drop-down list (**A,** dropped down in lower panel) saves screen space but will not work if the screen form will be printed to paper for data collection. The option group (**B**) requires more screen space, but will work if printed.

should be imported directly into the study database to avoid the cost and potential transcription errors of reentering data. Computer systems can almost always produce comma-separated-value (csv) files or fixed-column-width text files that the database software can import. In clinical trials, this type of batch-uploaded information is referred to as "non-CRF data" (1).

Data Management Software

The **back end** of a study database consists of the data tables themselves. The **front end** (or interface) consists of the online forms used for entering, viewing, and editing the data. Study databases consisting of multiple data tables require relational database software (Table 19.1) to maintain the back-end data tables. If the data are collected on paper forms, entering the data will require transcription into online forms.

As discussed in Chapter 17, there are several tools, including SurveyMonkey, Zoomerang, Qualtrics, QuesGen, and REDCap, for developing online surveys to e-mail to study participants or post on a website. All these tools provide several question format options, skip logic, and the capability to aggregate, report on, and export survey results. Some statistical packages, such as Statistical Analysis System (SAS), have developed data entry modules. Integrated desktop database programs, such as Microsoft Access and Filemaker Pro, also provide extensive tools for the development of on-screen forms.

TABLE 19.1 SOME SOFTWARE USED IN RESEARCH DATA MANAGEMENT

Spreadsheet

Microsoft Excel
Apple Numbers
Google Sheets[a]
Apache OpenOffice Calc[a]

Statistical Analysis

Statistical Analysis System (SAS)
Statistical Package for the Social Sciences (SPSS)
Stata
R[a]

Integrated Desktop Database Systems

Microsoft Access (for Windows only)
Filemaker Pro

Relational Database Systems

Oracle
SQL Server
MySQL[a]
PostgreSQL[a]

Integrated Web-Based Platforms for Research Data Management

Research Electronic Data Capture (REDCap—hosted by many academic institutions[a])
QuesGen (primarily academic, vendor hosted)
MediData RAVE (primarily nonacademic corporate, vendor hosted)
Oracle InForm (nonacademic corporate, company hosted)
Datalabs EDC (corporate, vendor hosted)
OnCore
OpenClinica
EpiInfo[a]

Online Survey Tools

SurveyMonkey
Zoomerang
Qualtrics

[a]Free.

Many research studies use integrated, web-enabled, research data management platforms, such as REDCap (Research Electronic Data Capture), which was designed specifically for clinical research by an academic consortium based at Vanderbilt University. It enables researchers to build and manage surveys, data entry forms, and databases. REDCap, which is available to investigators at many academic institutions, is an outstanding "do-it-yourself" tool for beginning investigators. It also provides access to a repository of data collection instruments. However, options for customization and advanced functionality are limited. A REDCap database consists of a single table with one column for every field in the database and one row for every data collection event, and can be exported easily into statistical packages. REDCap does not permit detailed tracking of a large and variable number of repeated measurements per study participant, and it cannot do sophisticated data validation or reporting, nor can it be queried as can a relational database (see below).

Full-featured, web-based research data management platforms, such as QuesGen, MediData RAVE, or Oracle InForm, can accommodate complex data structures and provide sophisticated data validation, querying, and reporting. The companies that provide these tools also provide support and configuration assistance.

■ EXTRACTING DATA (QUERIES)

Once the database has been created and the data entered, the investigator will want to organize, sort, filter, and view ("query") the data. **Database queries** are used for monitoring data entry, reporting study progress, and analyzing the results. The standard language for manipulating data in a relational database is called **Structured Query Language or SQL** (pronounced "sequel"). Many relational database programs also provide a graphical interface for building queries. The R statistical program supports SQL but also offers an alternative set of commands in the dplyr library (11).

A query can join data from two or more tables, display only selected fields, and filter for records that meet certain criteria. Queries can also calculate values based on raw data fields from the tables. Figure 19.7 shows the results of a query from the infant jaundice database that filtered for boys examined in February and then calculated their ages in months and their BMIs . (The query also used a sophisticated table-lookup function to calculate growth curve percentile values for the child's BMI.) One of the tenets of the relational database model is that operations on tables produce table-like results; thus, the result of a query that joins two tables, displays only certain fields, selects rows based on special criteria, and calculates certain values still looks like a table. The data in Figure 19.7 are easily exported to a statistical analysis package.

ParticipantID ▾	ExDate ▾	AgeMonths ▾	Sex ▾	ExWght ▾	ExHght ▾	BMI ▾	Zscore ▾	ZPerc ▾
3625	2/10/2015	59	M	19.2	114	14.75	-0.63	26.4
2569	2/13/2015	60	M	25.0	113	19.58	2.34	99.0
2497	2/18/2015	61	M	20.5	121	14.02	-1.41	7.9
5305	2/23/2015	60	M	20.5	116	15.21	-0.18	42.9
4430	2/23/2015	59	M	35.0	105	31.75	4.38	100.0
5310	2/24/2015	60	M	19.6	115	14.78	-0.59	27.8
3031	2/26/2015	59	M	15.5	102	14.94	-0.45	32.6

Record: I◄ ◄ 5 of 7   ► ►I ►*   ⧊ No Filter   Search

■ **FIGURE 19.7** A query in datasheet view that filtered for boys examined in February and calculated age in months and BMI. The query also used a sophisticated table-lookup function to calculate growth curve percentile values for the child's body mass index (BMI). For ParticipantID 4430, the 100th percentile value associated with the BMI of 31.75 should have triggered investigation of the outlier as a possible data entry error.

Identifying and Correcting Errors in the Data

The entire data management system (data tables, data entry forms, and queries) should be tested using dummy data. For clinical trials that will be used in an FDA submission, this is a regulatory requirement (12).

Once data collection begins, values that are outside the preset permissible range should not get past the data entry process. However, the database should also be queried for missing values and outliers (extreme values that are nevertheless within the range of allowed values). If data are collected by investigators at different locations, means and medians should be compared across investigators and sites. Substantial differences by investigator or site can indicate systematic differences in measurement or data collection.

Many data entry systems are incapable of doing cross-field validation, which means that the data tables may contain field values that are within the allowed ranges but inconsistent with one another. For example, it would be highly unlikely for a 5-year-old who weighed 35 kg to be only 105 cm tall. Although the weight and height values are both within the allowed ranges, the weight (extremely high for a 5-year-old) is inconsistent with the height (extremely low for a 5-year-old). Such an inconsistency can be identified using a query like the one in Figure 19.7.

Missing values, outliers, inconsistencies, and other data problems that are identified by queries should be communicated to the study staff, who can respond by checking original source documents, interviewing the participant, or repeating the measurement. If the study relies on paper source documents, any resulting changes to the data should be highlighted (eg, in red ink), dated, and signed. As discussed later in this chapter, **electronic databases should maintain an audit log of all data changes.**

Data editing is an iterative process; after errors are identified and corrected, editing procedures should be repeated until very few important errors are identified. At this point, for some studies, the edited database may be declared final or "locked" and no further changes are permitted (1).

■ ANALYSIS OF THE DATA

Analyzing the data often requires creating derived variables based on the raw values in the database. For example, continuous variables may be made dichotomous (eg, a new variable called "BMIge25" can be defined as a BMI ≥ 25 kg/m^2), new categories created (eg, antibiotics grouped by type), and calculations made (eg, pack years defined as number of packs of cigarettes per day $\times$ years of smoking). Missing data should be handled consistently. "Don't know" may be recoded as a special category, combined with "no," or excluded as missing. If the study uses database software, queries can be used to derive the new variables prior to export to a statistical analysis package. That said, many investigators are more familiar with statistical packages than database programs and prefer to calculate derived variables after export.

■ CONFIDENTIALITY AND SECURITY

An investigator is obligated ethically and legally to protect participants' confidentiality. If participants are clinic or hospital patients, their identifying information is also protected under the Privacy Rule of the Health Insurance Portability and Accountability Act (HIPAA). To ensure confidentiality, the database should assign each participant a unique participant identifier (eg, ParticipantID) that has no meaning external to the study database (ie, it should not incorporate the participant's name, initials, birth date, or medical record number)—and thus cannot be used on its own to identify the participant. If a database has multiple tables, personal identifiers should be kept in a separate table.

Study databases that contain personal identifiers must be maintained on secure servers accessible only to authorized members of the research team, each of whom will have a user ID and password. **Database fields that contain personal identifiers should not be exported.** Dedicated web-based research data management platforms such as REDCap and QuesGen allow designation of fields containing participant identifiers. Different user roles can allow or prohibit exporting, changing, or even viewing these specially designated fields.

The database system should audit all data entry and editing. Auditing allows determination of when a data element was changed, who made the change, and what change was made. This is a regulatory requirement for pharmaceutical and device trials (12). The study database also must be backed up regularly; the backup procedure should be tested periodically. Web-based data management platforms provide user validation, auditing, backups, and data security automatically.

At the end of the study, the original data, data dictionary, final database, and the study analyses should be stored securely. This allows the investigators to respond to questions about the integrity of the data or analyses, perform further analyses to address new research questions, and share data with others.

■ SUMMARY

1. The study **database** consists of one or more **data tables** in which the *rows* correspond to records (eg, study participants) and the *columns* correspond to fields (attributes of the records).

2. Identifying study participants with a **unique ParticipantID** that has no meaning external to the study database enables the "delinking" of the study data from personal identifiers to maintain confidentiality. Databases that contain personal identifiers must be stored on secure servers, with access restricted and audited.

3. Accommodating a variable number of **repeated measurements per study participant**, such as lab results or medications, **requires normalization** of the measurement data into separate tables in which each row corresponds to a measurement rather than an individual study participant.

4. The study database may also store **administrative data such as call logs, exam schedules, and reimbursement records**.

5. The **data dictionary** specifies the name, data type, description, and range of allowed values for all the fields in the database.

6. The **data entry system** is the means by which the data tables are populated, usually by electronic data capture using online forms.

7. A spreadsheet or statistical package is adequate only for the simplest study databases; **complex databases require the creation of a relational database** using database management software based on Structured Query Language (SQL).

8. Database **queries sort and filter the data** as well as calculate values based on raw data fields. Queries are used to monitor data entry, provide reports on study progress, and format the results for analysis.

9. Loss of the database must be prevented by **regular backups** and by storing and **securing a final copy of the database** for future use.

REFERENCES

1. Prokscha S. *Practical Guide to Clinical Data Management*. 3rd ed. CRC Press; 2012.
2. Newman TB, Liljestrand P, Jeremy RJ, et al. Outcomes among newborns with total serum bilirubin levels of 25 mg per deciliter or more. *N Engl J Med*. 2006;354(18):1889-1900.
3. Codd EF. A relational model of data for large shared data banks. *Commun ACM*. 1970;13(6):377-387.
4. Date CJ. *An Introduction to Database Systems*. 8th ed. Pearson/Addison Wesley; 2004.
5. FDA. Collection of Race and Ethnicity Data in Clinical Trials (10/26/2016). Accessed March, 20, 2021. https://www.fda.gov/regulatory-information/search-fda-guidance-documents/collection-race-and-ethnicity-data-clinical-trials
6. NHAMCS. Sample 2020 Emergency Department Patient Record. Accessed March, 20, 2021. https://www.cdc.gov/nchs/data/nhamcs/2020-NHAMCS-ED-PRF-sample-card-508.pdf
7. NINDS. Common Data Elements. Accessed March, 20, 2021. https://www.commondataelements.ninds.nih.gov/
8. NCI. NIH CDE Repository. Accessed March, 20, 2021. https://cde.nlm.nih.gov/home/
9. FDA. CDER Data Standards Program. Accessed March, 20, 2021. https://www.fda.gov/drugs/electronic-regulatory-submission-and-review/cder-data-standards-program
10. CDISC. The Clinical Data Interchange Standards Consortium Study data tabulation model. 2012. Accessed March, 20, 2021. http://www.cdisc.org/sdtm
11. Wickham H, Grolemund G. *R for Data Science: Import, Tidy, Transform, Visualize, and Model Data*. 1st ed. O'Reilly; 2016.
12. DHHS. Guidance for industry: computerized systems used in clinical trials. May, 2007. FDA. Use of Electronic Records and Electronic Signatures in Clinical Investigations Under 21 CFR Part 11 — Questions and Answers; June 2017. Accessed March, 20, 2021. https://www.fda.gov/regulatory-information/search-fda-guidance-documents/use-electronic-records-and-electronic-signatures-clinical-investigations-under-21-cfr-part-11
13. Lowenstein DH, Alldredge BK, Allen F, et al. The prehospital treatment of status epilepticus (PHTSE): design and methodology. *Control Clin Trials*. 2001;22:290-309.
14. Alldredge BK, Gelb AM, Isaacs SM, et al. A comparison of lorazepam, diazepam, and placebo for the treatment of out-of-hospital status epilepticus. *N Engl J Med*. 2001;345(9):631-637.

APPENDIX 19A
Exercises for Chapter 19.
Data Management

1. The PHTSE (Pre-Hospital Treatment of Status Epilepticus) Study (13, 14) was a randomized blinded trial of lorazepam, diazepam, or placebo in the treatment of prehospital status epilepticus. The primary endpoint was termination of convulsions by hospital arrival. To enroll patients, paramedics contacted base hospital physicians by radio. The following are base hospital physician data collection forms for two enrolled patients:
   a. Display the data from these two data collection forms in a two-row data table.
   b. Create a nine-field data dictionary for the data table in exercise 1a.
   c. The paper data collection forms were completed by busy base hospital physicians who were called from the emergency department to a radio room. What are the advantages and disadvantages of using an on-screen computer form instead of a paper form? If you designed the study, which would you use?

PHTSE

Base Hospital Physician Data Collection Form

PHTSE Subject ID :

Study Drug Administration | 189

Study Drug Kit #: | A322

Date and Time of Administration :   3 / 12 / 94   17 : 39
                                                    (Use 24 hour clock)

Transport Evaluation
Seizure Stopped
Time Seizure Stopped   17 : 44
                                   (Use 24 hour clock)

Final ("End-of-Run") Assessment
Time of Arrival at Receiving Hospital ED: 17 : 48
                                             (Use 24 hour clock)

On arrival at the receiving hospital:
[X] 1 Seizure activity (active tonic/clonic convulsions) continued
[   ] 0 Seizure activity (active tonic/clonic convulsions) stopped
    Verbal GCS
    [   ] 1   No Verbal Response
    [   ] 2   Incomprehensible Speech
    [   ] 3   Inappropriate Speech
    [   ] 4   Confused Speech
    [   ] 5   Oriented

PHTSE

Base Hospital Physician Data Collection Form

PHTSE Subject ID :

Study Drug Administration

| 410 |

Study Drug Kit #:

| B536 |

Date and Time of Administration :   12 / 01 / 98   01 : 35
(Use 24 hour clock)

Transport Evaluation
[X]Seizure Stopped
Time Seizure Stopped   01 : 39
(Use 24 hour clock)

Final ("End-of-Run") Assessment
Time of Arrival at Receiving Hospital ED: 01 : 53
(Use 24 hour clock)

On arrival at the receiving hospital:
[ ] 1 Seizure activity (active tonic/clonic convulsions) continued
[X] 0 Seizure activity (active tonic/clonic convulsions) stopped
    Verbal GCS
    [ ] 1   No Verbal Response
    [ ] 2   Incomprehensible Speech
    [ ] 3   Inappropriate Speech
    [X] 4   Confused Speech
    [ ] 5   Oriented

---

2. The data collection forms in exercise 1 include a question about whether seizure activity continued on arrival at the receiving hospital (which was the primary outcome of the study). This data item was given the field name *HospArrSzAct* and was coded 1 for yes (seizure activity continued) and 0 for no (seizure activity stopped). Interpret the average values for *HospArrSzAct* as displayed below:

	HospArrSzAct	
	(1 = Yes, seizure continued; 0 = No, seizure stopped)	
	N	*Average*
Lorazepam	66	0.409
Diazepam	68	0.574
Placebo	71	0.789

CHAPTER 20

Writing a Proposal for Funding a Research Study

Steven R. Cummings, Deborah G. Grady, and Alka M. Kanaya

As noted in Chapter 2, developing a research study begins with a statement of the research question. This should be followed by a one-page outline of the study plan (Appendix 1), which can be circulated to obtain advice from mentors, colleagues, and experts. When we teach courses in designing clinical research, the students produce a five- to seven-page study plan that includes most of the important elements of the study—the background, design, participants, measurements for the predictor, outcome and potential confounding variables, sample size and power estimates, and any human subject concerns.

A **protocol** is a detailed written plan of the study. Writing the protocol forces the investigator to organize, clarify, and refine all the elements of the study, and this enhances the scientific rigor and the efficiency of the project. Even if the investigator does not require funding for a study, a protocol is necessary for guiding the work and for obtaining ethical approval from the institutional review board (IRB). A **proposal** is a document written for the purpose of obtaining funds from a granting agency. It includes descriptions of the study's aims, significance, research approach, and human subjects concerns, as well as the budget and other administrative and supporting information required by the agency.

This chapter describes how to write a proposal that will be most likely to be successful at receiving funding. It focuses on original research proposals that use the format suggested by the National Institutes of Health (NIH), but submissions to most other funding agencies (such as the Department of Veterans Affairs, Centers for Disease Control and Prevention [CDC], Department of Defense [DOD], Agency for Healthcare Research and Quality [AHRQ], and private foundations) require a similar format. Excellent advice on writing an application, preparing budgets, and submitting proposals is available on the NIH website (https://grants.nih.gov/grants/how-to-apply-application-guide.html).

■ WRITING PROPOSALS

The task of preparing a proposal requires several months of organizing, writing, and revising. The following steps can help the project get off to a good start.

- **Decide where the proposal will be submitted.** Every funding agency has its own unique areas of interests, processes, and requirements for proposals. Therefore, the investigator should start by deciding where the proposal will be submitted, determining the limit on amounts of funding, and obtaining specific guidelines about how to craft the proposal and deadlines for that particular agency. The NIH is a good place to start, at http://grants.nih.gov/grants/oer.htm. Areas of interest can be identified through the websites of individual NIH institutes and other funders that describe their priorities. Additional information about current areas of interest can be obtained by talking with program officers at the NIH institutes, whose contact information and areas of responsibility are listed on NIH Funding Opportunity Announcements, as well as on institute and foundation websites.

- **Organize a team and designate a leader.** Most proposals are written by a team of several people who will eventually carry out the study. This team may be small (just the investigator and their mentor) or large (including collaborators, a biostatistician, a fiscal administrator, research assistants, and support staff). The team should include—or have access to—the main expertise needed for designing and conducting the study.

- The **principal investigator** (PI) of the team assumes the responsibility for leading the effort and has the ultimate authority and accountability for the study. The PI must exert steady leadership during proposal development, delegating responsibilities for writing and other tasks, setting deadlines, conducting periodic meetings of the team, ensuring that all necessary tasks are completed on time, and taking charge of the quality of the proposal. The PI is often an experienced scientist whose knowledge and wisdom are useful for design decisions and whose track record with previous studies makes it more likely that a study will be successful, thereby increasing the probability that it will be funded.

- That said, the NIH encourages **new investigators** to apply for grants as PIs, has special funding opportunities for them, and often gives preference to funding their proposals if they are early stage (http://grants.nih.gov/grants/new_investigators/). The NIH defines new investigators as scientists who have not yet been the PI of an NIH research grant; **early stage investigators** are within 10 years of their terminal research degree or clinical training. First-time PIs are most likely to be funded if they have some experience carrying out research, under the guidance of a senior scientist and with funding provided by that individual, through a career development award, or after receiving small institutional or foundation grants. **A track record in publishing, including first authorships on original research papers, provides evidence that a new investigator has the potential to be a successful independent scientist and is prepared and able to lead a research team.**

- A first-time PI should include coinvestigators on the grant application with a history of successful research in the area of interest to provide guidance about the conduct of the study and improve the chances of a favorable review and funding. Although there is usually only one PI per proposal, the NIH allows more than one if they bring different, but complementary expertise, and their distinct roles and responsibilities are defined (http://grants.nih.gov/grants/multi_pi/overview.htm).

- **Follow the guidelines of the funding agency.** All funding sources provide written guidelines that the investigator should read before starting to write the proposal. This information includes the types of research that will be funded, along with detailed instructions for organizing the proposal, page limits, and the maximum amount of funding that can be requested. However, these guidelines do not contain everything that the investigator should know about the operations and preferences of the funding agencies. Early in the development of the proposal, it is a good idea to discuss the plan with an individual at the agency who can comment on whether the agency is interested in the planned research and clarify the scope and detail of the proposal. The NIH, other federal agencies, and private foundations have scientific administrators (often called **program officers**) who help investigators design their proposals to be more responsive to the agency's funding priorities. The relevant program officer should be contacted by e-mail or telephone to clarify the agency's guidelines, interests, and review procedures. Subsequently, meeting with the program officer (say, at a scientific conference or by visiting the agency headquarters) is a good way to establish a working relationship that promotes fundable proposals.

- **Make a checklist of the required details and review it repeatedly** before submitting a proposal. An otherwise excellent proposal may be rejected for lack of adherence to specified guidelines—a frustrating and avoidable experience. Most university grant managers have checklists that they review before submission of a proposal, but following the agency guidelines is the responsibility of the PI.

- **Establish a timetable and meet periodically.** A schedule for completing the writing tasks keeps gentle pressure on team members to meet their obligations on time. In addition to addressing the scientific components specified by the funding agency, the timetable should take into account the administrative requirements of the institution where the research will take place. Universities often require a time-consuming review of proposed space, budget, and subcontracts before a proposal can be submitted, so the *real* deadline to complete a proposal may be several days or even weeks before the agency deadline. Leaving these details to the end can precipitate a last-minute crisis that damages an otherwise well-done proposal. A timetable works best if it specifies deadlines for written products and if everyone participates in setting their own assignments. The timetable should be reviewed during periodic meetings or conference calls of the writing team to check that the tasks are on schedule and the deadlines are still realistic.

- **Find model proposals.** It is extremely helpful to look at recent proposals that were funded by the agency that will be evaluating the application: They illustrate both the content and the format of good proposals. An investigator can often find inspiration for new ideas and prepare a proposal that is clearer, more logical, and more persuasive. Similarly, it's worthwhile to review written criticisms of previous proposals to the agency—whether successful or not—to identify what matters to the scientists who will be reviewing the proposal. These examples can often be obtained from the Office of Sponsored Research at the investigator's institution or from colleagues who are PIs of similar studies.

- **Work from an outline.** Begin by setting out the proposal in outline form (Table 20.1) to help organize the tasks that need to be done. If several people will be working on the grant, the outline should include who is responsible for writing each part of the proposal. A common roadblock to creating an outline is believing that the entire research plan must be completed before starting to write the first sentence. The investigator should put this notion aside by letting thoughts flow onto paper, thus creating the raw material for editing, refining, and getting specific advice from colleagues.

- **Review and revise repeatedly.** Writing a proposal is an iterative process; there are usually many versions, each reflecting new ideas, advice, and additional data. Beginning early in the process, drafts should be reviewed critically by colleagues who are familiar with the subject matter and the funding agency. Particular attention should go to the significance and innovativeness of the research, the validity of the design and methods, how well the proposal is organized, and the clarity of the writing. It is better to have sharp and detailed criticism before a proposal is submitted than to have it rejected because of failure to anticipate and address problems. When the proposal is nearly ready for submission, the final step is to review it for internal consistency, adherence to agency guidelines, and grammatical, formatting, and typographical errors. Sloppy writing implies sloppy work and less-than-competent leadership and detracts significantly from otherwise good ideas.

■ ELEMENTS OF A PROPOSAL FOR A MAJOR GRANT

The elements of a proposal for a major research grant such as an NIH R01 are set out in Table 20.1. Applications for other types of NIH grants and contracts, and from other funding institutions, are similar, but may require less information or a different format. The investigator should review the guidelines of the agency that will receive the proposal.

The Beginning

A descriptive and concise title will provide the first impression—and a lasting reminder—of the overall research goal and design of the study. For example, the title "A randomized trial of

TABLE 20.1 MAIN ELEMENTS OF A PROPOSAL, BASED ON THE NIH MODEL

Title
Project summary or abstract
Administrative parts
    Budget and budget justification
    Biosketches of investigators
    Institutional resources
Specific aims (usually one page)
Potential impact
Research strategy (usually 12 pages)
    Significance
    Innovation
    Approach
      Overview
      Justification (rationale for the planned research and preliminary data)
      Study participants
        Selection criteria
        Design for sampling
        Plans for recruitment
        Plans to optimize adherence and complete follow-up
      Study procedures (if applicable)
        Randomization
        Blinding
      Measurements
        Main predictor variables (intervention, if a clinical trial)
        Outcome variables
        Potential confounding variables
      Statistics
        Approach to statistical analyses
        Hypotheses, sample size, and power
      Content and timing of study visits
      Data management and quality control
      Timetable and organizational chart
      Limitations and alternative approaches
Human subjects
Bibliography
Appendices and collaborative agreements

NIH, National Institutes of Health.

MRI-guided high frequency ultrasound vs. sham ultrasound for treating symptomatic fibroids" summarizes the research question, study design, and population. Avoid unnecessary phrases like "A study to determine the …."

The **project summary or abstract** should begin with the research aims and rationale, then set out the design and methods, and conclude with a statement of the impact of the potential study findings. The abstract should be informative to persons working in the same or related fields, and understandable to a scientifically literate lay reader. Most agencies restrict the abstract to a limited number of words or lines, so it is best to use efficient and descriptive terms. Because the abstract may be the *only* page read by some of the reviewers, as well as serving as a convenient reminder of the specifics of the proposal for everyone else, it must therefore stand on its own, incorporating all the main features of the proposed study and describing the strengths and potential impacts persuasively.

The Administrative Parts

Almost all agencies require an administrative section that includes a **budget, budget justification, and institutional resources,** which include a description of the qualifications of personnel, the resources of the investigator's institution, and access to equipment, space, and expertise.

The budget section should be organized according to guidelines from the funding institution. The NIH, for example, has a prescribed format that requires a detailed budget for the first 12-month period and a summary budget for the entire project (usually 2 to 5 years). The detailed 12-month budget includes the following categories of expenses: personnel (including names and positions of all persons involved in the project, the percent of time each will devote to the project, and the dollar amounts of salary and fringe benefits for each individual); consultant costs; equipment; supplies; travel; patient care costs; alterations and renovations; consortium/contractual costs; and other expenses (eg, the costs of telephones, mail, conference calls, copying, illustration, publication, books, and fee-for-service contracts).

Preparing the budget should not be left until the last minute. Many elements require time (eg, to get good estimates of the cost of space, equipment, and personnel). Universities employ knowledgeable administrators whose job is to help investigators prepare budgets and budget justifications and the other administrative parts of a proposal. The best approach is to notify this administrator as soon as possible that you plan to submit a proposal and schedule regular meetings or calls to review progress and the timeline for finishing the administrative sections. An administrator can begin working as soon as the outline of the proposal is formulated, recommending the amounts for budget items and helping to ensure that the investigator does not overlook important expenses. Institutions have regulations that must be followed and deadlines to meet, and an experienced administrator can help the investigator anticipate their institution's rules, pitfalls, and potential delays. The administrator can also be very helpful in drafting the text of the sections on budget justification and institutional resources, and in collecting the biosketches, subcontracts, appendices, and other supporting materials for the proposal.

The need for the amounts requested for each item of the budget must be fully explained in a budget justification. Personnel comprise most of the overall cost of a typical clinical research project, so the need and specific responsibilities for each person must justify the requested percent effort. Complete but concise job descriptions for the investigators and other members of the research team should leave no doubt in the reviewers' minds that the estimated effort of each person is essential to the success of the project.

Reviewers are often concerned about the percentages of time committed by key members of the research team. Occasionally, proposals may be criticized because key personnel have only a very small commitment of time listed in the budget—and many other commitments—implying that they may not be able to devote the necessary energy to the proposed study. More often, the reviewers may balk at percentages that are inflated beyond the requirements of the job description. If they are not convinced by the justification for budgeted items, reviewers can recommend that the item be cut or reduced.

Even the best-planned budgets will change when the study is carried out. In general, once a grant is awarded, the investigator is allowed to spend money in different ways from those specified in the budget, provided that the changes are modest and the expenditures are related to the aims of the study. When the investigator wants to move money across categories or make a substantial ($>25\%$) change in the effort of key investigators, they may need to get approval first. Agencies generally approve reasonable requests for rebudgeting so long as the investigator is not asking for an increase in total funds.

The NIH requires a biosketch for all investigators and consultants who will receive funding from the grant. Biosketches are five-page resumes that follow a specified format, including a personal statement about how the investigator's experience is relevant to conducting the study; a list of education, training, and employment; a limited number of publications and honors; and relevant research grants and contracts.

The section of the proposal on institutional resources available to the project may include computer and technical equipment, access to specialized imaging or measurement devices, office and laboratory space, and resources available to facilitate participant recruitment, data collection and management, and specimen storage. The resources section often draws on boilerplate descriptions from previous proposals or from material supplied by the investigator's institution, center, or laboratory.

Specific Aims

The **specific aims** are statements of the research question(s) using concrete terms to specify the desired outcome of the research project. This section of an NIH proposal is limited to a single page. Because many reviewers pay the most attention to this page, it should be written carefully and revised repeatedly as the proposal is developed.

A common pattern is to begin with two or three short paragraphs that summarize the background information: the research question and why it's important, the studies that have been done and how they haven't solved the problem, and the approach to answering the question in the proposed study. This is followed by a concise statement of the specific aims, expressed as tangible descriptive objectives and, whenever possible, as testable hypotheses.

The aims are presented in a logical sequence that the investigator tailors to the planned study. They may begin with cross-sectional aims for the baseline period followed by aims related to follow-up findings. Or they may begin with aims that address pathophysiologic mechanisms and end with those that address clinical or public health outcomes. A pattern that works well for career development awards begins with qualitative aims that use focus groups to design a key instrument or develop an intervention, followed by quantitative aims with predictors, outcomes, and hypothesis tests (this is often called "mixed methods research"). Yet another pattern is to start with the most important aim to highlight it; this has the advantage of giving the primary aim first place in all other sections of the proposal, such as sample size and power.

The Specific Aims section often ends with a short final paragraph that concisely sums up the potential impact of the study findings on knowledge of health and disease, clinical practice, public health, or future research. The goal is to make a compelling case that will lead the members of the review committee, including those who were not primary or secondary reviewers (and may have read just this section), to review the proposal favorably.

Research Strategy

The current NIH format limits most types of proposals to 12 pages for presenting the research strategy, in three sections:

- The **significance** section, typically two to three pages, describes how the study findings would advance scientific understanding, address an important problem or a barrier to progress in the field, improve clinical practice or public health, or influence policy. This section should state the magnitude of the problem, summarize what has been accomplished, define problems or gaps with current knowledge, and show how the proposed study will advance the field.
- The **innovations** section, typically one to two pages, points out ways the proposed study represents an advance from prior research on the topic, such as by using new measurement methods, discovering new mechanisms of disease, enrolling different or larger populations, identifying new treatments, or taking new approaches to data analysis. NIH guidelines focus on how the research will shift current research or clinical practice paradigms by employing innovative concepts, methods, or interventions. That said, many funded clinical studies result in only incremental improvements and refinements in concept, methods, or interventions. Our advice is to describe the novel features of the research accurately, without overstating claims that the study will change paradigms or use wholly innovative methods.
- The **approach** section (formerly termed "methods") is typically seven to nine pages long. It provides the details of study design and conduct, and receives close scrutiny from reviewers. NIH guidelines suggest that the approach section be organized by specific aims, and that it include the components and approximate sequence in Table 20.1. This section starts with a concise overview of the approach, sometimes accompanied by a schematic diagram or table,

to orient the reader (Table 20.2). The overview should state the study design and give a brief description of the study participants, the main measurements, any intervention, length of follow-up, and main outcome(s).

The approach section typically includes a brief rationale for the research, supported by **preliminary data**—previous research by the investigator's team suggesting that the proposed study will be successful. Emphasis should be placed on the importance of the previous work and on the reasons that it should be continued or extended. Results of pilot studies that support the feasibility of the study matter for many proposals, especially when the research team has limited previous experience with the proposed methods or when there may be doubts about the feasibility of the proposed procedures or recruitment of participants. This is an opportunity to show that the investigator and team have the experience and expertise necessary to conduct the study.

Other components of the approach section have been discussed earlier. The **study participants** section (Chapter 3) should define and provide a rationale for inclusion and exclusion criteria, specify the sampling method, describe how the study participants will be recruited and followed, and ensure the reviewers that the investigators can enroll the desired number of study participants. Plans for optimizing adherence to the study intervention (if applicable) and study visits should be provided.

The approach section should include a description of **important study procedures**, such as randomization and blinding. Study measurements (Chapter 4) should describe how predictor, outcome, and potential confounding variables will be measured and at what point in the study these measurements will be made, as well as how interventions will be applied and how the main outcome will be ascertained and measured.

The **statistics** section usually begins with the plans for analysis, organized by specific aim. The plan can be set out in the logical sequence; for example, first the descriptive tabulations and then the approach to analyzing associations among variables. This is followed by a discussion of sample size and power (Chapters 5 and 6) that should begin with a statement of the null hypothesis for the aim that will determine the sample size for the study. Estimates of sample size and power rely on assumptions about the magnitude of associations (effect sizes) that are likely to be detected and the precision of the measurements that will be made. These assumptions

TABLE 20.2 STUDY TIMELINE FOR A RANDOMIZED TRIAL OF THE EFFECT OF TESTOSTERONE ADMINISTRATION ON RISK FACTORS FOR HEART DISEASE, PROSTATE CANCER, AND FRACTURES

	SCREENING VISIT	RANDOMIZATION VISIT	3 MONTHS	6 MONTHS	12 MONTHS
Medical history	X	–	–	–	X
Blood pressure	X	X	X	X	X
Prostate examination	X	–	–	–	X
Prostate-specific antigen	X	–	–	–	X
Blood lipid levels	–	X	X	X	X
Markers of inflammation	–	X	–	–	X
Bone density	–	X	–	–	X
Markers of bone turnover	–	X	X	–	X
Handgrip strength	–	X	X	X	X
Adverse events	–	–	X	X	X

must be justified by citing published literature or preliminary work. It is often useful to include a table or figure showing how variations in the effect size, power, or other assumptions influence the sample size to demonstrate that the investigator has made reasonable choices. Most NIH review panels attach considerable importance to the statistics section, so it is a good idea to involve a statistician in writing this component and add one to the list of investigators if the statistical methods are complex.

It is helpful to include a table that lists study visits or participant contacts, the timing of visits, and what procedures and measurements will occur at each visit. Such a table provides a concise overview of all study activities (Table 20.2). Descriptions of quality control and data management (Chapters 18 and 19) should address how the study data will be collected, stored, and edited, along with plans for maximizing data quality and security.

The proposal must provide a realistic work plan and timetable, including dates when each major phase of the study will be started and completed (Figure 20.1). Similar timetables can be prepared for staffing patterns and other components of the project. For large studies, an organizational chart describing the research team can indicate levels of authority and accountability, lines of reporting, and show how the team will function.

Although not required, it can be helpful to include a discussion of the limitations of the proposed research and alternative approaches. Rather than ignore potential flaws, an investigator may decide to address them explicitly, discussing the advantages and disadvantages of the various trade-offs in reaching the chosen plan. Pointing out important challenges and potential solutions can turn criticisms of the application into strengths. It is a mistake to overemphasize these problems, however, for this may lead a reviewer to focus disproportionately on the weaker aspects of the proposal. The goal is to reassure the reviewer that the investigator has anticipated the major problems and developed a realistic and thoughtful approach to dealing with them.

Final Components of a Major Proposal

The human subjects section is devoted to the ethical issues raised by the study and addresses issues of informed consent, safety, privacy, and confidentiality (Chapter 7). This section has been expanded by the NIH to include plans to inform potential participants of the risks and benefits, and to obtain their consent to participate. It also describes the inclusion and exclusion criteria; plans for inclusion of individuals across the lifespan, women, and minority groups; and justification for exclusion of any of these groups. There are additional requirements for clinical trials, including a detailed recruitment and retention plan, study timeline, and data and safety monitoring plan, as well as separate sections describing the intervention, masking, allocation, outcome measures, statistical design and power, and dissemination plan. Although there are no page limits for these human subjects sections, the investigator should be concise.

The bibliography sends a message about the investigator's familiarity with the field by being comprehensive and up-to-date—not simply an exhaustive and unselected list. Each reference

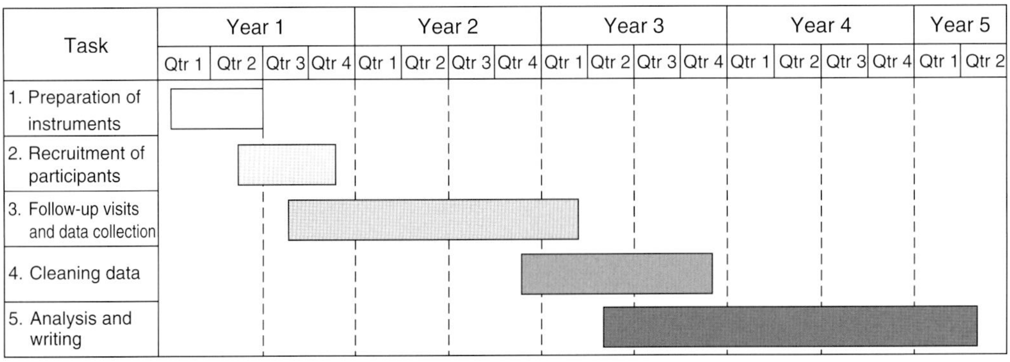

Task	Year 1				Year 2				Year 3				Year 4				Year 5	
	Qtr 1	Qtr 2	Qtr 3	Qtr 4	Qtr 1	Qtr 2	Qtr 3	Qtr 4	Qtr 1	Qtr 2	Qtr 3	Qtr 4	Qtr 1	Qtr 2	Qtr 3	Qtr 4	Qtr 1	Qtr 2
1. Preparation of instruments																		
2. Recruitment of participants																		
3. Follow-up visits and data collection																		
4. Cleaning data																		
5. Analysis and writing																		

■ **FIGURE 20.1** A hypothetical timetable for preparing a proposal.

should be cited accurately; errors in citations or misinterpretation of the work will be regarded negatively by reviewers familiar with the field.

For some types of proposals, appendices can be useful for providing detailed technical and supporting material mentioned briefly in the text. However, to avoid the use of appendices to circumvent page limits for proposals, NIH limits their use. Appendices for NIH grants may only include data collection instruments (such as questionnaires) and blank consent/assent forms. Primary and secondary reviewers are the only review committee members who receive the appendices. Therefore, everything important must be summarized in the main proposal.

The proposed use and value of each consultant should be described, accompanied by a signed letter of agreement from the individual and a copy of their biosketch. Other **letters of support**, such as those from persons who will provide access to equipment or resources, should also be included. An explanation of the programmatic and administrative arrangements between the applicant organization and any collaborating institutions and laboratories should be accompanied by letters of commitment from responsible officials addressed to the PI.

■ CHARACTERISTICS OF GOOD PROPOSALS

A good proposal for research funding has several attributes. First is the **scientific quality of the research strategy**: It must be based on a good research question, use a design and approach that are rigorous and feasible, and have a research team with the experience, skill, and commitment to carry it out. Second is **clarity of presentation**; a proposal that is concise, engaging, well-organized, formatted attractively, and free of errors reassures the reader that the conduct of research is likely to be of similarly high quality.

The members of a scientific review committee are often overwhelmed by a large stack of proposals to evaluate, so a project's merits must stand out even with a quick or cursory reading. A **reviewer's understanding of the proposal can be enhanced by following an outline based on the specific aims, putting text into short sections with meaningful subheadings, and breaking up long stretches of text with tables and figures.** Current NIH guidelines recommend starting paragraphs with a **topic sentence** in **bold type** that makes the key point, allowing harried reviewers to understand the essential elements of the proposal by scanning topic sentences. Include enough detail to convince an expert reviewer of the significance and sophistication of the proposed work, while still engaging the larger number of reviewers less familiar with the area of investigation.

Most reviewers are put off by overstatement and other heavy-handed forms of grantsmanship. Proposals that exaggerate the importance of the project or overestimate what it can accomplish will generate skepticism. Writing with enthusiasm is good, but the investigator should be realistic about the limitations of the project. Reviewers are adept at identifying potential problems in design or feasibility.

When the proposal is just about finished—but at a time when changes are still possible—ask a few colleagues with expertise in the field who have not been involved in the proposal's development to read it and make comments and suggestions. It is also useful to have someone with excellent writing skills provide advice on style and clarity. Finally, **always read a printed copy of the proposal before submitting it**: Do not just rely on spell- and grammar-check programs to catch all the typographical errors.

■ FINDING SUPPORT FOR RESEARCH

Investigators should be alert to opportunities to conduct good research without formal proposals for funding. For example, beginning researchers may analyze data sets that have been collected by others or receive small amounts of support from a senior investigator or department to carry out small studies. Conducting research without funding of a formal proposal is quicker and simpler, but has the disadvantage that the projects are limited in scope. Furthermore, academic institutions often base decisions about career advancement in part on a scientist's success in garnering funding for research.

There are four main categories of funds for medical research:

- The government (notably NIH, but also the Department of Veterans Affairs, Centers for Disease Control and Prevention, Agency for Healthcare Research and Quality, Department of Defense, and many other federal, state, and county agencies);
- Foundations, professional societies (such as the American Heart Association and the American Cancer Society) and individual donors;
- Corporations (notably pharmaceutical and device manufacturing companies); and
- Intramural resources (eg, the investigator's university).

Getting support from these sources is a complex and competitive process that favors investigators with experience and tenacity: Beginning investigators are well advised to find a mentor with these characteristics. In the following sections, we focus on several prominent funding sources.

National Institutes of Health Grants and Contracts

The NIH offers many types of grants and contracts. The **R awards** (R01 and smaller R03 and R21 awards) support research projects conceived by investigators on topics of their choosing or written in response to a publicized request by one of the institutes at NIH (see www.nimh.nih .gov/research-funding/grants/research-grants-r.shtml). The **K awards** (K23, K01, and K08 and locally awarded K12 and KL2 awards) are an excellent resource that provide salary support for training and career development of junior investigators, as well as modest support for research (see https://researchtraining.nih.gov/programs/career-development). There are several different sections in K grant applications that are scored and influence the overall impact (Table 20.3).

Institute-initiated proposals are designed to stimulate research in areas designated by NIH advisory committees and take the form of either Requests for Proposals (RFPs) or Requests for Applications (RFAs). In response to an RFP, the investigator contracts to perform specific research activities determined by the NIH. By contrast, under an RFA, investigators conduct research in a topic area defined by the NIH, but they choose their specific research questions and study designs. RFPs use the *contract* mechanism to reimburse the investigator's institution for the costs involved in achieving the planned objectives, whereas RFAs use the *grant* mechanism to support activities that are more open-ended.

After being submitted, an application goes through a review process that includes an initial administrative review by NIH staff, **peer review** by a group of scientists, recommendations about funding by the institute advisory council, and the final decision about funding by the institute director. Grant applications are usually reviewed by one of many NIH **study sections**, groups of scientific reviewers with specific areas of research expertise drawn from research institutions around the country. A list of the study sections and their current membership is available on the NIH website.

The NIH process for reviewing and funding proposals is described at https://grants.nih.gov/ grants/referral-and-review.htm. When an investigator submits a grant application, it is assigned by the NIH Center for Scientific Review (CSR) to a particular study section (Figure 20.2). Proposals are assigned to a primary and two or more secondary reviewers who each rate the application from 1 to 9 for **significance, innovation, approach, investigators, and environment**, as well as providing a summary rating of the likely **overall impact** of the study. An overall impact score of "1" indicates an exceptionally strong application with essentially no weaknesses, and a "9" is an application with serious weaknesses and few strengths. The assigned reviewers' ratings are revealed to the study section, and proposals with scores in the better half are discussed with the entire committee; the remainder are "triaged" (not discussed), with a few deferred to the next application cycle 4 months later pending clarification of points that were unclear. After discussion, the assigned reviewers again propose ratings (the scores may have changed as a result of the discussion) and all committee members then provide scores by secret ballot. These

TABLE 20.3 CAREER DEVELOPMENT "K" GRANT APPLICATION SCORED SECTIONS

SCORED SECTIONS	SUGGESTED LENGTH	REVIEWER CONSIDERATIONS
Candidate	1 page	• Does the candidate have potential to develop into an independent researcher? • Are prior training and experience appropriate? • Is there evidence of commitment to the research program? • Is there evidence of productivity (papers, abstracts, grants)?
Career development plan and career goals/objectives	2-3 pages	• Will plan help candidate develop significantly to become independent? • Is the content, scope, phasing, and duration of the training plan appropriate for candidate?
Research plan	7-8 pages	• Is the approach of significant scientific and technical merit? • Is the plan appropriate to candidate's stage of research and useful to develop the necessary skills from the training plan? • Is the research relevant to the candidate's career objectives?
Mentor(s)/mentoring team	0.5-1 page	• Are the mentors qualified and experienced to provide the needed training to the candidate? • Do the mentors have complementary skills? • Is there adequate description of the mentor's roles for training objectives?
Institutional commitment	1 page	• Is there clear commitment from the institution that the required minimum of the candidate's effort will go toward research and training? • Is the institution's commitment to the training of the candidate strong? • Are the research facilities and training opportunities appropriate and adequate?

are averaged and then multiplied by 10 to yield an overall score from 10 (best) to 90 (worst). For R01 grants, NIH converts the overall impact score to a percentile, which ranks the proposal relative to the others that have been reviewed by that study section in its past three review meetings. The final impact score (or percentile) of the application is used by each institute to prioritize funding decisions.

The investigator should decide in advance, with advice from senior colleagues, which study section would be the best choice to review the proposal. **Study sections vary a great deal not only in topic area but also in the expertise of the reviewers and in the quality of competing applications.** Investigators can request up to three study section(s) they would like their proposal to be sent to (or not), though there is no guarantee that their suggestions will be followed.

In addition to assigning each grant application to a particular study section, the CSR also assigns it to a particular *institute* (or center) at NIH, which can also be preselected by the investigator. Each institute then funds the grants assigned to it, in order of priority score tempered by an advisory council review and sometimes overridden by the Institute's director (Figure 20.3). Proposals from new investigators who are early stage and have not yet received NIH research funding are funded at somewhat more favorable percentile cutoffs than those from established investigators. Institutes sometimes arrange to share funding if an application is of interest to more than one.

After an application has been reviewed, the investigator receives written notification of the study section's action. This **summary statement** includes the score and detailed comments and criticisms from the committee members who reviewed the application.

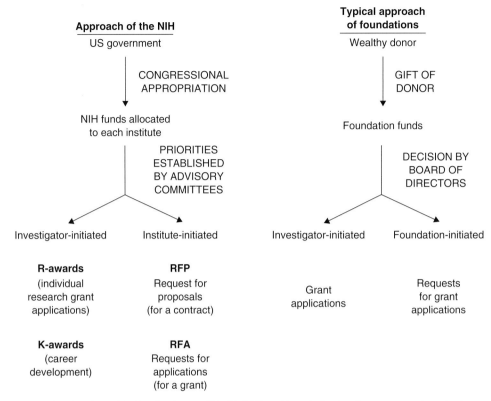

Approach of the NIH
US government

CONGRESSIONAL
APPROPRIATION

NIH funds allocated
to each institute

PRIORITIES
ESTABLISHED
BY ADVISORY
COMMITTEES

Investigator-initiated   Institute-initiated

R-awards   **RFP**
(individual   Request for
research grant   proposals
applications)   (for a contract)

K-awards   **RFA**
(career   Requests for
development)   applications
                               (for a grant)

**Typical approach
of foundations**
Wealthy donor

GIFT OF
DONOR

Foundation funds

DECISION BY
BOARD OF
DIRECTORS

Investigator-initiated   Foundation-initiated

                                   Requests
Grant   for grant
applications   applications

■ **FIGURE 20.2** Overview of National Institutes of Health (NIH) and foundation funding sources and mechanisms.

NIH applications that are not funded, as is often the case for first submissions, can be revised and resubmitted once. If the reviewers' initial criticisms and scores suggest that the application can be improved, then a revised version may have good chance of obtaining funding when resubmitted. (It may be more difficult to raise reviewers' enthusiasm if they indicate that the proposal lacks innovation or significance.) Program officers from the relevant institute attend the study section meetings, so it is important to discuss the review with them, especially because the written comments are often drafted before the meeting and may not reflect all the issues discussed by the study section.

Investigators need not make all the changes suggested by reviewers, but they should make revisions that will satisfy the reviewer's criticisms wherever possible and justify any decision not to do so. NIH limits responses to reviews to a single page Introduction describing the changes that have been made in the revised proposal. **A good format for the Introduction is to summarize each major criticism from the summary statement in bold or italic font and address it with a concise statement of the consequent change in the proposal.**

Investigators may also submit the proposal again (and again) as a new application, with no connection to the previous score or reviews. The proposal should, of course, be updated and may also need to be revised. Investigators should check with NIH staff or regulations if they are uncertain about how to submit a proposal again (https://grants.nih.gov/grants/policy/resubmission_q&a.htm).

Grants from Foundations and Professional Societies

Most **private foundations** (such as the Robert Wood Johnson Foundation) restrict their funding to specific areas of interest. Some disease-based foundations and professional societies (such as the American Heart Association and American Cancer Society) also sponsor research programs,

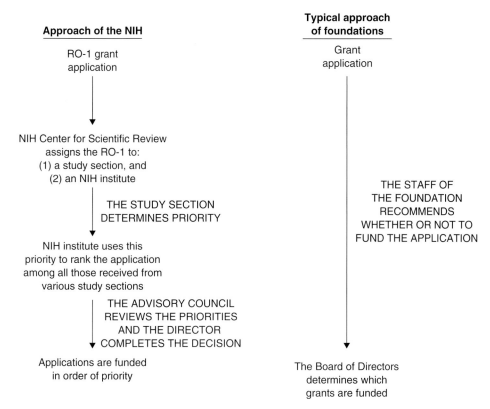

■ **FIGURE 20.3** National Institutes of Health (NIH) and foundation procedures for reviewing grant applications.

many of which are designed to support junior investigators. The total amount of research support is far smaller than that provided by the NIH, and most foundations have the goal of using this money to fund projects that have topics or methods that are unlikely to be funded by the NIH. A few foundations offer career development awards focused on specific areas, such as quality of health care. The Foundation Center (http://candid.org/) maintains a searchable directory of foundations and contact information, along with advice about how to write effective proposals. Decisions about funding follow procedures that vary from one foundation to another, but usually occur rapidly (Figure 20.3). The decisions are often made by an executive process rather than by peer review; typically, the staff of the foundation makes a recommendation that is ratified by a board of directors.

To determine whether a foundation might be interested in a proposal, an investigator should consult with his mentors and check the foundation's website, which describes the goals and purposes of the foundation and often lists projects that have been funded recently. If it appears that a foundation might be an appropriate source of support, it is best to **contact a staff member** to describe the project, determine potential interest, and obtain guidance about how to submit a proposal. Many foundations ask that investigators first send a letter describing the background and principal goals of the project, the qualifications of the investigators, and the approximate duration and cost of the research. If the letter is of sufficient interest, the foundation may request a more detailed proposal.

Research Support from Industry

Corporations that make drugs and devices are a major source of funding, especially for randomized trials of new treatments. The largest form of industry support for clinical research is through contracts to clinical sites for enrolling participants into multicenter trials that test new drugs and devices. These large trials are usually run by the corporate sponsor, often through a contract with a **clinical research organization (CRO)**; such trials are occasionally designed and managed by an academic coordinating center.

Contracts for enrolling participants in clinical trials generally pay each site a fixed fee for each participant. The trial closes enrollment when the desired study-wide goal has been met. An investigator may sometimes enroll enough participants to receive funding that exceeds the actual costs, in which case the institution retains the surplus (which can sometimes be used to support other research projects), but the institution will lose money if too few participants are enrolled to cover the expenses of the trial. **Before deciding to participate in these multisite trials, investigators should be certain that the contract and protocol can be approved by the institution's administrative offices and IRB in time to enroll enough participants before recruitment closes.**

Industry funding, particularly from marketing departments, is often channeled into topics and activities intended to increase sales of the company's product. The findings in an industry-managed trials are often analyzed by their own statisticians and manuscripts drafted by their medical writers who may spin the message of papers to promote that product (Chapter 7). If investigators participate in manuscripts from industry-sponsored trials, they should be vigilant that the analyses are rigorous and that the paper presents the results objectively. Ideally, multicenter industry-sponsored studies would have Steering or Publications Committees composed largely or entirely of the investigators/members who are not employees of the sponsor.

Some companies accept applications **for investigator-initiated studies**, such as small projects, about the effects or mechanisms of action of a treatment or epidemiologic studies about conditions of interest to the company. They may supply the drug or device and a matching placebo for a clinical trial proposed by an investigator. In general, the investigator analyzes the data and writes the manuscripts from these studies.

Intramural Support

Universities and research institutions have **intramural research funds** for their own investigators. Grants from these funds are generally limited to relatively small amounts, but they can be available much more quickly (weeks to months)—and to a higher proportion of applicants—than those from the NIH or private foundations. Intramural funds may be restricted to special purposes, such as pilot studies that may lead to external funding or the purchase of equipment. Such funds are often earmarked for junior faculty and provide a unique opportunity for a new investigator to acquire the experience of leading a funded project. Guidelines for submitting proposals for intramural funding vary substantially, and investigators should speak with university administrators before submitting a proposal.

■ SUMMARY

1. **A proposal is an expanded version of a written plan for a study** (the protocol) that is used to request funding. It also contains budgetary, administrative, and supporting information required by the funding agency.
2. A new investigator working on a research proposal should begin by **getting advice from senior colleagues** about the research question they will pursue and the choice of funding agency. The next steps are to study that agency's written guidelines and to contact a scientific administrator in the agency for advice.
3. The process of writing a proposal, which often takes much longer than expected, includes **organizing a team** with the necessary expertise; **designating a PI**; **outlining a proposal** to conform strictly to agency guidelines; **establishing a timetable** for written products; **finding a model proposal**; and **reviewing progress** at regular meetings. The proposal should be reviewed by knowledgeable colleagues, revised often, and polished at the end with attention to detail.

4. The **major elements of a proposal** include the abstract (summary); the administrative parts centered around the budget, budget justification, biosketches and institutional resources; the very important specific aims; and the research strategy with its significance, innovations, and approach sections, including previous research by the investigator.

5. A good proposal requires a **good research question, study plan, and research team**, as well as a clear presentation: The proposal should follow a logical outline that indicates the advantages and disadvantages of trade-offs in the study plan. Subheadings, tables, and diagrams should be used to highlight the merits of the proposal so they will not be missed by a busy reviewer.

6. There are **four main sources of support** for clinical research:
   a. The **NIH and other governmental sources** are the largest providers of support, using a system of peer and administrative review that moves slowly but funds a wide array of grants and contracts for research and for career development.
   b. **Foundations and societies** are often interested in promising research questions that are not in the usual scope of NIH funding and have review procedures that are quicker but specific to the foundation.
   c. **Pharmaceutical and medical device companies** are a large source of support, mostly for trials of new drugs and medical devices. Some companies offer investigator-initiated grants on topics related to the condition or the company's treatment.
   d. **Intramural funds** from the investigator's institution tend to have favorable funding rates for getting small amounts of money quickly, and they are an excellent first step for pilot studies and new investigators.

APPENDIX 20A
Exercises for Chapter 20. Writing a Proposal for Funding Research

1. After the Specific Aims, what are the three major sections of the Research Strategy?
2. In reviews of NIH grant proposals, what are the four criteria, besides environment, that receive numerical ratings (from 1 to 9) that are used to develop an overall impact score for the grant proposal?
3. Consider a study that plans to compare three types of measurements of blood pressure—an automatic inflatable cuff, a wristwatch, and using an app on a mobile phone. The blood pressures would be collected in over 50,000 people age 20 years or older from the entire United States who have volunteered to participate in online research studies about cardiovascular disease. The investigator plans to determine blood pressure and variability in blood pressure from each device and then follow-up to collect data about incident strokes and about fatal strokes from the medical records of these participants.

   a. Write one to two sentences for each of two or three Specific Aims for this study.
   b. Write a brief Innovations section that describes at least two novel features of the study.
4. Name at least three sources of grant support for research, besides the NIH. (Ideally, these sources should be applicable to your line of research.)

Answers to the Exercises at the Ends of Chapters

Chapter 1　Getting Started: The Anatomy and Physiology of Clinical Research

1a. This is an internal validity inference (because it refers to the women in this study) that is probably valid. However, it could be invalid if something other than Early Limited Formula (ELF) caused the difference in breastfeeding rates (eg, if the control intervention adversely affected breastfeeding), if self-reported breastfeeding does not reflect actual breastfeeding, or if the association occurred by chance. (A significant *P* value does not rule out this possibility; and in fact, this positive finding was not replicated in a later, larger study [Flaherman VJ, Narayan NR, Hartigan-O'Connor D, Cabana MD, McCulloch CE, Paul IM. The effect of early limited formula on breastfeeding, readmission, and intestinal microbiota: A randomized clinical trial. *J Pediatr*. 2018;196:84-90 e1].)

1b. This is an external validity inference (because it involves generalizing outside the study) that may be valid. However, in addition to the threats to internal validity (which also threaten external validity), it is likely that women giving birth in community hospitals and in other parts of the country might respond differently to the intervention, or that other clinicians providing the ELF might carry out the intervention differently from the way it was done in the original study, or that the benefits might not last as long as 6 months.

1c. This is an external validity inference that goes far beyond the population and intervention that were studied and is probably not valid. It not only involves generalizing to other mothers and newborns in other locations but also includes newborns who have not lost 5% of their body weight; expands the intervention from early, limited formula to providing formula without limitation; and asserts broad, vague health benefits that, although reasonable, were not examined in the ELF study.

2a. This is a cohort study of whether watching wrestling on television predicts subsequent fighting among Winston-Salem high school students.

2b. This is a case-control study of whether the duration of breastfeeding is associated with reduced risk of ovarian cancer among Chinese women who have breastfed at least one baby.

2c. This is a cross-sectional study of the relationship between self-reported saturated fat intake and sperm concentration in Danish men being examined for military service.

2d. This is a randomized trial of whether left atrial occlusion (vs. no occlusion) reduces the incidence of stroke or systemic embolism in adults with atrial fibrillation undergoing cardiac surgery for another reason.

　　Each of these four sentences is a concise description that summarizes the entire study by noting the design and the main elements of the research question (key variables and intended sample). For example, in exercise 2a the design is a cohort study, the predictor is watching wrestling on television, the outcome is fighting, and the intended sample is high school students in Winston-Salem.

Chapter 2   Conceiving the Research Question and Developing the Study Plan

1. The process of going from a research question to a study plan is often iterative. One might begin with an answer like: "A cross-sectional study to determine whether marijuana use is associated with health status among young adults." The possibility that "marijuana use" is related to "health status" seems important, but the question as stated is still too vague to judge whether the study is feasible, novel, and ethical. How will marijuana use and health status be measured, and in what target population? Also, it will be difficult to establish causality in a cross-sectional design—does marijuana use lead to worse health or vice versa?

   A more specific version that could better meet the FINE criteria (feasible, important, novel, and ethical) might be: **"A cohort study to determine whether daily marijuana use among college juniors is associated with the number of illness-related visits they make to the student health service in the next year as compared with nonusers."**

2. In the case of the association between acetaminophen and asthma, the observation that acetaminophen use and asthma prevalence have both increased worldwide and biologic plausibility related to depletion of reduced glutathione by acetaminophen lead to all studies being interesting and relevant; as more studies are done, they become less novel.

   Study #1: A **case-control study** to compare the self-reported frequency of acetaminophen use among adults with asthma symptoms seen in South London general practices (the cases), with the frequency reported by randomly selected adults without such symptoms from the same general practices (the controls). Case-control studies are often a good way to start investigating possible associations (Chapter 9). This study was made feasible because it was part of a larger population-based case-control study of asthma investigating the effects of dietary antioxidants. Asthma was associated with acetaminophen use, with an odds ratio of 2.4 (95% confidence interval [CI], 1.2 to 4.6) among daily users. The study was ethical because it was an observational study that did not put the participants at risk (Shaheen SO, Sterne JA, Songhurst CE, Burney PG. Frequent paracetamol use and asthma in adults. *Thorax.* 2000;55:266-270).

   Study #2: A multinational **cross-sectional study** of parent-reported allergic symptoms (asthma, hay fever, and eczema) among 6- to 7-year-old children that included questions about use of acetaminophen in the previous year and usual use for fevers in the first year after birth. This study (which included 205,487 children ages 6 to 7 years from 73 centers in 31 countries) would not have been feasible if it had not been part of the more general International Study of Asthma and Allergies in Childhood (ISAAC) study. This illustrates the importance of seeking existing data or existing studies when investigating a new research question (Chapter 16). The authors found a strong dose-response relationship between current use of acetaminophen and wheezing, and an odds ratio of 1.46 (95% CI, 1.36 to 1.56) for wheezing and a "yes" answer to the question: "In the first 12 months of your child's life, did you usually give paracetamol [acetaminophen] for fever?" (Beasley R, Clayton T, Crane J, et al. Association between paracetamol use in infancy and childhood, and risk of asthma, rhinoconjunctivitis, and eczema in children aged 6-7 years: analysis from Phase Three of the ISAAC programme. *Lancet.* 2008;372:1039-1048).

   Study #3: A **randomized double-blind trial** of the effect of acetaminophen (12 mg/kg) versus ibuprofen (5 or 10 mg/kg) on hospitalizations and outpatient visits for asthma over 4 weeks among febrile children 6 months to 12 years old who were being treated for asthma at enrollment. A randomized trial is generally the least feasible design, because of the expense and logistics involved. In addition, as evidence of a potential adverse drug effect accumulates, randomized trials to confirm it become less ethical. In this situation, investigators did a retrospective analysis of data on the subset of children with asthma in the

Boston University Fever Study, a randomized double-blind trial that had completed enroll-ment in 1993. They found that children randomized to acetaminophen had greater risks of outpatient visits for asthma but not hospitalizations (Lesko SM, Louik C, Vezina RM, Mitchell AA. Asthma morbidity after the short-term use of ibuprofen in children. *Pediatrics.* 2002;109:E20).

3. Share your answer with colleagues!

Chapter 3   Choosing the Study Participants: Specification, Sampling, and Recruitment

1a. This sample of eleventh graders may not be well suited to the research question if the antecedents of smoking take place at an earlier age. A target population of greater interest might be students in middle school. Also, the accessible population (students at this one high school) may not adequately represent the target population, because the causes of smoking differ in various cultural settings. The investigator might do better to draw her sample from several high schools selected randomly from the whole region. Most impor-tant, the sampling design (calling for volunteers) is likely to attract students who are not representative of the accessible population in their smoking behavior.

1b. The unrepresentative sample could have resulted from random error, but this would have been unlikely unless it was a very small sample. For example, in a sample of only 10 partici-pants, a 7:3 disproportion would occur fairly often as a result of chance; in fact, the prob-ability of selecting at least 7 girls in a total sample of 10 from a large class that is 50% girls is about 17% (plus another 17% chance of selecting at least 7 boys). But if the sample size were 100 instead of 10, the probability of sampling at least 70 girls is < 0.01%. This demonstrates that the magnitude of the random component of sampling error can be estimated once the sample has been acquired (and reduced to any desired level by enlarging the sample size).

   The unrepresentative sample could also have resulted from systematic error. The large proportion of females could have been due to different rates of participation among boys and girls. The strategies for preventing nonresponse bias include the spectrum of tech-niques for enhancing recruitment. The large proportion of females could also represent a technical mistake in enumerating or selecting the names to be sampled. The strategies for preventing mistakes include the appropriate use of pretesting and quality control proce-dures (Chapter 18).

2a. Random sample (probability). The main concern for generalizability will be nonresponse—it will be important to keep the questionnaire short and to provide some incentive to fill it out. (Possible nonresponse bias is an issue for all sampling schemes discussed in this question.)

2b. Stratified random sample (probability), with a threefold oversampling of women, perhaps because the investigator anticipated that fewer women would attend the concert.

2c. Systematic sample (nonprobability). Although perhaps convenient, this systematic sam-pling scheme would lead to underrepresentation of both members of couples. Also, at least theoretically, the vendor in the box office could manipulate which patrons receive tickets ending in 1.

2d. Cluster sample (probability). This may be convenient, but the clustering needs to be accounted for in analyses, because people who sit in the same row may be more similar to one another than concertgoers selected randomly. This could be a particular problem if the music was louder in some rows than others.

2e. Consecutive sample (nonprobability). Consecutive samples are usually a good choice, but people who arrive early for concerts may differ from those who arrive later, so several con-secutive samples selected at different times would be preferable.

2f. **Convenience sample** (nonprobability). This scheme will miss participants who bought tickets by mail. In addition, people who come to concerts in groups could be over- or underrepresented.

2g. **Convenience sample** (nonprobability). This sampling scheme is not only biased by the whims of the investigator, it may run into nonresponse by patrons who are unable to hear the invitation.

3a. The **target population** (to which the authors wished to generalize) was the U.S. population of children under 5 years of age at the time of the study. We know this because the authors used nationwide survey data to estimate the burden of human metapneumovirus (HMPV) disease in the United States. Of course, it would be of great interest to generalize to future years as well, and many readers will do so without a second thought. However, especially for infectious diseases whose frequency varies annually, generalizing beyond the years of the study is an additional, potentially fragile, inference.

3b. The **accessible population** (the population from which they drew their participants) was children <5 years old living in the counties surrounding the three study sites (Cincinnati, Nashville, and Rochester, NY) and obtaining care from the study sites. Presumably these cities were selected because of their proximity to the investigators. It is not clear how representative they are of other areas in the United States with respect to the frequency of HMPV infection.

3c. The sampling scheme was a **convenience sample**. The choice of days of the week (which is not specified) could have led to some bias if, for example, parents of children with milder respiratory symptoms over the weekend wait until Monday to bring them to see a doctor and HMPV symptoms are more or less severe than those of other viruses. On the days when the investigators were enrolling participants, they may have tried to get a consecutive sample (also not specified), which would have helped to control selection bias. The reason for restriction to certain months of the year is not provided, but was presumably because the authors believed almost all HMPV cases would occur during these months.

3d. The observations were **clustered by geographic area**, which would need to be accounted for statistically. The more different the estimates were among cities, the more this would widen the confidence intervals. Intuitively, this makes sense. Very different rates by city would lead one to wonder how different the estimate would have been if other cities had been included, and we would expect to see this uncertainty reflected in a wider confidence interval.

A more subtle level of clustering occurs by year. Again, if there is a lot of year-to-year variation in the incidence of HMPV, then if the desire is to generalize to future years (rather than just to estimate what the incidence was in the years studied), clustering by year would need to be accounted for statistically. Annual variation in incidence rates would also lead to a wider confidence interval.

Chapter 4 Planning the Measurements: Precision, Accuracy, and Validity

1a. Dichotomous
1b. Continuous
1c. Dichotomous
1d. Nominal
1e. Discrete numerical
1f. Ordinal
1g. Continuous
1h. Nominal
1i. Dichotomous

Power is generally increased by using an outcome variable that contains ordered information. For example, power would be greater if education were examined as highest year or total number of years of schooling rather than categorized as having or not having at least a college degree. Similarly, use of body mass index as a continuous outcome would offer more power (contain more information) than the presence or absence of obesity, or the intermediate choice of underweight/normal weight/overweight/obese, which is an ordinal variable.

2a. This is a source of **systematic error** because of instrument variability. The 10-kg weight used to calibrate the scale needs to be replaced, or else the scale will underestimate the weight of babies systematically in future measurements. Note, however, that if the same scale were used to weigh all of the babies, the study would still give an unbiased answer to the question of how well intake of fruit juice at 6 months predicts body weight at 1 year.

2b. This is a problem with **precision** most likely because of instrument variability. The excessive variability could be observer error (especially if the scale is not digital), but more likely the scale or its batteries need replacing.

2c. This situation can **cause both imprecision and systematic error.** Imprecision will result from variation in the degree to which babies squirm on the scale or the effect of that squirming. Systematic error will result from the observer's hold on the baby altering the observed weight; this might tend to increase or decrease the observed weight, depending on how the observer holds the babies. This problem might be solved by having the mother calm the baby; an alternative that would work if a sufficiently accurate adult-sized scale were available would be to weigh the mother with and without the baby, and take the difference.

2d. This is primarily a problem with **precision**, because the numbers on the scale will vary around the true weight (if the scale is accurate). The problem is with the participants and has the same solution as 2c.

2e. This is mainly a problem with **precision**, because the babies' weights will vary depending on whether they ate or wet their diapers before the examination. This problem of participant variability could be reduced by giving the mothers instructions not to feed the babies for 3 hours before the examination and weighing all babies naked. If the observers vary in how they handle babies with wet diapers (some remove them, some change them, some do neither) there could also be observer variability.

3a. **Predictive validity:** The burnout scores predicted an outcome that we might expect to be associated with burnout.

3b. **Face validity:** People familiar with burnout agree that this seems like a reasonable approach to assessing burnout.

3c. **Construct validity:** This measure of burnout is responsive to circumstances that we would expect to affect burnout.

3d. **Criterion-related validity:** These two items agree closely with a well-accepted standard measure.

Chapter 5   Getting Ready to Estimate Sample Size: Hypotheses and Underlying Principles

1.   **Sample size** = the number of participants included in a research study. Sample size estimates should project the number of participants who will *complete* the study and have data available for analysis. For analytic studies, this can be estimated from the number required to be able to detect a given effect size (at the specified levels of alpha and beta).

Null hypothesis = a statement of the research hypothesis that indicates that there is no difference between the groups being compared.

Alternative hypothesis = a statement of the research hypothesis that indicates that there is a difference between the groups being compared.

Power = the likelihood of detecting a statistically significant difference between the groups being compared (with a given sample size and level of statistical significance) if the real difference in the population is equal to the specified effect size.

Level of statistical significance = the preset chance of (falsely) rejecting the null hypothesis if it is true.

Effect size = the minimum size of the difference in the two groups being compared that the investigator wishes to have a reasonable chance of detecting.

Variability = the amount of spread in a measurement, usually expressed as a standard deviation.

2a. **Neither.** This is a statistically significant result, and there is nothing to suggest that it represents a type I error.

2b. The sample size was small and very few participants would have developed lung cancer during the study. These negative results are almost certainly because of a **type II error**, especially given extensive evidence from other studies that smoking causes lung cancer.

2c. There is no prior epidemiologic or pathophysiologic reason to believe that alcohol use reduces the risk of developing diabetes; this result is likely because of a **type I error**. The investigator could have been more informative: $P < 0.05$ could be $P = 0.04$ or $P = 0.001$; the latter would reduce (though not rule out) the likelihood of type I error.

Chapter 6   Estimating Sample Size: Applications and Examples

1. H_0: There is no difference in the body mass index of stomach cancer cases and controls.
H_A (two-sided): There is a difference in the body mass index of stomach cancer cases and controls. Body mass index is a continuous variable and case-control is dichotomous, so a *t* test can be used.

$$Effect\ size = 1\ kg/m^2$$
$$Standard\ deviation = 2.5\ kg/m^2$$
$$E/S = 0.4$$

From Appendix 6A,
   If alpha (two-sided) = 0.05, beta = 0.20, then **100 participants are needed per group.**
   If alpha (two-sided) = 0.05, beta = 0.10 (power = 0.9), then **133 participants are needed per group.**
   If alpha (two-sided) = 0.01, beta = 0.20, then **148 participants are needed per group.**

Extra credit:
Here are the strategies suggested in Chapter 6:

a. **Use continuous variables**—body mass index is already being measured as a continuous variable and there is no way to make case-control status, which is dichotomous, into a continuous variable.

b. **Use a more precise variable**—both weight and height are fairly precise variables, so the standard deviation of body mass index is composed mostly of between-individual variation, which cannot be reduced. Careful standardization of height and weight measurements to reduce measurement error would still be a good idea, but this is not the best choice.

c. **Use paired measurements**—not applicable; "change" in body mass index would address a different research question.

d. **Use a more common outcome**—not applicable for case-control studies.

e. **Use unequal group sizes**—the number of controls can be increased, as it is easy to find participants without stomach cancer. For example, if the number of controls can be increased 4-fold to 240, one can use the approximation formula in Chapter 6,

$$n' = ([c + 1] \div 2c) \times n$$

where n' represents the "new" number of cases, c represents the control-to-case ratio (in this example, 4), and n represents the "old" number of cases (assuming one control per case). In this example,

$$n' = ([4 + 1] \div 8) \times 100 = 5/8 \times 100 = 63$$

which is almost the number of cases that are available. Thus, a study with 60 cases and 240 controls will have similar (slightly less) power compared with one that has 100 cases and 100 controls.

2. H_0: There is no difference in mean strength between the DHEA-treated and placebo-treated groups.

H_A: There is a difference in mean strength between the DHEA-treated and placebo-treated groups

> Alpha (two-sided) = 0.05; beta = 0.10
> Effect size = 10% × 20 kg = 2 g
> Standard deviation = 8 kg
> E/S = 0.25

Comparing the groups using a t test, and looking at Appendix 6A, go down the left column to 0.25, then across to the fifth column from the left, where alpha (two-sided) = 0.05 and beta = 0.10. Approximately **338 participants per group** would be needed. If beta = 0.20, then the sample size is 253 per group.

3. H_0: There is no difference in the mean change in strength between the DHEA-treated and placebo-treated groups.

H_A: There is a difference in mean change in strength between the DHEA-treated and placebo-treated groups.

> Alpha (two-sided) = 0.05; beta = 0.10
> Effect size = 10% × 20 kg = 2 kg
> Standard deviation = 2 kg
> E/S = 1.0

Looking at Appendix 6A, go down the left column to 1.00, then across to the fifth column from the left where alpha (two-sided) = 0.05 and beta = 0.10. Approximately **23 participants per group** will be needed.

4. H_0: There is no difference in frequency of left-handedness in dyslexic and non-dyslexic students.

H_A: There is a difference in frequency of left-handedness in dyslexic and non-dyslexic students.

> Alpha (two-sided) = 0.05; beta = 0.20
> Effect size = odds ratio of 2.0

Given that the proportion of non-dyslexic students who are left-handed (P_0) is about 0.1, the investigator wants to be able to detect a proportion of dyslexic students who are left-handed (P_1) that will yield an odds ratio of 2.0. The sample size estimate will use a chi-squared test, and one needs to use Appendix 6B. However, that appendix is set up for entering the two proportions, not the odds ratio, and all that is known is one of the proportions ($P_0 = 0.1$).

To calculate the value for P_1 for an odds ratio of 2, one can use the formula in Chapter 6:

$$P_1 = \frac{OR \times P_0}{(1 - P_0) + (OR \times P_0)}$$

In this example:

$$P_1 = \frac{2 \times 0.1}{(1 - 0.1) + (2 \times 0.1)} = \frac{0.2}{0.9 + 0.2} = 0.18$$

These proportions will be compared using the chi-squared test. If P_1 is 0.18 and P_0 is 0.1, then $P_1 - P_0$ is 0.08. Table 6B.2 in Appendix 6B reveals a **sample size of 318 per group**.

5. Although IQ tests typically have a standard deviation of 15, it is plausible that the distribution among medical students would be somewhat narrower. Standard deviation of IQ scores is about one-fourth of the "usual" range (which is 150 − 110 = 40 points), or 10 points.

Total width of the confidence interval = 6 (3 above and 3 below).

Standardized width of the confidence interval = total width ÷ standard deviation = 6/10 = 0.6.

Confidence level = 99%.

Using Table 6D, go down the W/S column to 0.60, then across to the 99% confidence level. **About 74 medical students' IQ scores** would need to be averaged to obtain a mean score with the specified confidence interval of ±3 points.

Chapter 7 Addressing Ethical Issues

1a. From an ethical perspective, the proposed study could certainly be done under the original informed consent if participants in the original study gave consent for future additional research, including DNA sequencing, or if participants gave broad consent to unspecified future research. The original consent, however, could have been ambiguous (eg, "may be shared with other researchers doing related research") or silent regarding future research. In that case the IRB could decide that the proposed secondary project falls within the scope of the original consent.

1b. A very strict interpretation of the original consent would preclude valuable secondary studies that could yield important knowledge about the disease, that do not harm the participants, and that would be prohibitively difficult if fresh biospecimens need to be collected. There are no additional medical risks in the proposed study. Genomic sequencing might be viewed differently from carrying out other laboratory studies on stored specimens, such as validating new biomarkers for diabetes or coronary artery disease. Participants could suffer stigmatization, loss of privacy, and discrimination if confidentiality is breached. Thus, appropriate confidentiality provisions need to be put into place.

There are several options for researchers to carry out the secondary study even if the original consent did not cover it. **The IRB could grant a waiver of informed consent,** following the appropriate criteria for such a waiver. More commonly, the **holders of the data and biospecimens remove overt identifiers,** such as medical record numbers, so that participants' specimens and data are linked by a numerical code, the key to which is destroyed or not shared with secondary researchers.

If the original consent, however, specifically said that specimens would not be shared with other researchers, it would be ethically problematic to remove overt identifiers and carry out the secondary research as described earlier.

1c. When researchers collect new biospecimens in a research project, it is prudent to **ask permission to collect and store additional blood to be used in future research studies.** Storing biospecimens allows future research to be carried out more efficiently than assembling a new cohort. **Tiered consent** is recommended: The participant is asked to consent (1) to the specific study (eg, in the original cohort study), (2) to other research projects on the same general topic (such as risk of coronary artery disease or stroke), or (3) to all other future research that is approved by an IRB and by a scientific review panel. To address the issues raised in exercise 1b, the participant might also be asked to consent specifically to research in which his or her DNA would be sequenced. The participant may agree to one, two, or all options. Of course, it is impossible to fully describe future research. Hence, consent for future studies is not really informed in the sense that the participant will not know the nature, risks, and benefits of future studies. The participant is being asked to trust that IRBs and scientific review panels will only permit future studies that are scientifically and ethically sound. The NIH is developing points to consider and sample language for consent to future use of biospecimens (see https://grants.nih.gov/grants/guide/notice-files/NOT-OD-21-131 .html).

2a. **Withholding drugs from the control group that are known to improve clinically significant outcomes would subject participants to unjustified harm** and would therefore be unethical. Even if participants would give informed consent to participate in such a placebo-controlled trial, an IRB should not approve such a study, because it violates the regulatory requirements that the risk-benefit balance be acceptable and that the risks be minimized.

2b. If all participants in the trial were treated with current standard-of-care chemotherapy, the participants could then be randomized to the new treatment or placebo. Alternatively, the investigators might try to identify a subgroup of patients for whom no therapy has been shown to prolong survival (the most clinically significant endpoint in cancer). For example, **patients whose disease has progressed despite several types of standard chemotherapy and who have no options that are proven effective could be asked to participate in a placebo-controlled trial of the experimental intervention.** This approach assumes that if the drug is active after other treatments have failed, it will also be active in previously untreated patients. It is, of course, also possible that a drug that does not work in refractory disease may be effective as first-line treatment. These study designs would have reduced power, compared to a placebo control.

3a. When clinical research is carried out in resource-poor countries by sponsors and investigators from better-resourced countries, there is a risk that research could take advantage of vulnerable participants and countries. The strongest ethical design would be to have the **feasibility study and subsequent trial run by a trusted humanitarian organization that** provides on-the-ground medical care in the host country, such as Médecins Sans Frontières, in collaboration with investigators in the host country who have no conflicts of interest. The host country government and nongovernmental service organizations should approve the study. To ensure that the host country and its residents receive some long-term benefit, there should be **agreement negotiated before the feasibility trial to provide meaningful access to the vaccine within the host country,** for example, by making a meaningful amount of vaccine available at affordable prices.

3b. During informed consent, the investigators must discuss: (1) **the nature of the study;** (2) the number and length of visits; (3) the **potential benefits and risks** of participation (in this case primarily stigma and discrimination if confidentiality is breached); (4) **alternatives** to participation in the trial, including HIV prevention measures that are or may become available outside the trial; (5) the voluntary nature of participation and the right to withdraw at any time; (6) protection of confidentiality consistent with state public health reporting requirements.

3c. Investigators need to present information in a manner that participants can understand. Participants with low health literacy will not be able to comprehend a detailed written consent form. It would be useful for the researchers to consult with community and advocacy groups on how to present the information such as by using videos or comic books. Extensive pretesting of translated and back-translated consent materials should be carried out. Furthermore, researchers should determine what misunderstandings about the study are common and develop the consent process to address them.

Furthermore, even though this is an observational study, researchers have an ethical obligation to provide information to participants about how to reduce their risk for HIV infection. There are both ethical and scientific reasons for doing so. Researchers have an ethical obligation to prevent harm to participants in their study. They may not withhold feasible public health measures that are known to prevent the potentially fatal illness that is the endpoint of the study. Such measures would include counseling, condoms, and referral to substance abuse treatment and needle exchange programs. Researchers must also invoke these measures to prevent harm to participants in the subsequent vaccine trial, even though these measures will reduce the power of the trial.

Chapter 8 Designing Cross-Sectional and Cohort Studies

1a. First, you would define inclusion and exclusion criteria and recruit a sample for your study, perhaps persons at least 70 years old with no previous history of hip fractures. Then you would measure serum vitamin B_{12} levels and other predictors of hip fracture on these participants (perhaps storing serum samples for later use; see further). For ethical reasons, you would want to treat (and probably then exclude) anyone you identified with clear-cut vitamin B_{12} deficiency. Then you would follow the participants for a period of time (say, 5 years) for the occurrence of hip fractures and analyze the association between B_{12} levels and incident hip fractures.

1b. An advantage of the prospective cohort design for studying vitamin B_{12} levels and hip fractures:

- Temporal sequence (ie, vitamin B_{12} levels measured in serum samples obtained before the hip fractures occur) helps establish a cause-effect relationship. People who fracture their hips might develop lower vitamin B_{12} levels *after* the fractures because they have reduced B_{12} intake, perhaps because of nursing home placement. (This would likely be an even greater problem for vitamin D levels, which are related to sun exposure.) Obtaining serum samples as soon as possible after the fractures would mitigate this concern. Disadvantages of the prospective cohort design:

- A prospective cohort study will require many thousands of participants to be followed for many years. It will therefore be expensive, and the findings would be delayed.

- During the long follow-up period, changes in diet and use of supplements may alter vitamin B_{12} levels so that baseline levels no longer reflect those at the time of the fracture. This may require repeated measurements of vitamin B_{12} during follow-up, adding to the complexity and expense of the study.

1c. A retrospective cohort study could be done if you could find a cohort with stored serum and with reasonably complete follow-up to determine who suffered hip fractures. The main advantage of this design is that it would be less time consuming and expensive. The major drawbacks are that measurements of vitamin B_{12} might be altered by long-term storage, and that measurements of potential confounders (such as physical activity and cigarette smoking) may not be available.

2a. Although the PRIDE study is a randomized trial, the report of the baseline examination is an (observational) **cross-sectional study**. Cross-sectional studies are often the first step in cohort studies or randomized trials.

2b. Although it is possible that depression increases urinary incontinence, it also seems plausible that **urinary incontinence could contribute to depression**. As we will discuss in Chapter 10, it is also possible that the association is due to bias, if depressed women were more likely to *report* incontinence episodes even if they did not have more of them, or to confounding if a third factor (eg, obesity) caused both depression and incontinence.

  A longitudinal (cohort) study could help by clarifying the time sequence of the association. For example, depressed and nondepressed women with little or no incontinence at baseline could be followed to see whether the depressed women *develop* more or worse incontinence over time. Similarly, women with different levels of urinary incontinence and with no history of depression could be followed to determine whether more incontinent women are more likely to become depressed. (Studying more than two levels of the incontinence [exposure] variable allows the investigators to see if there is evidence of a dose-response relation.) Finally, and most convincingly, the investigators could study *changes* in depression or incontinence, either naturally occurring or (ideally) as a result of an intervention, and see if changes in one preceded changes in the other. For example, do depressive symptoms improve when incontinence is successfully treated? Does (reported) continence improve when depression lifts?

Chapter 9 Designing Case-Control Studies

1. Using the cohort assembled in question 8.1c, the main way to improve efficiency would be to reduce the number of measurements of vitamin B_{12} levels. Instead of measuring B_{12} levels on the entire cohort at baseline (and treating and excluding those with very low levels), the investigators could draw and store blood for later analyses. They then could **do a nested case-control study**, in which B_{12} levels are measured on all hip fracture cases and a random sample of those who did not develop a hip fracture (the controls). Measuring levels in four to five controls per case gets close to maximum efficiency (see the formula under "Unequal Group Sizes" in Chapter 5) and would reduce the number of vitamin B_{12} assays compared with measuring them in all participants.

2a. The best choice is to **enroll all cases from a predefined cohort in a nested case-control study**. An age range (say, 30 to 75 years) and minimum criteria for diagnosis (eg, pathology) would be specified. If a sufficiently large cohort was not available, recent cases could be identified from tumor registries, limiting enrollment to those who can be contacted by telephone and who agree to participate. Selecting recent cases reduces the probability of bias that might result from studying only survivors (see further). Ideally, the investigators would interview surviving relatives of any deceased cases.

2b. The controls could be a random sample of all women between 30 and 75 years of age from the same cohort (for the nested case-control study) or from the counties covered by the tumor registries. Obtaining a random sample is more feasible if the population has been enumerated, as is in some European countries. In the United States, the random sample might need to be obtained using random-digit dialing (hence the need to restrict cases to those who have telephones).

2c. Because ovarian cancer requires intensive therapy and can be fatal, some cases may be unwilling to enroll in the study or may have died before they can be interviewed. If a family history of ovarian cancer is related to more aggressive forms of ovarian cancer, then the study might underestimate its relative risk, because those cases with a positive family history would be less likely to survive long enough to be included in the sample of cases.

If familial ovarian cancer has a better prognosis than other ovarian cancers, the opposite could occur.

Similarly, it is possible that healthy women who have a family member with ovarian cancer will be more interested in the study and more likely to enroll as controls. In that situation, the prevalence of family history of ovarian cancer in the control group will be artificially high, and the estimate of the risk for ovarian cancer because of family history will be falsely low. This problem might be minimized by not telling the potential control participants the exact research question or which cancer is being studied if it can be done ethically.

2d. Family history of ovarian cancer is measured by asking participants how many female relatives they have and how many of them have had ovarian cancer. **Recall bias** is a possible problem with this approach. Women with ovarian cancer, who may be concerned about the possibility of a genetic predisposition to their disease, may be more likely to remember or find out about relatives with ovarian cancer than healthy women who have not had reason to think about this possibility. This would cause the estimate of the association between family history and ovarian cancer to be falsely high.

In addition, women may confuse gynecologic cancers (cervical, uterine, and ovarian) as well as benign gynecologic tumors that require surgery. This may cause misclassification of exposure: some women without a family history of ovarian cancer will report having the risk factor and be misclassified. If misclassification of exposure occurs equally in the cases and controls, the estimate of the odds ratio for family history and ovarian cancer will be biased toward 1. If this type of misclassification is more common in cases (who may be more likely to misinterpret the type of cancer or the reason for surgery in relatives), then the estimate of the odds ratio for family history and ovarian cancer will be falsely high. Misclassification could be decreased by checking medical records of family members who are reported to have had ovarian cancer to verify the diagnosis.

Finally, it would be desirable to account for the *opportunity* for cases and controls to have a positive family history, because women with many aunts and older sisters have greater opportunity to have a positive family history than those smaller families or with only brothers or younger sisters. As discussed in Chapter 10, matching and stratification are two ways of dealing with this possibility.

2e. The simplest approach would be to dichotomize family history of ovarian cancer (eg, first-degree relatives or not) and use the odds ratio as the measure of association. The odds ratio approximates the relative risk because the outcome (ovarian cancer) is rare. A simple chi-squared test would then be the appropriate test of statistical significance. Alternatively, if family history were quantified (eg, proportion of first- and second-degree female relatives affected), one could create an ordinal categorical variable for strength of family history and look for a dose-response, computing odds ratios at each level of exposure. Finally, a genome-wide association study (GWAS) could identify genes that were more common in cases than controls, but this would require large sample sizes.

2f. The **case-control design** is a reasonable way to answer this research question despite the problems of sampling bias, recall bias, and misclassification noted previously. One alternative would be a large cohort study; however, because ovarian cancer is so rare, a cohort design to answer just this specific question is probably not feasible. A retrospective cohort study, in which data on family history were already collected systematically, would be ideal, if such a cohort could be found.

3a. Cases could be younger drivers (perhaps 16 to 20 years old) who were involved in crashes, and controls could be friends or acquaintances they identify who have not had a car crash. It would be important to exclude friends with whom they play video games to avoid over-matching. Random-digit dialing would likely be less successful as a strategy for identifying controls, given the high prevalence of cellular phones in this age group. Cases and controls could also be identified if the investigator had access to the records of an automobile insurance company. An argument could be made that cases and controls should be matched for sex, given that both playing video games and crashing cars are more common in young men. The exposure would be measured using a questionnaire or interview about video game use. It would be important to ask about video games that do not involve driving as well as about those that do, because causal inference would be enhanced if the association were specific, namely, if there was an effect for use of driving/racing games, but not for shooting or other games.

3b. For intermittent exposures hypothesized to have a short-term effect, like use of a video game just before driving, **a case-crossover study** is an attractive option. As in exercise 3a, cases could be younger drivers who were involved in crashes. In a case-crossover study there are no controls, just control time periods. Thus, case drivers would be asked about use of racing video games just before the trip that included the crash and also about control time periods when they did not crash. The time period just before the crash is compared in a matched analysis with other time periods to see if racing video game use was more common in the precrash period than in other time periods.

Chapter 10   Estimating Causal Effects Using Observational Studies

1a. There are four reasons why the observed association between dietary fruit and vegetable intake and CHD may not represent the causal effect:

- **Chance.** The finding that people with CHD ate fewer fruits and vegetables may have been due to random error. As discussed in Chapter 5, the *P* value allows quantification of the magnitude of the observed difference compared with what might have been expected by chance alone; the 95% confidence interval shows the range of values consistent with the study results. All else being equal, the smaller the *P* value and the further the null value is from the end of the confidence interval that is closer to it, the less plausible it is that chance is the entire explanation for an observed association.

- **Bias.** There may have been a systematic error (a systematic difference between the research question and the way the study plan was carried out) with regard to the sample, predictor variable, or outcome variable. For example, the sample may be biased if the controls were patients at the same health plan as the cases, but were selected from those attending an annual health maintenance examination, because such patients may be more health conscious (and hence eat more fruits and vegetables) than the entire population at risk for CHD. The measurements of the exposure (diet) could be biased if, for example, people who have had a heart attack are more likely to recall poor dietary practices than controls (recall bias), or if unblinded interviewers asked the questions or recorded the answers differently in cases and controls. Finally, the measurement of the outcome (CHD) could be biased if, for example, those who ate more fruits and vegetables had doctors who were more (or less) aggressive about pursuing a diagnosis of CHD.

- **Effect-cause.** It is possible that having a heart attack changed people's dietary preferences, so that they ate fewer fruits and vegetables than they did before the heart attack. It seems more likely, however, that the scare from having a heart attack might make people eat more fruits and vegetables; this would tend to make eating fruits and vegetables appear to be less beneficial at preventing CHD than it really is. The possibility of effect-cause can often be addressed by designing the study to examine the historical sequence—for example, by asking the cases and controls about their previous diet rather than their current diet, or (better yet) nesting the case-control study in an existing cohort with prerecorded dietary information.

- **Confounding.** There may be other differences between those who eat more fruits and vegetables and those who eat fewer, and these other differences may be the actual cause of their differing rates of CHD. For example, people who eat more fruits and vegetables may also exercise more (see part 1b).

1b. Possible approaches to controlling for confounding by exercise are summarized in the following table:

Method	Possible Plan	Advantages	Disadvantages
Design Phase			
Specification	Enroll only people who report no regular exercise	Simple	Will limit the pool of eligible participants, making recruitment more difficult. The study may not generalize to people that do exercise.
Matching	Match each case to a control with similar exercise level	Eliminates the effect of exercise as a predictor of CHD, often with a slight increase in the precision (power) to observe diet as a predictor	Requires extra effort to identify controls to match each case. Will waste cases if there is no control with a similar exercise level. Eliminates the opportunity to study the effect of exercise on CHD.
Opportunistic study	Find an external influence on fruit and vegetable intake not otherwise associated with CHD (an instrument)	If a suitable instrument can be found, has the potential to control for both measured and unmeasured confounders	Often it is hard to find strong and convincing instruments.
Analysis Phase			
Stratification	For the analysis, group the participants into three or four exercise strata	Easy, comprehensible, and reversible	Can only reasonably evaluate a few strata and a few confounding variables. Will lose some of the information contained in exercise measured as a continuous variable by switching to a categorical variable, and if categories are too broad, this may result in incomplete control of confounding.
Statistical adjustment (modeling)	Use a multivariable model (eg, logistic regression or the Cox model) to control for exercise as well as other potential confounders	Can reversibly control for all the information in exercise as a continuous predictor variable, while simultaneously controlling for other potential confounders such as age, race/ethnicity, diabetes, hypertension, and smoking	The statistical model might not fit the data, resulting in incomplete control of confounding and potentially misleading results. For example, the effect of diet or physical activity may not be the same in smokers and nonsmokers. The important potential confounders must have been measured in advance. Sometimes it is difficult to understand and describe the results of the model, especially when there are interactions or the variables are not dichotomous.

In addition to these strategies for controlling confounding in observational studies, there is another approach: Designing a randomized trial. However, such a trial would likely need to estimate the causal effect of an intervention designed to encourage fruit and vegetable intake, rather than the intake itself.

It is also worthwhile to seek lines of evidence that support causality, including a **dose-response relationship** (decreasing odds of CHD with increasing fruit and vegetable intake), a **biologic mechanism**, such as evidence that there are components of fruits and vegetables (eg, antioxidants) that protect against atherosclerosis, and **consistency** across multiple populations and study designs, such as evidence from ecologic studies that CHD is much less common in populations that eat more fruits and vegetables.

2. This is an example of **conditioning on a collider**, or shared effect: The study included only infants with fever, which can be caused by both urinary tract infections and ear infections. Because uncircumcised boys were much more likely to have a urinary tract infection, they were more likely to have that as the cause of their fever, rather than an ear infection (ie, uncircumcised boys were overrepresented among those without ear infections because they were also overrepresented among those with urinary tract infections).

3. The association between maternal acetaminophen use and asthma in offspring could be examined in a cohort study, in which mothers were asked about acetaminophen use during pregnancy, and offspring were followed for the development of asthma. Investigators would look for evidence that **maternal genotype modifies the effect of maternal acetaminophen exposure on asthma in the children (interaction)**, with a stronger association between exposure and outcome among those predicted to be most genetically susceptible. In fact, such results have been reported (Shaheen SO, Newson RB, Ring SM, Rose-Zerilli MJ, Holloway JW, Henderson AJ. Prenatal and infant acetaminophen exposure, antioxidant gene polymorphisms, and childhood asthma. *J Allergy Clin Immunol*. 2010;126(6): 1141-1148 e7).

Chapter 11   Designing Randomized Blinded Trials

1a. The main advantage of using change in the biomarker (a continuous variable) as the primary outcome of the trial is a **smaller sample size and a shorter duration** to determine whether the treatment reduces the level of the marker. The main disadvantage is the **uncertainty of whether change in the level of the marker** induced by the treatment means that the treatment **will reduce** the incidence of the clinically far more important outcome, developing **dementia**.

1b. The main advantage of using clinical diagnosis of dementia as the primary outcome of the trial is that it is a **more meaningful** outcome that could improve clinical practice for prevention of dementia. The **disadvantage is that such a trial would likely be large, long, and expensive**, given that clinical dementia tends to develop slowly over time and occur in a small number of participants.

2a. To maximize your study team's ability to follow up and retain participants, **baseline collection of data should include information about how to contact the participant, a close friend, a family member, or a health care provider.**

2b. To enable others to evaluate the generalizability of the study sample, you could **collect baseline information about participants'** demographic characteristics (such as their age, race/ethnicity, and sex or gender), their general health status, and the degree of cognitive impairment they have at baseline.

2c. To guide assessment of the efficacy of treatment, you should **administer all efficacy outcome measures at baseline,** such as cognitive function tests or other measures of the impact of cognitive impairment on the participants' daily lives.

2d. To pave the way for future subgroup analyses, **you might collect baseline data on risk factors or possible effect modifiers for the outcome,** such as hypertension, family history of dementia, or presence of the ApoE4 allele. These variables might identify participants with the highest rate of the outcome who could then be examined in subgroups.

2e. One way to maximize the potential usefulness of your trial data to answer future unanticipated research questions is to collect data, for example, about potential risk factors for dementia, and **store biologic specimens** such as serum or plasma to allow future measurement of factors, such as genotypes of enzymes that metabolize the drug, that could influence the efficacy of the treatment. You could also ask colleagues if they want to propose simple ancillary measures such as extra questionnaires to administer at baseline that could allow exploration of other research questions in the trial sample.

3a. You will need to **enroll enough individuals with the ApoE4 allele** to have power for future analyses comparing the effects of huperzine among participants who have the allele versus those who do not. This will require you to screen for the presence of the ApoE4 allele at baseline and enrich enrollment of candidates with the allele so that they make up the necessary minimum threshold proportion of your total trial sample. Stratified blocked randomization could be used to make sure that there are similar numbers of participants with the ApoE4 genotype in the treatment and the placebo groups.

3b. On the one hand, this could **provide clinically useful information** if it turns out that huperzine has a very different efficacy profile based on ApoE4 genotype. On the other hand, this process **will make the trial more complicated.** Assessing ApoE4 genotype before enrollment will delay randomization and raise issues that include how to counsel participants about the results. It will be more challenging and expensive to enrich the trial sample with individuals with the ApoE4 allele, rather than enrolling participants regardless of allele status provided that they meet eligibility criteria. The greater complexity of your randomization scheme will also make it more challenging to prepare and package study medication and placebo for each stratum. As a result, for an initial trial conducted when it is still unclear whether huperzine has any efficacy for slowing the progression of dementia, you might decide not to explore differential effects based on ApoE4 allele status.

4a. This approach involves little effort or expense, but it is unlikely to result in accurate detection of gastrointestinal symptoms that could be the result of huperzine. First, at the end of a longer term trial, **participants may not accurately recall** gastrointestinal symptoms that they experienced early on in the study. Also, participants may not be the best judge of **whether their gastrointestinal symptoms were caused** by the use of study medication.

4b. This approach would likely result in **underreporting** of gastrointestinal symptoms, because **participants may not remember** to mention these symptoms even if they are encouraged to do so at the start of the trial. And similar to approach #1, this approach might lead to underreporting of gastrointestinal symptoms if participants **do not attribute** their symptoms to use of study medication.

4c. This approach would be more likely to yield consistent information about the experience of diarrhea, nausea, and vomiting. Some reported symptoms might not be related to use of study medication, but **your research team could compare rates and severity of reported symptoms between the huperzine and placebo** groups to assess whether there is greater frequency or severity of symptoms in participants assigned to huperzine.

4d. This approach might detect participants' gastrointestinal symptoms but also detect many other symptoms or adverse health issues experienced by participants in the course of the trial. This would have the benefit of allowing you **to assess for other unanticipated adverse effects** of huperzine. Responses to this open-ended question could subsequently be classified and categorized for data analysis. On the other hand, if it is important to you to quantify the burden of gastrointestinal symptoms associated with huperzine, you should consider questioning participants specifically about diarrhea, nausea, and vomiting, in addition to asking a more general open-ended question about symptoms and health conditions.

5. As an interim monitor, you might find it useful to request information about the **severity or duration** of the gastrointestinal symptoms to gauge whether the harms of this potential side effect might outweigh the potential benefits for cognitive function. You might also be interested in the **characteristics of the participants who developed symptoms** to assess whether this side effect occurred only in a specific subgroup that

could be excluded from the trial in the future. You could recommend that the investigators incorporate new questions about prior history of gastrointestinal symptoms (such as a history of irritable bowel syndrome) into their future screening procedures to prevent enrollment of participants who may be more likely to develop severe symptoms in response to study therapy.

6. The main **disadvantage** of intention-to-treat analysis is that it **includes participants who did not comply with the randomized treatment**, and who therefore reduce the apparent magnitude of any effect that is observed for the whole randomized group. However, the disadvantages of using as-treated rather than intention-to-treat analysis are potentially even greater. Because **participants who do not comply with the intervention usually differ** from those who do comply in important but unmeasured ways, as-treated analysis **no longer has a true randomized comparison** and may incorrectly conclude that the huperzine is efficacious.

7. The conclusion that huperzine works better in younger participants, based on a subgroup analysis, may be wrong because the result **may be due to chance**. The probability of finding a "significant" treatment effect in a subgroup when there is not a significant treatment effect overall increases with the number of subgroups tested; it is not clear how many subgroups were tested to find this "significant" effect. The claim that the treatment is efficacious in participants younger than age 60 years implies that the treatment was not efficacious—or even had the opposite effect—in older participants. This result should also be reported and tested statistically for age-related modification of the effect of huperzine on cognitive impairment. The investigators should avoid concluding that huperzine is efficacious in the subgroup of younger participants if this subgroup analysis was performed post hoc rather than **specified in advance based on a biologic basis**, if a large number of subgroups were tested, and if the P value for effect modification (interaction) between the effect of treatment and age is not statistically significant.

Chapter 12   Alternate Interventional Study Designs

1a. A trial that compared HairStat to placebo would offer the **simplest study, require the smallest sample size**, and therefore be the least expensive design. This trial design could provide clear evidence that HairStat is better than placebo. However, this design has disadvantages if finasteride is already widely available as a treatment for male pattern baldness, as some participants would be tempted to use finasteride during the trial. Even in a double-blind study, if HairStat were effective in reducing baldness, men who were assigned to placebo might be more likely to use finasteride than men assigned to HairStat, and this could prevent the trial from detecting the benefit of HairStat. The investigators could **instruct men in both groups to avoid using finasteride**, but some men might be reluctant to enroll in the trial knowing that they will not be able to use finasteride, a medication with demonstrated efficacy.

1b. An advantage of comparing HairStat to finasteride is that if finasteride is commonly used for male pattern baldness, the trial will **answer a clinically important question**: whether there is any evidence of different efficacy. The investigators should first decide if they think HairStat is more efficacious than finasteride. If so, a **comparative efficacy trial** that could demonstrate potential superior efficacy of HairStat would be the best choice to compare HairStat to finasteride. If the investigators think that HairStat is just as good as finasteride, but will be much cheaper, they should consider a **noninferiority trial**. In this case, they must take care to use a trial design that is very similar to that used to document the efficacy of finasteride (inclusion criteria, dose, duration of treatment, outcome measures) and must conduct the trial to ensure that there is minimal nonadherence and loss to follow-up. A major drawback of a noninferiority trial is that the sample size is likely to be much larger than that required for a placebo-controlled trial.

1c. An advantage of a placebo-controlled trial of HairStat that enrolled only men who had previously tried and failed finasteride is that it would avoid the challenges posed by options a and b above. **Participants would not be tempted to use finasteride**, and there would be no clinical reason to compare the efficacy of HairStat to finasteride in this population. However, a disadvantage is that it **may be more difficult to recruit a sufficient number of men** who had already tried and failed finasteride. Furthermore, people who have problems tolerating one medication may also be more likely not to tolerate another, even if the medications have different mechanisms of action. So, the investigators may find that the frequency or severity of medication tolerability issues may be higher in this trial of HairStat than had been reported with finasteride, even though in a less selected population the adverse event profiles of the two drugs might be similar.

1d. A factorial design that includes a placebo has the advantages of comparing each treatment to a placebo and (if planned with adequate statistical power) testing whether the combination of treatments is better than either one alone. The disadvantages of this approach are the larger size and greater cost and complexity of the trial.

1e. An advantage of a crossover trial is that it might be appealing to potential participants, because it would allow all participants to have some exposure to each of the study medications. In addition, because each participant acts as his own control, the sample size would be smaller than for a parallel group trial. However, this approach has disadvantages if the effects of medication persist for a substantial amount of time after it is discontinued. In that case, continued hair growth in the first few months after change from HairStat to finasteride (or vice versa) might be attributed to the wrong medication.

2a. A classic, individual-level randomized trial might seem to be the simplest approach to evaluating the effects of the dietary change intervention on weight. However, the nature of the intervention makes it difficult, even impossible, to deliver the intervention to some but not all employees in the same office. For example, any educational posters posted in office common areas would be visible to all employees, regardless of the intervention group to which they were assigned. For that reason, a clinical trial that randomizes employees at the individual level is probably not feasible for this type of intervention that takes place at the workplace level.

2b. Advantages of this approach are that it maximizes exposure of all employees and offices to the intervention and also has the benefit of simplicity in outcomes analysis. After collecting information about preintervention employee weight, the company could roll out the dietary intervention across all office sites simultaneously and then assess change in employee weight 6 months later. **Without a comparison group**, however, it would be difficult to determine whether any observed change in employee weight (or lack thereof) was specifically attributable to the intervention. For example, if employee weight remained the same (or even slightly increased), the company might conclude incorrectly that the intervention offered no benefit for weight control, when it is possible that the employees would have gained more weight if no intervention had been implemented. Some of the limitations of this design might be overcome by using an **interrupted time series analysis approach**, in which the analysis considered the preintervention trends in employee weight and extrapolated to the likely trajectory of their weight if no intervention were implemented.

2c. This approach has the advantage of allowing the intervention to be gradually introduced to all company offices, and from that perspective might be more conducive to the company's goal of promoting weight loss among all its overweight or obese employees. However, a disadvantage is that this approach assumes that intervention effects are equivalent regardless of the month in which the intervention is initiated. In reality, **there might be underlying temporal trends** in employee weight (eg, a tendency for employees to gain weight during the winter months rather than the fall or spring months) that could invalidate the findings.

2d. This approach has the advantage of allowing for rigorous assessment of changes in employee weight in offices that were randomly selected to implement versus not implement the intervention. The main disadvantage is that **a large number of offices would need to be randomized** to ensure that the trial was adequately powered, given that the primary unit of analysis would be the office, rather than the individual employee. Outcome analyses might also be complicated by differences in the size of offices (and thus the weight given to each in outcome analysis).

Chapter 13   Designing Studies of Medical Tests

1a. The best way to sample patients for a diagnostic test is generally to **sample those at risk of a disease before it is known who has the disease** and who does not. In this case, sampling women who present to a clinic or emergency department with abdominal pain consistent with PID would probably be best. Comparing the ESRs of women hospitalized for PID with those of a healthy control population would be the worst approach, because both the spectrum of disease and especially the spectrum of nondisease are not representative of the groups in whom the test would be used clinically. (Those hospitalized for PID probably have more severe disease than average, and healthy volunteers are much less likely to have high ESRs than women with abdominal pain because of causes other than PID.)

1b. If those assigning the final diagnosis used the ESR to help decide who had PID and who did not, both the **sensitivity and specificity might be falsely high**. The more those assigning the diagnosis relied on the ESR, the greater the bias (called "incorporation bias") in the study.

1c. The best answer is that **you should not use any particular cut point** for defining an abnormal result. Rather, you should display the trade-off between sensitivity and specificity using a ROC curve and present likelihood ratios for various ESR intervals (eg, <20, 20 to 49, ≥50 mm/hour) rather than sensitivity and specificity at different cutoffs. This is illustrated by the following table, which can be created from the information in the question:

ESR	PID	NO PID	LIKELIHOOD RATIO
<20	10%	50%	0.20
20-49	15%	35%	0.43
≥50	75%	15%	5.00
Total	**100%**	**100%**	

The ROC curve could also be used to compare the ESR with one or more other tests such as a white blood cell count. This is illustrated in the following hypothetical ROC curve, which suggests that the ESR is superior to the WBC for predicting PID:

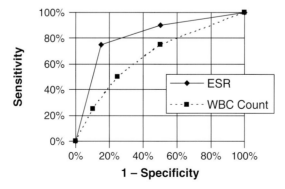

2a. This problem illustrates the common error of **excluding people from the numerator without excluding them from the denominator**. Although it is true that there were only 10 children with "unexpected" abnormalities, the denominator for that yield must be the number of children in whom abnormalities would be considered unexpected, that is, those with normal neurologic examinations and mental status. This is probably a much smaller number than 200. For example, suppose that only 100 of those sent for a CT scan had both a normal mental status and no neurologic findings. In that situation, the yield would be 10 of 100, or 10%—twice as high.

2b. **Many of these "abnormalities" may be findings of little or no clinical significance.** Unless the "abnormality" leads to changes in management and there is some way to estimate the effects of these management changes on outcome, it will be very hard to know what yield is sufficient to make the CT scan worth doing. It would be better to use "intracranial injury requiring intervention" as the outcome in this study, although this will require some consensus on what injuries require intervention and some estimate of the effectiveness of these interventions for improving outcome.

2c. The first advantage of studying the effects of the CT scan on clinical decisions is the ability to examine **possible benefits of normal results.** For example, a normal CT scan might change the management plan from "admit for observation" to "send home." In diagnostic yield studies, normal results are generally assumed to be of little value. Second, as mentioned earlier, abnormal CT scan results might not lead to any changes in management (eg, if no neurosurgery was required and the patient was going to be admitted anyway). Studying effects of tests on clinical decisions helps to determine **how much useful new information** they provide, beyond what is already known at the time the test was ordered. Evidence that a test affects clinical decisions is necessary but not sufficient evidence that it improves outcome. (Tests can, after all, lead to clinical decisions that do not improve outcome, such as the further evaluation of patients with false-positive results.)

3a. If only children who had a CT scan are included, the study will be susceptible to **partial verification bias**, in which sensitivity is falsely increased and specificity is falsely decreased, because children without focal neurologic abnormalities (who are either "false negatives" or "true negatives") will be underrepresented in the study.

3b. If children with head injuries who did not have a CT scan are included and assumed not to have an intracranial injury if they recover without neurosurgery, then the study will be susceptible to **differential verification bias** ("double gold standard bias"), which will tend to increase both sensitivity and specificity if some intracranial injuries resolve without neurosurgery.

Chapter 14   Qualitative Approaches in Clinical Research

1. Mistrust of medicine and research among Black American populations has been examined by many investigators, which provides the basis for launching a **descriptive study** of mistrust among Black immigrant subpopulations. This would be the best design, as it leverages existing knowledge while leaving opportunity for further exploration. For example, a descriptive study would build on insights from previous studies in designing interview guides and structure deductive analytical approaches. Given the lack of previous research on mistrust within immigrant Black populations, an **exploratory study design** would be acceptable, but not ideal. An exploratory design postulates that the phenomena under study are largely unknown. A **comparative qualitative study** is appropriate when investigators can articulate anticipated findings based on previous research. As presented, there is not sufficient evidence to justify such a design, which would be appropriate if more information about migration experiences and mistrust was available.

2. **Answer b is the best choice. Focus groups** are appropriate when investigators want to find out how a group discusses and makes sense of a particular issue or question. They are not a strategy for increasing the number of research participants, as the group is the unit of analysis, not the number of individuals. Focus groups can sometimes create an environment in which participants feel freer to express opinions, but they can also have the opposite effect:

Individuals may be reluctant to offer opinions that differ from those expressed by other group members.

3. **Inductive analysis** was most appropriate for the Trials Knowledge study, which was exploring a study question that had not been examined previously. The interview protocol encouraged respondents to raise new topics and provide insights that investigators had not anticipated. Data analysis thus used a "bottom-up" approach to identify new findings. In the Deimplementing study, investigators used **key informant interviews** to understand stakeholders' response to medical home policies. Key informants have deep knowledge of the study topic and their interviews lend themselves to **deductive analyses** that build on the topics in the interview guide. The Deimplementing study was the more likely of the two to combine both types of analyses. Analysis started with a deductive analysis of questions asked during key informant interviews and continued with inductive analysis to pursue unanticipated issues raised in response to these questions. In contrast, the Trials Knowledge presented few opportunities for deductive analysis because the study focus was so novel.

Chapter 15   Community-Engaged Research

1a. A **modest level of community involvement** includes approaches in which community organizations and members **help with discrete tasks**, such as translation of recruitment materials, or participant outreach through mailings, promotional events, and short talks. Community engagement studios can also be created for project-specific input on the protocol or other important aspects of the study.

> Advantages: Community partners can provide local knowledge about beliefs and attitudes regarding research participation, breast cancer screening, and experience with using community health workers, which may create a more acceptable intervention. The program may be more sustainable over time and more generalizable to other immigrant Asian groups.

> Challenges: It takes time and effort to build trust with community partners. The investigator will need to budget adequate support for the partner(s) to help with each task. The timeline for the project will need to be addressed and agreed upon by all parties.

1b. A **more substantial level of community involvement** would include input on the study design and methods, as well as (often) assistance with its implementation. A community advisory board can be created early in the planning period to provide suggestions throughout the study.

> Advantages: Having more substantial community engagement in research projects builds community capacity for research, can help with longer term sustainability of the program, and can be more impactful for health equity.

> Challenges: It takes time and effort to develop substantial levels of commitment from community partners. This level of community partnership should be delineated with a Memorandum of Understanding (MOU) or a research subcontract and may require substantial budgetary support. There should be clear communication about the goals of the project with a timeline that is feasible for all partners.

Chapter 16   Research Using Existing Data or Specimens

1. Some possibilities:
   a. Analyze data from the **National Health and Nutrition Examination Survey (NHANES)**. These national population-based studies are conducted periodically, and their results are available to any investigator at a nominal cost. They contain data that include variables

on self-reported clinical history of gallbladder disease and the results of abdominal sonography.

b. Analyze **Medicare data** on frequency of gallbladder surgery in patients more than 65 years of age in the United States, or National Hospital Discharge Survey data on the frequency of such surgery for all ages. Both data sets contain a variable for race. Denominators could come from census data. Like NHANES, these are very good population-based samples, but have the problem of answering a somewhat different research question (ie, What are the rates of surgical treatment for gallbladder disease?). This may be different from the actual incidence of gallbladder disease because of factors such as surgical access and utilization.

2a. The main advantages are that using CHS data in a **secondary data analysis was quick, easy, and inexpensive**—especially compared with the time and expense of planning and conducting a large cohort study. In addition, the research fellow has since developed an ongoing collaboration with the investigators in CHS and has been able to add more sophisticated measures of kidney function to CHS as ancillary studies.

2b. In some cases, the secondary data set does not provide optimal measures of the predictor, outcome, or potential confounding variables. It is important to be sure that the data set will provide reasonable answers to the research question before investing the time and effort required to obtain access to the data. A further drawback is that it can be difficult to obtain data from some studies—the investigator generally needs to write a proposal, find a collaborator who is a coinvestigator on the study, and obtain approval from the study's steering committee and sponsor.

3. There have been several large randomized controlled trials of the effect of estrogen and selective estrogen receptor modulators on various disease outcomes, including cancer, cardiovascular events, and thromboembolic events. These trials include the Women's Health Initiative randomized trials, the Breast Cancer Prevention trial, the Multiple Outcomes of Raloxifene Evaluation trial, and the Raloxifene Use for the Heart trial. The best place for this investigator to begin would be to **determine if estrogen can be measured in stored frozen sera** and, if so, **determine if any of these large trials have stored sera** that could be used for this measurement. The best design for this question is a **nested case-control or case-cohort study**. The investigator will likely need to write a proposal for this ancillary study, obtain approval from the trial's steering committee and sponsor, and obtain funding to make the measurements, a relatively inexpensive prospect because most of the costs of the study have already been covered by the main trial.

4a. The investigator might assemble a cohort of diabetic patients treated at the health system who had a positive coronavirus test, infer exposure to SGLT2 inhibitors using prescribing orders, and conduct a **retrospective cohort study** to analyze the association between SGLT2 inhibitors and hospitalization or death from COVID-19. **Confounding by indication**, however, may pose a major threat to causal inference because diabetic patients prescribed SGLT2 inhibitors may be very different from other diabetic patients (eg, more severe diabetes, and better insurance), and those differences also might be associated with COVID-19 severity. The investigator could attempt a **propensity score analysis** (matching or weighting on factors that predict SGLT2 use to improve comparability of the exposed and unexposed groups), but differences in factors not measured well in EHR data, such as socioeconomic status, are likely to cause residual confounding.

4b. A simple descriptive analysis might simply count the total number of prescribing orders placed for an SGLT2 inhibitor by month and plot that value over time. This would be simplest to do, but would only give a very preliminary result because it lacks a denominator. If many people lost their employment and insurance as a result of the pandemic, numbers of prescriptions could also decline for that reason.

To refine the analysis, the investigator might track individual diabetic patients in the cohort (perhaps limiting to patients due a refill or for whom medication intensification appears warranted, and adjusting for other patient characteristics) and describe the likelihood that a prescribing order for an SGLT2 inhibitor would be placed as a function of time. An interrupted time series analysis of, for example, prescriptions per 100 diabetic patients per month might be undertaken to account for a dynamic baseline trend (eg, increasing SGLT2 inhibitor use before the pandemic) to demonstrate the "interruption" from the pandemic and the news report.

Chapter 17   Designing, Selecting, and Administering Self-Reported Measures

1. Some problems with the question are:
   - There is no definition of how big a "drink" is.
   - There is no way to respond if the participant is drinking > 6 drinks per day.
   - The question assumes that the amount is the same each day. It does not specify days of the week: People commonly drink more on weekends than on weekdays.
   - It assumes the person drinks every day; if someone typically has 3 to 4 drinks per week, it is unclear how they should answer.
   - It would be better to specify a particular time frame (eg, in the past 7 days).

2a. Which of the following statements best describes how *often* you drank alcoholic beverages during the past year? An alcoholic beverage includes wine, liquor, or mixed drinks. Select one of the eight categories:

◯ Every day	◯ 2-3 times per month
◯ 5-6 days per week	◯ About once a month
◯ 3-4 days per week	◯ < 12 times a year
◯ 1-2 days per week	◯ Rarely or not at all

2b. During the past year, *how many* drinks did you *usually* have on a *typical day when you drank alcohol*? A drink is about 12 oz of beer, 5 oz of wine, or 1.5 oz of hard liquor. _____ drinks

2c. During the past year, what is the *largest number* of alcoholic drinks you can recall drinking *during one day*? _____ drinks

2d. About how old were you when you first started drinking alcoholic beverages? _____ years old (If you have never consumed alcoholic beverages, write in "never")

2e. Was there ever a period when you drank quite a bit more than you do now?
    ◯ Yes
    ◯ No

2f. Have you ever had what might be considered a drinking problem?
    ◯ Yes
    ◯ No

3. Advantages and disadvantages include:
   - Obtaining data through interviews requires more staff training and time than a self-administered questionnaire and is therefore much more expensive.
   - Some participants may not like to tell another person the answer to sensitive questions in the area of sexual behavior, so they may be more likely to provide honest answers on a self-administered questionnaire.
   - Unless the interviewers are well trained and the interviews are standardized, the information obtained may vary because of differences in the way the questions are asked each time.
   - However, interviewers can repeat and probe in a way that can produce more accurate and complete responses in some situations than a self-administered questionnaire.

For example, they can assess whether respondents interpret "unprotected sexual intercourse" in the way that is intended.
- A diary may allow a participant to provide specific information about the timing of unprotected sexual intercourse, allowing more precise quantification of the frequency of this behavior.
- However, a diary may be burdensome for participants to keep over time; depending on the participants' motivation, they may stop filling it out after only a short period.

4a. The population that was used to develop and pretest the ICBP questionnaire (private practice orthopedic patients) is different from the target population of your study (low-income older adults). You may need to pretest the questionnaire in individuals who are more similar to your target respondents to assess whether the content and wording are comprehensible and appropriate.

4b. In a sample of patients with severe enough back pain to seek surgical consultation, the observed range for this measure seems low (maximum of 24, whereas the highest possible score is 40). This suggests lower variability of scores derived from this measure, with responses skewed toward lower impact.

4c. This is a relatively low Cronbach's alpha, suggesting poor internal consistency of the measure. Some of the items may not be that related to each other, raising concern about whether it is appropriate to combine all items into a single composite score.

4d. Because the BPI is another established measure of the severity and impact of pain, one would expect to see some correlation between scores on the BPI and the ICBP. Lack of correlation raises concerns about the ICBP's construct validity—that is, whether it is measuring what it is designed to measure.

Chapter 18   Study Implementation and Quality Control

1a. Not much! But here are some steps that might help:
- Identify all missing and out-of-range values and recheck the paper forms to make sure that the data were entered correctly.
- Retrieve missing data from participants' charts (for any variables recorded in the chart).
- Collect missing interview data from surviving participants (but this will not help among those who died or whose responses might have changed over time).
- Make a special effort to find participants who have been lost to follow-up to at least get a telephone interview with them.
- Obtain vital status, using the National Death Index or a company that helps find people.

1b. Some ways to reduce missing data in the next study are:
- Collect less data (and focus instead on the completeness and quality of more limited data).
- Check any paper forms on site immediately after collecting the data to be certain that all items are complete and accurate.
- Use interactive data entry with built-in checks for missing, out-of-range, and illogical values.
- Develop procedures for direct entry or abstraction of data into an electronic database, to decrease error associated with transfer of data from paper forms to the database.
- Review the database shortly after data entry, so that missing data can be collected before the participant leaves the hospital (or dies).
- Periodically tabulate the distributions of values for all items during the course of the study to identify missing values, out-of-range values, and potential errors.
- Hold periodic team meetings to review progress and emphasize the importance of complete data.

2. Other tasks for study start-up include:
- Developing and revising the data forms and database, as well as **testing the database** using dummy or mock data.
- Developing and **pretesting any interview scripts** or guides that will be used to screen participants.
- **Training and certifying the research assistants** or coordinators to carry out the study measurements and procedures for this study.
- **Mock study visits** to troubleshoot the flow of visit procedures and evaluate the length of study visits.

Chapter 19   Data Management

1a.

Subject ID	Kit Number	Admin Date	Admin Time	SzStopPre Hosp	SzStop PreHospTime	HospArr Time	HospArr SzAct	HospArr GCSV
189	A322	3/12/1994	17:39	0		17:48	1	
410	B536	12/1/1998	01:35	1	01:39	0.1:53	0	4

1b.

Field Name	Data Type	Description	Validation Rule
SubjectID	Integer	Unique subject identifier	
KitNumber	Text(4)	Four-character Investigational Pharmacy Code	
AdminDate	Date	Date study drug administered	
AdminTime	Time	Time study drug administered	
SzStopPreHosp	Yes/no	Did seizure stop during prehospital course?	
SzStopPreHospTime	Time	Time seizure stopped during prehospital course (blank if seizure did not stop)	
HospArrTime	Time	Hospital arrival time	
HospArrSzAct	Yes/no	Was there continued seizure activity on hospital arrival?	Check against SzStopPreHosp
HospArrGCSV	Integer	Verbal GCS on hospital arrival (blank if seizure continued)	Between 1 and 5

1c. Advantages of an on-screen form:
- No need for transcription from paper forms into the computer data tables
- Immediate feedback on invalid entries
- Programmed skip logic (if seizure stopped during prehospital course, computer form prompts for time seizure stopped; otherwise, this field is disabled and skipped)
- Can be made available via a Web browser at multiple sites simultaneously

  Disadvantages of an on-screen form:
- Hardware requirement—a computer workstation or tablet (or cell phone?)
- Some user training required

  Advantages of a paper form:
- Ease and speed of use
- Portability
- Ability to enter unanticipated information or unstructured data (notes in the margin, responses that were not otherwise considered, etc.)
- Hardware requirement—a pen
- User training received by all data entry personnel in elementary school

Disadvantages of a paper form:

- Requires subsequent transcription into the computer database
- No interactive feedback or automated skip logic
- Data viewing and entry limited to one person in one place

Although data entry via on-screen data collection forms has many advantages and we recommend it for most research studies, in this study it was impractical. Sometimes (increasingly rarely), the simplest, fastest, and most user-friendly way to capture data is still to use a pen and paper.

2. When coded with 0 for *no* or *absent* and 1 for *yes* or *present*, the average value of a dichotomous (yes/no) variable is interpretable as the proportion with the attribute. Of those randomized to lorazepam, 40.9% (27 of 66) were still seizing on hospital arrival; of those randomized to diazepam, 57.4% (39 of 68) were still seizing; and of those randomized to placebo, 78.9% (56 of 71) were still seizing.

Chapter 20   Writing a Proposal for Funding a Research Study

1. The three main sections for the Research Strategy section of an NIH grant proposal are Significance, Innovation, and Approach.
2. The four additional scored criteria for most NIH grants include Significance, Investigator(s), Innovation, and Approach. For NIH career development (K-series) grants, these criteria are: Candidate, Career Development Plan/Career Goals & Objectives, Research Plan, and Mentors.
3a. Some Specific Aims for this project could be:
- Determine the distribution and variability of multiple home blood pressure measurements by each of the devices.
- Evaluate the association between systolic blood pressure, diastolic blood pressure, and blood pressure variability and incident nonfatal and fatal stroke.
- Compare the strength of associations between mean blood pressure and stroke for each type of device.
3b. The Innovations section should highlight the new approaches used in the proposed research in contrast to the existing literature and other ongoing studies. These innovations may include:
- The use of innovative new measurements of blood pressure by a wearable device and mobile phone software.
- The use of web-based methods to conduct a study of blood pressure and cardiovascular outcomes.
- The large nationwide study population is innovative compared with studies based on volunteers visiting clinical sites.
- Other innovations may include advanced analytic methods in which you analyze repeated measurements of participant-uploaded data, automated digitally collected data, and/or electronic health records data that allow for complex trajectory analyses over time.
4. Other funding sources include foundations, medical societies, nonprofit organizations like the American Heart Association, other federal sources like the Patient-Centered Outcomes Research Institute (PCORI), investigator-initiated grants to industry, and intramural research support programs from your own institution.

Glossary

Terms that are *italicized* are defined elsewhere in the glossary. Citations indicate examples where studies are real and numbers approximately correct; others are illustrative.

A priori hypothesis. A term used to identify a hypothesis that is specified before data are analyzed—and preferably before the data were collected. For example, the investigators listed two *a prior* hypotheses in their grant proposal: First, that exposure to coal dust among men 45 to 64 years of age would be a risk factor for prostate cancer; and second, that among women whose husbands were 45 to 64 years of age, spousal exposure to coal dust would be a risk factor for endometrial cancer.

Absolute risk reduction. The amount by which a treatment reduces the *risk* of the outcome. It is defined as the risk in the untreated minus the risk in the treated; its reciprocal is the *number needed to treat*. (If the treatment increases risk, the risk reduction will be negative; it's easier in that situation to just switch the sign and call it the absolute risk increase. The reciprocal of an absolute risk increase is sometimes called the "*number needed to harm*.") For example, the Special Supplemental Food Program for Women, Infants, and Children (WIC) reduced the risk of low birth weight from 10% to 6%, a 4% absolute risk reduction. (Buescher PA, Larson LC, Nelson MD, Lenihan AJ. Prenatal WIC participation can reduce low birth weight and newborn medical costs: a cost-benefit analysis of WIC participation in North Carolina. J Acad Nutr Dietetics. 1993;93:163-166.)

Accessible population. The group of people to whom the investigator has access and who could be selected for and approached about participating in the study. For example, the accessible population for the study consisted of women with breast cancer who were treated at Longview Hospital from January 1, 2021, through June 30, 2024. See also *intended sample* and *target population*.

Accuracy. The degree to which a measurement corresponds to its true value; it is affected by (lack of) *bias* and by *precision*. For example, self-reported bodyweight is a less accurate measurement of actual bodyweight than one made with a calibrated electronic scale.

Active control trial (comparative efficacy trial). A clinical trial in which the *control* group receives an intervention that is known or believed to affect the outcome of interest. For example, investigators used an active control trial design to compare a new medication for joint pain with standard doses of nonsteroidal anti-inflammatory agents.

Adaptive clinical trial design. A clinical trial design that allows changes to the trial protocol based on *interim monitoring* and analyses of the results. For example, the adaptive trial design allowed for increasing the *sample size* and duration of recruitment if the intervention appeared to be efficacious in an interim analysis (but likely to need a larger sample size to have adequate power).

Adaptive randomization. A *randomization* technique aimed at ensuring balance of specified *covariates* among study groups. Randomization of each eligible participant is altered (adapted) based on the characteristics of participants who have already been enrolled. For example, in a study of a new treatment to prevent hospitalizations for asthma, adaptive randomization could be used to ensure that those with a history of requiring treatment with oral corticosteroids are more likely to be randomized to the study group that had a lower average risk of hospitalization at the time they were enrolled.

Adjustment. A general name for various statistical techniques used to account for the effects of one or more variables on an association between two other variables. For example, adjustment for maternal tobacco smoking reduced the magnitude of the association between maternal marijuana smoking and birth weight. See also *conditioning*.

Adverse events. Events that occur during a study (usually a clinical trial) that have an adverse effect on health or well-being. Adverse events are recorded in both the intervention and control groups and need not be associated with the intervention. For example, the most common adverse event during the study was upper respiratory symptoms.

Alpha. When designing a study, the preset maximum probability of committing a *type I error*, that is, rejecting the *null hypothesis* given that it is true. For example, by choosing an alpha of 0.05, the investigator set a maximum probability of 5% that her study would find a statistically significant association by chance alone between non-White race and the risk of colon cancer when there is not one in the target population. Also called the level of *statistical significance*.

Alternative hypothesis. The proposition, used in estimating *sample size*, that there is an association between the predictor and outcome variables in the population. For example, the study's alternative hypothesis was that teenagers who smoke cigarettes have a different likelihood of dropping out of school than those who do not smoke. See also *null hypothesis*.

Analytic study. A study that looks for *associations* between two or more variables. For example, the investigator did an analytic study of whether height was correlated with blood pressure in medical students. See also *descriptive study*.

Ancillary study. A study that adds one or more predictors or outcomes to another study that was designed originally without that measurement. For example, consider a randomized trial of the effect of a new medication for inflammatory bowel disease that had banked serum obtained at baseline from participants. An ancillary study might use those serum samples to test whether a *biomarker* predicts response to the medication.

Association. A quantifiable relation between two variables. For example, the study found an association between male sex and risk of cognitive impairment among 60- to 69-year-olds, with a risk ratio of 1.3.

As-treated analysis. An analysis of clinical trial data in which participants' outcomes are analyzed according to the treatment (intervention or control) they received, rather than the one to which they were assigned randomly. For example, consider a randomized trial that compared surgery (tympanostomy and drainage tube placement) with medical management (antibiotics) for recurrent otitis media in children. In an as-treated analysis of the study, participants assigned randomly to the medical management group who underwent surgery would be included in the surgical group, whereas those assigned randomly to the surgical group who did not undergo surgery would be included in the medical management group. See also *per-protocol analysis* and *intention-to-treat analysis*.

Bayesian analysis. An approach to data analysis, named for Reverend Thomas Bayes, that uses accumulated knowledge about the likelihood of the research hypothesis when making inferences from the study results. For example, in a Bayesian analysis that incorporated results from prior trials of a similar procedure, the investigators concluded that a new surgical treatment had a 95% chance of reducing 5-year mortality among patients with early-stage pancreatic cancer by 10% or more. See also *frequentist analysis*.

Bayesian trial. A trial that assumes a prior distribution for the efficacy of a treatment, which is then modified by the study results to generate a revised, *posterior distribution* of efficacy. A Bayesian trial may not have a fixed sample size; rather, it continues until there is sufficient likelihood that the treatment is efficacious, inefficacious, or neither. For example, assume a previous trial of a treatment showed a 30% reduction in the risk of cardiovascular (CV) outcomes, albeit with some uncertainty, for example, that there was a 10% chance that the treatment was not efficacious. If a subsequent Bayesian trial of the same treatment finds that CV risk is reduced by 25% after enough participants have been enrolled, that might lead to a *posterior probability* that the treatment has a 99% chance of reducing CV risk by at least 20% and a 90% chance that treatment reduces CV risk by at least 25%.

Before-after study (or trial) design. A study that compares an outcome before and after an intervention is applied (sometimes called a pre-post design). For example, investigators compared the rate of catheter-associated urinary tract infections in the intensive care unit before and after an intervention to reduce inappropriate catheter use.

Beneficence. A basic principle of research ethics that requires that the scientific knowledge to be gained from the study outweigh the inconvenience and risk experienced by research participants, and that risks be minimized. For example, asking participants to undergo very risky interventions, such as exposure to COVID-19 virus in vaccine challenge trials, may violate the ethical principle of beneficence.

Beta. When designing a study, the preset maximum probability of committing a *type II error*, that is, failing to reject the *null hypothesis* given that it is false. This measure is only meaningful in the context of an *effect size*. For example, because colon cancer is rare (about 20 cases per 100,000 middle-aged people each year), if an investigator specifies a beta of 0.20 and (a two-sided) *alpha* of 0.05, she would need about 25,000 participants per group in a trial to show that daily aspirin use (compared with placebo) halves the 10-year risk of colon cancer. Put another way, if aspirin had exactly that effect, a study of 25,000 per group would have a 20% chance of failing to reject the null hypothesis of no difference (at alpha = 0.05). See also *power*.

Between-groups design. A study design that compares the characteristics or outcomes of participants in two (or more) different groups. For example, the investigator used a between-groups design to compare in-hospital mortality rates among patients treated in intensive care units that had round-the-clock on-site intensivists with mortality rates among patients treated in units that used electronic monitoring of patients by intensivists from a central hub. See also *within-group design*.

Bias. A systematic error in a measurement, or in an estimated association, because of a shortcoming in a study's design, execution, or analysis. For example, because of a bias in the way participants remembered their exposure to toxic chemicals, patients with leukemia were more likely to report prior use of insecticides than were controls.

Biomarker. An objective, quantifiable characteristic of a biologic process. For example, serum CA-125 levels are often used as a biomarker during follow-up of women with ovarian cancer. . See also see *intermediate marker*.

Blinding. The process of ensuring that participants, treating clinicians, and/or investigators are unaware of the group (eg, intervention or control) to which participants are assigned, usually in the context of a randomized trial (also called masking, especially in ophthalmologic studies). For example, by using identical placebo pills and keeping the list of participant assignments off-site, both the participants and the investigators (including research assistants) were blinded to which participants were treated with the active medication.

Blocked randomization. A method of assigning participants to an intervention in blocks (groups) of a prespecified size (eg, four or six) to ensure that similar numbers of participants are assigned to the intervention and control groups. Often used in multicenter studies in which the investigators want the total numbers of intervention and control participants to be similar at each site. For example, patients within each clinic were randomly assigned to either the treatment or control groups in blocks of six, ensuring that the number of participants per group would differ by no more than three. See also *stratified blocked randomization*.

Bonferroni correction. A technique to reduce the likelihood of *type I errors* by dividing the overall *alpha* in a study by the number of hypotheses tested. For example, because the investigators were testing four different hypotheses, they used Bonferroni correction to reduce alpha for each hypothesis from 0.05 to 0.0125.

Bootstrapping. A method of estimating a parameter of interest by taking repeated random *samples* (with replacement) from a data set. Because each of these samples will have slightly different estimates of the parameter(s) of interest, bootstrapping can be used to create *confidence intervals* and other indicators of the variability of the estimates. For example, an investigator who used backward stepwise logistic regression to select variables for a *clinical prediction model* could employ that procedure multiple times using bootstrapping to estimate the 95% confidence interval for the sensitivity and specificity of the resulting rule.

Calibration.
1. The process of ensuring that an instrument gives a consistent reading; usually done by measuring a known standard and then adjusting (calibrating) the instrument accordingly. For example, the scale for neonates was calibrated monthly by weighing a 3-kg block of steel.
2. The extent to which predicted probabilities of an event match the observed probabilities. Calibration is often displayed visually using a graph in which predicted probabilities are on the *X*-axis and observed probabilities on the *Y*-axis. For example, the American College of Cardiology's pooled cohort equations are often used to estimate the 10-year risk of cardiovascular events to guide statin treatment decisions. However, these equations may not be well calibrated for more contemporary cohorts, overestimating the risk of future cardiovascular events.

Carryover effect. The residual influence of an *intervention*, if any, after it has been stopped. For example, because of carryover effects, bone density may not return to baseline levels for years after a course of bisphosphonate treatment.

Case. A participant who has, or who develops, the outcome of interest. For example, cases were defined as those diagnosed with malignant melanoma from 2018 to 2022 in San Diego County. See also *control*.

Case series. A (generally descriptive or hypothesis-generating) study of a series of people diagnosed with a specific disease, sometimes treated a particular way. For example, a case series of patients who underwent cataract surgery performed by physician assistants reported that all had satisfactory outcomes.

Case-cohort study. A research design in which participants who develop a disease (or other outcome) are selected as cases during follow-up of a larger *cohort* and then compared with a random *sample* of the overall cohort. For example, a case-cohort study enrolled a cohort of 2000 men with early prostate cancer and compared levels of androgens and vitamin D from samples obtained at baseline among those who died of prostate cancer during follow-up (the cases) with levels in a random sample of the entire cohort.

Case-control study. A research design in which cases who have or develop a disease (or other outcome) are compared with controls who do not. For example, a case-control study compared the average weekly consumption of nuts and seeds among cases of diverticulitis seen in an emergency room with consumption among controls who had other gastrointestinal diagnoses.

Case-crossover study. A type of *case-control study* in which each case serves as his own control, and the value of a time-dependent exposure in the period before the outcome occurred is compared with its value during one or more control periods. This design is susceptible to recall bias and is therefore most useful when an exposure can be ascertained objectively. For example, a case-crossover design was used to determine whether patients who presented to an emergency room with a pulmonary embolism were more likely to have flown on an airplane within the previous 48 hours than during the same times a week before.

Categorical variable. A variable that can have only one of several possible values. For example, the investigator transformed her measurements of reported educational level into a categorical variable with four values: less than high school, high school or some college, college degree only, or any postgraduate education. See also *continuous variable*, *dichotomous variable*, *nominal variable*, and *ordinal variable*.

Causal effect. For a dichotomous exposure and outcome at an individual level, a *counterfactual* comparison of whether an outcome would occur in someone with the exposure of interest compared with what would have happened had he not been exposed; best estimated in a randomized blinded trial. At a population level, it is the average of all the individual causal effects. For example, the investigator estimated the average causal effect of aspirin on the risk of developing melanoma by randomly assigning half of the participants to take aspirin—and half a matching placebo—and following them for 20 years with periodic skin exams. Casual effects can be defined in an analogous fashion for categorical and continuous variables.

Cause-effect. The concept that a predictor is responsible for producing an outcome—or increasing the likelihood of an outcome's occurrence. The purpose of many *observational studies* is to demonstrate cause-effect, though this is difficult to do unless the cause (eg, a treatment) is assigned randomly. For example, the investigator performed a *multivariable analysis* hoping to determine whether there was a cause-effect relation between drinking alcohol (the cause) and pancreatic cancer (the effect) while controlling for possible confounding variables. See also *causal effect*, *confounding*, and *effect-cause*.

Censoring. In *longitudinal* studies, the lack of complete information about the outcome in study participants who were lost to follow-up, stopped being at risk, or did not have the event of interest before the study ended. The time to an event or survival time is not known in censored participants, just that it is greater than their follow-up time. For example, in a study of risk factors for uterine cancer, participants were censored at the time of hysterectomy.

Certificate of confidentiality. A document issued by a federal agency that prohibits disclosure of individually identifiable data to anyone not associated with a research study without a participant's consent (including by subpoena or court order). For example, a certificate of confidentiality protected the investigators from being required to provide data to enforcement agencies from their study of amphetamine use.

Chi-squared test. A *statistical test* that compares two (or more) proportions to determine if they are significantly different from one another. For example, a study determined whether the risk of dementia was similar among people who exercised at least twice a week (vs. those who exercised less frequently) by comparing those risks statistically with a chi-squared test.

Classification and Regression Tree (CART). See *recursive partitioning*.

Clinic-based control. In the context of a *case-control study*, the selection of control patients from the same clinics (or practices) from which the cases were chosen. For example, the investigator used clinic-based controls in her study of whether running on pavement for at least 2 miles per week was associated with radiographic osteoarthritis of the knee.

Clinical data managers. The specialists who create data entry forms, manage and monitor the data collection process, and format and extract the data for analysis, usually for clinical trials preparatory to application for regulatory approval of a drug or device. For example, a clinical data manager might become a millionaire by blowing the whistle on detected research improprieties.

Clinical prediction model. An algorithm that combines several predictors, including the presence or absence of various signs and symptoms and the results of medical tests, to estimate the probability of a disease or outcome. For example, the investigators developed a clinical prediction model for the diagnosis of wrist fracture among postmenopausal women based on information about prior fractures, the characteristics of the fall (if any), and physical examination of the forearm.

Clinical trial. A research design in which participants receive one of (at least) two different *interventions*. Usually (and preferably), the interventions are assigned randomly, thus the term "randomized clinical trial." For example, the investigator performed a clinical trial to determine whether prophylactic treatment with penicillin reduced the risk of bacterial endocarditis among patients with abnormal heart valves who were undergoing dental procedures. See also *randomized blinded trial*.

Closed-ended question. A question that prompts the respondent to choose from among two or more prespecified response options. For example, the participant was not sure how to respond to the closed-ended question about religious preference because she was a Deist, which was not one of the listed options. See also *open-ended question*.

Close-out. The time in a study when participants make final visits or data collection activities end. For example, study close-out procedures specified that, after the last study visit, all participants should be sent the results of all lab tests completed during the study.

Cluster randomization. A technique in which groups of participants, known as clusters, are assigned randomly to different treatments, rather than having each participant assigned randomly as an individual. For example, in a study of the effects of noise reduction on recovery from cardiac surgery, the investigator used cluster randomization to assign intensive care units in 40 different hospitals to either a "postoperative quiet" intervention or a "usual care" control.

Cluster sampling. A sampling technique in which participants are selected in groups (clusters) rather than as individuals, most often used for convenience when sampling large populations. For example, an investigator interested in determining the prevalence of drug abuse used cluster sampling to enroll 300 patients. First, she identified potential participants by choosing 10 three-digit prefixes (eg, 285-, 336-) within an area code; then she used random-digit dialing to find 30 willing participants within each three-digit cluster.

Codebook. A list of the thematic and other codes developed during a qualitative research project. The codebook includes a definition of each code, as well as the conceptual relationships among codes, often depicted in a hierarchical or tree structure. For example, the codebook contained terms about physician-patient communication during clinical interactions, such as Com_Active, Com_Disengaged, and Com_Go WithTheFlow, each of which included a definition and examples to illustrate how each code should be applied.

Coding. See *thematic coding*.

Coefficient of variation (CV). A measure of the *precision* of a measurement, obtained by dividing the *mean* of a series of measurements performed on a single sample by the *standard deviation* of those measurements. Sometimes, the CV is obtained for values at the middle and the extremes of the measurement. For example, the lab determined that its coefficient of variation for serum estradiol levels was 10% in a sample from a perimenopausal woman (in whom the estradiol level was very low), but only 2% in a younger woman.

Cohort study. A *prospective cohort study* involves enrolling a group of participants (the cohort), performing some baseline measurements, and then following them forward in time to observe outcomes; a *retrospective cohort study* involves identifying a group of participants (the cohort) in whom the measurements have already been made, and in whom the follow-up has already occurred. Some cohort studies have both features. For example, an investigator did a cohort study of whether the results of an emotional intelligence test administered when soldiers enlisted in the U.S. Army were associated with the likelihood of developing posttraumatic stress disorder (PTSD), including PTSD diagnosed during military service before the study began as well as during a subsequent follow-up period.

Cointervention. In a clinical trial, an *intervention*—other than the one being studied—that occurs after randomization and that affects the likelihood of the outcome. Cointerventions that occur at different rates in the study groups can *bias* the outcome and make it difficult to ascribe causality to the intervention being studied. For example, a study comparing the effect of carotid artery stenting (vs. surgery) on subsequent strokes was hard to interpret because the participants in the stent group were also more likely to receive long-term anticoagulation.

Collider. See *conditioning on a shared effect.*

Common data models. A specification for structuring a data table or set of tables—often with a standard set of variable names, and standard units for continuous variables and standard value sets for categorical variables—so that data from different sources can be combined and analyzed. For example, systolic blood pressure (SBP) data collected from OMRON home monitor and a iHealth home monitor systems may have different variable names (sbp vs. sysbp) and date/time formats (date = "12/3/21 03:05:44" vs. dt = 03dec2021); these formats can be standardized into a common data model for blood pressure (eg, SBP, date= "12/03/2021") for easier computation across sources, but some information may be lost (eg, time of day).

Community advisory board. An approach in which community representatives from different disciplines are convened early in a study and provide ongoing input and feedback on many aspects of the research project. For example, a community advisory board for a new study investigating the social determinants of cardiovascular health in the Bangladeshi community will provide input on the measures to collect, methods for community engagement and recruitment, how to disseminate culturally relevant results to the community, and future research questions that may evolve from the current study.

Community engagement studio. A panel of community stakeholders who provide timely feedback for specific aspects of a research project. For example, an investigator studying interventions to improve breast cancer screening among Vietnamese American populations will benefit from input about the proposed research design and implementation from different members of the Vietnamese community in an engagement studio, including breast cancer patients and their caregivers, health care workers, and other local leaders.

Community outreach. A modest intensity and common strategy used to engage community members by providing them with information about the need and rationale for a proposed research study, often used to help in recruitment and retention. For example, investigators may do community outreach by giving educational talks about a new study that they are conducting about dementia prevention in older immigrant communities to raise awareness about the problem.

Community-based participatory research. A fundamental approach to community-engaged research in which the community stakeholders participate in all aspects of the research, with shared authority and governance between the academic and community partners. For example, the Asian American Network for Cancer Awareness, Research and Training project is a long-term, collaborative, community-based participatory research to promote cancer awareness and prevention among academic researchers and community partners in San Francisco.

Community-engaged research. A research orientation in which the project is designed to meet the needs of the community, with varying degrees of collaboration between academic investigators and community stakeholders. For example, for questions like how to improve breast cancer screening rates in communities that have low screening rates, a community-engaged research project would benefit from local knowledge and input.

Comparative efficacy trial. See *active control trial.*

Comparative study. In qualitative research, a study that aims to determine how study sites or participants are similar, as well as to identify important differences. For example, the investigator did a comparative study that looked at why a work-based program for weight management enrolled nearly half of those who were eligible at one site, but fewer than 10% of those eligible at another site. See also *descriptive study* and *exploratory study.*

Complex hypothesis. A *research hypothesis* that has more than one *predictor* or *outcome variable.* Complex hypotheses should be avoided, because they are difficult to test statistically. For example, the investigators reformulated their complex hypothesis ("That a new program in case management would affect length of stay and the likelihood of readmission") into two *simple hypotheses* ("That a new program in case management would affect length of stay" and also "That a new program in case management would affect the likelihood of readmission").

Composite outcome. Outcomes that are composed of multiple related events or measures; usually, the first occurrence of any of the events during the study is counted. For example, a composite outcome for cardiovascular disease might include death from a cardiovascular cause, as well as hospital admission for myocardial infarction, stroke, coronary revascularization, or heart failure.

Conceptual adequacy. The extent to which a measurement instrument appropriately and comprehensively reflects a concept or characteristic of interest. For example, an investigator tested the conceptual adequacy of a newly developed measure by assessing whether a small group of respondents understood its meaning in the way that it was intended.

Conceptual equivalence. The extent to which a measure of a characteristic or concept has a similar meaning across different populations or groups. For example, pretesting of a questionnaire measure of depression suggested potential problems with its conceptual equivalence in Mexican Americans, because respondents interpreted questions about "feeling blue" differently based on positive associations with the color blue.

Concordance. A measure of (exact) agreement between two (or more) observers about the occurrence of a phenomenon. For example, the concordance between radiologists A and B was 96% for the presence of a lobar pulmonary infiltrate, but only 76% for cardiomegaly. See also *kappa.*

Conditioning. The process of examining the associations between two or more other variables at fixed levels of a "conditioned-on" variable. (Conditioning can also refer to how a study's selection criteria were chosen; see the following entry.) *Specification, matching, stratification,* and *multivariable adjustment* are the most common ways of conditioning on a variable. For example, the investigator found no association between cocaine use and the risk of syphilis after conditioning on the number of sexual partners in the previous 6 months.

Conditioning on a shared effect. A source of *bias* in which an association (often an inverse one) is introduced between two variables, both of which cause an effect (thus the term "shared effect," also known as a *collider*), by conditioning on that effect. This bias can occur because of who was selected for the study or how the data were analyzed. For example, because of conditioning on a shared effect (total screen time), there is an inverse association between watching television and gaming among children who average at least 6 hours per day of screen time: Those who spend more time watching television spend less time playing videogames. But that would not mean that watching more television would reduce gaming time!

Confidence interval. A term that is often misunderstood, a confidence interval (CI) is best thought of as a measure of *precision*: The narrower a CI, the more precise the estimate. For example, for the same *risk ratio* of 3.2, a 95% CI of 2.9 to 3.5 indicates a much more precise estimate than a 95% CI of 1.5 to 6.8.

CIs are closely related to *statistical significance*. A 95% CI (approximately) includes the range of values that were not statistically significantly different (at a significance level of $1 - 95\% = 0.05$) from what was observed. For example, a risk ratio of 3.2 with a 95% CI of 0.9 to 11 would not be statistically significant at an alpha of 0.05, because the interval includes "no effect" (a risk ratio of 1.0).

CIs are often erroneously interpreted as direct statements about *posterior probability* (eg, that there is a 95% probability that the true value is contained within the 95% CI). This is incorrect because posterior probability depends on other information besides what was found in the study. CIs are also commonly misinterpreted as being bar-shaped (such that all values in the interval are equally likely), but they are actually bell-shaped (such that values near the ends of the interval are less likely). See also *alpha* and *P value*.

Conflicts of interest. A researcher's primary interests should be providing valid answers to important scientific questions and protecting the safety of participants. Conflicts of interest arise when researchers have other interests that conflict with those goals and might lead to *bias* in the research, impair its objectivity, or undermine public trust. For example, an investigator who serves on the scientific advisory board of a company that developed a new device to measure anxiety would have a conflict of interest if asked to review a manuscript about an alternative device.

Confounder. See *confounding*.

Confounding. An epidemiologic phenomenon in which the measured association between a predictor and an outcome variable differs from their causal effect because of another variable—called the confounder—that causes (or is in the causal pathway to) the predictor and the outcome. For example, part of the apparent association between pressure ulcers and in-hospital mortality is confounded by underlying health status, because patients with pressure ulcers have worse underlying health. See also *directed acyclic graph* (DAG) and *effect modification*.

Confounding by indication. A specific form of confounding in which one of the indications for a treatment is the confounder; usually occurs in observational studies of the association between a treatment and an outcome. For example, the reviewers of an observational study were concerned that the reported association between a new treatment for bipolar disorder and increased suicide risk might have occurred because patients with more severe underlying disease had been selectively treated with the new medication.

Confounding variable. See *confounding*.

Consecutive sample. A study *sample* in which the participants are chosen one after another until the *sample size* is achieved. Usually used to refer to the intended sample, it may also refer to the actual sample when performing medical records reviews, because informed consent may not be required. For example, the investigators performed consecutive sampling to review the charts of the first 100 patients with rheumatoid arthritis seen in the rheumatology clinic, beginning January 15, 2020.

Construct validity. A term that describes how well a measurement corresponds to the theoretical definitions of the trait (the "construct") that is being measured. For example, a measurement of social anxiety was thought to have construct validity, because there were substantial differences in its values among people whose friends described them as "fun-loving" and "extroverted" as compared with those who were described as "shy" and "unlikely to go to parties." See also *content validity* and *criterion-related validity*.

Contamination. The undesirable process by which some or most of the effects of an intervention also affect participants in the control group. For example, a study of the effects of whether teaching children to count backward improved their overall arithmetic skills was plagued by contamination, because the children in the intervention group couldn't resist teaching that skill to their friends in the control group. In this situation, a better design would have used *cluster randomization*.

Content validity. A term that describes how well a measurement represents several aspects of the phenomenon being studied. For example, a measurement of insomnia was thought to have content validity because it measured total amount of sleep, episodes of nighttime awakening, early morning awakening, energy on arising for the day, and daytime sleepiness. See also *construct validity* and *criterion-related validity*.

Continuous variable. A measurement that, in theory, can have an infinite number of possible values. In practice, the term is often used for numeric measurements that have "many" (some say 10 or more, others say 20 or more) possible values. For example, systolic blood pressure was measured as a continuous variable in mm Hg using a mercury sphygmomanometer. See also *categorical variable*, *dichotomous variable*, and *discrete variable*.

Control.

1. A participant who does not have the outcome of interest and is therefore a member of a comparison group to which those with the outcome (the cases) are compared. For example, for a study of risk factors for peptic ulcer disease, controls were selected from patients hospitalized during the study period with a nongastrointestinal diagnosis. See also *case*.
2. An inactive treatment (eg, a *placebo*) or comparison treatment (eg, usual care) received by participants in a clinical trial who did not receive the study intervention; in that context, control is also used to refer to a participant who received the alternative treatment. For example, the controls were given placebo tablets that looked identical to the active drug. See also *intervention*.
3. Used as a verb, attempting to prevent an undesired situation or event. For example, in an observational study to determine the causal effect of participation in after-school activities on the risk of suicide in teens, the investigator used logistic regression to control for possible confounders such as age, race/ethnicity, sex, and use of illicit drugs. See also *adjustment* and *conditioning*.

Controlled before-after study. A study design that measures outcomes in two groups of participants concurrently before and after an intervention. For example, in a controlled before-after study, the change in rate of injuries to children in automobile crashes before and after the introduction of child car seat laws was compared in states that instituted such laws and those that did not.

Convenience sample. A group of participants who were selected for a study because they were relatively easy to access. For example, the investigator used a convenience sample of patients from her clinic to serve as controls for her case-control study of risk factors for meningioma.

Coordinating center. The group of investigators and staff that has the organizational, communications, data management, and statistical expertise to ensure that all sites in a multicenter study meet recruitment goals, use the same study procedures, and produce comparable data that can be combined in the analysis of the results. For example, the coordinating center collected data from the four study sites to prepare for analyses.

Correlation coefficient. A statistical term that indicates the degree to which two continuous measurements are related linearly, such that a change in one measure is associated with a proportional change in the other. Often abbreviated as r. For example, height and weight were correlated in a sample of middle-aged women with $r = 0.7$.

Count variable. A variable that has a countable number of values that can be expressed as a positive integer. For example, the number of people living in a household is a count variable.

Counterfactual. Contrary or opposite to what actually happened. For example, if Violet was chronically exposed to hair dyes, her counterfactual would be not having that exposure. As applied to causal reasoning, it is an approach to estimating a *causal effect* by comparing outcomes of actual exposures with what they would have been under the opposite ("counterfactual") exposures. For example, a counterfactual approach to estimating the effect of poverty on violent crime in a city would project violent crime rates assuming there were no poor people in that city and then compare those rates with what they would be if everyone in that city were poor.

Covariate. A characteristic—other than the treatment in a clinical trial, the main predictor variable in an analytic study, or the outcome in any study—of study participants. Sometimes called a covariable. For example, in a cross-sectional study that looked at whether excessive exposure to cellphone screens was a predictor of self-reported insomnia, covariates included age and use of caffeine, alcohol, and sedative medications.

Cox model. Also called the Cox proportional hazards model. A multivariable statistical technique that measures the individual effects of one or more predictor variables on the rate (hazard) at which an outcome occurs, accounting for differing lengths of follow-up among participants. For example, using a Cox proportional hazards model, a study reported that men were about twice as likely as women, and Blacks about 3 times as likely as Whites, to develop strokes, adjusting for age, blood pressure, and diabetes, as well as length of follow-up. See also *logistic regression model*.

Credible interval. A way to summarize the *posterior distribution* of a treatment effect, based on the study results and a given *prior distribution*. Often, but not necessarily, the *highest posterior density interval*. For example, in a study of a weight loss drug, if the 95% credible interval is from –1.5 to –4.6 kg, there will be a probability of 0.95 that the effect of the drug lies between those two numbers.

Criterion-related validity. A term that describes how well a measurement correlates with other ways of measuring the same phenomenon. For example, a measurement of depression in adolescents was thought to have criterion-related validity, because it had a high correlation with scores on the Beck depression inventory. See also *construct validity* and *content validity*.

Crossover.
1. A term used to describe a participant, usually in a clinical trial, who starts out in one group (say, usual care) and switches to the other group (say, active treatment) during the study. Most commonly occurs when the active treatment involves a procedure. For example, 15% of participants with prostate cancer who were assigned initially to watchful waiting were crossovers who received radiation therapy or surgery during the trial.
2. More generally, any change from one exposure level to another over time. For example, in a *case-crossover study* of the risk factors for skateboard injuries in an emergency department, participants were asked whether they had watched skateboarding videos on the day they were injured as well as during the previous day to see if there had been a crossover in that exposure from one day to the next.

Crossover study. A research design in which all the participants from one treatment (or control) group are switched to the other group, usually at the midway point of the study. Sometimes, there is a *washout period* between the two phases. This design, which enables all participants to receive the active treatment, is only useful for conditions that return to baseline after treatment. For example, patients with attention-deficit hyperactivity disorder were involved in a crossover study comparing a new drug with a placebo for the treatment of symptoms.

Cross-sectional study. A research design in which participants are selected and measurements made at one point in time (or within a limited period), usually to estimate the *prevalence* of an exposure or a disease. For example, the prevalence of myopia was estimated in a cross-sectional study of 1200 college students in Berkeley, California.

Cumulative incidence. See *incidence*.

DAGs. See *directed acyclic graph*.

Data dictionary. A table of variable names with corresponding data types, formats, labels, allowed values, and descriptions. For example, the investigator consulted the data dictionary because she had forgotten that a "4" in the field named "education" was used to indicate "some college."

Data entry system. The on-screen forms used to enter study data, as well as the routines for importing data from sources such as electronic health records (EHRs) and measurement devices. For example, one component of a data entry system might be a web-based questionnaire that can be completed on a tablet computer.

Data management software. The system used to store, manage, and validate a study's data. For example, the study used Research Electronic Data Capture (REDCap), which was made available at no cost for data management by the investigator's institution.

Data table. A table of data in which rows represent *records* and columns represent *fields* or attributes. For example, each row in a table of participants would represent a different study participant; the columns would be unchanging attributes, like date of birth, of those participants.

Data use agreement. A contractual arrangement that governs the sharing of clinical data among institutions, including the information to be shared and the purpose of the agreement. Most institutions have templates that can be used, as well as rules that designate who can sign such agreements. For example, the data use agreement specified that no protected health information except age, sex, and race/ethnicity would be included in the data set, and that the data would be used as part of a collaborative research study called "Factors associated with nursing home placement among adults with cognitive dysfunction."

Database query. An instruction that uses the SQL (pronounced "sequel") language for selecting specific *records* from one or several tables and displaying *fields* from those records. A simple query takes the form SELECT (fields desired) FROM (table(s) that contains those fields) WHERE (the conditions that define the records you want). For example, SELECT LastName FROM Participants WHERE FirstName = "Freddie" would yield a list of last names for all study participants named Freddie—and no one else.

Deduction. An analytical approach in which examples are examined in a top-down fashion in light of a prespecified theory or hypothesis. For example, investigators used deduction to examine how clinic leadership implemented a new health care delivery policy, paying careful attention to the techniques used for change management and employee training. See also *induction*.

Deidentified data. Data that have been stripped of any information that might identify the study participant. This term has specific legal meaning in the Health Insurance and Portability and Accountability Act, referring to removal of 18 identifiers. Deidentified data derived from health care delivery may be used for research with fewer legal barriers than identified data. For example, the investigators obtained a data set with deidentified data from the local school system to study whether performance on a test of fine motor skills in kindergarteners affected subsequent reading comprehension among third graders.

Dependent variable. See *outcome variable*.

Descriptive study.
1. In quantitative research, a study that does not look for associations, test hypotheses, or make comparisons. For example, the investigator performed a descriptive study of the prevalence of obesity among preschool children. See also *analytic study*.
2. In qualitative research, a situation in which there is enough knowledge to focus on an area, but not yet enough for a comprehensive protocol, such as when an investigator wishes to adapt a research instrument or protocol to a new target population. For example, the investigator did a descriptive study that looked at why a work-based program for weight management that had worked at another site enrolled fewer than 10% of the anticipated number of participants. See also *comparative study* and *exploratory study*.

Diagnostic test study. A study that looks at how much, if at all, the results of a medical test affect the likelihood of a given diagnosis in a patient. For example, a diagnostic test study was designed to determine whether serum bicarbonate levels were useful in the diagnosis of sepsis among patients with fever.

Dichotomous variable. A variable that can have only one of two values, such as yes/no or alive/dead. For example, the examiner dichotomized systolic blood pressure into hypertensive ($\geq$140 mm Hg) or not. See also *categorical variable* and *continuous variable*.

Difference-in-differences. An analytic approach in which the differences in the change in an outcome variable are compared between the *intervention* and *control* groups, where change is usually measured as the difference between the variable's final and initial values. For example, to study the effect of ultraviolet (UV) disinfection of hospital rooms, investigators used a difference-in-differences analysis to estimate the effect of the UV intervention compared to a standard cleaning protocol on changes in the rates of hospital-acquired infections.

Differential misclassification bias. A general term for the situation in which a measurement varies systematically by the status of the participant, usually by whether the participant is a case or a control; it most commonly occurs with recalled exposures. For example, because cases of adult celiac disease were more likely to recall childhood exposures to wheat-containing products as children than their siblings who had grown up in the same household, the investigators suspected that there was *recall bias*, one type of differential misclassification bias. See also *nondifferential misclassification bias*.

Differential verification bias. A *bias* that occurs in studies of diagnostic tests when different *gold standards* (which do not always give the same answers) are applied to different participants, depending at least in part on the result of the test being studied. For example, in a study of prostate-specific antigen (PSA) screening for prostate cancer in men, those with high PSA levels received prostate biopsies, whereas those with normal PSA levels were followed clinically; this raised the concern that differential verification bias falsely increased the sensitivity, and decreased the specificity, of PSA screening in men with indolent prostate cancer.

Directed acyclic graph (DAG). A schematic representation of how investigators believe the variables in a study are related causally to one another. For example, a DAG connecting risk-taking behavior, injection drug use, human papillomavirus (HPV) infection, and cervical cancer might look like:

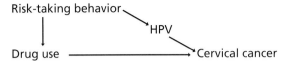

In this DAG, HPV infection causes cervical cancer and—because it also shares a common cause (risk-taking behavior) with injection drug use—it can confound an apparent association between injection drug use and cervical cancer.

Discrete variable. A type of variable that takes on only integer values, either positive or negative. Many continuous variables are treated as discrete variables. For example, change in weight in the past year was recorded to the nearest pound, a discrete variable. See also *count variable* and *continuous variable*.

Discrimination. The ability of a test or decision rule to separate the tested population into those in which the condition of interest is more likely or less likely. A test has perfect discrimination if it always provides more abnormal results in those who have the condition compared with those who do not. Discrimination can be measured as the area under a *receiver-operating characteristic curve*. For example, a phrenologist claimed to be able to estimate the likelihood of syphilis by feeling bumps on the heads of French nobility, but when subjected to rigorous evaluation, his discrimination was no better than chance alone, inferior to that of the court jester.

Dose-response. The phenomenon by which the greater the exposure (dose), the greater the magnitude or likelihood of the outcome (response). If an exposure is protective, then the greater the exposure, the lower the likelihood of the outcome. For example, a study reported a dose-response relation between sun exposure and numbers of melanocytic nevi (moles).

Double gold standard bias. See *differential verification bias*.

Double-cohort study. A study design in which participants are enrolled into one of two distinct cohorts, often by occupation within an industry, that have different levels of an exposure. For example, a double-cohort study was used to compare the risks of plantar fasciitis among cooks (who stand for most of their shifts) versus cashiers (who sit) in the fast food industry.

Dropout. A study participant in whom outcome status cannot be ascertained, often because of refused follow-up. Sometimes this also includes participants who drop out because they died during the study. For example, there were 17 dropouts in a study of insomnia: 8 because of refusal of continued participation, 6 because of death, and 3 because of the development of dementia. See also *censoring*.

Ecologic fallacy. The situation in which there is an association when populations are compared, but not when individuals are compared. For example, there is an association between the overall proportion of households in a country that have washing machines and life expectancy, but that is an ecologic fallacy, because having a washing machine does not increase life expectancy in individuals.

Effect modification. The condition in which the strength of the association between a predictor and an outcome is affected by a third variable (often called the effect modifier). For example, the investigators found that the effects of poverty on stroke risk differed by race, such that poverty had stronger association with stroke in Blacks than in Whites. Effect modification depends on the underlying *risk model*. See also *confounding* and *interaction*.

Effect size. In the context of *sample size* planning, a measure of how big a difference (or the size of an association) the investigator wishes to detect between the groups that will be compared. More generally, the actual size of that difference or association after the study is completed. For example, the investigators based their sample size estimates on an effect size of a 20 mg/dL difference in mean blood glucose levels in the two groups.

Effect-cause. The situation in which an outcome causes the predictor, rather than vice versa. For example, although a case-control study observed that exposure to inhaled bronchodilators was associated with an increased risk of interstitial lung disease, the most likely explanation was effect-cause, namely that patients with interstitial lung disease were more likely to have been treated (erroneously) with inhalers. See also *cause-effect*.

Effectiveness. Although there is no standard definition of this term, we use it to refer to a measure of how well an *intervention* works in actual practice, as opposed to how well it works in a randomized trial. For example, because clinical trials have found that tissue plasminogen activator (tPA) reduces morbidity and mortality from stroke in several trials performed in urban settings, the investigators studied its effectiveness in 25 rural emergency rooms. See also *efficacy*.

Efficacy. Although there is no standard definition of this term, we use it to refer to a measure of how well an *intervention* worked in a clinical trial, as opposed to how well it would work in actual practice. For example, a clinical trial reported that tissue plasminogen activator (tPA) had an efficacy of 25% in reducing morbidity and mortality among patients with acute stroke. See also *effectiveness*.

Entry criteria. See *selection criteria*.

Epidemiologist. A clinical researcher, broken down by age and sex. For example, one or more of the authors (but we are not saying which!).

Epidemiology. The science of determining the frequency and determinants of diseases or other health outcomes in populations. For example, a study investigated the epidemiology of handgun violence in inner cities.

Equipoise. Genuine uncertainty or controversy about which arm of a randomized trial is superior, such that the investigators believe that participants will not be harmed if they allow their care to be determined by randomization. For example, there was equipoise among experts and clinicians as to whether guided imagery would be efficacious for the treatment of asthma.

Equivalence study. A study whose purpose is to show that two (or more) treatments have similar outcomes; usually, one of the treatments is new and the other is known to be efficacious. For example, an equivalence study design was used to compare two antibiotics (new drug A with old drug B) for the treatment of urinary tract infections.

Ethnography. A method for documenting the social interactions and behaviors of a group, team, organization, or community to provide a rich, holistic analysis of culture. For example, an ethnographic study shadowed surgical residents to explore how they learned to make sense of different kinds of errors.

Exclusion criteria. A list of attributes that prevent a potential participant from being eligible for a study. For example, the exclusion criteria for the study were prior treatment with an antidepressant medication in the previous 2 years, current use of alpha-blockers or beta-blockers, and an inability to read English at the sixth-grade level. See also *inclusion criteria*.

Exempt from IRB review. Studies that do not require institutional review board (IRB) review, such as surveys and interviews, as well as secondary analyses of deidentified existing records and specimens. For example, the proposed survey of medical students to determine how well prepared they felt to conduct end-of-life discussions was determined to be exempt from IRB review.

Expedited IRB review. Certain studies that pose minimal risk to participants may undergo expedited review by a single member of an institutional review board (IRB) rather than the full committee. For example, a study that involved taking nasal swabs from participants to ascertain viral infections received expedited IRB review.

Experiment. See *clinical trial*.

Exploratory study. In qualitative research, a study of a topic about which little-to-nothing is known, such as an unusual clinical finding or the unexpected failure of an intervention. Research protocols are often revised extensively during such a study. For example, the investigator did an exploratory study that looked at why a new work-based program for weight management enrolled fewer than 10% of the anticipated number of participants. See also *comparative study* and *descriptive study*.

Exposure. A term used to indicate that a study participant has an attribute thought to be related to the outcome. For example, in a study to determine factors associated with gastrointestinal bleeding, exposure to aspirin was defined as taking an average of one or more aspirin tablets (of any size) a week during the previous 6-month period. See also *protective factor* and *risk factor*.

External validity. The degree to which the conclusions in a study apply to people and events outside the study. For example, the reviewers of a submitted manuscript—which had concluded that mortality from hemorrhagic strokes was greater in those under 50 years of age—raised concerns about its external validity because the *sample* came from a quaternary care center that specialized in the treatment of intracranial aneurysms. Synonymous with generalizability.

Fabrication. Making up data or results and recording or reporting them. For example, fabrication of data is less likely when an investigator works in a group where many people have access to, and oversight of, raw data and data analyses.

Face validity. A term that describes how well a measurement appears to measure a phenomenon, based on whether it seems reasonable. It is generally not a very reliable method for assessing validity. For example, a measurement of popularity in adolescents was regarded as having face validity, because it included items that the investigators thought would differentiate the popular students from those who were not. See also *construct validity*, *content validity*, and *criterion-related validity*.

Factorial trial. A clinical trial of two (or more) treatments (eg, A and B), sometimes with two unrelated outcomes, in which participants are assigned randomly to receive active treatment A and placebo B, active treatment B and placebo A, both active treatments A and B, or both placebos A and B. For example, the investigator performed a factorial trial to determine whether long-term use of beta-carotene and aspirin affected the risk of gastrointestinal cancer.

False-negative result.

1. A test result that is falsely negative in a patient who has the condition being tested for. For example, though the patient had biopsy-proven breast cancer, her mammogram was interpreted as being normal; this was a false-negative result.
2. A study result that fails to detect an effect in the *sample* (ie, the study result was not *statistically significant*) that is present in the population. For example, though subsequent studies showed that cigarette smoking increases the risk of stroke, an early case-control study failed to find a significant effect ($P = 0.23$); this was a false-negative result.

False-positive result.

1. A test result that is falsely positive in a patient without the condition being tested for. For example, in a patient who did not have breast cancer or develop it during 6 years of follow-up, the mammogram was interpreted as showing cancer; this was a false-positive result.
2. A study result that detects an effect in the *sample* (ie, the study result was *statistically significant*) that is not present in the population. For example, though subsequent studies showed that cigarette smoking does not increase the risk of Parkinson's disease, an early case-control study had a false-positive result suggesting that it did ($P = 0.03$).

Falsification. Manipulating research data, materials, equipment, or procedures or changing or omitting data or results, so that the research record misrepresents the actual findings. For example, a publication by Andrew Wakefield suggesting that a vaccine against measles, mumps, and rubella (MMR) was associated with an increased risk of autism in children was retracted because of falsification of data. (Rao TS, Andrade C. The MMR vaccine and autism: Sensation, refutation, retraction, and fraud. *Indian J Psychiatry*. 2011;53(2):95-96.)

Falsification tests. Tests of the robustness of research findings that specify hypotheses that, if falsified, would lead to concerns that the main research results were biased. For example, if a study found that use of nonsteroidal anti-inflammatory drugs (NSAIDs) increased the risk of asthma (perhaps because of their effects on prostaglandins), falsification tests could see whether NSAIDs also increased the risk of medical conditions not thought to be related to prostaglandins (like urinary tract infections) or whether the association with asthma showed (the expected) dose-response relation.

Field. An attribute recorded in a database column. For example, bodyweight would be a likely field in a study of blood pressure.

Financial conflicts of interest. Financial arrangements (such as patents, stock, stock options, and monetary payments) that might lead to *bias* in the design and conduct of a study, overinterpretation of positive results, or failure to publish negative results. For example, an investigator who holds stock options in a company that manufactures the study drug in a clinical trial for which he is the principal investigator has a financial conflict of interest.

Focus group. A group interview involving a small number of participants chosen for their ability to provide input on a research topic. For example, the investigator conducted focus groups in health care providers and patients to explore their feelings about the hospital's plan to ban sugar-sweetened beverages.

Foreign key. A *field* (column) in a database table that is the primary key for a different table, allowing the two tables to be linked together. For example, ParticipantID would be a foreign key in an Exams table that links back to a Participants table, and ProviderID could be a foreign key in a Participants table that links to a Provider table.

Framework analysis. A *deductive* analytical approach in which data from case studies are arranged in tabular format, with study concepts in rows and case studies in columns. For example, the investigators used framework analysis to compare how different clinics responded to a new policy initiative.

Frequentist analysis. A common approach to study design and data analysis in which the investigators determine the *P value* for the test statistic for the study results and compare it to *alpha*, the preset level of statistical significance. It is based on how frequently those results would occur under the *null hypothesis* of no effect; it does not use any prior information about the likelihood of the result (eg, from other studies of similar research questions). For example, in a frequentist analysis, the investigators concluded that a new surgical treatment reduced 5-year mortality among patients with early-stage pancreas cancer by 10% ($P = 0.003$). See also *Bayesian analysis*.

Generalizability. See *external validity*.

Ghost authors. People who make substantial contributions to a research manuscript, abstract or other publication, but are not listed as authors, often to obscure the role of a sponsor in designing, analyzing, or writing up the study. For example, an employee of the company that developed the study medication was a ghost author because she wrote the manuscript reporting the results of the pivotal clinical trial, but her name was not included in the author list.

Gold standard. An unambiguous method of determining whether a patient has a disease or outcome. For example, the gold standard for the diagnosis of hip fracture required confirmation by a board-certified radiologist who had reviewed all radiologic images of the involved hip.

Good clinical practice. Guidelines for high-quality research developed for clinical trials that test drugs requiring approval by the U.S. Food and Drug Administration (FDA) or other regulatory agencies; defined as "an international ethical and scientific quality standard for designing, conducting, recording, and reporting trials that involve the participation of human participants." For example, the investigator ensured that the study staff followed the requirements of good clinical practice by preparing a thorough operations manual and checking their work frequently.

Grounded theory. An *inductive* method of qualitative research that uses data to develop new theory. Coding leads to the discovery of themes, which are then analyzed and developed into new theoretical propositions. For example, based on what the investigators observed in an intensive care unit, grounded theory was used to develop a theoretical understanding of the experience of in-hospital death.

Guest author. People who are listed as authors on research manuscripts, abstracts, or other publications despite having made only trivial contributions. Also known as honorary authorship. For example, a well-known expert in the field was asked to be a guest author because the investigator thought a journal editor would be more likely to send the submitted manuscript for external review.

Hazard rate. An epidemiologic term that measures the instantaneous *rate* at which an outcome occurs in a population. For practical purposes, it is almost always estimated as the rate of an outcome. For example, the hazard rate for developing coronary artery disease among women ages 50 to 59 years was estimated as 0.008 per year.

Hazard ratio. The ratio of the *hazard rate* in those with an exposure divided by the hazard rate in those who are not exposed; it is almost always estimated from a proportional hazards (Cox) model. For example, the hazard ratio for developing coronary artery disease was 2.0 comparing men ages 50 to 59 years with women in the same age group.

Health Insurance Portability and Accountability Act (HIPAA). A U.S. law that protects individually identifiable information collected in the process of routine health care, billing, or administration (see *protected health information*). Under the rule, individuals must sign an authorization for the use of protected health information in a research project. For example, HIPAA authorization from patients was required before individually identifiable information from the electronic health record could be used to study the genetics of Alzheimer's disease.

Health literacy. The degree to which individuals have the capacity to access, process, and understand basic health information. For example, a consultant suggested replacing the word "axilla" with "armpit" and the word "emesis" with "vomiting" to make the study questionnaire comprehensible to those with average levels of health literacy.

Healthy user effect. *Confounding* that arises in an observational study because those who do a particular activity, or use a particular product, may be healthier than nonusers, so they appear to have better outcomes. For example, healthy people may be more likely to use a device that tracks physical activity than those who are less healthy. Because of the healthy user effect, an evaluation of outcomes might show reduced cardiovascular mortality among users of the device—even if the device itself had no effect.

Heterogeneity. A situation in which the *association* between a predictor and an outcome is not uniform, either among different studies or among different subgroups of participants. For example, there is substantial heterogeneity among studies that have looked at the effects of postmenopausal estrogen on mood and cognition, with some studies showing positive effects, some adverse effects, and some no effect. See also *homogeneity*.

Highest posterior density interval. The narrowest way to summarize a given proportion of the *posterior distribution* of a treatment effect. (For the technically inclined, the smallest distance on the X-axis of a posterior distribution curve that corresponds to the given proportion, thus identifying the interval with the highest probability density.) For example, in a study of weight loss drug, if the highest 95% posterior density interval is from -1.5 to -4.6 kg, there is a probability of 0.95 that the effect of the drug lies between those two numbers and no other 95% *credible interval* would be narrower.

Homogeneity. A situation in which the *association* between a predictor and outcome is uniform in different studies. For example, there is homogeneity among reasonably sized studies that have looked at the effects of smoking on lung cancer: All have found a substantially increased risk among smokers. See also *heterogeneity*.

Hospital-based controls. In the context of a *case-control study*, the selection of control patients from the same hospital(s) from which the cases were chosen. For example, in her study of whether eating processed meats was associated with upper gastrointestinal cancer, the investigator used hospital-based controls selected from patients who had nonmalignant gastrointestinal diseases and who were treated at the same hospital as the cases.

Hypothesis. A general term for a statement of belief about what the study will find. For example, the study hypothesis was that chronic use of antiepileptic medication was associated with an increased risk of oral cancer. See also *null hypothesis* and *research hypothesis*.

Immortal time bias. A *bias* that arises when survival (or other time-to-event data) is compared in a way that does not accurately reflect person-time at risk. So-named from studies whose design (usually the definition of exposed and unexposed, or treated and untreated groups) made it impossible for some participants to die during a period they nonetheless got credit for surviving. For example, consider a study that compared mortality after hospital discharge between elderly patients who did and did not fill their discharge prescriptions within 14 days. The time from discharge to filling a prescription (eg, at 10 days) was "immortal" because no one who filled a prescription at 10 days could have died in the previous 9 days. Thus, failing to account for immortal time bias would make filling prescriptions look more beneficial than it really was.

Incidence. The proportion of participants who develop an outcome during the follow-up period; sometimes called the incidence proportion or cumulative incidence. For example, the investigators found that pregnant vegetarians had a lower incidence of preterm delivery than pregnant women who ate meat.

Incidence rate. The *rate* at which a disease or outcome occurs in a group of participants previously free of that disorder. Usually calculated as the number of new cases of the outcome divided by the *person-time* at risk. For example, the incidence rate of myocardial infarction was 35 per 1000 person-years in middle-aged men, about twice the rate (17 per 1000 person-years) in middle-aged women.

Incidence-density sampling. Within a *nested case-control study*, a technique to sample controls when an important exposure changes with time; thus, the exposure needs to be measured at a similar time in both cases and controls. For example, a nested case-control study to determine whether use of antihistamine medications, which varies seasonally, increases the short-term risk of hip fractures (presumably because of an increased risk of falling) used incidence-density sampling of controls, such that a control's use of an antihistamine was measured during the same month that a hip fracture occurred in a case.

Inclusion criteria. A list of attributes required of the potential participants for a study. For example, the inclusion criteria for a study were people ages 18 to 65 years who lived in San Francisco and had no prior history of depression. See also *exclusion criteria.*

Incorporation bias. A *bias* that can occur when an index test is evaluated by comparing it with a *gold standard* that incorporates the result of the index test, thus making the index test look more useful than it really is. For example, a study of lipase levels as a test for pancreatitis was likely affected by incorporation bias because the investigators used a consensus definition of pancreatitis as the gold standard, one element of which was an abnormal lipase level.

Independent.

1. The condition in which two variables do not influence each other. For example, the investigators determined that dietary consumption of nuts and serum glucose levels were independent: there was no evidence in their study that nut consumption affected glucose levels, or vice versa.
2. An effect that one variable has on another variable that does not depend upon (ie, "is independent of") a third variable. For example, because she was concerned that maternal education and breastfeeding were associated with one another, the investigator adjusted for maternal education to estimate the independent effect of breastfeeding on language skills at age 2 years.

Independent variable. See *predictor variable.*

Index test. The test being evaluated in a study of a diagnostic or prognostic test. Results on the index test are compared with a *gold standard* for a diagnostic test or with what actually happened to the study participants for a prognostic test. For example, the index test of abdominal ultrasonography was compared with the gold standard of pathologic findings for the diagnosis of appendicitis.

Induction. An analytical approach in which theory or a hypothesis is derived in a bottom-up fashion from reviewing empirical evidence. For example, investigators observed hospitalized patients to develop a new theory of the experience of death. See also *deduction.*

Inference. The process of drawing conclusions based on observations in a *sample*. For example, because twice as many cases of bladder cancer as controls reported drinking well water ($P = 0.02$) in an analysis that adjusted for other known causes of bladder cancer (such as tobacco smoking and exposure to dyes), the investigators made the inference that consumption of well water doubles the risk of bladder cancer.

Informed consent. The process of telling potential research participants about the key elements of a research study, what their participation will involve, the potential risks and benefits of the study, alternatives to participating in the study, and obtaining their consent to participate in research. For example, the institutional review board required revision of the informed consent form for the study because it was confusing and failed to disclose important risks of the treatment.

Institutional review board (IRB). A committee (sometimes called an independent ethics committee, ethical review board, committee on human research, or research ethics board) that reviews research proposals to ensure that the research is ethically acceptable and that the welfare and rights of research participants are protected. The IRB has the authority to disapprove or require modifications of research proposals. For example, the university IRB refused to approve the study because it did not provide enough protections for participant privacy.

Instrument bias. *Bias* in a measurement because an instrument consistently over- or underestimates its true value. For example, because of instrument bias, measurement of the volume of air expired was underestimated consistently because of an air leak.

Instrument variability. Differences in repeated measurements because of variations in the instrument making the measurement. For example, bone density of the proximal femur may vary depending on the position of the hip, leading to instrument variability in the measurement.

Instrumental variable. A variable that is associated with the *predictor variable*, but not otherwise associated with the *outcome variable*. It therefore can be used to indirectly estimate the effect of the predictor on the outcome. For example, investigators found marked regional differences in the use of a new influenza vaccine, so they were able to use region of residence as an instrumental variable to study the effect of the influenza vaccine on mortality in older adults.

Intended sample. The group of participants the investigator intended to include in a study, as described in the study protocol. For example, the intended sample for the study consisted of women with breast cancer who were seen initially for treatment on a Monday or Thursday at Longview Hospital (the days that the investigator or her research staff were available) and who were within 6 weeks of their original diagnosis, during the period from January 1, 2021, through June 30, 2021. See also *accessible population* and *sample*.

Intention-to-treat analysis. In a randomized trial, the process of comparing participants based on the group to which they were assigned randomly, even if this is not the same as the treatment they received. This is the most rigorous form of analysis. For example, the investigators performed an intention-to-treat analysis to determine whether random assignment to receive 6 months of psychotherapy improved symptoms of anxiety compared with random assignment to a control group that received a pamphlet about stress reduction. See also *as-treated analysis* and *per-protocol analysis*.

Interaction. A concept long used synonymously with *effect modification*, but that now implies that the effect modifier is a cause of the outcome. For example, the investigators reported that there was an interaction among smoking, asbestos exposure, and lung cancer, such that asbestos caused a greater increase in the risk of lung cancer among smokers than among nonsmokers.

Interaction term. In a *multivariable analysis*, such as linear or logistic regression, an interaction term is used to estimate the "extra" effects on an outcome that result from the combination of the effects of two or more predictor variables, apart from their individual effects. Interaction terms, which are easiest to understand for *dichotomous* predictor variables (which have the values of 0 or 1), depend on the underlying model of risk. For example, under a multiplicative *risk model*, if male sex increases the risk of bladder cancer 2-fold and cigarette smoking increases the risk 5-fold, then men who smoke should have 10 times (2×5) the risk of women who do not. Including an interaction term (eg, male sex [value = 1] $\times$ smoking [value = 1] = 1) in the model could be used to determine the effects—either a greater or lesser than 10-fold increased risk—that result from the combination of male sex and smoking.

Intercoder reliability. The degree to which two (or more) individuals apply the same tags or codes to data. For example, the intercoder reliability was greater for the code "mentioned a helpful staff member" than for "described personal confusion."

Interim monitoring. Monitoring the data in a clinical trial intermittently as they are collected to determine if the study should be stopped early or the protocol altered to protect participant safety. For example, during a trial of three antiarrhythmic drugs (vs. placebo) to suppress ventricular ectopy in survivors of myocardial infarction, interim monitoring found that mortality in the intervention groups was much higher than in the placebo group—and the trial was stopped. (Echt DS, Liebson PR, Mitchell, LB, et al. Mortality and morbidity in patients receiving encainide, flecainide, or placebo—the cardiac arrhythmia suppression Trial. *N Engl J Med*. 1991;324:781-788, and The Cardiac Arrhythmia Suppression Trial II Investigators. Effect of the antiarrhythmic agent moricizine on survival after myocardial infarction. *N Engl J Med*. 1992;327:227-233.)

Intermediate marker. A measurement that is associated with a clinical outcome, but changes in the marker have not (yet) been demonstrated to change that outcome. For example, a study found that serum levels of S100B were an intermediate marker for depression, as levels were higher in women with depression than among controls. See also *mediator* and *surrogate marker*.

Internal consistency. The extent to which different items in a multi-item measure produce responses that correlate with each other. For example, a questionnaire would have high internal consistency if all of the questions that were designed to measure the same general construct produced similar scores.

Internal validation. Validation (most often of a *clinical prediction model*) on a sample of participants from the same *accessible population* as was used to derive the model. For example, developers of a clinical prediction model for neonatal sepsis developed the model using half of the cases from their nested case-control study and then performed internal validation in the other half of cases.

Internal validity. The degree to which a study's conclusions reflect what happened in the study. For example, the investigators used an automated sphygmomanometer to measure blood pressure on three occasions at baseline and again at the end of the study to bolster the internal validity of their conclusion that meditation was no more efficacious than reading poetry at reducing elevated systolic blood pressure. See also *external validity*.

Interpretation. In qualitative research, the empirical analysis of qualitative data that emphasizes a holistic understanding of social phenomena in their contextual richness. For example, when analysts interpret interviews, they use their judgment to identify key points and produce a narrative of the patient's experiences.

Interrupted time series design. A kind of *regression discontinuity* (and *opportunistic*) study design in which time is the running variable, such that the probability of treatment or exposure changes suddenly at one point in time. For example, investigators used an interrupted time series design to study the effect of recalibration of bilirubin testing instruments in Kaiser Permanente of Northern California hospitals and found an abrupt 60% drop in the use of phototherapy for neonatal jaundice following recalibration. (Kuzniewicz MW, Greene DN, Walsh EM, McCulloch CE, Newman TB. Association between laboratory calibration of a serum bilirubin assay, neonatal bilirubin levels, and phototherapy use. *JAMA Pediatr.* 2016;170(6):557-561.)

Intervention. In a randomized trial, the active treatment that participants receive. For example, in a randomized trial of psychotherapy for the treatment of anxiety, the intervention consisted of 6 months of weekly 1-hour sessions with a licensed psychologist that emphasized cognitive-behavioral approaches. See also *control* (second definition).

Justice. A basic principle of research ethics which requires that the benefits and burdens of research be distributed fairly. For example, carrying out clinical trials of new chemotherapy drugs only among people with insurance to pay for the tests required in the research may violate the ethical principle of justice if uninsured patients cannot get access to potential cutting-edge treatments.

Kappa. A statistical term that measures the degree to which two (or more) observers agree whether a phenomenon occurred, beyond that expected from the *marginals*. Varies from –1 (perfect disagreement) to 1 (perfect agreement). For example, the kappa comparing how well two pathologists agreed about the presence of cirrhosis in a sample of liver biopsy specimens was 0.55.

K-fold cross validation. A method of validating an estimate of a model's performance that may have been inflated by overfitting. For example, in a 10-fold cross validation, the sample would be divided into ten groups. Ten separate models would be derived, each time leaving out one of the tenths. Estimates of model performance are based on the predicted and observed values in the 10 different left-out groups.

Level of statistical significance. See *alpha*.

Likelihood ratio. A term used to describe the quantitative effects of a diagnostic test result on the likelihood that a patient has the disease (or outcome) being tested for. It is defined as the likelihood of that test result in a patient *with* the disease divided by the likelihood of that result in a patient *without* the disease (the mnemonic is WOWO: with over without). A likelihood ratio that is positive increases the likelihood of the disease; one that is negative reduces that likelihood. Tests with categorical (or continuous results) have likelihood ratios for each possible result. For example, for the diagnosis of iron deficiency anemia, the likelihood ratio is 52 for a serum ferritin level ≤15 µg/L, whereas the likelihood ratio is 0.08 for a serum ferritin level ≥100 µg/L. (Guyatt G, Oxman AD, Ali M, Willan A, Mcllroy W, Patterson C. Laboratory diagnosis of iron deficiency anemia. *J Gen Intern Med.* 1992;7(2):145-153.)

Likert scale. A set of answers (often five) to a question that provides a similarly spaced range of choices. For example, the potential answers to the question "How likely are you to return to this emergency room for care?" were placed on a Likert scale as follows: Very likely, Somewhat likely, Neither likely nor unlikely, Somewhat unlikely, Very unlikely.

Limited data set. Under the *Health Insurance and Portability and Accountability Act* (HIPAA), a data set that has been deidentified and stripped of all identifiers specified in HIPAA, with the exception of dates (eg, dates of service provided by a health system), age, and zip codes. A limited data set may be distributed for a particular approved use, as specified in a *data use agreement* signed by the proposed user. For example, to study the impact of the COVID-19 pandemic on health care utilization, a researcher might receive access to a limited data set from a health insurer.

Logistic regression model. A statistical technique used to estimate the effects (expressed as *odds ratios*) of one or more predictor variables on a dichotomous outcome variable, adjusting for the effects of other predictor and confounding variables. For example, in a logistic regression model, men were about twice as likely as women, and Blacks about 3 times as likely as Whites, to develop strokes, adjusting for age, blood pressure, and diabetes.

Longitudinal. A term used to describe studies or measurements that are done over time—in that sense, the opposite of *cross-sectional*. For example, a cohort study of the annual incidence of cataracts among people who started corticosteroid treatment would be longitudinal.

Marginals. A general term for the row and column totals of a table of dichotomous or categorical data. For example, looking at the marginals in a 2 × 2 table evaluating how well two pathologists agreed on the diagnosis of skin cancer showed that the first pathologist found cancer in 25% of specimens, compared with 18% for the second pathologist.

Masking. See *blinding.*

Matching. The process of selecting participants in one study group to be similar in certain attributes to another study group. For example, in a case-control study of the risk factors for brucellosis, controls were matched to cases by age (within 3 years), sex, and county of residence. As another example, in a cohort study of the effects of seat belt use on the risk of serious injury or death in automobile crashes, those who used seat belts were compared with other occupants of the same car who did not use seat belts, thus matching for attributes such as type of crash, time of day, and speed. See also *overmatching.*

Maturation effect. The tendency for people to learn and improve over time. Maturation can result in improvement after an intervention even if the intervention itself is not efficacious. For example, the accuracy of reading electrocardiograms improved in medical students who did or did not receive online training because of the maturation effect.

Mean. The average value of a *continuous variable* in a sample or population; calculated as the sum of all the values of that variable divided by the number of participants. For example, the mean serum cholesterol level in a sample of middle-aged women was 187 mg/dL. See also *median* and *standard deviation.*

Measurement error. The situation in which the *precision* or *accuracy* (or both) of a measurement is less than perfect. There is at least some measurement error for most variables in a study (except possibly vital status). For example, to reduce measurement error, the investigator in a study of neonatal hearing used a 2-kg stainless steel weight to calibrate the scale weekly.

Median. The value of a variable that divides a sample or population into two halves of (approximately) equal size; equivalent to the 50th percentile. Often used when a continuous variable has a few very high (or very low) values that would overly influence the mean value. For example, the median annual income in a sample of 548 physicians was $275,000. See also *mean* and *standard deviation.*

Mediation. The process by which a treatment or exposure causes an outcome as a result of changing another cause of the outcome; that second, intermediate, cause is called the *mediator*. For example, investigators wished to study whether improvements in birth weight that occurred as a result of providing an income supplement were mediated by improved maternal nutrition.

Mediator. A variable that is caused by the *predictor* of interest and that causes the *outcome*; it accounts for at least part of how the predictor causes the outcome. For example, in studying the overall causal effect of obesity on the risk of stroke, the investigators did not adjust for diabetes, because they believed that diabetes was a mediator, in that obesity increases the risk of diabetes which in turn increases the risk of stroke.

Memo. A short essay that identifies emerging topics of interest and guides ongoing data collection in a qualitative study. For example, the investigator prepared a memo that discussed why they changed the protocol to begin asking all participants about prior histories of seeing a loved one die in a hospital.

Memorandum of Understanding (MOU). A document that specifies the scope of work, including expected products and tasks ("deliverables") and a general timeline, that is created and signed by both parties. For example, the investigator's academic institution and the community organization with which they were working prepared and signed an MOU to provide structure for the collaboration, including relevant milestones and payments for each stage of the project.

Mendelian randomization. A technique for enhancing causal inference by taking advantage of the random inheritance of genes that cause or affect susceptibility to a risk factor or treatment. For example, the likelihood of a causal relationship between maternal use of acetaminophen and asthma in children was enhanced by the observation that the association was significantly greater in mothers with the T1 genotype of glutathione S-transferase, an enzyme involved in the detoxification of an acetaminophen metabolite. (Shaheen SO, Newson RB, Ring SM, Rose-Zerilli MJ, Holloway JW, Henderson AJ. Prenatal and infant acetaminophen exposure, antioxidant gene polymorphisms, and childhood asthma. *J Allergy Clin Immunol.* 2010;126(6):1141-8.e7.)

Meta-analysis. A process for combining the results of several studies with similar predictor and outcome variables into a single summary result. For example, a meta-analysis of nine studies found that high birth weight was associated with about a 20% greater risk of developing asthma.

Meta-regression. A statistical technique for analyzing how selected characteristics of a study affect its results. For example, a meta-regression analyzed 30 randomized trials of statin medications to see whether older age predicts lower efficacy, while adjusting for other study characteristics like the proportion of participants who were male and rates of concurrent aspirin use.

Minimal clinically important difference. The smallest difference (or change) in an instrument score that is meaningful, based on how well it corresponds to a clinical outcome or metric; often determined before the study and used in estimating the *sample size*. For example, an insomnia treatment program resulted in a small increase in sleep quality score that was below the threshold for a minimal clinically important difference.

Minimum necessary data. The smallest number of data elements necessary to complete a specific approved research project, as defined under the *Health Insurance and Portability and Accountability Act*. For example, an institutional review board may approve use of previously collected electronic health record data without the consent of patients, but only the minimum necessary data should be extracted and used for the project.

Misclassification. A measurement error for a *categorical* (or *dichotomous*) *variable* in which participants with one value of the variable are counted (misclassified) as having another value. For example, investigators were worried that because medical records were incomplete, some participants who really had fallen during their hospitalization were misclassified as not having had a fall. See also *differential misclassification bias* and *nondifferential misclassification bias*.

Missing data. Data that were not collected during a study, whether at baseline or during follow-up. Usually refers to data that were collected on some—but not all—participants, rather than data that were not collected at all. For example, the investigator was concerned that the relatively large proportion (34%) of participants who had missing data on alcohol use may have biased her study of the risk factors for falls.

Multiple cohort study. A cohort study that enrolls two or more distinct groups of participants (the *cohorts*) and then compares their outcomes. Often used in studies of occupational exposures, in which the cohorts being compared are either exposed to a potential risk factor or not. For example, the investigators performed a multiple cohort study of whether exposure to cosmic rays during airplane flights is associated with an increased risk of hematologic malignancies; the investigators studied four cohorts: pilots and flight attendants (who would be exposed to cosmic rays) and ticket agents and gate attendants (who would not). See also *double-cohort study*.

Multiple hypothesis testing. The situation in which an investigator studies more than one—and usually many more than one—hypotheses in a study, thereby increasing the risk of making a *type I error* unless the level of *statistical significance* is adjusted. For example, although the investigator reported a statistically significant ($P = 0.03$) association between use of supplemental vitamin C and cognitive decline, her results were criticized because she did not account for the effect of multiple hypothesis testing—the study had looked at more than 30 nutritional supplements. See also *Bonferroni correction*.

Multivariable analysis. A general term for the statistical techniques used to adjust for the effects of one or more potential *confounding* variables on the association between a predictor and outcome. For example, using multivariable analysis, the study found that consumption of two or more alcoholic drinks a day was associated with an increased risk of cognitive decline, adjusting for age, sex, education, baseline cognitive function, and smoking.

Natural experiment. A type of *opportunistic study design* in which exposure to a treatment or risk factor is likely to be random, or at least unassociated with determinants of outcome, thereby facilitating estimates of causal effects. For example, the opening of American Indian–owned casinos has been used as a natural experiment to study the effects of additional income on a wide variety of outcomes. (The effects are generally favorable!)

Negative predictive value. See *predictive value, negative.*

Nested case-control study. A study in which the *cases* and *controls* are selected from a (larger) defined *cohort* or from among previously enrolled participants in a cohort study. This design is usually used when it is too expensive to make certain measurements in all the participants in the cohort. For example, the investigators planned a nested case-control study to determine whether relative cytokine levels on newborn screening blood spots were associated with the development of cerebral palsy; levels would be measured in samples from all infants with cerebral palsy and a random sample of 1% of controls.

Nested double (or multiple) cohort study. A study in which separate *cohorts* of exposed and unexposed (or differentially exposed) participants are sampled from a larger cohort. For rare exposures, nested multiple cohort studies are more efficient than following the entire cohort. For example, within a large health care system, outcomes of those who had hip replacements with metal-on-polyethylene implants could be compared with those who received ceramic-on-polyethylene implants.

No-cost extension. The period after a study's funding has ended during which surplus budgeted funds can be spent to complete or extend the work described in the study award. For example, a 6-month no-cost extension was approved by the National Institutes of Health (NIH) so that the investigators could complete their data analyses and manuscript preparation.

N-of-1 design. A *crossover trial* that enrolls only one person; also called single patient trials. A patient is randomly assigned for a set period of time to a blinded treatment or to placebo (or a different active treatment), then crossed over to the alternative intervention for the same duration of time. For example, a clinician and patient used an N-of-1 trial to determine if trigger point injections with lidocaine were more effective than saline for pain relief.

Nominal variable. A *categorical variable* for which there is no intrinsic order. For example, religious affiliation (Buddhist, Christian, Hindu, Jewish, Moslem, other, none) was coded as a nominal variable. See also *ordinal variable.*

Nondifferential misclassification bias. A type of *bias* that is not affected by whether a participant was a case or control (or occasionally, by whether a participant was exposed or not exposed). Nondifferential misclassification tends to make associations harder to find because it reduces apparent differences between groups. For example, although recall of past exposure to antibiotics was imperfect in both cases and controls, the bias appeared to be nondifferential, in that a review of medical records indicated that both groups had similar inaccuracies. See also *differential misclassification bias.*

Noninferiority margin. A prespecified difference in *efficacy* between two treatments, often called delta (Δ), that is small enough to allow an investigator to conclude that the new treatment is not significantly inferior to a standard treatment. For example, in a noninferiority trial of a new anticoagulant (compared with warfarin) to prevent strokes among patients with atrial fibrillation, the noninferiority margin was set at a difference in stroke rates of 1%.

Noninferiority trial. A clinical trial comparing a new treatment that has some advantages over an established treatment (eg, the new treatment is safer, less expensive, or easier to use), with the goal of demonstrating that the efficacy of the new treatment is not inferior to the established treatment. For example, a noninferiority trial of a new pain medication that does not cause drowsiness demonstrated that the new medication was not inferior to oxycodone for relief of postoperative pain.

Nonprobability sample. A *sample* in which the likelihood that a member of the accessible population is included cannot be defined. This applies to many if not most samples in clinical research. For example, the investigators enrolled a *convenience sample* of patients seen in their orthopedics practice whenever some-one was available to interview them, usually on days they were less busy; this is one kind of nonprobability sample. See also *probability sampling*.

Nonresponse bias. A type of *bias* in which failure to respond (eg, to a questionnaire) affects the results of a study. For example, the investigators were concerned about nonresponse bias in their study of the effects of illicit drug use on the risk of developing renal failure because the question about it was often left unanswered.

Normalization. A process for ensuring that a *relational database* adheres to certain rules that facilitate queries, enforce referential integrity, and reduce redundancy and internal inconsistencies. Normalization often entails converting repetitive columns in a wide table into separate rows in a narrow table. For exam-ple, consider an unnormalized database consisting of a Participant table that has *fields* (columns) for many laboratory tests, such as labID1, labresult1, labdate1, labID2, labresult2, labdate2, etc. Normalization would entail creating a new LabResult table with fields for the *primary key*, labID, labresult, and labdate, as well as for the *foreign key* that links back to participant-specific data (see Figure 19.3).

Null hypothesis. The form of the *research hypothesis* that specifies there is no difference in the groups being compared. For example, the null hypothesis stated that the risk of developing claudication would be the same in participants with normal lipid levels who were treated with a statin as in those treated with placebo.

Number needed to harm. The absolute number of people who need to receive a treatment in order to cause the occurrence of one outcome. Calculated as the reciprocal of the *risk difference*. For example, if the risk difference for venous thromboembolic events from use of estrogen is 0.3%, the number needed to harm is 333. See also *number needed to treat*.

Number needed to treat. The absolute number of people who need to receive a treatment in order to prevent the occurrence of one outcome. Calculated as the reciprocal of the *absolute risk reduction*. For example, when evaluating the benefits of the Special Supplemental Food Program for Women, Infants, and Children (WIC), the number needed to treat is about 25 pregnant women to prevent one low birth weight infant.

Numeric variable. A variable that can be quantified by a number. For example, body mass index (BMI) expressed in kg/m^2 is a numeric variable.

Observational study. A general term for a research design in which the investigators observe participants without any interventions; this term excludes randomized trials. For example, the examiners performed an observational study to determine the risk factors for melanoma.

Observer bias. The situation in which an investigator (or research assistant) makes a nonobjective assessment that is affected by her knowledge of one or more of the participant's attributes, such as whether the participant is a case or control, or was exposed or not exposed to a particular risk factor. For example, observer bias was apparently responsible for the finding that, based on an interview, Hispanic teenagers were more likely to be characterized as having issues with anger management than Asians, because a self-administered survey and a review of school records found no differences between the two groups.

Observer variability. Differences in repeated measurements of variable because of variations in the observer making the measurement. For example, examiners recording a participant's waist circumference may place the measuring tape at different levels of the abdomen, thereby causing observer variability in its measurement.

Odds. The *risk* of a disease (or other outcome) divided by (1 – risk). For example, if the lifetime risk of breast cancer among high-risk women is 20%, then the lifetime odds of developing breast cancer are 0.25 (0.20 ÷ 0.80). Risk and odds are similar for rare diseases (those that develop in less than about 10% of persons).

Odds ratio. The ratio of the odds of a disease (or other outcome) in those exposed to a risk factor divided by the odds of that disease in those not exposed. Also, the odds of an exposure in those with a disease (eg, among cases in a case-control study) divided by the odds of that exposure in those without that dis-ease (eg, among controls). The *risk ratio* and the odds ratio are similar when a disease is rare in both the exposed and the unexposed, because the odds and the risks of the disease are similar. For example, in a case-control study of end-stage renal disease (ESRD), which occurs in about 0.04% of the U.S. population per year, the odds ratio for non–insulin-dependent diabetes was 7, meaning that those with non–insulin-dependent diabetes were about 7 times as likely to develop ESRD as those without diabetes. (Perneger TV, Brancati FL, Whelton PK, Klag MJ. End-stage renal disease attributable to diabetes mellitus. *Ann Intern Med.* 1994;121:912-918.)

One-sample *t* test. A *statistical test* used to compare the mean value of a variable in a sample to a fixed constant. The most common type of one-sample *t* test is a *paired* t *test*, in which the sample mean for the difference between paired measurements (eg, on the same participant at different points in time) is compared with zero. For example, the investigators found that men gained a mean (± SD) of 4 ± 3 kg in weight during their residencies ($P = 0.03$, by one-sample *t* test). See also *two-sample* t *test*.

One-sided hypothesis. An *alternative hypothesis* in which the investigator is interested in evaluating the possibility of committing a *type I error* in only one of the two possible directions (eg, that a treatment causes either a greater risk or a lesser risk of the outcome, but not both). For example, the investigator tested the one-sided hypothesis that smoking was associated with an increased risk of dementia. See also *two-sided hypothesis.*

One-to-many. A relationship between "one" participant (or attribute) in a database that also has "many" measurements related to that participant (or attribute). For example, consider a study that includes data about serial measures of bodyweight in participants, each of whom has a primary care provider and a city of residence. Participant could be on the "one" side and bodyweight on the "many" side; city could be on the "one" side and participant (and provider) could be on the "many" side; and provider could be on the "one" side and participant could be on the "many" side. See also *relational database.*

Open-ended question. A question that is designed to elicit a free-form or open-text response. For example, the investigator asked an open-ended question ("What do you think is the greatest health threat facing our community?") to allow participants to answer in their own words. See also *closed-ended question.*

Operations manual. An expansion of the study protocol that generally includes the *protocol*, information on study organization and policies, and a detailed version of the methods section. For example, the operations manual specified that measurement of blood pressure should be done after the participant had been sitting quietly for 5 minutes.

Opportunistic study design. A term for a study design that arises in response to a particular opportunity. For example, the sharp distinction between what happens to drivers who have blood alcohol levels above or below the legal limit of 0.08% in Washington State led to an opportunistic study design (namely, a *regression discontinuity* design) to study the effect of punishment for drunk driving. The investigators compared the risk of repeat drunk driving offenses among drivers whose blood alcohol levels were just below—or at or just above—that legal limit. (Hansen B. Punishment and deterrence: evidence from drunk driving. *Am Econ Rev.* 2015;105(4):1581-1617.)

Optimistic prior distribution. A *prior distribution* in which a treatment is thought to be efficacious, usually within a narrow range, because several pertinent studies of the research question have been done. For example, the investigators studying the *efficacy* of a new drug that resembles metformin used an optimistic prior distribution; it was bell-shaped and centered on a 30% reduction in blood glucose levels, with most of the distribution between 20% and 40%.

Ordinal variable. A *categorical variable* whose values have a logical order. For example, patient satisfaction with their overall care was measured as an ordinal variable on a 5-point scale from very poor to very good. See also *nominal variable.*

Outcome. A general term for the endpoint(s) of a study, such as death or the occurrence of a disease. For example, in a study of whether radiosurgery was beneficial for patients with solitary brain metastasis, participants were followed for the outcomes of death or placement in a skilled nursing facility.

Outcome variable. The formal definition of the outcome for each participant. For example, in a study of the effects of different types of exercise on bodyweight and body composition, the outcome variables were defined as the change in weight in kg from baseline to the final measurement after 1 year, and the change in waist circumference in cm during that same period.

Overdiagnosis. Diagnosis of a disease that would never have affected the patient if it had not been diagnosed. For example, one risk of prostate cancer screening is overdiagnosis; this risk increases with the age of the patient.

Overfitting. A problem that arises when investigators select the variables or cutoff points for a *multi-variable adjustment* model based partly on chance variation in the sample, leading to overly optimistic estimates of model performance. For example, reviewers suspected overfitting when the authors reported excellent performance of a model to predict recurrent vertebral fractures that was based on 4 of the 25 measured predictors and only 20 outcomes.

Overmatching. The situation in which matching beyond that necessary to control for *confounding* reduces the investigator's ability to determine whether a risk factor is associated with an outcome because the controls have become too similar to the cases. For example, in a study of risk factors for endocarditis among injection drug users, having cases suggest acquaintances who also injected drugs would likely lead to overmatching, because the cases and controls would likely use similar injection techniques and have similar sources of drugs.

***P* value.** The probability of finding an effect (more precisely, a value of the test statistic) as large or larger than that found in the study by chance alone if there is no effect in the population from which the sample was drawn (ie, the *null hypothesis* is correct). For example, if the null hypothesis is that drinking coffee is not associated with the risk of myocardial infarction, and the study found that the relative risk of myocardial infarction among coffee drinkers compared with nondrinkers was 2.0 with a *P* value of 0.10, there was a 10% probability of finding a relative risk of 2.0 or larger in the study if there was no association between coffee drinking and myocardial infarction in the population.

Paired measurements. Measurements closely linked with one another in some way, such as those done on different sides of the same person, different members of a twin pair, or (most commonly) the same participant at two different times, such as before and after an intervention. For example, in a study of the effect of an exercise program on glucose control among patients with type II diabetes, paired measurements of glycohemoglobin levels were made at baseline and again after 3 months of exercise.

Pairwise matching. Matching of one *control* to one *case* (or, less commonly, one exposed to one unexposed person) based on similar or identical values of the matching variable. It is used to control confounding by that variable. For example, in a case-control study of exposure to persistent organic pollutants as a risk factor for preeclampsia, each woman (case) with preeclampsia was matched to a woman (control) of the same age (within 2 years) and prepregnancy body mass index (within 3 kg/m^2) who did not develop preeclampsia.

Partial verification bias. (Also called verification bias, workup bias, or referral bias.) A *bias* in the assessment of the *accuracy* of a test that occurs when participants selectively undergo disease verification by *gold standard* testing based partly on the results of the study test itself, and only those who had the gold standard are included. For example, if a study of the accuracy of chest percussion to diagnose pneumonia included only patients who had a chest x-ray, and if those with dullness to percussion were more likely to get an x-ray, the sensitivity of percussion would be falsely increased, and specificity falsely decreased, because of partial verification bias.

Participant. Someone who takes part in a research study. The term "participant" is preferred over "subject" because it emphasizes that someone enrolled in a study is an active participant in advancing science, not merely a subject being experimented upon. For example, in a study of a new drug for treatment of insomnia, the participants are the (often sleep-deprived) people who are eligible for, and enroll in, the study.

Participant bias. See *recall bias.*

Participant identification number. A *field*, usually the leftmost column in the table of participants, that identifies each participant in a study database. For example, an investigator for a study that anticipated having about 250 participants used participant identification numbers that started at 101; all of them would be three digits long.

Participant variability. Differences in a repeated measurement because of variation in a participant. For example, transient moods and sleep adequacy affect cognitive performance, leading to participant variability in its measurement.

Peer review. Review of a protocol, proposal, or manuscript by peers of the investigator who prepared these documents. For example, proposals submitted for funding to the National Institutes of Health (NIH) undergo a peer review process in which scientists in the same field score the protocol using well-defined criteria. Similarly, manuscripts submitted to medical journals are peer reviewed by scientists who make suggestions about how to improve it and help the journal editors decide whether it should be published.

Per-protocol analysis. In a clinical trial, an analysis approach in which data from participants are only included if the participants adhered to the study protocol, which is typically defined as taking or using the study intervention as instructed. For example, in a randomized trial of surgery compared with physical therapy for treatment of severe osteoarthritis of the knee, a per-protocol analysis would include data only from participants in the surgery group who underwent surgery and from participants in the physical therapy group who were adherent to the physical therapy regimen. See also *intention-to-treat analysis* and *as-treated analysis*.

Person-time. The sum of the amounts of time each of the participants in a study or population is at risk, used as the denominator for calculation of *incidence rates*. It equals the number of participants who are at risk of an outcome multiplied by their average time at risk. For example, the total person-time of follow-up among the 1000 participants who had an average of 2.5 years at risk was a total of 2500 person-years, although 5% of the participants were followed for 1 month or less.

Phase I trial. An early phase, generally unblinded, uncontrolled trial of escalating doses of a new treatment in a small number of human volunteers to test its safety. For example, a phase I trial of a new drug for treatment of menopausal hot flashes would generally include a small number of volunteers (with or without hot flashes) who receive escalating doses of the drug to determine its effects on blood counts, liver and renal function, physical findings, symptoms, and other unexpected adverse events.

Phase II trial. A small randomized (and preferably blinded) trial to test the effect of a range of doses of a new treatment on side effects as well as on *biomarkers* or clinical outcomes. For example, a phase II trial of a new drug for treatment of hot flashes that has been shown to be safe in a *phase I trial* might enroll a small number of postmenopausal women with hot flashes, randomly assign them to two or three different doses of the new medication or placebo, and then follow them to determine the frequency of hot flashes, as well as side effects.

Phase III (pivotal) trial. A randomized (and preferably blinded) trial that is large enough to test the efficacy and safety of a new treatment. For example, if the optimal dose of a new treatment for hot flashes has been established in a *phase II trial* and the new treatment was acceptably safe, the next step would be a large phase III trial in which postmenopausal women with hot flashes are randomly assigned to the new treatment or placebo and followed for the occurrence of hot flashes and adverse effects.

Phase IV trial. A large study, which may or may not be a randomized trial, conducted after a drug is approved by a regulatory agency such as the U.S. Food and Drug Administration (FDA), often to determine the drug's safety over a longer term than typical in a *phase III trial*. For example, after a new drug for the treatment of menopausal hot flashes has been approved by the FDA, a phase IV trial might include women with less severe hot flashes than those included in the phase III trial.

Pilot study. A small study conducted to determine whether a full-scale study is feasible, as well as to optimize the logistics and maximize the efficiency of the full-scale study. For example, a pilot study of restorative yoga for the prevention of diabetes in patients with insulin resistance might aim to demonstrate the feasibility of measuring insulin resistance; refine and standardize the yoga intervention; and show that it is possible to recruit and randomize participants to yoga and control groups.

Placebo control. An inactive control that (ideally) is indistinguishable from the active drug or intervention used in a randomized blinded trial. For example, in a randomized, placebo-controlled trial of a new treatment for incontinence, the placebo should look, smell, taste, and feel the same as the new medication that is being tested.

Placebo effect. An effect of a treatment that cannot be attributed to any of its specific properties (and is therefore likely because of a participant's belief in that treatment). For example, administration of an inert substance to college students with chronic insomnia caused an increase in sleep duration because of the placebo effect.

Plagiarism. A type of *scientific misconduct* in which an investigator appropriates another person's ideas, results, or words without giving appropriate credit. For example, using another investigator's description of a new measurement method without appropriate attribution constitutes plagiarism.

Platform trial. An *adaptive clinical trial design* that has a single trial infrastructure and master protocol to support evaluation of multiple interventions, either simultaneously or sequentially. For example, I-SPY 2 is a platform trial that compares the efficacy of a series of novel drugs in combination with standard chemotherapy with standard therapy alone for the treatment of breast cancer.

Polychotomous categorical variables. *Categorical variables* with three or more categories. For example, ABO blood group, which includes types A, B, AB, and O, is a polychotomous categorical variable.

Population. A complete set of people with specified characteristics. For example, the population of eleventh graders in the United States could be sampled to estimate the prevalence of regular vaping.

Population-based sample. A *sample* of people who represent an entire population. For example, the National Health and Nutrition Examination Survey (NHANES), which provides data on a random sample of the entire population of the United States, is a population-based sample.

Positive predictive value. See *predictive value, positive.*

Postaward manager. A staff member who ensures that funds available to an investigator through grants or contracts are spent appropriately. For example, the postaward manager prepared a monthly report on study expenditures and remaining funds.

***Post hoc* hypothesis.** A hypothesis that is formulated after data have been analyzed. For example, in a study of the association between sleep quality and the risk of frequent falls, the hypothesis that insomnia increases the risk of falls only among men 75 years of age and older (but not in women or younger men) was a *post hoc* hypothesis developed by the investigators after they looked at the effects of various sleep disturbances in many age and sex subgroups.

Posterior distribution. The likelihoods of various levels of a treatment's efficacy, as determined from a study's result (usually from a clinical trial) and the *prior distribution*. Often summarized as a *credible interval* or *highest posterior density interval*. For example, the posterior distribution (95% credible interval) for the effect of a new angiotensin receptor blocker on the frequency of migraine episodes was expressed as a reduction of 15% to 40% from baseline. See also *Bayesian analysis.*

Posterior probability.

1. In the context of diagnostic testing, a probability estimate obtained by combining the prior probability (the initial probability of, say, a disease based on a patient's clinical characteristics) with additional information, such as from a medical test. For example, based on the presence of circulating virus during the pandemic and a patient's symptoms of fever and cough, a physician estimated that a patient's likelihood (prior probability) of having COVID-19 was 60%. A rapid antigen test was subsequently negative, and using the test characteristics, the posterior probability of COVID-19 was revised to 40%.
2. In a *Bayesian analysis* of study results, a probability estimate obtained by combining the prior likelihood of a treatment's efficacy with the results of a clinical trial. As an example, based on prior studies of the same treatment, an investigator believed there was a 70% prior probability that there would be at least a 30% increase in median survival with a particular treatment. After conducting the trial, which found that the treatment was beneficial, the posterior probability that the treatment causes at least a 30% increase in median survival rose to 95%.

Power. The probability of correctly rejecting the *null hypothesis* in a sample if the actual effect in the population is equal to a specified *effect size*. For example, suppose that exercise leads to an average reduction of 20 mg/dL in fasting glucose among diabetic women in the entire population. If an investigator set power at 90% and drew a sample from the population on numerous occasions, each time carrying out the same study with the same measurements, then in about 9 of every 10 studies the investigator would correctly reject the null hypothesis and conclude that exercise reduces fasting glucose levels. See also *beta.*

Practice-based research networks. Networks in which physicians from community settings work together to study research questions of interest. For example, a study from a practice-based research network of treatments for carpal tunnel syndrome in primary care practice showed that most patients improved with conservative therapy. This contrasted with previous literature from academic medical centers, which suggested that the majority of patients with carpal tunnel syndrome required surgery.

Preaward manager. A staff member who helps the investigators prepare and submit grant applications and budgets in accordance with institutional and regulatory requirements. For example, the preaward manager asked the *principal investigator* to share a draft budget justification at least 2 weeks before the grant application was due so there would be enough time to check that the budget amounts met the sponsor's requirements.

Precision. The degree to which the measurement of a variable is *reproducible*, having nearly the same value each time it is measured under the same conditions. For example, automated cell counters provide much more precise estimates of the absolute neutrophil count than those obtained by looking at white blood cells through a microscope. See also *accuracy*.

Preclinical study. Studies that occur before an intervention is tested in humans. Such studies might include cells, tissues, or animals. For example, the U.S. Food and Drug Administration requires preclinical studies in two different animal species to document safety before new drugs can be tested in humans.

Predictive validity. A term that describes how well a measurement represents the underlying phenomenon it is intended to measure, based upon its ability to predict related outcomes. For example, the predictive validity of a measurement of depression would be strengthened if it was associated with the subsequent risk of suicide.

Predictive value, negative. The probability that a person with a negative test result does not have the disease being tested for. For example, among men aged 62 to 91 years, the negative predictive value of a prostate-specific antigen (PSA) ≤4.0 ng/mL was about 85%. (Thompson IM, Pauler DK, Goodman PJ, Tangen CM, Lucia MS, Parnes HL, et al. Prevalence of prostate cancer among men with a prostate-specific antigen level < or =4.0 ng per milliliter. N Engl J Med. 2004;350(22):2239-2246.) See *prevalence, prior probability, sensitivity,* and *specificity*.

Predictive value, positive. The probability that a person with a positive test result has the disease being tested for. For example, in a population of men with a prevalence of prostate cancer of 15%, the positive predictive value of a prostate-specific antigen (PSA) >4.0 ng/mL is about 30%. See *prevalence, prior probability, sensitivity,* and *specificity*.

Predictor variable. In considering the *association* between two variables, the predictor variable occurs first or is more likely on biologic grounds to cause the other variable. For example, in a study to determine if obesity is associated with an increased risk of sleep apnea, obesity would be the predictor variable. In a randomized trial analyzed by intention to treat, the predictor variable is group assignment.

Preliminary data. Data collected before a study begins to provide information about the likelihood that the study will be successful. For example, the investigators gathered preliminary data about the effectiveness of their recruitment plan by contacting people who met the study's *inclusion* and *exclusion criteria*. They found that 15 of the 20 people contacted were enthusiastic about the study, suggesting that the study would be able to recruit its *sample size* of 400 participants.

Pre-post design. See *before-after study (or trial) design*.

Pretest. An evaluation of specific questionnaires, measures, or procedures that can be carried out by study staff before a study starts. Its purpose is to assess and improve the measure's functionality, appropriateness, or feasibility. For example, pretesting the data entry and database management system could be done by having study staff complete forms with missing, out of range, and illogical data to ensure that the data editing system identifies these errors.

Pretest probability. See *prior probability*.

Prevalence. The proportion of persons who have a disease or condition at one point in time. Prevalence is affected by both the *incidence* of a disease and duration of the disease. For example, the prevalence of systemic lupus erythematosus (SLE) is the proportion of people who have this condition at a specific point in time; it would increase if the incidence of SLE increased or if a (noncurative) treatment improves survival with SLE.

Primary hypothesis. The main hypothesis for a research study, used to determine the *sample size* and other study details. For example, the primary hypothesis for the study was that a new treatment for elevated C-reactive protein levels would reduce the risk of cardiovascular events during 5 years of follow-up among smokers when compared with a matching placebo.

Primary key. The *field* (column) in a database table that identifies each *record* (row) of a table. Every table should have a primary key. For example, the primary key in an Exam table might be called ExamID. See also *foreign key*.

Primary outcome. The outcome measure that reflects the main research question, guides calculation of *the sample size*, and sets the priority for efforts to implement the study. For example, the primary outcome of a randomized trial of treatment of outpatient COVID-19 infection was admission to a hospital or death.

Principal investigator (PI). The person who has ultimate responsibility for the design and conduct of a study, and the analysis and presentation of the study findings. Some studies have coprincipal investigators who each have specific responsibilities. For example, the institutional review board asked to speak with the study's PI because some members had questions about the protocol.

Prior distribution. The estimated likelihoods of various levels of a treatment's *efficacy*, as estimated before a study's result is known. For example, an optimistic prior distribution for the effect of a new angiotensin receptor blocker was a reduction of 35% ± 15% (mean ± standard deviation) in the frequency of migraine episodes, based on prior studies of another angiotensin receptor blocker. See also *Bayesian analysis* and *posterior distribution*.

Prior probability.

1. The likelihood that someone has a disease (or another attribute) before being tested for it; this is sometimes called the pretest probability. For example, the prior probability of bacterial pneumonia among adults who present to an emergency room with fever and cough is 12%. See *posterior probability*.
2. The likelihood of a treatment effect as estimated before the study result is known. For example, the investigator estimated that the prior probability was about 50% that a new type of drug-eluting stent for peripheral vascular disease would reduce the risk of poststent claudication by at least 25%. See *Bayesian analysis* and *prior distribution*.

Probability sampling. A random process, usually using a table of random numbers or a computer algorithm, to guarantee that each member of a population has a specified chance of being included in the *sample*, thereby providing a rigorous basis for making *inferences* from the sample to the population. For example, an observation from a probability sample of 5% of persons with chronic obstructive pulmonary disease (COPD) based on hospital discharge diagnoses from all hospitals in California should provide reliable findings about risk factors for rehospitalization and death.

Professional conflicts of interest. Nonfinancial incentives, such as professional reputation and intellectual commitment to an idea that may cause *bias* in favor of a preconceived result of research. For example, an investigator who has spent his entire career trying to prove that treatment with vitamin B_6 reduces the risk of coronary heart disease may have a conflict of interest if he is on a panel creating recommendations for vitamin B_6 intake.

Propensity score. The estimated probability that a study participant will have a specified value of a predictor variable, most often the probability of receiving a particular treatment. Controlling for the propensity score (eg, by *matching, stratification,* or *multivariable analysis*) is one method for dealing with *confounding by indication*: Instead of adjusting for all factors that might be associated with the outcome, the investigator creates a multivariable model to predict receipt of the treatment. Each participant is then assigned a predicted probability of treatment (the propensity score), which can then be used as the only confounder when estimating the association between the treatment and the outcome. For example, the investigators used a propensity score to adjust for the factors associated with the use of aspirin to determine the association between aspirin use and colon cancer.

Proposal. A document that includes a study protocol, budget, and other administrative and supporting information that is written for the purpose of obtaining funding from a granting agency. For example, the National Institutes of Health (NIH) evaluates proposals for funding multiple types of research.

Prospective cohort study. A study design in which a defined group (the *cohort*) of study participants has baseline values of predictor variables measured and then is followed over time for specific outcomes. For example, the Nurses' Health Study is a prospective cohort study of risk factors for common diseases in women. The cohort is a sample of registered nurses in the United States and the outcomes have included cardiovascular diseases, cancer, and mortality.

Protected health information. Individually identifiable health information. Federal health privacy regulations (called HIPAA regulations after the *Health Insurance Portability and Accountability Act*) require researchers to maintain the confidentiality of protected health information, such as names and medical record numbers, in research. For example, protected health information should not be stored on flash drives or sent via regular e-mail.

Protective factor. An attribute thought to be related to a decreased likelihood of developing an outcome. For example, greater serum high-density lipoprotein (HDL) cholesterol levels are a protective factor for cardiovascular disease. See also *exposure* and *risk factor*.

Protocol. The detailed written plan for a study. For example, the study protocol for a study specified that only participants who could understand English at the eighth-grade level were eligible for participation.

Psychometric adequacy. The extent to which a self-reported measure demonstrates robust psychometric characteristics within a population. For example, the researcher confirmed the psychometric adequacy of the questionnaire by confirming that it had high test-retest reliability and construct validity in the target population. See also *psychometric characteristics*.

Psychometric characteristics. Performance characteristics of a self-reported measure that provide information about its adequacy, relevance, and usefulness. Common types of psychometric characteristics include variability, reliability, validity, and norming. For example, the investigator did not use the Female Sexual Function Questionnaire in her study of transgender women, because its psychometric characteristics had not yet been evaluated in this target population.

Psychometric equivalence. The extent to which a self-reported measure shows similar psychometric characteristics in a new or different population. For example, a depression questionnaire was shown to have good reliability and validity in college-educated respondents, but the investigator was concerned about its psychometric equivalence in respondents with lower literacy levels.

Publication bias. A distortion of the published literature that occurs when published studies are not representative of all studies that have been done, usually because positive results (eg, those showing a treatment is efficacious) are submitted and published more often than negative results. For example, publication bias was suspected by authors of a meta-analysis that found that six small positive studies, but only one large negative study, had been published.

Purposeful sampling (or selection). A *sampling* method in which study participants are selected in a systematic, nonprobabilistic fashion that is designed to explore the research topics of interest. For example, in a study of the patient-centered medical home, researchers interviewed a purposeful sample of clinic administrators and frontline personnel to examine how the policy was implemented and deimplemented.

Quality control. The processes to ensure that the conduct of a study, including enrollment, measurements, laboratory procedures, and data management and analysis, is of the highest quality. For example, the investigators controlled the quality of data collection by preparing explicit written procedures for all study measurements in an operations manual and intermittently observing study staff to make sure they followed them.

Quality improvement. A term for efforts made by health providers and administrators to improve the quality of the care they deliver. These activities—especially if they are instituted for nonresearch purposes—may not require informed consent or approval by an institutional review board. For example, a hospital might undertake a quality improvement effort to reduce central line infections by creating automated reminders for staff to change the lines' dressings on a regular basis.

Quasi-experimental (quasi-randomized) design. A not-particularly-rigorous study design that compares the effect of an intervention on an outcome that was measured before and again after the intervention was implemented. For example, in a quasi-experimental trial, investigators compared reading ability before and after giving elementary schoolchildren a tablet computer. See *before-after study*.

Query. A command or instruction to a *relational database* to select or manipulate the data. For example, the study coordinator wrote a query to select names and contact information for all study participants who were due for a follow-up visit in the next 2 months that had not yet been scheduled.

Questionnaire. A measurement instrument consisting of a series of questions to obtain information from study participants. Questionnaires can be either self-administered or administered by study staff. For example, the 2014 Block Food Frequency Questionnaire asks about usual intake of 127 food items to assess intake of multiple nutrients and food groups.

Random error. A departure of a measurement or an estimate from the true value because of chance variation. Random error can be reduced by averaging repeated measurements and by increasing the *sample size*. For example, if the true prevalence of the use of fish oil by persons with coronary disease in the population is 20%, a study that enrolls 100 participants might find that exactly 20% use fish oil, but just by random error, the proportion is likely to be a bit higher or lower than that.

Random sample. A *sample* drawn by enumerating the units of the *accessible population* and selecting a subset at random. For example, a random sample of persons with cataracts at an investigator's clinic would require that the investigator list all the patients with cataracts and use computer-generated random numbers to select the sample. See also *probability sampling* and *sampling frame*.

Randomization. The process of randomly assigning eligible participants to one of the study groups in a randomized trial. The number of treatment groups and the probability of being assigned to any group are determined before randomization begins. Although eligible participants are usually assigned to two study groups with equal (50%) probability, random assignment can be made to any number of study groups with any predetermined probability. For example, in a study comparing two treatments with a placebo control, randomization could be to three groups, with 30% assigned to each of the two active treatment groups and 40% assigned to placebo.

Randomized blinded trial. A study design in which eligible participants are randomly assigned to the study groups with predetermined probability and study group assignment is not known to investigators, participants, or other staff involved in the study. In addition, outcomes are ascertained without knowledge of group assignment. For example, a randomized blinded trial of a new pill for treatment of diarrhea would require that eligible participants be randomly assigned to the new pill or an identical placebo pill (usually with 50% chance of being assigned to each group) and that the investigators, participants, and study staff not know if a participant is taking the active medication or placebo.

Randomized quality improvement trial. A study that implements a quality improvement intervention via random assignment in some settings and then compares process and health outcome data between those settings to ensure that quality of care improves (without unintended consequences) before implementing the intervention fully. For example, clinical leadership might believe that vaccination rates can be increased by sending patients a letter encouraging vaccination signed by their health care provider. They conduct a randomized quality improvement trial by sending the letter to a random half of eligible patients and measuring whether vaccination rates increase.

Randomized registry trial. A randomized trial conducted within an ongoing *registry*. For example, consider a registry that follows all patients who receive a particular medical device for 5 years to collect data about outcomes and complications. An investigator may conduct a randomized registry trial by enrolling patients at the time they receive the device, randomly assigning them to receive a new versus older surgical technique, and then using the registry to collect outcomes.

Rate. A measure of *risk* over time, defined as the number of participants who develop an outcome divided by the *person-time* at risk. For example, the rate of developing cirrhosis among patients with nonalcoholic steatohepatitis (NASH) was 7 per 1000 person-years. See also *hazard rate*.

Rate ratio. A ratio of the *rate* of an outcome in the exposed (or treated) to the rate in the unexposed (or untreated). Rate ratios are preferable to *risk ratios* when follow-up is unequal among participants because they account for any differences in the length of time at risk. For example, use of a checklist when inserting a central line reduced the rate of bloodstream infections from 5.9 to 3.8 per 1000 catheter-days, a rate ratio of 3.8/5.9 = 0.64. (Wichmann D, Belmar Campos CE, Ehrhardt S, et al. Efficacy of introducing a checklist to reduce central venous line associated bloodstream infections in the ICU caring for adult patients. *BMC Infect Dis.* 2018;18(1):267.)

Recall bias. A specific type of *bias* in which a participant's recollection of his exposure to a risk factor is influenced by another factor, especially by whether the participant is a case or a control. For example, recall bias was thought to be the reason why cases of amyotrophic lateral sclerosis were more likely than controls to recall exposure to insecticides.

Receiver-operating characteristic (ROC) curve. A graphical technique to quantify the accuracy of a diagnostic test and illustrate the trade-off between *sensitivity* and *specificity* at different thresholds for considering the test positive. The curve displays the rates of true positives (sensitivity) on the *Y*-axis and the corresponding rates of false positives (1 − specificity) on the *X*-axis at several cut points for considering the test positive. The area under the ROC curve (AUROC), which ranges from 0.5 for a useless test to 1.0 for a perfect test, is a useful summary of the overall accuracy of the test. For example, the area under the ROC curve for the diameter of the appendix as measured with an abdominal ultrasound scan was about 0.85 to diagnose appendicitis in children between the ages of 5 and 15 years. (Pedram A, Asadian F, Roshan N. Diagnostic accuracy of abdominal ultrasonography in pediatric acute appendicitis. *Bull Emerg Trauma.* 2019;7(3):278-283.)

Record. A row in a *relational database* table (best identified by a *primary key*) that includes information about a specific person, transaction, result, or event. For example, a Participants table might have one record for each participant in the study, with StudyId as its primary key, as well as other information such as date of birth and gender as fields.

Recruitment. The process of identifying and enrolling eligible *participants* in a study. Recruitment methods vary depending on the nature of the study. For example, recruitment for the study included identifying eligible patients in specialty clinics, and advertising in fliers, newspapers, and social media sites.

Recursive partitioning. A *multivariable analysis* technique for classifying people according to their risk of an outcome; unlike techniques that require a model, such as logistic regression, it does not require any assumptions about the forms of the relationships between predictor variables and outcome. Rather, it creates a classification tree that includes a series of yes/no questions, called a Classification and Regression Tree (CART). For example, using recursive partitioning, investigators determined that emergency department patients ages 20 to 65 years who had abdominal pain but who did not have loss of appetite, fever, or rebound tenderness were at low risk of acute appendicitis. See *clinical prediction model* and *overfitting*.

Referential integrity. A database property that forbids the creation of a so-called "orphan record," which is a *record* on the "many" side of a *one-to-many* relationship that lacks a corresponding record on the "one" side. It also prevents deletion of a record on the "one" side unless all corresponding records on the "many" side have been deleted. For example, when an investigator tried to delete Participant #243 from the Participants table, he received an error message because that participant had data in other tables. Frustrated, rather than appreciative, he seethed, "Curse you, referential integrity!"

Registry. A database of persons with a certain disease or who underwent a certain procedure. Studies can be conducted using registries by collecting outcome data as part of the registry, or by linking registry data to other sources, such as cancer registries or the National Death Index. For example, the San Francisco Mammography Registry obtains data on all women who undergo mammography at the three largest mammography centers in San Francisco; investigators have linked it with local cancer registries to estimate mammography accuracy.

Regression discontinuity design. An *opportunistic study design* that is possible when an underlying "running" variable determines or strongly influences whether people are treated (or exposed) and there is a cutoff above which treatment is much more or less likely. For example, the effect of admission to a Neonatal Intensive Care Unit (NICU) on breastfeeding at 6 months was studied using a regression discontinuity design comparing newborns whose gestational age was just above or below 35 weeks (the running variable), which was the cutoff for eligibility for admission to a Mother-Baby unit rather than the NICU.

Regression to the mean. The tendency for outlying (very high or very low) values to be closer to the population mean when repeated. For example, in a group of children selected for a study based on having systolic blood pressures above the 95th percentile, because of regression to the mean, the majority of children were observed to have lower blood pressures at the first follow-up visit, even though they had not yet received any treatment.

Relational database. A database that consists of interrelated tables with multiple ("many") measurements recorded for each ("one") participant or attribute. A table in a relational database is said to be on the "many" side of a *one-to-many* relationship when it contains a field (see *foreign key*) that links repeated measurements of a variable back to the *field* to which they apply. For example, the infant jaundice database described in Chapter 19 is a relational database.

Relative risk. See *risk ratio*.

Reliability. See *precision*.

Representative sample. A *sample* of people enrolled in a study that represents the *accessible population*. For example, the investigators selected a representative sample of the accessible population of men with elevated prostate-specific antigen (PSA) levels in a health plan by obtaining a list of all such men and reviewing medical claims data from a random sample of 5%.

Reproducibility. The degree to which repeated measures of the same characteristic or phenomenon give the same result when the characteristic or phenomenon has not changed. For example, a baby scale gives highly reproducible results if each time it weighs a standard 3-kg weight, the result is 3.000 kg. Note that reproducibility is not the same as *accuracy*; the scale would also give highly reproducible results if each time the result was, say, 3.047 kg.

Reproducibility study. A study in which the reproducibility of a measurement is the main research question, typically performed by comparing the results of a measurement done multiple times by the same person or machine (intraobserver reproducibility) or the results of the same measurement done by different persons or machines (interobserver reproducibility). For example, the investigators had two research assistants code answers to an open-ended question to do a reproducibility study of their coding.

Research hypothesis. A statement by the investigator that summarizes the main elements of the study, including the *target* (or *accessible*) *population*, the *predictor* and *outcome variables*, and an anticipated result. For statistical purposes, the research hypothesis is stated in a form that establishes the basis for tests of statistical significance, generally including a *null* and *alternative hypothesis*. For example, the research hypothesis was that prostatectomy for the treatment of prostate cancer would be associated with at least a 40% increase in the risk of urinary incontinence compared with radiation therapy.

Research misconduct. See *scientific misconduct*.

Research proposal. See *proposal*.

Research question. The question a research project is intended to answer. A good research question should include the predictor and outcome of interest and the population that will be studied. Research questions generally take the form of "Is A associated with B in population C?" or (for a clinical trial) "Does A cause B in population C?" For example, "Does regular use of dental floss reduce the risk of coronary events in adults with diabetes?"

Respect for persons. A basic principle of research ethics which recognizes that all people have the right to make their own decisions about research participation. It requires investigators to obtain voluntary informed consent from participants (or to protect those whose ability to do so is compromised), to allow them to discontinue participation at any time, and to protect their privacy. For example, the Tuskegee Syphilis Study violated the ethical principle of respect for persons because participants in the study were not informed that they were in a research study and did not give informed consent.

Response rate. The proportion of eligible participants who respond to a questionnaire or an item on it. A low response rate can decrease the internal validity of the study and *bias* the outcome. For example, in a survey of high school students, a response rate of 20% to a question on marijuana use would suggest the result is not likely to be a valid estimate of the true rate of use. See also *missing data*.

Retrospective. Literally, "looking backward," a term used inconsistently (and often disparagingly) for studies in which the outcomes occurred before the investigator decided to do the study or before the predictor variables were measured. For example, in a retrospective *case-control study* of hat-sharing as a risk factor for head lice, an investigator might send a questionnaire about hat-sharing to the families of children diagnosed with head lice and to a sample of controls who had not been so diagnosed.

Retrospective cohort study. A *cohort study* in which assembly of the cohort, baseline measurements, and follow-up happened in the past. For example, to describe the natural history of thoracic aortic aneurysms, an investigator conducting a retrospective cohort study in 2022 could obtain data from radiology records of patients who had a new diagnosis of aortic aneurysm in 2017 and use hospital discharge records and the National Death Index to determine which patients subsequently had a ruptured aortic aneurysm or died before 2022.

Risk. The probability that an event will happen. For example, the risk of being struck by lightning in the United States is about 1 in 500,000 each year (https://www.cdc.gov/disasters/lightning/victimdata.html). See *incidence*.

Risk difference. The *risk* for an outcome in one group minus the risk in a comparison group. For example, if the risk for venous thromboembolic events among women who are current users of estrogen is 5/1000 (0.5%) and the risk among those who never used estrogen is 2/1000 (0.2%), the risk difference among women using estrogen compared to nonusers is 3/1000 (0.3%). See also *number needed to harm* and *number needed to treat*.

Risk factor. An attribute thought to be related to an increased likelihood of developing an outcome. For example, female sex is a risk factor for multiple sclerosis. See also *exposure* and *protective factor*.

Risk model. The assumed way that *exposures* affect the *risk* of an *outcome*. The most common risk models are additive (in which exposures are modeled to have consistent effects on *risk differences*) or multiplicative (in which exposures are modeled to have consistent effects on *risk, rate, hazard,* and *odds ratios*).

For example, the investigators used logistic regression, a multiplicative risk model, to study the effects of age, exercise, leg strength, and the use of alcohol and sleep medications on the risk of having an injurious fall and found that use of alcohol multiplied the odds of an injurious fall by 2.7, which was also approximately the effect of a 5-year increase in age.

Risk ratio (relative risk). The *risk* for an outcome in one group divided by the risk in a comparison group. For example, if the risk for venous thromboembolic events among women who are current users of estrogen is 5/1000 (0.5%) and the risk among those who never use estrogen is 2/1000 (0.2%), the relative risk among women using estrogen compared with nonusers is 2.5. See also *hazard ratio* and *odds ratio*.

Risk set. In a *case-control study* that uses *incidence-density sampling*, a risk set consists of the participants at risk of the outcome who had not yet become a case when a case was diagnosed and are therefore eligible to be selected as controls. For example, to determine whether use of oral fluconazole during pregnancy affected the risk of spontaneous abortions, investigators did an incidence-density case-control study, in which for each case of a spontaneous abortion, the risk set included women who had reached that point in pregnancy without a spontaneous abortion. (Bérard A, Sheehy O, Zhao JP, et al. Associations between low- and high-dose oral fluconazole and pregnancy outcomes: 3 nested case-control studies. *CMAJ.* 2019;191(7):E179-E187.)

Run-in period. In a clinical trial, a brief period during which eligible participants take either the placebo or the active intervention; only those who achieve a certain level of adherence, tolerate the intervention, or have a beneficial effect on an intermediate outcome are eligible for the main trial. For example, in the Cardiac Arrhythmia Suppression Trial, only those who had a satisfactory reduction in premature ventricular contractions on active medication during the run-in period were randomized to continue medication or switch to placebo.

Sample. The subset of the *accessible population* that participates in a study. For example, in a study of a new treatment for asthma, in which the *target population* is all children with asthma and the accessible population is children with asthma in the investigator's town this year, the sample is the children in the investigator's town this year who enroll in the study.

Sample size. Either the estimated number of participants needed for a study to be successful or the number of participants enrolled in a study. For example, the investigator estimated that she needed to have a sample size of 54 participants to have 90% power to detect a doubling in the risk of aggressive behavior among third-grade boys exposed to violent video games; the actual study had a sample size of 58 children.

Sampling. The process of selecting participants to enroll in a study when the number of eligible participants is larger than the estimated sample size. For example, the investigator's sampling scheme involved rolling a die to select, on average, one-sixth of the eligible participants, namely those in whom she rolled a six. See also *cluster sampling*, *consecutive sample*, *convenience sample*, *probability sampling*, *stratified random sampling*, and *systematic sample*.

Sampling bias. See *selection bias*.

Sampling frame. A list of everyone in the *accessible population* who might be included in a study. For example, the sampling frame consisted of all the members of the Topeka Health Plan at least 18 years of age who had been diagnosed with narcolepsy in the previous year.

Scale. A common approach to measuring abstract concepts by asking multiple questions that are scored and combined into a scale. For example, the SF36 scale for measuring quality of life asks 36 questions that yield 8 scales related to functional health and well-being. (SF stands for "short form.") See also *Likert scale*.

Scientific misconduct. A general term for intentionally defrauding the scientific community, including research misconduct (*fabrication* and *falsification* of data and *plagiarism*), as well as *guest* and *ghost authorship*, and *conflict of interest* that is not disclosed or managed. For example, the investigator's institution judged that she was guilty of scientific misconduct because she failed to disclose an equity interest in the company that made the medical device she was studying.

Secondary data analysis. Use of existing data to investigate research questions other than the ones for which the data were originally collected. Secondary data sets may include previous research studies, medical records, health care billing data, and death certificates. For example, data from a study of whether a multiple risk factor intervention reduced the risk of coronary heart disease were used in a secondary data analysis to determine the association between serum cholesterol levels and mortality among those screened for the study.

Secondary hypothesis. An additional hypothesis (or, more commonly, hypotheses) for a research study, for which the study may have less power than for the *primary hypothesis*. For example, a secondary hypothesis for the study was that a new treatment for elevated C-reactive protein levels would reduce the risk of cardiovascular mortality during 5 years of follow-up among smokers when compared with a matching placebo.

Secondary research question. Questions other than the primary *research question*, often including additional predictors or outcomes. For example, if the primary research question is to determine the association between alcohol consumption in pregnant women and low birth weight infants, a secondary question might be to determine the association between alcohol consumption and anemia during pregnancy.

Selection bias. A systematic error that causes the *sample* of persons selected for a study to not represent the target population; sometimes called "selection bias." For example, there would be sampling bias if the participants in a study of factors that affect prognosis in scleroderma had all been cared for at an academic medical center; they are likely to have more severe disease—and perhaps better access to care—than typical scleroderma patients.

Selection criteria. A list of the attributes that participants must have to be eligible to participate in a study, including the *inclusion* and *exclusion criteria*. These criteria may vary if participants are enrolled in different groups, such as in case-control or double-cohort studies. For example, the selection criteria for a study of a new medication for gout included age between 20 and 75 years, at least one episode of physician-diagnosed gout in the previous 12 months, a serum uric acid level of at least 6 mg/dL, and no prior history of allergies to similar medications.

Self-reported measure. A measurement instrument that involves direct report by a participant about the phenomenon of interest, such as a questionnaire, structured interview, diary, or log. For example, the investigator was reluctant to use a self-reported measure of participant weight, because of concerns that some participants would not know or would underreport their actual weight.

Sensitivity. The proportion of participants with disease in whom a test is positive ("positive in disease," or "PID"). In general, sensitivity is greater for more advanced disease. For example, compared with pathology results on biopsy, the sensitivity of a serum prostate-specific antigen (PSA) test result ≥4.0 ng/mL is about 20% for the detection of prostate cancer; in other words, one in five men with prostate cancer will have a PSA of 4.0 ng/mL or greater. For the detection of high-grade prostate cancer, the sensitivity of PSA ≥4.0 ng/mL is about 50%, meaning that about half of men with high-grade prostate cancer will have a PSA of 4.0 ng/mL or greater. See also *likelihood ratio*, *negative predictive value*, *positive predictive value*, and *specificity*.

Sensitivity analysis. Using different methods (eg, alternate definitions of predictor or outcome variables, different statistical tests) to determine if the results of the primary analysis are robust. For example, in a *meta-analysis* of clinical trials of the effect of selective serotonin reuptake inhibitors on depression, in a sensitivity analysis, the investigator might include only blinded trials that had at least 90% follow-up to demonstrate that the results are robust when the analysis is restricted to high-quality trials.

Sensitivity to change. The extent to which a measurement instrument is able to detect meaningful changes in the underlying construct it is designed to measure. For example, a new (and shorter) questionnaire about anxiety showed limited sensitivity to change, because even when participants experienced a marked improvement in the severity of their anxiety when ascertained using a standard instrument, their scores on the new questionnaire showed little change.

Shared effect. An effect that has more than one cause. Shared effects are important because *conditioning* on (adjusting for) them can introduce spurious associations between their common causes. For example, vomiting is a shared effect of early pregnancy and gastroenteritis. If investigators studied causes of vomiting in young women, they might find that early pregnancy seemed to protect against gastroenteritis.

Simple hypothesis. A hypothesis with only one *predictor variable* and one *outcome variable*. For example, the investigator rephrased a complex hypothesis about the effects of vitamins on gastrointestinal diseases into the simple hypothesis that people with levels of 25-hydroxy vitamin D $<$ 20 ng/mL are more likely to develop diverticulitis.

Simple random sample. A *sample* that is chosen from the *sampling frame* using a random process in which every participant has the same probability of being selected. For example, the investigators identified all children from 5 to 10 years of age who had been seen in a local emergency room in the prior 6 months, assigned each one a random number between 0 and 1, and then selected those whose random number was 0.5 or less.

Skeptical prior distribution. A *prior distribution* in which a treatment is not thought to be efficacious, usually within a narrow range, often because pertinent studies of the research question have not been done in humans. For example, the investigators studying the efficacy of a new type of glucose-lowering drug used a skeptical prior distribution; it was bell-shaped and centered on a 0% reduction in blood glucose levels and extended from a 20% reduction to a 20% increase.

Snowball sampling. A *sampling* method in which investigators ask participants and stakeholders to suggest other individuals for a study. For example, the investigators used snowball sampling when they asked a nurse who had been interviewed to suggest other staff from her unit to participate in the study.

Specific aims. In a research *proposal*, brief statements of the goals of the research. For example, one specific aim of a randomized trial of the effect of testosterone on bone mineral density in men might be: "To test the hypothesis that, compared with men assigned to receive a placebo patch, those assigned to receive the testosterone patch will have less bone loss during 3 years of treatment."

Specification. A design phase strategy to cope with a *confounder* by specifying a value of that confounder as an *inclusion criterion* for the study. For example, in a study of the effect of pacifier use on the risk of sudden infant death syndrome, the investigator might use specification to include only formula-fed infants in the study. If a decreased risk of sudden death was found in pacifier users, it could not be because they were more likely to be breastfed.

Specificity. The proportion of participants without the disease being tested for in whom a test is negative ("negative in health," or "NIH"). For example, compared with pathology results on biopsy, the specificity of a serum prostate-specific antigen (PSA) test result of $>$4.0 ng/mL is about 90% for the detection of prostate cancer; in other words, 90% of men without prostate cancer will have a PSA $\leq$4.0 ng/mL. See also *likelihood ratio*, *negative predictive value*, *positive predictive value*, and *sensitivity*.

Spectrum bias. The situation in which the *accuracy* of a test is different in the *sample* than it would have been in the population because the spectrum of disease (which affects sensitivity) or nondisease (which affects specificity) in the sample differs from that in the population in which the test will be used. For example, because of spectrum bias, a new serum test designed to diagnose esophageal cancer was found to be relatively accurate in a study of patients with advanced esophageal cancer compared to healthy medical students, but performed poorly when used in elderly patients with undiagnosed difficulty swallowing.

Split sample validation. A method used to avoid *overfitting* by dividing a *sample* into two groups and deriving a clinical prediction rule or other model in one group of participants and validating it in the other group. For example, a rule to predict future neonatal jaundice using data available during the birth hospitalization was derived using 80% of the births and validated on the remaining 20%.

Standard deviation. A measure of the variability (spread) in a *continuous variable*; it equals the square root of the *variance*. For example, the investigator reported that the mean age in the cohort of 400 men was 59 years, with a standard deviation of 10 years.

Standard error (of the mean). An estimate of the *precision* of the *mean* of a *continuous variable* in a *sample*; it depends on both the standard deviation and the (square root of the) sample size. (The 95% confidence interval extends approximately two standard errors from the mean in each direction.) For example, the investigator reported that the mean age in a cohort of 400 men was 59 years, with a *standard deviation* of 10 years and a standard error of 0.5 years.

Standard operating procedures. A set (or sets) of written guidelines describing how the study will be conducted. For example, the study protocol, operations manual, statistical analysis plan, and data and safety monitoring plan outline the standard operating procedures for a clinical study.

Standardization. Specific, detailed instructions for how to perform a measurement designed to maximize *reproducibility* and *precision* of the measurement. For example, in a study that measures blood pressure, standardization of the measurement could include instructions on preparing the participant, what size cuff to use, where to place the cuff, how high to inflate and deflate the cuff, and which sounds indicate systolic and diastolic blood pressure.

Standardized effect size. A term used in *sample size* planning when a continuous variable is being compared between groups. It is defined as the expected difference between the mean values in the two groups divided by its standard deviation; the quantity is unitless. For example, in a study comparing hemoglobin levels in 80- to 89-year-olds with those 90 years of age and older, the investigator expected the mean hemoglobin level in the 80- to 89-year-olds to be 13.7 g/dL; the mean level in those over 90 to be 13.2 g/dL; and the standard deviation in both groups to be 1.2 g/dL. Thus, the standardized effect size for the comparison of the two groups would be $0.5 \div 1.2 = 0.42$.

Statistical program. A program, such as Stata, SAS, SPSS, or R, used to analyze and visualize data. Unlike spreadsheet programs, the columns in these programs have dedicated variable names, labels, types, and formats, as well as a programming language that allows users to enter commands interactively or store a sequence of commands in a program for later execution. For example, the investigator decides to use R to analyze the study's data because it was free to the public.

Statistical significance. The claim that a research result comparing two or more groups would have been unlikely to have occurred if the *null hypothesis* (of no difference between groups) were true, suggesting that *random error* is an unlikely explanation for the findings. This claim is almost always made by comparing the *P* value for the result (actually, for the test statistic for the result) with a preset threshold, called *alpha*. For example, suppose those randomly assigned to receive a new treatment for nonalcoholic steatohepatitis had less progression of liver disease than those in the placebo control group ($P = 0.02$) and alpha had been set at 0.05. The investigators could conclude that the results reached statistical significance and infer that the treatment was efficacious.

Statistical test. A way to evaluate data to provide quantitative evidence to refute (or fail to refute) a specific hypothesis, usually a *null hypothesis*. Different types of data (eg, continuous, dichotomous) use different statistical tests. For example, the investigators used a statistical test called the *chi-squared test* to compare the proportions of men and women who believed that COVID-19 vaccinations were effective.

Steering committee. In a multicenter study, a committee that provides overall governance for the study. It is generally composed of the *principal investigators* of each study site, investigators and staff from the *coordinating center*, and representatives of the sponsor. For example, the study's steering committee decided whether proposed *ancillary studies* should be conducted.

Stepped wedge trial. A variation of *cluster randomization* in which a cluster or a group of clusters is randomized, not to intervention or control, but to the order in which they begin the intervention. After a baseline period of data collection, clusters randomly begin the intervention at set time intervals (called steps) and continue the intervention until the end of the trial. For example, investigators used a stepped wedge trial design to study the effect of a wearable device that encouraged hand washing in 12 units in a skilled nursing facility.

Stratification. An analysis phase strategy for controlling *confounding* by segregating the study participants into groups (strata) according to the levels of a potential confounder and analyzing the association between the predictor and outcome separately in each stratum. For example, in a study of the association between exercise and the risk of developing osteoarthritis, not exercising regularly might be associated with an increased risk of osteoarthritis because many people who don't exercise are obese, and obesity increases osteoarthritis risk. To minimize the potential confounding effect of obesity, participants were stratified by their body mass index, and the analyses were carried out separately in those who were normal weight, overweight, or obese at baseline.

Stratified blocked randomization. A randomization procedure designed to ensure that equal numbers of participants with a certain characteristic (usually a *confounder*) are randomly assigned to each of the study groups. Randomization is stratified by the characteristic of interest; within each stratum, participants are randomly assigned in blocks of predetermined size. For example, in a trial of a drug to prevent fractures, a history of vertebral fracture is such a strong predictor of the outcome and of response to many treatments that it would be best to ensure an equal number of participants with and without prior vertebral fractures in each of the study groups. Therefore, the investigators used stratified blocked randomization to divide participants into two strata (those with vertebral fractures and those without such fractures); within each stratum, randomization was carried out in blocks of 6 to 10 participants.

Stratified random sampling. A *sampling* technique in which potential participants are stratified into groups based on characteristics, such as age, race, or sex, and a *random sample* is taken from each stratum. The strata can be weighted in various ways. For example, the investigators used stratified random sampling in a study of the prevalence of pancreatic cancer in California to oversample racial and ethnic minorities.

Study plan. A description of the intended study that specifies its essential elements, including the hypothesis, design, sample, primary measurements, and intervention (if relevant), to determine its feasibility, importance, and novelty and to ensure that it will be ethical. For example, a research question about whether nutrition affects muscle function in the elderly might be developed into a study plan for a randomized placebo-controlled trial to test the effect of 4 weeks of 1600 IU of vitamin D daily on quadriceps muscle power in healthy people aged 80 years or older.

Study start-up. The period of study activity before the first participant is enrolled or the first data elements are collected. Depending on the study design, this may include finalizing the budget, developing and signing any necessary contracts, defining staff positions, hiring and training staff, obtaining institutional review board approval, writing the operations manual, developing and testing data forms, developing and testing the study database, and planning participant recruitment. For example, the investigators did not realize how much study start-up work was required before the first participant could be enrolled, which delayed enrollment by more than 3 months.

Subgroup analysis. Comparisons between groups in a subset of the study participants. For example, in a randomized trial of the effect of a selective estrogen receptor modulator (SERM) on recurrence of breast cancer, the investigators performed subgroup analyses of the effect of treatment by stage of cancer, comparing the effects of the SERM to placebo among women with stage I, stage II, and stage III disease.

Subject. See *participant*.

Suppression. A type of *confounding* in which the confounder diminishes the apparent association between the predictor variable and the outcome variable because it is associated with the predictor but affects the outcome in the opposite direction. For example, an association between smoking and skin wrinkles could be missed ("suppressed") in a study if smokers were younger and confounding by age was not controlled.

Surrogate marker (or surrogate outcome). A measurement that is associated with—and is sometimes substituted for—a meaningful clinical outcome because treatment-related changes in the surrogate marker occur more quickly (or in more participants). Surrogate markers should be *mediators* of most of the effect of the treatment on the outcome. For example, increased CD4 lymphocyte counts in patients with human immunodeficiency virus (HIV) infection are often used as a surrogate marker for the efficacy of antiretroviral drugs because they predict a lower risk of opportunistic infections. However, there are also examples where a beneficial change in a potential surrogate marker has not improved clinical outcome. For example, although treatment with torcetrapib had beneficial effects on serum levels of low-density lipoprotein cholesterol and high-density lipoprotein cholesterol—both of which are often regarded as surrogate markers for atherosclerosis progression—it increased mortality and cardiovascular morbidity. (Barter PJ, Caulfield M, Eriksson M, et al. Effects of torcetrapib in patients at high risk for coronary events. *N Engl J Med.* 2007; 357:2109-2122.) See also *intermediate marker*.

Survey. A *cross-sectional study* in a specific population, usually involving a questionnaire. For example, the National Epidemiologic Survey on Alcohol and Related Conditions enrolled a representative sample of adults in the United States and surveyed them about present and past alcohol consumption, alcohol use disorders, and utilization of alcohol treatment services.

Survival analysis. A statistical technique used to compare times to an outcome (not necessarily survival) among groups in a study. For example, in a randomized trial of the effect of coronary artery bypass surgery compared with percutaneous coronary angioplasty for the prevention of myocardial infarction and death, survival analysis could be used to compare time from starting treatment to either of those outcomes in the two groups.

Systematic error. See *bias*.

Systematic review. A review of the medical literature that uses a systematic approach to identify all studies of a given research question, clear criteria to include a study in the review, and standardized methods to extract data from the included studies. A systematic review may also include a *meta-analysis* of the study results. For example, the investigator did a systematic review of all studies that tested whether zinc supplements reduced the risk of developing colds.

Systematic sample. A *sample* that is drawn by specifying the *sampling frame*, from which a subset is selected using a prespecified—but not random—process. For example, the investigators identified all children between 5 and 10 years of age who had been seen in a local emergency room in the prior 6 months, and then selected a systematic sample of every other child. It has no advantages—and several disadvantages—compared with a *simple random sample*.

_t_ test (or Student's _t_ test). A statistical test used to determine whether the *mean* value of a *continuous variable* in one group differs significantly from that in another group. For example, among study participants who were treated with two different antidepressants, a *t* test could be used to compare the mean depression scores after treatment in the two groups (an unpaired two-sample *t* test) or the mean change from baseline to after treatment in the two groups (a paired two-sample *t* test). See also *one-sample* t *test* and *two-sample* t *test*.

Target population. A large set of people defined by clinical and demographic characteristics, to which the study investigator wishes to generalize the results of a study. For example, the target population for a study of a new treatment for asthma in children at the investigator's hospital might be children with asthma throughout the world.

Test-result-based sampling. A *sampling* scheme for studies of diagnostic test *accuracy* in which participants with different test results (eg, positive or negative) are sampled separately, so that the proportions with specific results are set by the investigator rather than occurring naturally. This is often done to save the cost of follow-up tests. For example, to determine the *sensitivity* and *specificity* of a urine dipstick for diagnosing urinary tract infections, investigators sent a urine sample for culture (the gold standard) in everyone who had a positive dipstick, but only in a random sample of 20% of those with a negative dipstick.

Thematic coding. Marking sections of qualitative data with tags or codes—which typically are compiled in a *codebook*—to indicate how they relate to research concepts. For example, analysts used thematic coding to identify passages in which respondents spoke about health literacy.

Thematic (or data) saturation. The situation in which ongoing data collection and analysis have not yielded new conceptual or theoretical insights. For example, the investigators concluded that the study had reached thematic saturation when coding data from the last three interviews did not generate any new themes.

Time series design. A *within-group design* in which measurements are made before and after each participant (or a whole community) receives an intervention. This design eliminates most *confounding* because each participant serves as his own control. However, within-group designs are susceptible to *maturation effects*, *regression to the mean*, and secular trends. For example, using a time series design, fasting blood glucose levels were measured among a group of patients with diabetes before starting an exercise program and again after the program was completed to determine if exercise lowered fasting glucose levels. See also *within-group design*.

Translational research. Research that aims to translate scientific findings to improve health. Translational research may aim to test basic science findings from the laboratory in clinical studies in patients (often called "bench-to-bedside research") or to apply the findings of clinical studies to improve health in populations (often called "bedside to population research"). For example, a study to determine whether a genetic defect that causes congenital deafness in mice has a similar effect in humans would be a bench-to-bedside study, while a study to determine whether a statewide effort to screen newborns with a test that measures cortical response to sound to detect hearing loss improves school performance would be a bedside to population study.

Treatment. See *intervention*.

Triangulation. The comparison of multiple types of data (from interviews, observations, or quantitative data) to enhance the nuance, accuracy, or credibility of a finding. For example, after performing interviews and direct observations, the investigators used triangulation to gain a fuller understanding of how different members of the operating room team responded to the time-out process.

Truth-telling. A basic principle of research ethics that requires investigators to tell the truth and not withhold important relevant information, exaggerate potential benefits, or minimize potential risk to potential participants. For example, the ethical principle of truth-telling is violated when investigators focus on the potential benefits—and minimize discussion of the potential risks—in a consent discussion with a potential participant in a trial of a new cancer treatment.

Two-sample _t_ test. A statistical test used to compare the _mean_ value of a _continuous variable_ in a sample with its mean value in another sample. For example, the investigators found that participants treated with olive oil supplements gained a mean of 10 mg/dL in high-density lipoprotein cholesterol levels during the study as compared with an increase of 2 mg/dL among those treated with placebo ($P = 0.14$, by two-sample _t_ test). See also _one-sample_ t _test_.

Two-sided hypothesis. An _alternative hypothesis_ in which the investigator is interested in evaluating the possibility of committing a _type I error_ in both possible directions (eg, that a treatment causes a greater risk or a lesser risk of the outcome). For example, the investigator tested the two-sided hypothesis that use of anxiolytic medications was associated with an increased or decreased risk of dementia. See also _one-sided hypothesis_.

Type I error. An error in which a _null hypothesis_ that is actually true is rejected because of a statistically significant result in a study (ie, the _P value_ is $\leq$ _alpha_). For example, a type I error occurs if a study of the effects of dietary carotene on the risk of developing colon cancer (with alpha set at 0.05) concludes that carotene reduces the risk of colon cancer ($P < 0.05$) when there is actually no association. See also _false-positive result_.

Type II error. An error in which a _null hypothesis_ that is actually false is not rejected in a study (ie, the _P value_ is $>$ _alpha_). For example, a type II error occurs if a study fails to reject the _null hypothesis_ that dietary carotene has no effect on the risk of colon cancer ($P > 0.05$) when carotene actually does reduce the risk for colon cancer. See also _false-negative result_.

Undue influence. Situations that might pressure participants to enroll in research against their will or better judgment, such as excessive payments or enrolling prisoners or the investigator's students as research participants. For example, offering prisoners early parole if they participate in research constitutes undue influence.

Uninformative prior distribution. A _prior distribution_ that expresses no belief about the probable magnitude of a treatment effect—and that all treatment effects within a given range are equally likely—usually because pertinent studies of the research question have not been done. For example, the investigators studying the effect of a novel antihypertensive drug on serum creatinine levels in a trial used an uninformative prior distribution; it was rectangular in shape and extended from a 40% increase to a 40% decline in creatinine levels.

Validity. The degree to which a measurement represents the phenomenon of interest. For example, the score on a questionnaire measurement of sleep disruption is valid to the extent that it measures sleep disruption as ascertained, say, from a recording made in a sleep lab.

Variability. The amount of spread in a measurement, usually expressed as its _standard deviation_. For example, if change in bodyweight produced by a diet ranges from substantial weight gain to substantial weight loss, the change is highly variable. See also _variance_.

Variable. A measurement that can have different values. For example, use of injection drugs is a variable because it can have several different values, such as never, past only, or current. See also _categorical variable_, _confounding variable_, _continuous variable_, _count variable_, _dichotomous variable_, _discrete variable_, _nominal variable_, _ordinal variable_, _outcome variable_, and _predictor variable_.

Variance. A measure of the spread of continuous values in a population or sample. It is calculated by determining the _mean_ value, then summing the squared differences from that mean for each value, and finally by dividing that sum by the number of values. (In a sample, the variance is determined by dividing the sum by the number of values minus one.) Variance does not have much intuitive meaning, but its square root is the *standard deviation*. For example, the variance of heights on a men's professional basketball team was 92 cm^2 (equivalent to a standard deviation of 9.6 cm).

Verification bias. See *partial verification bias*.

Visual analog scale. A *scale* (usually a line) that represents a continuous spectrum of answers, from one extreme to the other. Typically, the line is 10 cm long and the score is measured as the distance in centimeters from the lowest extreme. For example, a visual analog scale for the severity of pain might present a straight line with "no pain" on one end and "unbearable pain" on the other end; the study participant marks an "X" at the spot that best describes the severity of his pain.

Vulnerable research participants. Those who might be at greater risk for being used in ethically inappropriate ways in research, such as children and prisoners, as well as persons who have difficulty understanding the risks and benefits of research or are subject to undue influence. For example, people with advanced dementia are vulnerable research participants.

Wait-list design. A clinical trial design in which participants are randomized to receive the intervention at the start of the trial or to a wait-list control group that receives the intervention at the end of a defined period of time. For example, investigators used a wait-list design to study the effect of pelvic muscle training on the frequency of urinary incontinence.

Washout period. In a *crossover study*, the period between two treatments (or between the treatment and control) that allows the effects of the first treatment to wear off so the outcome measure can return to baseline. For example, in a crossover trial comparing a diuretic medication to placebo for treatment of high blood pressure, the investigator might specify a 1-month washout period.

Within-group design. A study design in which measurements are compared in a single group of participants, most often at two (or more) different times. This design eliminates *confounding* by factors that do not change with time because each participant serves as his own control. However, within-group designs are susceptible to learning effects, *regression to the mean*, and secular trends. For example, using a within-group design, vital capacity was measured among a group of patients with pulmonary sarcoidosis before starting an exercise program and after the program was completed to determine if it improved with exercise. See also *between-groups design*, *one-sample t test*, and *time series design*.

Z test. A *statistical test* used to compare proportions to determine if they are statistically significantly different from one another. Unlike the *chi-squared test*, which is always two-sided, the Z test can be used for one-sided hypotheses. For example, a one-sided Z test can be used to determine if the proportion of prisoners who have tattoos is significantly greater than the proportion of free-living persons who have them. In contrast, a two-sided Z test (or a chi-squared test) could be used to determine if the proportion of prisoners who have tattoos is significantly different (ie, smaller or larger) than the proportion not in prison who have them.

Index

Note: Page numbers followed by *f* indicate figures; those followed by *g* indicate glossary; those followed by *t* indicate tables.